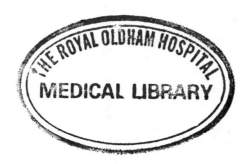

EVIDENCE-BASED DIAGNOSIS IN PRIMARY CARE

PRACTICAL SOLUTIONS TO COMMON PROBLEMS

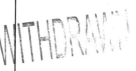

EVIDENCE-BASED DIAGNOSIS IN PRIMARY CARE

PRACTICAL SOLUTIONS TO COMMON PROBLEMS

Edited by

Andrew Polmear MA MSc FRCP FRCGP

Former Senior Research Fellow, The Trafford Centre for Graduate
Medical Education and Research, University of Sussex; former
General Practitioner, Brighton and Hove, UK

Foreword by

Paul Glasziou MRCGP FRACGP PhD
Professor of Evidence-Based Medicine, University of Oxford, Oxford, UK

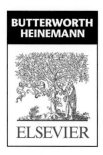

Edinburgh   London   New York   Oxford   Philadelphia   St Louis   Sydney   Toronto   2008

BUTTERWORTH
HEINEMANN
ELSEVIER

© 2008, Elsevier Limited. All rights reserved.
First published 2008

ISBN: 978 0 7506 4910 0

British Library Cataloguing in Publication Data
A catalogue record for this book is available from the British Library.

Library of Congress Cataloging in Publication Data
A catalog record for this book is available from the Library of Congress.

Note
Knowledge and best practice in this field are constantly changing. As new research and experience broaden our knowledge, changes in practice, treatment and drug therapy may become necessary or appropriate. Readers are advised to check the most current information provided (i) on procedures featured or (ii) by the manufacturer of each product to be administered, to verify the recommended dose or formula, the method and duration of administration, and contraindications. It is the responsibility of the practitioner, relying on their own experience and knowledge of the patient, to make diagnoses, to determine dosages and the best treatment for each individual patient, and to take all appropriate safety precautions. To the fullest extent of the law, neither the Publisher nor the Editor assumes any liability for any injury and/or damage to persons or property arising out of or related to any use of the material contained in this book.

The Publisher

your source for books,
journals and multimedia
in the health sciences
www.elsevierhealth.com

Working together to grow
libraries in developing countries

www.elsevier.com | www.bookaid.org | www.sabre.org

ELSEVIER   BOOK AID
            International   Sabre Foundation

The
publisher's
policy is to use
**paper manufactured
from sustainable forests**

Printed in China

Contents

PART ONE: Symptoms

PART TWO: Disorders

Foreword

Uncertainty is one of the unavoidable difficulties of clinical practice. We can curse it, or try to ignore it, but the best approach – taken by this book – is to make uncertainty explicit. This exposure to the daylight of probabilistic reason makes the demons of uncertainty less threatening. More importantly, it is an aid to better decision making and hence to better care of our patients. It won't make diagnostic uncertainty go away, but will help make it manageable.

This approach works best when the probabilities are based on good quality research. Though not always possible, we should use what is in the literature – and use subjective estimates (based on experience) when no evidence is available. This is better than ignoring probability altogether. However, most textbooks of clinical diagnosis are written as if uncertainty did not exist. For example, a recent review of 10 major textbooks of clinical skills and diagnosis revealed that most rarely or never made the (in)accuracy of symptoms, signs and tests explicit – 2 of the 10 provided partial information (King, EBM Journal 2005: 131–132). That is a shame, as research has helped separate out the good signs from the myths, and provided estimates of how accurately that allows us to interpret the good signs. This book by Polmear and colleagues is an exception and does make excellent use of the research base we have.

The general approach taken in this book is an excellent one. The differential diagnosis includes not just a list, but tells us – quantitatively where possible – what is common and what is serious. Then for the signs and symptoms, likelihood ratios for positive and negative results are given. Readers unfamiliar with these concepts might want to work through the Introduction section first. Finally, the chapters give us some 'red flags' – elements of the history or examination that should alert us to the possibility of serious disease. These are vital for general practice: much of the time we see minor illness, but we need to recognise when a patient does not have the usual, more benign causes.

While the range of presenting problems is limited, the ones covered are common in practice, and are those fraught with uncertainty and pitfalls. When seeing a patient with headache, do you worry about having missed something important (or worse still sending everyone off to the revolving door of the CT scanner)? The analysis and evidence given in this chapter will be of great assistance – in particular, the lists and data on 'red flags' to watch for are superb.

Evidence-based practice has paid most attention to treatment decisions; diagnosis has been the Cinderella of evidence. There is a change now occurring though. Of particular note is that the Cochrane Collaboration has recently taken up the issue and started reviews of diagnostic accuracy. I am sure more will follow. Among these initiatives, this book will stand as a milestone in diagnostic reasoning, and I am sure readers will be amply rewarded by a careful and repeated read.

Paul Glasziou,
Professor of Evidence-Based Medicine,
University of Oxford, 2008

Preface

This book arose out of the realisation that the process of diagnosis is one of asking, whether consciously or unconsciously, a series of questions; and that the diagnosis can be reached with greater accuracy if those questions are answered in a way that combines the doctor's intuitive understanding with knowledge of the research evidence.

Considerable evidence to inform those answers is now available but, to the author's knowledge, it has not previously been assembled in an accessible and comprehensive fashion that is relevant to primary care. Examples exist from secondary care but they are based on prevalences where the chance of disease is much higher than in primary care, where expertise is greater and investigations more readily available, and they often do not address the poorly defined symptoms that are the stuff of general practice.

General practice is well suited to an approach to diagnosis that uses the evidence to shift probabilities. As Marshall Marinker has pointed out, the GP lives with uncertainty, explores probabilities and tries to reduce danger.[1] This is in contrast to the specialist who chases down possibilities, however unlikely, in the search for a secure diagnosis.

The structure of each chapter attempts to reproduce the thought processes of the GP when consulted by a patient with that complaint. This process usually takes the form of:

1. This is probably x because that's the most likely cause in this patient (but it could be y or z . . .).
2. Yes – the initial history sounds like x.
3. Yes – checking out x in more detail seems to confirm it.
4. Is there anything else it could be that it would be disastrous to miss?

Of course, if, in step 2 or 3, the clinical assessment does not confirm x, the GP repeats the process for y or z.

The application of a statistical approach is more than one of refining an intuitive estimate of the probability of disease that is roughly correct. General practitioners tend to think that a positive test means that the patient does have the disease in question. Sometimes it does. Laboratory errors aside, an unequivocally raised thyroid stimulating hormone (TSH) is proof of hypothyroidism. But most tests do not carry this degree of certainty. The finding of crackles in the lung of a patient in whom pneumonia is suspected has a positive likelihood ratio (LR) of only 2.[2] If the initial probability of pneumonia was 10%, the finding of crackles only raises this to 18%. The absence of crackles (LR– 0.8) only reduces the probability of pneumonia to 8%. Yet few of us who have practised as GPs, without the benefit of immediate chest X-rays, can deny that we have diagnosed pneumonia because of crackles or ruled it out because we have found the chest to be clear.

A second way in which the use of evidence alters the way a practitioner works is that it reasserts the importance of the history and the examination, before an investigation can be interpreted. A positive throat swab for beta-haemolytic group A streptococci may be only 85% sensitive and 50% specific for active streptococcal infection.[3] Consider the implications of this for an adult patient presenting with a sore throat but no exudates, no lymphadenopathy and no fever, who therefore has a probability of streptococcal infection of 3%.[3] A positive swab (LR+ 1.7) only raises this to 5% while a negative swab (LR– 0.3) reduces it to 1%. However, if the patient has fever, exudates and lymphadenopathy, the probability of streptococcal infection is 42%. A positive swab raises this to 55% while a negative one lowers it to 18%. The swab result is meaningless without reference to the clinical picture.

The interpretation of an investigation in the light of clinical judgement is not new to experienced clinicians. We have always been ready to dismiss a test result as a false positive when we are convinced that the patient does not have the disease and as a false negative when we are convinced the disease is present.

The use of a statistical approach does not mean that there is no place for clinical judgement. An individual patient may have some characteristic which alters the probability of disease that is not considered in the likelihood ratios quoted. Wicki and colleagues in Geneva found that the most accurate diagnosis of pulmonary embolism came from a combination of a scoring system and clinical judgement.[4]

The evidence base for diagnosis in primary care is patchy. Often statistics are only available for the small group of patients referred to secondary or tertiary care; or the authors find themselves resorting to the opinions of experts, or indeed of themselves, because stronger evidence is lacking. Where formal clinical prediction rules, or decision rules, have been formulated, they have rarely been assessed for their impact on clinical practice.[5] These reservations are important and the reader should understand why the statistics quoted may not apply to the consultation in which they are trying to apply them.

The likelihood ratio for a diagnostic test in a study is only applicable to a consultation in general practice if:

(a) the patient is similar to the patients in the study; and

(b) the expertise and understanding of the doctors are the same.

In using studies from secondary care a further problem arises. Not only do the patients in the study represent only the most extreme end of the spectrum, with a much higher probability of disease, but also the clinical features that are most useful in primary care may have been 'used up' by the time the patient reaches secondary care, so that in the secondary care study the feature appears useless. An example is the referral of patients with chest pain to a chest pain clinic. Since they all have chest pain, the presence of chest pain is useless in distinguishing those with coronary artery disease from those without. However, in primary care, the complaint of chest pain is the most useful pointer towards coronary heart disease.

For these reasons, the authors have tried to give enough information about the evidence quoted for the reader to be clear whether it applies to the situation in hand.

Despite these reservations, where reliable evidence is found it is expressed, above all, as likelihood ratios, since only they permit the clinician to estimate the post-test probabilities for an individual patient.

Sometimes, clinicians will, quite rightly, dispense with all the tests recommended. This might be because, in the patient in front of them, the probability of disease is so low that, if a test were to prove positive, they would dismiss it as a false positive. Alternatively, the probability of disease might be so high, or the seriousness of a disease so great, that the clinician would refer a patient to a specialist regardless of the test result. Tests are only useful in those patients in whom they could affect the management plan.

This volume covers only a limited number of symptoms and disorders. They have been selected because they pose problems with which GPs need help and because evidence with which to provide that help could be found fairly readily. The search for evidence has not been conducted with the thoroughness of a systematic review. If a well-conducted systematic review or guideline was found, the search might stop there. Only if adequate secondary sources were not found would a search for primary research be made.

The editor plans a second volume to cover further topics.

I am conscious that the book is UK based and that some of the recommendations may be inappropriate in other healthcare settings.

GPs who are new to the idea of using likelihood ratios have asked whether I really expect them to calculate probabilities during the consultation; and, if not, what use do I think this book has. I suggest the following uses:

(a) Some situations occur so commonly that I think that a knowledge of the pre-test probabilities and likelihood ratios would be useful during the consultation. An example is the use of the throat swab in the example above.

(b) Other more complex situations call for reflection at the end of the surgery or the day, as the GP decides on a diagnostic management plan for the patient. There is then time to look up the pre-test probability for that patient, decide on questions to ask, signs to seek and investigations to perform at the next consultation.

(c) Finally I think that a study of the evidence gathered in this book can teach the reader some general points about diagnosis:

■ that while some diagnoses are obvious at a glance, others require a calculation of pointers for, and against, each possibility

- that most features of the clinical assessment, referred to here as 'tests', alter the probability of the suspected diagnosis only modestly
- that, in making a diagnosis, *all* aspects of the clinical assessment that could contribute must be assessed, both positive and negative
- that a test is only worth performing if it would provide useful information. If a result would be dismissed if it did not fit with the suspected diagnosis, there was no point in performing it; and
- that tests must be performed properly in order to function reliably. The test for postural hypotension that is not continued for long enough, or a limb whose circulation is casually examined, can lead to a missed diagnosis.

The final and most ambitious thought behind the book is that the doctor who comes to an explicit estimate of diagnostic probabilities can share that estimate with the patient rather than merely give an opinion which the patient can accept or reject; and the doctor and patient together can then make an informed decision about the need for investigation and further management.[6]

Andrew Polmear, 2008

REFERENCES

1. Marinker M. *Looking and leaping.* In: Marinker M, Peckham M, eds. Clinical futures. London: BMJ Books, 1998.

2. McGee S. *Evidence-based physical diagnosis.* Philadelphia: Saunders, 2001.

3. Komaroff AL. *Sore throat and acute infectious mononucleosis in adult patients.* In: Black ER, Bordley DR, Tape TG, Panzer RJ, eds. Diagnostic strategies for common medical problems, 2nd edn. Philadelphia: American College of Physicians, 1999:229–242.

4. Wicki J, Perneger T, Junod A, et al. *Assessing clinical probability of pulmonary embolism in the emergency ward.* Arch Intern Med 2001;161:92–97.

5. Reilly B, Evans A. *Translating clinical research into clinical practice: impact of using prediction rules to make decisions.* Ann Intern Med 2006;144:201–209.

6. Epstein R, Alper B, Quill T. *Communicating evidence for participatory decision making.* JAMA 2004;291:2359–2366.

Acknowledgements

I am deeply indebted to the following:

At Butterworth-Heinemann, Alison Taylor, Kim Benson, Joannah Duncan and Catherine Jackson; and Heidi Harrison, who refused to accept my resignation from the job when things were tough.

The librarians of the Sussex Postgraduate Medical Centre, now the Audrey Emerton Centre, Royal Sussex County Hospital, Brighton for retrieving so many articles with such goodwill.

Alan Schwartz of the Department of Medical Education at the University of Illinois at Chicago, whose on-line Diagnostic Test Calculator I used for the calculation of sensitivities, specificities, likelihood ratios and post-test probabilities.

Richard Vincent, who encouraged and enabled me to enter academic medicine.

Lady Helen Trafford, who encouraged me while I worked at the Trafford Centre for Graduate Medical Education and Research, both with grants and with personal support.

My tutors at the Oxford University Masters Programme in Evidence-Based Health Care, especially David Sackett, and Kate Sears; and Martin Dawes who first showed me that the positive predictive value of a test can be very different from what you might expect from its sensitivity and specificity, because it all depends on the prevalence of the condition.

Above all, Alex Khot, who persuaded me to start writing and whose ideas, as we worked together on writing *Practical General Practice*, shaped not only that book but this one as well; and my wife Margaret, who at times couldn't decide if this was work or a hobby but who really understood that it was both and gave me the space to pursue it.

Disclaimer

List of contributors

EDITOR

Andrew Polmear MA MSc FRCP FRCGP
Former Senior Research Fellow, The Trafford
Centre for Graduate Medical Education and
Research, University of Sussex and former
General Practitioner, Brighton and Hove, UK

CONTRIBUTORS

Acute respiratory infections

Sharon Sanders BSc Pod, MPH
Senior Research Officer, Discipline of General
Practice, University of Queensland Medical
School, Queensland, Australia

Jenny Doust BMBS FRACGP
Senior Research Fellow in Clinical Epidemiology,
Discipline of General Practice, University of
Queensland Medical School, Queensland,
Australia

Chris Del Mar MA MD MB BChir FRACGP
FAFPHM
Dean of Health Sciences and Medicine, Bond
University, Gold Coast, Queensland, Australia

Breast problems, neck pain and rectal bleeding (with Andrew Polmear)

David Lewis MBBS, FRCSEd, MRCGP
General Practitioner, Watford, UK

Dizziness, rhinorrhoea and tinnitus

Ahmed Issa MBChB MSc MD
General Practitioner, Heart of Birmingham
Teaching Primary Care Trust, UK

Guy Houghton MA MB FRCGP
GP Associate Dean, West Midlands Deanery.
Research Fellow, University of Staffordshire, UK

Food allergy

Sukhmeet Singh Panesar MB BS
Doctor, North Middlesex University Hospital
NHS Trust, London, UK

Aziz Sheikh BSc MSc MBBS MD FRCP FRCGP
DCH DFFP
Professor of Primary Care Research &
Development, Allergy and Respiratory Research
Group, Division of Community Health Sciences:
GP Section, University of Edinburgh, UK

Haematuria

Steven McKie Kane-ToddHall BM BCh MA
MRCGP DFFP DRCOG Dip.Ther.
General Practitioner, Redcar, UK

Haemoptysis

Hilary Pinnock MD MB ChB MRCGP
Clinical Research Fellow, Allergy and Respiratory
Research Group, Division of Community Health
Sciences: GP Section, University of Edinburgh.
Principal in General Practice, Whitstable Health
Centre, Kent, UK

Palliative care

Geoff Mitchell MBBS PhD FRACGP FAChPM
Associate Professor, Discipline of General
Practice, University of Queensland Medical
School, Queensland, Australia

Tremor

Alex Khot MA MB BChir DCH
General Practitioner, East Sussex, UK

Vaginal discharge

Jackie Cassell MSc MRCP DipGUM DFFP FFPH
Senior Lecturer in Clinical Epidemiology,
Brighton and Sussex Medical School, University
of Sussex and Brighton University, UK

All other chapters were written by the editor.

Helen Mitchell MA FRCOG DipGUM DFFP
Consultant Physician in Sexual and Reproductive
Health, Mortimer Market Centre, Camden
Primary Care Trust, London, UK

List of abbreviations

A

ABI	ankle brachial index
ABPM	ambulatory pressure monitoring
AC	air conduction
ACE	angiotensin-converting enzyme
ACR	American College of Rheumatology
ACS	acute coronary syndrome
AD	Alzheimer's disease
ADA	American Diabetes Association
A&E	accident and emergency (department)
AF	atrial fibrillation
AIDS	acquired immune deficiency syndrome
AMI	acute myocardial infarction
AMTS	Abbreviated Mental Test Score
AN	acoustic neuroma
ANA	anti-nuclear antibodies
ANDI	abnormalities of normal development and evolution
AOM	acute otitis media
AP	anteroposterior
APT	atopy patch test
APTT	activated partial thromboplastin time
AST	aspartate transaminase
AV	atrioventricular
AXR	abdominal X-ray

B

BC	bone conduction
BDD	body dysmorphic disorder
BHS	British Hypertension Society
BMI	body mass index
BMJ	British Medical Journal
BNP	brain natriuretic peptide
BP	blood pressure
BPH	benign prostatic hypertrophy
BPV	benign positional vertigo
BV	bacterial vaginosis

C

CFS	chronic fatigue syndrome
CFU	colony forming unit
CHD	coronary heart disease
CHF	congestive heart failure
CI	confidence interval
CIN	cervical intraepithelial neoplasia
CKD	chronic kidney disease
CNS	central nervous system
COPD	chronic obstructive pulmonary disease
CRC	colorectal cancer
CRP	C-reactive protein
CRPS	complex regional pain syndrome
CSF	cerebrospinal fluid
CT	computerised tomography
CTZ	chemoreceptor trigger zone
CVA	cerebrovascular accident
CVD	cardiovascular disease
CXR	chest X-ray

D

DE	duct ectasia
DEXA	dual energy X-ray absorptiometry
DMARD	disease-modifying antirheumatic drug
DP	dorsalis pedis
DRE	digital rectal examination
DSM	Diagnostic and Statistical Manual of Mental Disorders
DU	duodenal ulcer
DVT	deep vein thrombosis

E

ECG	electrocardiogram
ED	(1) emergency department; (2) erectile dysfunction
ELISA	enzyme-linked immunosorbent assay
EMA	endomysial antibody
ENT	ear, nose and throat
EP	ectopic pregnancy
EPDS	Edinburgh Postnatal Depression Scale
ERF	established renal failure
ESR	erythrocyte sedimentation rate
ET	essential tremor

F

FAP	familial adenomatous polyposis
FBC	full blood count
FESS	functional endoscopic sinus surgery
FEV_1	forced expiratory volume in 1 second
FH	fetal heart
FM	fibromyalgia
FSH	follicle stimulating hormone
FT_3	free tri-iodothyronine
FT_4	free thyroxine
FVC	forced vital capacity

G

GABHS	Group A beta-haemolytic streptococcus
GAD	generalised anxiety disorder
GCA	giant cell arteritis
GDS	Geriatric Depression Scale
GFR	glomerular filtration rate
GI	gastrointestinal
GORD	gastro-oesophageal reflux disease
GP	general practitioner
γGT	gamma-glutamyl transferase
GTN	glyceryl trinitrate
GU	gastric ulcer

H

HADS	Hospital Anxiety and Depression Scale
Hb	haemoglobin
hCG	human chorionic gonadotrophin
HIV	human immunodeficiency virus
HNPCC	hereditary non-polyposis colorectal cancer
HRCT	high resolution computerised tomography
HRT	hormone replacement therapy
HTA	Health Technology Assessment
HVS	high vaginal swab

I

IBD	inflammatory bowel disease
IBS	irritable bowel syndrome
ICD	International Classification of Diseases
IFG	impaired fasting glycaemia
IgA	immunoglobulin A
IgE	immunoglobulin E
IgG	immunoglobulin G
IGT	impaired glucose tolerance
IHS	International Headache Society
IM	intramuscular
IPPS	International Prostate Symptom Score
IU	International Units
IUD	intrauterine device
IVU	intravenous urogram

J

JVP	jugular venous pressure

K

KUB	X-ray of kidneys, ureters and bladder

L

LBBB	left bundle branch block
LFT	liver function test
LH	luteinising hormone
LR	likelihood ratio
LUTS	lower urinary tract symptoms
LV	left ventricular
LVF	left ventricular failure

M

MAOI	monoamine oxidase inhibitor
MCH	mean corpuscular haemoglobin
MCHC	mean corpuscular haemoglobin concentration
MCL	mid-clavicular line
MCV	mean cell volume
ME	myalgic encephalomyelitis
MI	myocardial infarction
MMSE	Mini Mental State Examination
MRC	Medical Research Council
MRI	magnetic resonance imaging
MSU	midstream urine
MVP	mitral valve prolapse

N

NICE	National Institute for Health and Clinical Excellence
NIHL	noise-induced hearing loss
NNT	number needed to treat
NNTest	number needed to test
NPV	negative predictive value
NSAID	non-steroidal anti-inflammatory drug
NTproBNP	N-terminal proBNP

O

OCD	obsessive-compulsive disorder
OR	odds ratio
OSA	obstructive sleep apnoea
OSAHS	obstructive sleep apnoea/hypnoea syndrome

P

PA	(1) pernicious anaemia; (2) posteroanterior

PaO$_2$	partial pressure of oxygen in arterial blood
PCR	polymerase chain reaction
PD	Parkinson's disease
PDM	periductal mastitis
PE	pulmonary embolus
PEFR	peak expiratory flow rate
PEG	percutaneous endoscopic gastrostomy
PHN	post-herpetic neuralgia
PMR	polymyalgia rheumatica
PND	postnatal depression
PPI	proton pump inhibitor
PPV	positive predictive value
PSA	prostate specific antigen
PT	posterior tibia
PTSD	post-traumatic stress disorder
PU	peptic ulcer
PV	plasma viscosity
PVD	peripheral vascular disease

R

RAST	radioallergosorbent testing
RCT	randomised controlled trial
RF	rheumatoid factor
RLS	restless legs syndrome
RR	relative risk

S

SAH	subarachnoid haemorrhage
SDS	Severity of Dependence Scale
SLE	systemic lupus erythematosus
SNHL	sensorineural hearing loss
SPECT	single photon emission computed tomography

SPT	skin prick test
SSRI	selective serotonin reuptake inhibitor
STD	sexually transmitted disease
STI	sexually transmitted infection
SVT	supraventricular tachycardia

T

T$_3$	tri-iodothyronine
T$_4$	thyroxine
TB	tuberculosis
TFT	thyroid function test
TGN	trigeminal neuralgia
TIA	transient ischaemic attack
TMJ	temporomandibular joint
TSH	thyroid stimulating hormone
tTGA	tissue transglutaminase antibody

U

UC	ulcerative colitis
U&Es	urea and electrolytes
URTI	upper respiratory tract infection
USS	ultrasound scan
UTI	urinary tract infection

V

VC	vomiting centre
VQ	ventilation–perfusion
VT	ventricular tachycardia
VTE	venous thromboembolism

W

WBC	white blood cell (count)
WHO	World Health Organization

Introduction

INTRODUCTION TO THE STATISTICS USED IN THE BOOK

The key to understanding the statistics of diagnosis is the 2 by 2 table:

	Disease present	Disease absent
Test positive	a	b
Test negative	c	d

- If you want to summarise how good a test is you need to know its **accuracy**: $(a + d/a + b + c + d)$. This answers the question: *what proportion of tests give the correct result?*

More useful are:
- Its **sensitivity** $(a/a + c)$. This answers the question: *what proportion of people with the condition does the test pick up?* A high sensitivity means that a negative result virtually rules out the disease. A low sensitivity means you get a lot of false negatives. Perhaps the easiest way to think of it is that a test with high sensitivity is one that detects most of the cases. Another way of thinking of it is as the true positive rate: the ratio of true positives to the total number in the study with the disease (true positives and false negatives).
- Its **specificity** $(d/b + d)$. This answers the question: *what proportion of normals have a negative test?* A high specificity means that a positive result strongly confirms the disease. A low specificity means you get a lot of false positives. Perhaps the easiest way to think of it is that a test with high specificity is one that pulls in few non-cases. Another way of thinking of it is as the true negative rate: the ratio of true negatives to the total number in the study without the disease (true negatives and false positives).

The difficulty of gaining an intuitive understanding of sensitivity and specificity is shown by the number of ways different authors have tried to help clinicians understand them. David Sackett and colleagues suggest the method of SnNouts and SpPins.[1] When a test has a high **Sen**sitivity, a **N**egative rules the diagnosis **out**. When a test has a high **Sp**ecificity, a **P**ositive rules the diagnosis **in**.

My own preference is to think of highly sensitive tests as good screening tests: they pick up all those with the disease but usually lots of normals as well. Highly specific tests are good diagnostic tests: if it's positive, the patient is much more likely to have the disease than before the test.

From these, or from the 2 by 2 table, can be calculated:
- **The false negative rate** $(c/a + c)$. This answers the question: *how often will the disease be missed by this test?* It is 1 minus the sensitivity.
- **The false positive rate** $(b/b + d)$. This answers the question: *how often will the disease be diagnosed by this test in those who do not have it?* It is 1 minus the specificity.

However, clinicians do not usually want to know how good a test is. They want to know what the test result tells them about the probability that their patient has, or has not, got the condition in question. The simple ways to express this are:
- **The positive predictive value** $(a/a + b)$. If the test is positive, this is the probability that the patient has the disease.
- **The negative predictive value** $(d/c + d)$. If the test is negative, this is the probability that the patient does not have the disease.

Unfortunately, there is a problem with this simple approach. These calculations will only apply to a specific patient if that patient shares the same characteristics as the patients in the studies from which those results were derived. A Dutch study has shown that the probability that a patient with a new severe headache of sudden onset is having a subarachnoid haemorrhage is 25%.[2] This is likely to be true of patients in England since the incidence of subarachnoid haemorrhage is similar. It would not be true in Finland, where the incidence is higher and so the probability would be above 25%. It would not be true in Saudi Arabia, where the incidence is lower and so would be the probability in any one patient.

The way round this is to exploit the fact that, while the predictive values are dependent on the prevalence of the condition, the sensitivity and specificity are not. From them can be calculated the likelihood ratios, which indicate how many times more likely it is that there will be a certain test result in a patient with the disease compared to a patient without the disease. It is calculated as follows:

- **Likelihood ratio for a positive result (LR+) = sensitivity/1 minus specificity**. It is the proportion of people with the disease who have a positive test, divided by the proportion without the disease who have a positive test. It is easier to remember as the true positive rate (or sensitivity) divided by the false positive rate. A high LR+ is associated with a high specificity.

- **Likelihood ratio for a negative result (LR−) = 1 minus sensitivity/specificity**. It is the proportion of people with the disease who have a negative test, divided by the proportion without the disease who have a negative test. It is easier to remember as the false negative rate divided by the true negative rate (or specificity). A low LR− is associated with a high sensitivity.

These ratios do not have huge intuitive appeal but they become more meaningful if you realise that an LR+ of 10 or more is very interesting in confirming a diagnosis. If the probability of the condition was 50% before the test, a positive test with an LR+ of 10 increases it to 90%. An LR− of 0.1 is equally interesting. If the probability of the condition before the test was 50% it means that a negative result reduces that probability to 10%. An LR of 1 means that the test has been useless.

In order to use the likelihood ratio, the clinician needs to know, or guess, the pre-test probability. From that, and the likelihood ratio, the post-test probability can be found.

- **Pre-test probability = $a + c/n$ (where $n = a + b + c + d$)**. It answers the question: *what is the prevalence of this disease in the group of people under consideration?* The likelihood ratio is then applied to this probability to produce the post-test probability:

- **Post-test probability**. This answers the questions: *If the test is positive, what is the probability that the patient has this disease? If the test is negative, what is the probability that, nevertheless, the patient has the disease?* The post-test probability for a positive test is the same as the positive predictive value (PPV), provided the prevalence is the same in the population being tested and the population on whom the test was assessed. However, the post-test probability for a negative test is not the same as the negative predictive value (NPV). It is 1 − NPV.

The calculation is not simple but it can be done by using statistical software if your computer is handy (e.g. on http://araw.mede.uic.edu/cgi-bin/testcalc.pl or http://www.cebm.utoronto.ca), or by using a nomogram (see pp. xxiii–xxiv). Figure 1 gives the example of the probability of hypothyroidism being present in a patient who presents in primary care in the UK with chronic fatigue. It is 1.5% (see left-hand column). Imagine that the GP finds a number of clues in favour of hypothyroidism in the history and examination which, together, have an LR+ of 18 (middle column). By drawing a line through those two points and extending it, the post-test probability can be read off (right-hand column). It is 22%.

Similarly, a negative history and examination carries an LR− of 0.1, which gives a post-test probability of virtually zero.

McGee has suggested a simple way in which the post-test probability can be estimated without recourse to the nomogram or to the formula.[3] It only works if the pre-test probability is between 10% and 90%. The clinician needs to remember the effect of only three benchmark likelihood ratios:

- 2, 5 and 10 for an LR+

- 0.5, 0.2 and 0.1 for an LR−.

They will alter the pre-test probability by 15%, 30% and 45% respectively.

For example, if the pre-test probability of a disease is 50% and a test, with an LR+ of 5, is positive, the post-test probability is 50% + 30% = 80%.

Conversely, if the test, with an LR− of 0.2, is negative, the post-test probability is 50% − 30% = 20%.

The 95% confidence interval (CI) is the range within which there is a 95% chance that the true

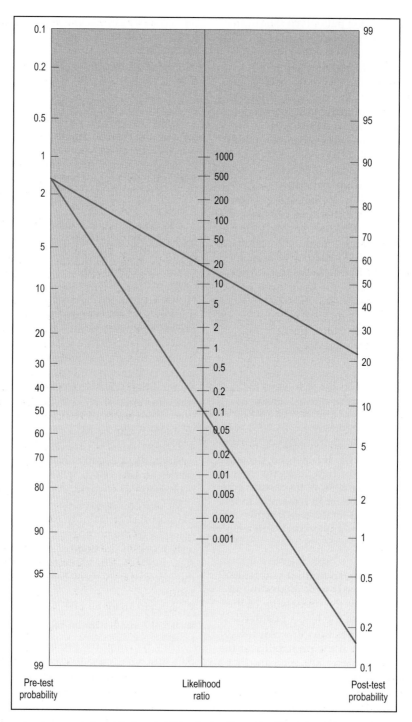

Figure 1 Nomogram showing pre- and post-test probabilities in the diagnosis of hypothyroidism.

answer for the whole population lies. The larger the sample, the narrower the confidence interval is likely to be.

In the example above, the post-test probability following a negative test is zero with a 95% confidence interval of 0 to 1%. The diagnosis has not been ruled out, merely made more unlikely. The probability that hypothyroidism is present despite the negative history and examination is now <1% in 19 out of 20 patients.

A final concept to explain is the *number needed to test*, which, to avoid confusion with the *number needed to treat* (NNT), I propose should be called the NNTest. It is the number of people who need to be tested to achieve one positive diagnosis. It is 1/PPV. For instance, when screening middle-aged Caucasian women for diabetes, it is found that 2% of those who have a fasting glucose <6 mmol/L have diabetes when a 2-hour glucose level is estimated.[4] The NNTest for the 2-hour glucose in this context is therefore 100/2 = 50. It is, of course, dependent on the prevalence of the disease in the population being tested.

It is important that readers are aware of several cautions in the use of the statistics in this book.

1. There is a paucity of good quality research on diagnosis. Statistics given may be based on small numbers. The apparent precision of an LR+ of 18, or 118, should not hide the fact that its confidence interval may be wide and a subsequent study may change its value considerably.

2. Some of the data used are derived from secondary care because there are no results from primary care. This causes three main problems:

    (a) Pre-test probabilities in a hospital outpatient clinic will be very different from those in a GP's surgery, unless the GP refers every patient who presents with that condition. In practice, GPs screen out the majority of patients who do not have the condition in question, giving higher pre-test probabilities in secondary care.

    (b) The usefulness of a test may change as a patient moves from primary to secondary care. A patient with early meningitis in primary care may have fever and headache but no neck stiffness and may well not be admitted. When neck stiffness develops hours later, the patient is admitted. A primary care study would show the danger

of dismissing the diagnosis of meningitis because of the absence of neck stiffness. A hospital study would show that most patients with meningitis do have neck stiffness and that its absence is useful in excluding the diagnosis. This is called **spectrum bias.**

    (c) The accuracy of a test varies according to who uses it. Fundoscopy in the diagnosis of diabetic retinopathy may be a more valuable tool in an ophthalmic clinic than in the GP's surgery. Likelihood ratios derived from the administration of a test by an expert cannot necessarily be applied to primary care. This is called **observer variation.** Sometimes an attempt will have been made to test whether the clinicians in a study interpreted the results of a test in the same way. The degree of agreement is expressed as **kappa**, where a kappa of 1.0 means that agreement was complete and a kappa of 0.0 means that the degree of agreement was no better than would be expected by chance. A kappa >0.6 suggests good agreement and a kappa >0.8, very good agreement. However, even if all the clinicians in a study agree, and they are all specialists in the field, that is no guide to whether GPs would interpret the results in the same way.

Other points the reader should be aware of:

(a) Spectrum bias may also affect a primary care population. Pre-test probabilities may depend on age, sex, race and other factors not taken into account by the studies used. And those same factors may alter the likelihood ratios because some tests show sensitivities and specificities that are specific to one or other subgroup within the primary care population.[5]

(b) The pre-test probabilities given are summary figures for groups of patients. The clinician can refine that figure to fit the patient in question. The pre-test probability of hypothyroidism in patients presenting with chronic fatigue is 1.5%. It will be higher in females and in older patients and much higher in patients with a history of irradiation for thyroid disease.

(c) The use of a likelihood ratio converts the pre-test probability to the post-test probability. That post-test probability becomes the new pre-test probability if the patient undergoes another test. Numerous likelihood ratios can be applied in sequence in this way, *but only if the tests are independent of each other*. The LR+ of the two physical signs, lid retraction and lid lag, in hyperthyroidism cannot be applied one after the other since they share the same underlying pathophysiology. The finding of lid retraction means that lid lag is more likely to be present as well. Use only the LR of the more powerful predictor of the two signs.

REFERENCES

1. Sackett D, Straus S, Richardson W, et al. *Evidence-based medicine: how to practice and teach EBM, 2nd edn.* London: Churchill Livingstone, 2000.

2. Linn FHH, Wijdicks EFM, van der Graaf Y, et al. *Prospective study of sentinel headache in aneurysmal subarachnoid haemorrhage.* Lancet 1994;344: 590–593.

3. McGee S. *Simplifying likelihood ratios.* J Gen Intern Med 2002;17: 646–649.

4. Larrson H, Ahren B, Lindgarde F, et al. *Fasting blood glucose in determining the prevalence of diabetes in a large, homogeneous population of Caucasian middle-aged women.* J Intern Med 1995;237:537–541.

5. Goehring C, Perrier A, Morabia A. *Spectrum bias: a quantitative and graphical analysis of the variability of medical diagnostic test performance.* Stat Med 2005;23:125–135.

THE STRUCTURE OF THE BOOK

The book is divided into three parts:

Introduction, in which the structure of the book and the statistics used are described.

Part 1: Symptoms, in which certain symptoms commonly encountered in primary care are discussed. Where a symptom is the only avenue which would lead a clinician to a diagnosis, that diagnosis is included here. Where the symptom is only one of several avenues by which the clinician might arrive at a diagnosis, confirmation of that diagnosis is discussed under *Disorders*.

Part 2: Disorders, in which some of the common disorders encountered in primary care, which have not been dealt with in Part 1, are discussed.

The core of each chapter is composed of a statement of the initial (pre-test) probability of the condition followed by a guide to what features of the history, examination and investigations alter that probability.

If the topic is a symptom, this core will comprise the following steps:

1. The prevalence of that symptom is given, both in the population and in those who consult in primary care. This gives the GP an idea of the size of the problem. It is especially useful to know the prevalence of a symptom if, like depression or vomiting in bulimia, it is often missed or hidden.

2. The initial (pre-test) probabilities of the causes of that symptom are given; that is, the probabilities of the different possible diagnoses based solely on their frequency.

3. Different features of the history and examination are listed, with, if available, their ability to alter the probabilities of the possible diagnoses. This ability will be expressed as a likelihood ratio. Each feature of the history and examination is a 'test' which, once it has been performed and provided the evidence exists, permits the estimation of a post-test probability, using its likelihood ratios (LRs).

   If there are a number of possibilities, this section will be divided into two parts: step 1, in which an initial diagnosis is made; and step 2, in which that initial diagnosis is checked in more detail.

4. Investigations will be listed, if appropriate, with their operating characteristics, i.e. their sensitivities, specificities and likelihood ratios. If post-test probabilities are also given, sensitivities and specificities may be omitted for lack of space. The reader can calculate them from the LRs if desired.

If the topic is a disorder, a similar structure is used but the initial (pre-test) probabilities are those of the disorder, not of the symptoms. They are given in three settings:

1. The probability of the disorder in the general population.

2. The probability of the disorder in those who consult in primary care. This probability will be higher than that in the general population, since

those attendees are, on the whole, unwell and so more likely to have any given disorder.

3. The probability of the disorder in those who present with a particular symptom, e.g. the probability of asthma in those who complain of wheeze.

In addition to this core, other parts of the chapter will discuss issues of definition, problems such as those of the quality of evidence, difficulties of defining a gold standard, and other issues specific to that chapter.

Almost every chapter starts with a summary of the key points and a diagnostic strategy and ends with an example. These examples have several functions. They show the formal application of evidence to a specific diagnostic problem, conscious as I am that many clinicians are used to functioning in a more intuitive way. They also show how the evidence can be used less formally and even how it can be legitimately ignored if the situation demands it. Above all, they aim to show how diagnosis involves the marriage of a clinical art with the evidence of research. The changing probabilities in the examples are shown on nomograms for the benefit of those who function visually rather than mathematically.

The examples do not describe real doctors or patients. They are, however, true to life.

Occasionally a chapter will follow very little of the structure outlined above. Palliative care, for instance, is a topic too important to omit but which could not be shoehorned into the standard format.

An explanation of the way the text is formatted

● Round bullets are used to signify statements of fact.

■ Square bullets are used to separate items in a list. Lists may also be signalled by numerals or by (a), (b) and (c) if that seems appropriate.

✴ Asterisks are used to give instructions.

Boxes are used to separate material from the rest of the text, which might otherwise have got lost.

Likelihood ratios are given to two significant figures only. More than two figures would give an impression of precision which would be spurious.

Each chapter is written with a particular structure so that readers can find their way around easily. There is no suggestion that every consultation should be structured in this way or that the wording used in the book should be used with the patient. Clinicians consult in their own special way and each consultation follows its own unique path. That is the art of consultation which this book hopes to support by giving both advice and the best available evidence behind that advice.

NOMOGRAM FOR THE ESTIMATION OF POST-TEST PROBABILITIES

To estimate the post-test probability of a condition

1. Decide on the pre-test probability, i.e. how likely it is that the patient has the condition before you do the test. The test may be an aspect of the history, of the examination or an investigation.

2. Look up the likelihood ratios for that test. If the test is positive, use the positive likelihood ratio (LR+); if negative, use the negative likelihood ratio (LR−).

3. Mark the pre-test probability on the left-hand scale (Fig. 2). Draw a line from that mark

through the likelihood ratio for the test, until it reaches the right-hand scale.

4. Read off the post-test probability.

5. If more than one test has been performed, and the tests are independent of each other, their likelihood ratios may be used in sequence, using the post-test probability of one as the pre-test probability of the next. Alternatively, the likelihood ratios may be multiplied together and applied in a single manoeuvre.

6. If the 95% confidence intervals for the likelihood ratio are given, note how much the post-test probability would change if the likelihood ratio were at one or other end of that range.

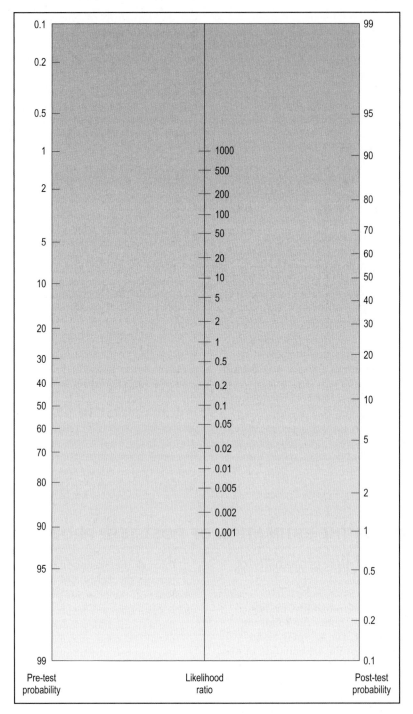

Figure 2 Nomogram for the estimation of post-test probabilities.

PART ONE

Symptoms

Altered bowel habit

1

The referral of all patients who present in primary care with altered bowel habit would overload any gastroenterology service. Referral, therefore, has to be based on an assessment of the probability of serious disease.

A PRACTICAL APPROACH

* Check for red flags for colorectal carcinoma:
  - alteration in bowel habit towards looser or more frequent stool
  - older age, or a family history of colorectal cancer
  - abdominal pain, blood in the stool, or weight loss.
* Check for pointers towards other conditions – medications, lifestyle changes, other physical or mental conditions.
* If there are no pointers towards serious disease, check for irritable bowel syndrome (IBS) using the Rome II criteria. If positive, explain that IBS is the likely diagnosis, but check the haemoglobin and check endomysial antibodies if the patient does not respond to treatment.

Background

• Changes in bowel habit are common in the general population. A survey of 2336 adults in North Lincolnshire, UK, found that 8.6% reported a change in the number of bowel movements in the previous 6 months and 9.7% reported a change in consistency.[1]

• Lower gastrointestinal (GI) symptoms are more common in patients with GI cancer than in those without, especially among younger patients,[2] but they are still common in the well population.

• Patients themselves act as a filter; over 80% of patients with lower bowel symptoms do not report them to their general practitioner.[3] However, that still leaves a sizeable proportion of the population that does present. For this reason, current UK guidelines attempt to separate out those in whom urgent referral is justified from those at lower risk.[4]

Initial probabilities and diagnostic pointers

No study has followed patients from presentation in primary care with altered bowel habit to final diagnosis. The figures that follow, therefore, are based on less direct methods.

When there is altered bowel habit without further differentiation:

■ *Irritable bowel syndrome* (IBS). The prevalence in the general population is as high as 11.5%.[5] The dominant symptom is abdominal pain or discomfort but it may be associated with a change, in either direction, of stool frequency or form. See *Irritable bowel syndrome*, page 423.

■ *Colorectal cancer*. Although altered bowel habit without further qualification is still quoted in textbooks as a symptom of colorectal cancer, the details of the alteration matter. A cross-sectional study from Cheshire, of patients referred because of distal colonic symptoms, examined the predictive power of different symptoms, comparing the number with cancer in those with each symptom to the number with cancer in those without that symptom.[6] For altered bowel habit, the following figures were found: LR+ 1.2 (95% CI 1.1 to 1.3);

LR– 0.5 (95% CI 0.3 to 0.8). This means that, if the patient reports altered bowel habit, the probability of colorectal cancer is increased from the baseline of 4.2% in this whole group to 5% (95% CI 5% to 5%). If absent, the probability falls to 2% (95% CI 1% to 3%). If the patient reports altered bowel habit which alternates between constipation and diarrhoea, the probability of cancer is not significantly changed from the baseline of 4.2%. See *Colorectal carcinoma*, page 366.

These figures, however, may be significantly inflated by selection bias. A case-control study from Exeter found that the probability of colorectal carcinoma in a patient with diarrhoea was only 0.94% and with constipation was 0.42%[7] (see *Colorectal carcinoma*, p. 366).

Main possibilities when there is a change towards looser, more frequent stool:

■ *Coeliac disease.* A UK study found a population prevalence of 1% (95% CI 0.4% to 1.3%). It is more common in certain groups of patients: it may be found in 3.3% of those with a diagnosis of IBS; in 4.7% of those with iron deficiency anaemia; and in 3.3% of those presenting with fatigue. Endomysial antibody testing has high sensitivity (>86%) and specificity (100%) for the condition.[8] See *Coeliac disease in adults*, page 361.

■ *Inflammatory bowel disease* (IBD). No figures are available for the pre-test probability of IBD in those presenting with more frequent or looser stool. The prevalence in the general population in Europe is 0.2%.

■ *Colorectal cancer.*

(a) The Cheshire study (above)[6] found the following figures for a change to looser stool: LR+ 1.9 (95% CI 1.5 to 2.4); LR– 0.7 (95% CI 0.6 to 0.9). These change the patient's baseline risk of cancer of 4.2% to 8% (95% CI 6% to 10%) if present and 3% (95% CI 3% to 4%) if absent.

(b) If the change is to more frequent stool, the results are similar: LR+ 1.8 (95% CI 1.5 to 2.1); LR– 0.5 (95% CI 0.4 to 0.7). These give post-test probabilities of cancer in the Cheshire study of 7% (95% CI 6% to 8%) and 2% (95% CI 2% to 3%) respectively. *Warning:* the likelihood ratios for looser and more frequent stool should not be applied sequentially to achieve a probability of cancer of 15%. They are unlikely to be independent of each other. A patient who has an alteration of bowel habit to looser *and* more frequent stool should be assumed to have a probability of cancer that is no more than 8%.

(c) The presence of other pointers in the history and examination increases the probability of colorectal carcinoma (see *Colorectal carcinoma*, p. 366).

■ Other causes of malabsorption.

■ Pancreatic disease.

■ Diverticular disease.

■ Anxiety disorders.

■ Drugs (e.g. colchicine, non-steroidal anti-inflammatory drugs (NSAIDs), alcohol, laxatives, magnesium-containing preparations).

Main possibilities when there is a change towards harder, less frequent stool:

■ *Causes of intestinal obstruction, including colorectal carcinoma.* This symptom increases the probability of colorectal cancer significantly over that in the general population but less than other colonic symptoms. The Cheshire study[6] of referred patients gave the following figures: LR+ 0.3 (95% CI 0.1 to 0.8); LR– 1.1 (95% CI 1.0 to 1.1). These give post-test probabilities of cancer of 1% (1% to 4%) if present and 5% (4% to 5%) if absent. However, the probability of colorectal cancer in a patient with a change to more constipated stool is still 20 times higher than the probability of cancer in the general population (annual incidence 0.05%). A policy of watchful waiting may be justified unless there are other pointers towards cancer (see *Colorectal carcinoma*, p. 366).

■ Other abdominal pathology, e.g. appendicitis, acute pelvic inflammatory disease, cholecystitis).

■ Recent decrease in physical activity.

■ Recent change in diet.

■ Hypothyroidism.

■ Drugs, e.g. codeine, tricyclic antidepressants, verapamil.

■ Faulty bowel habit.

■ Depression.

The significance of a history of altered bowel habit in the diagnosis of colorectal cancer is *increased* if it is associated with other warning features: increasing age, male sex, a family history of colorectal cancer, abdominal pain, rectal bleeding, weight loss and an erythrocyte sedimentation rate (ESR) >20.[9]

How does a family history of colorectal cancer alter these probabilities?

See *Colorectal cancer*, page 367.

Examination

Examination, including abdominal and rectal examination, for tenderness and masses is considered important, although no studies have assessed its value in primary care.

Is a search for occult blood worthwhile?

See *Colorectal cancer*, page 369.

Example

A man aged 55 presents with a history that his bowel habit has changed over the last month with a few days of looser stool alternating with a few days of constipation. He has felt some intermittent gripping central abdominal pain but there has been no blood in the stool. There are no other pointers towards a diagnosis and examination is normal.

The GP's assessment is that colorectal carcinoma is possible but unlikely. She knows that in secondary care, patients with altered bowel habit and no other pointers have a probability of carcinoma of 4%. The probability of carcinoma in a patient with altered bowel habit in primary care will be lower; the one study that has addressed this question suggests it is between 0.5% and 1%. This patient's age and sex raise the risk but not hugely. However, no more likely diagnosis presents itself. She has tested him against the Rome criteria for irritable bowel syndrome but he does not meet those criteria.

She decides to check the full blood count and ESR and, if the blood tests are normal, to see him in 2 weeks, to see if time will resolve the issue. If it has not, she knows she will refer him but not urgently, unless he proves to be anaemic.

REFERENCES

1. Summerton N, Mann S, Sutton J, et al. *Developing clinically relevant and reproducible symptom-defined populations for cancer diagnostic research in general practice using a community survey.* Fam Pract 2003; 20:340–346.

2. Curless R, French J, William G, et al. *Comparison of gastrointestinal symptoms in colorectal carcinoma patients and community controls with respect to age.* Gut 1994;35:1267–1270.

3. Thompson M, Heath I, Ellis B, et al. *Identifying and managing patients at low risk of bowel cancer in general practice.* BMJ 2003;327:263–265.

4. NICE. *Referral guidelines for suspected cancer.* London: National Institute for Health and Clinical Excellence, 2005. Online. Available: www.nice.org.uk.

5. Hungin A, Whorwell P, Tack J, et al. *The prevalence, patterns and impact of irritable bowel syndrome: an international survey of 40 000 subjects.* Aliment Pharmacol Ther 2003;17: 643–650.

6. Selvachandran S, Hodder R, Ballal M, et al. *Prediction of colorectal cancer by a patient consultation questionnaire and scoring system: a prospective study.* Lancet 2002;360: 278–283.

7. Hamilton W, Round A, Sharp D, et al. *Clinical features of colorectal cancer before diagnosis: a population-based case-control study.* Br J Cancer 2005;93:399–405.

8. Simon C, Everitt H, Birtwistle J, et al. *Oxford handbook of general practice.* Oxford: OUP, 2002.

9. Muris J, Starmans R, Fijten G, et al. *Non-acute abdominal complaints in general practice: diagnostic value of signs and symptoms.* Br J Gen Pract 1995;45:313–316.

Bleeding in early pregnancy

2

KEY FACTS

- Women with light bleeding without pain in the first 8 weeks of pregnancy can be reassured that their chance of miscarriage is no greater than normal.
- Women with bleeding that is more than light or who bleed after 8 weeks have a chance of a viable pregnancy that is about 50%.
- The GP's clinical assessment that the pregnancy is viable only increases that probability to about 75% while an assessment that it is not viable reduces it to about 25%.
- Clinical judgement is therefore not sufficiently reliable to decide whether the pregnancy is viable, although the finding of a small uterus, heavy bleeding, bleeding with clots and bleeding that is increasing, do make it more likely that the pregnancy is non-viable. The exception to this is the small number of cases in which the os is open or there are products of conception in the vagina.
- Doppler ultrasound of the fetal heart proves that the pregnancy is viable, if the heart sounds are heard. An absent fetal heart means that more sensitive ultrasound is needed.
- Clinical assessment of possible ectopic pregnancy is even less reliable than the assessment of suspected miscarriage. Once the suspicion is raised (by pain that is moderate or severe, by shoulder tip pain or faintness, by abdominal tenderness, rebound tenderness, guarding or rigidity, by uterine or adnexal tenderness or cervical excitation), admission is needed unless clear evidence of intrauterine pregnancy is found: an open os, products of conception in the vagina or a fetal heartbeat.

A PRACTICAL APPROACH

- ★ Ask whether bleeding is increasing, about the passage of clots, about pain.
- ★ Examine abdominally and vaginally to assess the uterine size and tenderness, the state of the os, and whether products of conception are present.
- ★ Look for the fetal heart with a handheld Doppler or abdominal ultrasound.
- ★ Refer all to an early pregnancy assessment unit for transvaginal ultrasound and human chorionic gonadotrophin (hCG) assessment, unless the pregnancy is clearly viable (because the fetal heart has been detected), or because the miscarriage is complete (because products of conception have been passed and the bleeding is lessening).
- ★ Refer as a suspected ectopic pregnancy if:
  - ■ pain is more than mild, or is felt in the shoulder tip, or
  - ■ there is at least one episode of fainting, or
  - ■ there is abdominal tenderness, rebound tenderness, guarding or rigidity, or
  - ■ there is cervical excitation or adnexal tenderness unless the os is open or products of conception are found or the fetal heart has been detected.

Prevalence and initial probabilities

Twenty per cent of recognised pregnancies bleed in the first half of pregnancy. Half of those which present to a doctor miscarry,[1] although many others do not present because the patient considers the bleeding to be trivial (see below). Other pregnancies will be lost having been unrecognised (estimate 8–22%) while further pregnancies will miscarry having never been reported to the medical services (estimate 10%).

Pregnant women often bleed lightly in the first 8 weeks of pregnancy and do not consult because they do not consider it serious. A US study of 151 pregnant women[2] found that 9% bled for at least a day in the first 8 weeks. The bleeding was typically lighter than a normal period and tended to occur around the time when a period would have been expected; 14% of these pregnancies with bleeding subsequently miscarried, which was not significantly greater than the miscarriage rate in those with no prior bleeding (i.e. with no bleeding other than as part of the miscarriage). Bleeding that stops then restarts may be more ominous. Both women in the US study with this pattern subsequently miscarried.

Urgent admission may be required, because of heavy blood loss or pain or because products of conception are lodged in the os. If so, no further diagnosis is required in primary care.

In *less urgent cases*, the initial probabilities in a woman presenting in primary care with bleeding in the first 16 weeks of pregnancy are:[3]
■ viable pregnancy (threatened miscarriage) 47%
■ non-viable pregnancy 23%; either:
  (a) incomplete abortion (now called retained products of conception), or
  (b) missed abortion (now called early fetal loss)[4]
■ miscarriage has already happened (complete miscarriage) 25%
■ ectopic pregnancy 4%
■ hydatidiform mole 1%.

Questions to consider

1. Is the pregnancy viable?
2. If not, is the miscarriage complete?
   with two subsidiary questions:
   ■ is a speculum examination necessary and
   ■ how reliable is the assessment of the fetal heart?
3. Could this be an ectopic pregnancy?
4. Could this be a hydatidiform mole?

1. Can the GP distinguish clinically between a viable and a non-viable pregnancy?

Traditionally, vaginal bleeding in the first trimester in the absence of other features represents a threatened miscarriage. The occurrence of pain and the finding of an open os confirms that the miscarriage is inevitable. The finding of a uterus that is not enlarged, or only slightly enlarged with a closed os and bleeding that is decreasing suggests a complete miscarriage. However, the clinical assessment is not reliable in the diagnosis of these conditions. Two studies have been helpful in reaching this conclusion. They come from different settings and give differing results and so will be discussed separately.

First, a study in primary care in the Netherlands[3] found that a few features assist the GP's decision but only slightly:
■ *Bleeding that is stable* reduces the probability that the pregnancy is viable with an odds ratio (OR) of 0.4 (95% CI 0.2 to 0.8). *Increasing bleeding* is a more powerful predictor of miscarriage with an OR of 0.1 (95% CI 0.0 to 0.3). In other words, stable bleeding roughly doubles the probability of miscarriage while increasing bleeding increases the probability of miscarriage 10-fold. Bleeding that is decreasing does not alter the probabilities either way.
■ A history of *passing blood clots* does not alter the probabilities but a history of not having done so increases the probability that the pregnancy is viable (OR 2.2 (95% CI 1.0 to 4.6)).
■ The finding of *blood in the vagina* increases the probability that the pregnancy is not viable (OR 0.4 (95% CI 0.2 to 0.8)) but the absence of blood does not affect the probabilities either way.
■ *Vaginal examination*, to assess whether the os is open or closed, is the most commonly used guide to whether a miscarriage is inevitable. In this study it was not found useful (although only 57% of GPs performed a vaginal examination).

The best results from the history and examination gave the figures in Table 2.1.

The most strongly positive clinical results will therefore increase the probability of viability from 47% to 70% and the most strongly negative results will decrease the probability of viability to 28%. These changes are not enough to encourage a GP to decide whether a pregnancy is viable on clinical grounds. When the GPs in the study made their own decisions on clinical grounds, without the benefit of the above

Table 2.1 Value of the features of the history and examination outlined in the text in the assessment of bleeding in early pregnancy[3]

Probability of viability before the assessment	Clinical assessment	Likelihood ratio (95% CI)	Probability of viability after the assessment (95% CI)
47%	Viable	2.6 (1.8–3.7)	70% (62–77%)
	Not viable	0.4 (0.3–0.6)	28% (22–34%)

Follow each row from left to right to see how the GP's assessment alters the probability that the pregnancy is viable.

Table 2.2 Value of the vaginal examination in the assessment of bleeding in early pregnancy[6]

Clinical features in the assessment of the viability of the pregnancy		Probability that the pregnancy is viable before the examination	Likelihood ratio (95% CI)	Probability (95% CI) that the pregnancy is viable after the examination
Condition of the os	Open	50%	Infinitely low (0–0.1)	0% (0–8%)
	Closed	50%	1.3 (1.2–1.3)	56% (55–57%)
Products of conception in the vagina	Found	50%	Infinitely low (0–0.3)	0% (0–20%)
	Not found	50%	1.1 (1.1–1.1)	52% (52–53%)

Follow each row from left to right to see how each finding alters the probability of a viable pregnancy.

knowledge, they performed even worse with an LR+ of only 1.5.

Second, a study from secondary care in Hong Kong among Chinese patients[5,6] found different results, with the vaginal examination of more value, but only in those unusual cases when the os was found to be open. The finding of an open os or of products of conception in the vagina were diagnostic of a non-viable pregnancy but were uncommon: their absence did not make the pregnancy more likely to be viable (Table 2.2).[6]

Logistic regression showed that the most useful features in shifting the probabilities towards the pregnancy *not* being viable were as shown in Table 2.3.[6]

It is interesting to note that, contrary to accepted teaching, abdominal pain was of no value in predicting the viability of the pregnancy. However, the presence of vomiting made it more likely that the pregnancy was viable.

The overall performance of the clinical assessment was as shown in Table 2.4. This table shows that if the clinician thought the pregnancy was not viable, it was almost certainly not viable. But if the clinician thought it was viable, there was still a 29% chance that it was not.

The better performance of these clinicians than those in the Dutch study[3] is likely to be because they were gynaecologists, working in good lighting with proper facilities, and because they took a full history and examined every patient digitally and by speculum. In practice, the difficulty they had in diagnosing a viable pregnancy means that they too could not dispense with further investigations.

2. Can the GP distinguish clinically between a complete and incomplete miscarriage?

In the Dutch study the clinical examination was poor at distinguishing the two (Table 2.5). In other words, if the GP thought the miscarriage was complete it probably wasn't (only 43% were). However, the diagnosis of incompleteness was usually right.

Table 2.3 The most useful features in the diagnosis of a non-viable pregnancy[6]

Initial probability that the pregnancy is not viable	Clinical feature	Likelihood ratio (95% CI)	Probability that the pregnancy is not viable after assessment
50%	A history of a passage of clots	4.5 (3.2–6.4)	82%
	No history of clots	0.6 (0.6–0.7)	37%
50%	Vaginal bleeding is increasing	3.6 (2.7–4.9)	78%
	Vaginal bleeding not increasing	0.6 (0.6–0.7)	37%
50%	Vaginal bleeding at least as heavy as a normal period	2.3 (1.8–3.0)	70%
	Bleeding less than a normal period	0.7 (0.6–0.8)	41%

Caution. These likelihood ratios cannot be used sequentially to estimate a final post-test probability because they are not independent of each other.

Table 2.4 The clinical assessment in the diagnosis of the viability of a pregnancy[5]

Probability that the pregnancy is viable before assessment	Clinical assessment	Likelihood ratio (95% CI)	Probability that the pregnancy is viable after assessment (95% CI)
50%	Pregnancy viable	2.5 (2.2–2.8)	71% (69–74%)
	Pregnancy not viable	0.01 (0.00–0.04)	1% (0–4%)

Table 2.5 Clinical assessment of whether a miscarriage is complete[3]

Probability that the miscarriage is complete	Clinical assessment	LR+	Probability that the miscarriage is complete (95% CI)
25%	Complete	2.2	43% (37–49%)
	Incomplete	0.3	10% (6–16%)

Subsidiary questions

Is a speculum examination necessary?

No. Traditional teaching is that a speculum examination is necessary (in addition to a digital vaginal examination) in order to detect non-uterine causes of bleeding. A study of the value of speculum examination in an A&E department in 236 women with bleeding in early pregnancy[7] found that it only altered the diagnosis in 4.2% and only altered the management in 1.3%. In none of these cases was pathology found that was unrelated to the pregnancy. It was only of value in cases where the diagnosis was uncertain following digital vaginal examination: usually to demonstrate an open os, products of conception

or amniotic fluid. It is even less likely to be of value in the less than ideal setting of a home visit and can be omitted in primary care unless a history of bleeding prior to the pregnancy suggests a cause other than the pregnancy, or a finding on digital examination needs visualisation.

Is fetal heart detection by ultrasound in primary care reliable in the diagnosis of a viable pregnancy?

Detection of the fetal heart (FH) using a handheld Doppler machine will detect 73% of viable pregnancies from the 10th week. If the FH is heard, the patient can be reassured (LR+ infinitely high). However, an absent FH, while reducing the probability of viability (LR– 0.3), does not exclude it. This is even more true in the 9th week when only 24% of viable pregnancies will be detected.[8] *If using the Doppler, the patient should be warned in advance that a negative result does not mean that the pregnancy is not viable.*

Much more useful is visualisation of fetal heart movements with abdominal ultrasound. Its use in women with bleeding in UK primary care by a trained GP or nurse gave a sensitivity of 97.3% and a specificity of 97.7% (LR+ 42; LR− 0.03) for the detection of a viable pregnancy.[9] If the few cases in which it was not clear to the operator whether or not there were fetal heart movements were excluded, sensitivity reached 100%. In addition, visualisation allowed the diagnosis of molar pregnancy and of severe fetal abnormalities.

Once the diagnosis of inevitable miscarriage has been made, a decision is still needed about whether to evacuate the uterus or to manage expectantly.[10] That is a management, not a diagnostic, matter and so is not discussed here.

3. Could this be an ectopic pregnancy (EP)?

Pre-test probability: 1–2% of reported pregnancies.[11,12] Ectopic pregnancy is found in 8–13% of women who present to US emergency departments in the first trimester with pain or bleeding.[13,14] The presence of risk factors (a previous ectopic pregnancy, tubal infection or surgery, use of an intrauterine device (IUD)) increases that risk, but their absence is not useful in eliminating it. About half are missed at first presentation.[15]

The clinical picture as traditionally described is of unilateral or midline lower abdominal or pelvic pain and slight red or brown vaginal loss in a woman who has missed a period and has some of the symptoms of early pregnancy. More severe episodes of pain may occur associated with syncope and/or with shoulder tip pain on lying down. Examination reveals tenderness and guarding in the lower abdomen, more on the affected side, and a uterus that may be smaller than would be expected for the dates, with cervical excitation and occasionally a tender swelling in one fornix.

The problem with the traditional picture is that several studies have shown that individual features of the clinical examination have low power to predict EP. A study from Boston of women presenting to an emergency department in the first trimester with pain or bleeding found that three clinical features had predictive power but that, while statistically significant, they were not clinically very useful (Table 2.6).

A study from the Netherlands[16] has identified other features on abdominal examination that are more useful than the above (Table 2.7). A normal examination argues against EP while tenderness, especially rebound tenderness, and rigidity argue in favour of it. However, the negative likelihood ratios are not low enough to allow the GP to exclude the suspicion of EP, even when tenderness, rebound tenderness and rigidity are absent.

Attempts have been made to combine the above features.

A more detailed analysis of the Boston data found only three groups of patients in whom the history and examination reduced the risk of an ectopic pregnancy below 10%:[17]

1. *no risk factors and no, or only mild, pain*: post-test probability of EP 5.5% (95% CI 3% to 10%)
2. *moderate to severe pain but no risk factors, no cervical excitation and no peritoneal signs*:

Probability of EP before considering the clinical features	Feature	Presence or absence	Likelihood ratio (95% CI)	Probability of EP after considering the clinical features
13%	Pain and bleeding	Present	1.3 (1.04–1.5)	16%
		Absent	0.7 (0.45–1.01)	9%
	Cervical excitation	Present	2.2 (1.5–3.2)	25%
		Absent	0.7 (0.6–0.9)	9%
	Adnexal tenderness	Present	1.3 (1.05–1.62)	16%
		Absent	0.7 (0.5–1.02)	9%

Table 2.6 Value of three clinical features in the diagnosis of EP[13]

Table 2.7 Value of abdominal examination in the diagnosis of EP[16]

Probability of an EP before the abdominal examination	Feature	LR+ (95% CI)	Probability of an EP after the abdominal examination
30%	Abnormal examination	2.5 (1.9–3.2)	52%
	Normal	0.5 (0.4–0.6)	18%
	Tender	1.9 (1.3–2.8)	45%
	Not tender	0.8 (0.7–0.9)	26%
	Rebound tenderness	3.7 (2.0–6.7)	62%
	No rebound	0.8 (0.8–0.9)	27%
	Rigidity	8 (1.7–38)	78%
	No rigidity	0.95 (0.90–0.99)	29%

post-test probability of EP 8.5% (95% CI 5% to 15%)

3. *moderate to severe pain, cervical excitation but an open os*: post-test probability of EP 0% (95% CI 0% to 4%).

In the rest the post-test probability was 44% (95% CI 32% to 58%).

For a GP, only the finding of an open os reduces the risk sufficiently to ignore the possibility of EP; and so the categories are of very limited use. In this study, 57 out of 441 patients with bleeding had an EP. Only 5 out of the 441 patients fell into the third category, of whom none had an EP.

An emergency department study from California[14] proposed a different classification of risk. The authors found that patients presenting with pain and/or bleeding in early pregnancy could be classified as high, intermediate or low risk for EP as follows. The prevalence of EP was 7.7%:

■ *high risk*: peritoneal signs and/or cervical excitation: probability of EP 29% (95% CI 19% to 41%)

■ *intermediate risk*: pain (other than midline cramping) and/or uterine or adnexal tenderness, no fetal heart sounds on Doppler and no tissue in the os: probability of EP 7% (95% CI 5% to 10%)

■ *low risk*: those not included above: probability of EP <1% (95% CI 0% to 3%).

In other words, EP could only be excluded clinically with any reliability if there were no pain or tenderness, or there were fetal heart sounds or tissue in the os.

Again, this has reduced the proportion of women with pain or bleeding in the first trimester in whom the possibility of EP can be ignored, although this time to a slightly more useful 21%.

Is digital vaginal examination useful in the assessment of suspected ectopic pregnancy in primary care?

The answer from the Netherlands study[16] is no. The traditional diagnostic feature of an adnexal mass has no predictive power, presumably because a mass is rarely found, and, when it is found, it is more likely to be a corpus luteum than an EP. Furthermore, while a vaginal examination that is 'normal' helps to rule EP out (LR− 0.5 (95% CI 0.4 to 0.6)), and the finding of tenderness helps to rule it in (LR+ 2.4 (95% CI 1.4 to 4.0)), their likelihood ratios are too close to 1 to be clinically useful.

Conclusion

In conclusion, therefore, the evidence supports the old teaching: that if *anything* raises the suspicion of an EP the possibility should be pursued. Only in a woman with bleeding and no, or only mild, midline pain, with no risk factors for EP and no other pointers on examination, can the pregnancy be assumed to be intrauterine.

4. Could this be a hydatidiform mole?

Pre-test probability: 0.05% of reported pregnancies but 0.2% of pregnancies in patients from the Far East. A history of a previous mole raises the risk of recurrence to 1.3%.[18]

The clinical picture is of brown loss or bleeding in early pregnancy but this only occurs in about half.[19] The other half are asymptomatic when discovered on routine ultrasound scan. The uterus may be found to be larger than expected for dates (in 15%) and the patient may be more unwell than would be expected, with vomiting and weight loss (in 2%). However, the diagnosis is unlikely to be made clinically even in those who are symptomatic, the patient being considered to be suffering from a threatened miscarriage which continues to bleed.

The diagnosis will be made, therefore, only when an ultrasound examination is performed because of continued vaginal bleeding.

The patient's perspective

Women find that uncertainty about whether their baby is alive adds to the stress of a miscarriage. They value the resolution of that uncertainty by ultrasound.[3]

Example

A 25-year-old woman presents with moderate bleeding 10 weeks into her first pregnancy. She thinks the bleeding is a little less than a normal period, and that the amount lost has stayed stable over the 2 days since it started. There is no pain.

The GP explains that a vaginal examination will pose no risk to the pregnancy but may help him to decide what is going on. He finds a uterus compatible with a 10-week pregnancy, a closed os and blood in the vagina.

The GP reckons that the various pointers towards a viable pregnancy (light loss, no clots) and away from one (loss is stable and blood is found in the vagina) cancel each other out. The probability of the pregnancy being viable is about where it was before, at 50%.

He explains to the patient that he wants to see if he can detect the fetal heart with a handheld Doppler, but warns her not to put too much store by this. If it's positive that's fine, but it may well be negative at this stage of the pregnancy, even though the fetus is alive and well. However, he cannot detect a fetal heart. The probability of a viable pregnancy has now dropped to 21% (Fig. 2.1).

The GP feels that it would be unfair to send the patient home for expectant management when he has access to abdominal ultrasound at the nearby polyclinic. The ultrasound fails to detect fetal heart movements. The probability of a viable pregnancy is now 1% (Fig. 2.2) and he refers her to the gynaecology team.

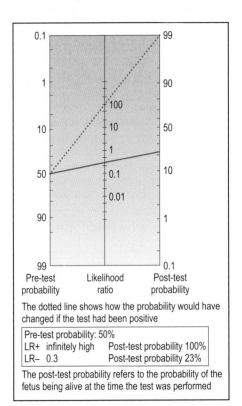

Pre-test probability | Likelihood ratio | Post-test probability

The dotted line shows how the probability would have changed if the test had been positive

Pre-test probability: 50%	
LR+ infinitely high	Post-test probability 100%
LR− 0.3	Post-test probability 23%

The post-test probability refers to the probability of the fetus being alive at the time the test was performed

Figure 2.1 The probability of miscarriage before and after the Doppler result in the example above.

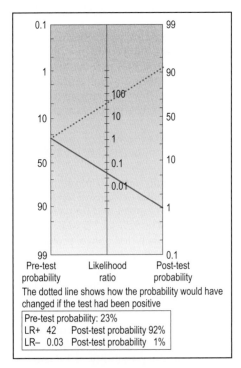

Pre-test probability | Likelihood ratio | Post-test probability

The dotted line shows how the probability would have changed if the test had been positive

Pre-test probability: 23%	
LR+ 42	Post-test probability 92%
LR− 0.03	Post-test probability 1%

Figure 2.2 The probability of miscarriage before and after the ultrasound result in the example above.

REFERENCES

1. Everett C. *Incidence and outcome of bleeding before the 20th week of pregnancy: prospective study from general practice.* BMJ 1997;315:32–34.

2. Harville E, Wilcox A, Baird D, et al. *Vaginal bleeding in very early pregnancy.* Hum Reprod 2003;18: 1944–1947.

3. Wieringa-de Ward M, Bonsel G, Ankum W, et al. *Threatened miscarriage in general practice: diagnostic value of history taking and physical examination.* Br J Gen Pract 2002;52:825–829.

4. Weeks A, Danielsson K. *Spontaneous miscarriage in the first trimester.* BMJ 2006;332:1223–1224.

5. Yip S, Sahota D, Cheung L, et al. *Accuracy of clinical diagnostic methods of threatened abortion.* Gynecol Obstet Invest 2003;56:38–42.

6. Chung T, Sahota D, Lau T, et al. *Threatened abortion: prediction of viability based on signs and symptoms.* Aust N Z J Obstet Gynaecol 1999;39: 443–447.

7. Hoey R, Allan K. *Does speculum examination have a role in assessing bleeding in early pregnancy?* Emerg Med J 2004;21:461–463.

8. Waterstone J, Campbell S. *Sensitivity of pocket Doppler fetal heart detectors in early pregnancy: a comparative study.* Br J Obstet Gynaecol 1993;100:189–190.

9. Everett C, Preece E. *Women with bleeding in the first 20 weeks of pregnancy: value of general practice ultrasound in detecting fetal heart movements.* Br J Gen Pract 1996;46: 7–9.

10. Ankum W, Wieringa-de Ward M, Bindels P. *Management of spontaneous miscarriage in the first trimester: an example of putting informed shared decision making into practice.* BMJ 2001;322:1343–1346.

11. Royal College of Obstetricians and Gynaecologists. *The management of tubal pregnancy: Green top guideline No. 21.* London: RCOG, 2004.

12. American College of Emergency Physicians. *Clinical policy: critical issues in the initial evaluation and management of patients presenting to the emergency department in early pregnancy.* Ann Emerg Med 2003;41: 123–133.

13. Kaplan B, Dart R, Moskos M, et al. *Ectopic pregnancy: prospective study with improved diagnostic accuracy.* Ann Emerg Med 1996;28:10–17.

14. Buckley R, King K, Disney J, et al. *History and physical examination to estimate the risk of ectopic pregnancy: validation of a clinical prediction model.* Ann Emerg Med 1999;34:589–594.

15. Della-Giustina D, Denny M. *Ectopic pregnancy.* Emerg Med Clin North Am 2003;21:565–584.

16. Mol B, Hajenius P, Engelsbel S, et al. *Should patients who are suspected of having an ectopic pregnancy undergo physical examination?* Fertil Steril 1999;71:155–157.

17. Dart R, Kaplan B, Varaklis K. *Predictive value of history and physical examination in patients with suspected ectopic pregnancy.* Ann Emerg Med 1999;33:283–290.

18. Khoo S. *Clinical aspects of gestational trophoblastic disease: a review based partly on 25-year experience of a statewide registry.* Aust N Z J Obstet Gynaecol 2003;43: 280–289.

19. Gemer O, Segal S, Kopmar A, et al. *The current clinical presentation of complete molar pregnancy.* Arch Gynaecol Obstet 2000;264:33–34.

3

Breast problems

Prevalence of breast symptoms

Women consult with breast problems at the rate of 19.2 presentations per 1000 women years in the UK[1] and at a similar rate in the USA.[2] In a study of 34 practices in South Wales from 1995 to 1996,[1] general practitioners recorded data from consultations with women aged over 17 in which a new breast symptom was presented. The number of patients recorded by individual practices was between 1.9 and 14.8 patients per GP per year. The mean age at presentation was 43.5 years (range 18–92 years). The average referral rate was 55%, rising with age from 49% for women aged 18 to 25 years to 73% for women aged over 65 years. Most complaints were of lumps or lumpiness, pain and discharge (Table 3.1). Other complaints included congenital abnormalities; extra nipples and breasts occur in 1% and 5% of men and women respectively.[3]

Relationship of breast symptoms to cancer

All breast complaints carry a risk of being related to breast cancer. In the US study[2] all four major symptoms carried a positive likelihood ratio of 10 or over (Table 3.2).

The effect of age on the risk of cancer

There is a clear increase in the incidence of breast cancer with increasing age. At the age of 30 a woman has a risk of developing breast cancer of 0.025% per year. By the age of 70 this has risen 20-fold to 0.5% per year.[4] However, the US study did not find that the patient's age when presenting with breast symptoms significantly affected the probability that her symptoms were due to cancer (Table 3.3). This may be an artefact because of the small numbers, or it may be that some other factor cancels out the expected rise in incidence. Perhaps more cancers in the older women are being detected on mammography.

Breast lumps

KEY FACTS

- The finding of a lump carries a likelihood ratio for cancer of 65.[2]
- The age of the patient is very significant when this likelihood ratio is used to calculate the probability of carcinoma. If the patient with a lump is a woman aged 70, her risk of carcinoma is raised from her annual risk of 0.5% to 33% by the fact that she has a lump. The same likelihood ratio raises the probability of carcinoma in a 30-year-old woman from 0.025% to only 7%, hence the stipulation in the UK guidelines that referral of women under 30 with a lump, but without other features of malignancy, is not urgent.[5]
- The same principle applies to men with a unilateral breast lump.
- The clinical examination cannot reliably distinguish benign from malignant lumps. The finding that a lump is large, fixed, hard and irregular increases the probability of carcinoma but does not rule it in. The finding that a lump is small, mobile and well-defined decreases the probability of carcinoma but does not rule it out.

A PRACTICAL APPROACH

* Refer all patients with a breast lump for specialist assessment for carcinoma unless:
  (a) it is an integral part of a symmetrical nodularity;[6] or
  (b) the patient is an adolescent girl where the lump is suggestive of asymmetrical nipple bud development; or
  (c) the patient is an adolescent boy where the lump is suggestive of asymmetrical gynaecomastia; or
  (d) the clinical picture overwhelmingly points to a diagnosis other than carcinoma, e.g. breast abscess in a lactating woman.

Initial (pre-test) probabilities

Benign:
- Cyst
- Fibroadenoma
- Mammary duct ectasia
- Intraduct papilloma

Carcinoma.

Breast lumps at special phases of life

Adolescence[7]

• Lumps in the male breast in adolescence are almost always due to gynaecomastia, with a peak incidence at age 13 or 14.

Table 3.1 Presenting symptoms and referral rates in South Wales[1]

Symptom	No. of presentations (%)	Number referred (%)
Breast lump	473 (46)	369 (78)
Lumpiness	165 (16)	72 (44)
Nipple discharge	56 (5)	36 (64)
Pain only	288 (28)	72 (25)
Other	38 (4)	15 (39)
Total	1020	564 (55)

Table 3.2 Symptoms of breast disease and the likelihood of cancer[2]

Symptom	No. of presentations	Proportion with cancer	LR+
Pain	169	1.2%	10
Mass	159	10.7%	65
Skin or nipple change	51	2.0%	16
Lumpiness	25	4.0%	14

Table 3.3 Relationship of age with cancer risk in patients presenting with breast symptoms[2]

Age at presentation	Number with cancer	Proportion with cancer
40–49	11	6.4%
50–59	6	4.4%
60–69	3	4.4%
70–79	3	8.3%

- Lumps in the female breast in adolescence peak between ages 16 and 20 years: 70% are fibroadenomas, 6% cysts, 12% due to abnormalities of normal development and evolution (ANDI). The commonest swelling in the early part of adolescence is asymmetrical development of the nipple bud.[8] Recognition of this is important since ill-advised biopsy may lead to failure of breast development.

Pregnancy and lactation[9]

- Mastitis/abscess is the most common.
- Galactocele and enlargement of axillary breast tissue are uncommon.
- Enlarging fibroadenoma and gigantomastia are rare.

Older women

- Women over 55 years old who have benign breast disorders usually suffer from non-specific nodularity; 25% of these will be associated with pain.[10]
- Cysts account for 8%, usually in patients under the age of 60. The use of postmenopausal hormone replacement therapy (HRT) increases the incidence of benign masses which are more usually associated with the second half of reproductive life, especially cysts and fibroadenomas.

Clinical history and examination in the assessment of the probability of malignancy[11]

History
- Duration
- Pain
- Change in size
- Relation to menstrual cycle
- Menstrual irregularity
- Past history of similar changes
- Risk factors for breast cancer: age, parity, age at first pregnancy, family history, hormone usage (HRT; contraception), smoking, a history of breast cancer in the other breast, a family history of breast cancer.

Examination
- The characteristics of the lump; its mobility, irregularity and consistency
- Tethering
- Distortion of the breast
- Nipple retraction or eczema.

Table 3.4 Characteristics of a breast lump and the likelihood of breast cancer[4]

Clinical characteristics of the lump	LR+
Fixed	2.4
Hard	1.6
Irregular	1.8
Diameter ≥2 cm	1.9

Questions to consider

Can benign and malignant lumps be reliably distinguished clinically?

No. The clinical features of the lump have traditionally been used to distinguish benign from malignant lesions, with a malignancy characteristically hard, irregular and fixed while benign lesions are soft, smooth and mobile. However, a study from the USA shows that these features are poor discriminators with likelihood ratios not far from 1 (Table 3.4).[4]

Furthermore, any two examiners often disagree over the results of an examination of the breast. A systematic review[4] found that the kappa for agreement between two examiners ranged from 0.22 to 0.59; i.e. in no studies was agreement good and in some it was poor. An examination that leads to different results in different hands cannot be used to distinguish patients who should be referred from those who should not.

One exception to this rule, that benign cannot be reliably distinguished from malignant clinically, is the bilateral induration found along the bottom edge of the breast in some older women. It forms a crescent of harder tissue and is due to compression of breast tissue by the weight of the breast. Referral is not needed.[12]

More detail about the value of the clinical assessment of a breast lump is provided by a study from Antwerp.[13] All patients referred because of a palpable lump were examined in the Department of Gynaecology. Only those lumps that were firmly circumscribed and mobile were declared to be clinically benign. The value of the clinical examination is shown in Table 3.5.

In some situations a sensitivity of 88% would be considered useful, but not in the assessment of possible breast cancer. In this study 11 out of 95 cancers were declared benign on examination, resulting in 12% of cancers being missed. The

Table 3.5 Value of the clinical examination in the detection of cancer[13]

Sensitivity	Specificity	LR+ (95% CI)	LR– (95% CI)
88%	71%	3.0 (2.2–4.1)	0.2 (0.1–0.3)

Table 3.6 Sensitivity of the examination according to tumour size and the patient's age and menopausal status[13]

Patient's characteristics		Sensitivity of the examination for cancer
Tumour size	Tumour <2 cm	80%
	Tumour >2 cm	94%
Patient's age	Age <40	66%
	Age >60	93%
Menopausal status	Premenopausal	70%
	Postmenopausal	93%

same study yielded interesting information about the effect of the size of the tumour, the patient's age and menopausal status, as shown in Table 3.6.

Examination of the older postmenopausal woman with a larger mass is more sensitive, but the proportion of cancers missed is still, even in skilled hands, too great for those judged to be benign not to be referred.

Should a woman be referred who has felt a lump but the examiner cannot?

In general, yes. The sensitivity of clinical breast examination, when used to *screen* for breast cancer, is only 54% (95% CI 48% to 60%).[4] This means that an individual examiner will miss almost half of breast cancers when examining the breast. Studies in which more time was spent examining the breast (at least 3 minutes per breast), and in which an explicit and correct technique was used, had higher sensitivities but these conditions are unlikely to be found in primary care (as opposed to dedicated screening clinics).

Should a women with a small, smooth, mobile soft breast lump be referred even if she is aged <25?

Yes. It is true that women aged 25 and under are at an age when their risk of fibroadenoma is at its peak, while their risk of breast cancer is at its lowest.[6] However, a fibroadenoma is not likely to disappear and will continue to give rise to anxiety. Referral, but not urgent referral, is recommended.

Should a woman be referred who has a lump in a nodular breast?

No studies have addressed this question. Consensus maintains that referral is unnecessary for young women with tender lumpy breasts and for older women with symmetrical nodularity. However, a woman with a new lump in pre-existing nodularity, or with asymmetrical nodularity that persists after menstruation, should be referred.[6]

How does a positive family history affect the probability that a woman has breast cancer?

The risk of cancer depends on the numbers of relatives with breast cancer, the closeness of their relationship, the age at which their cancer was diagnosed and whether a specific genetic mutation has been identified (Table 3.7) as well as other factors too detailed to include here.

Can a mass be ignored if the patient has had a recent normal mammogram?

No. Screening mammography has a sensitivity of 94% and specificity of 93% in women aged 50 to 69.[15] This gives an LR– of 0.06. Using data from California, this means that an asymptomatic

Table 3.7 Lifetime risk of breast cancer in a woman with a family history of breast or ovarian cancer: the main family combinations[14]

Category	Lifetime risk	Family history
High risk	≥30%	(a) One first and one second degree relative average age <50 (b) One first and two second degree relatives average age <60 (c) One first and three second degree relatives of any age
Moderate risk	17–29%	(a) One first degree relative aged <40 (b) One first and one second degree relative average age >50 (c) Two first degree relatives average age >50
Near population risk (previously called low risk)	3–16%	A family history less strong than those above
Population risk	<3%	No family history

Notes:
1. Relatives must be blood relatives on the same side of the family. A first degree relative is a parent, sibling or child. A second degree relative is a grandparent, grandchild, aunt, niece or half-sister.
2. 'Age' refers to the age at diagnosis.
3. Bilateral breast cancer counts as two relatives with cancer.
4. Ovarian cancer and male breast cancer are at least as powerful predictors as female breast cancer.
5. The finding of a specific BRCA mutation in a family increases the risk of breast cancer in all members (at least until their BRCA status is known). A genetic mutation in the BRCA1 gene or the BRCA2 gene carries a very high risk of breast cancer (50–80% lifetime risk) but is found in only 3% of women with breast cancer.[4]

woman in her sixties with a pre-test probability of breast cancer of 1.3% has a probability that she has breast cancer of 0.08% following a normal mammogram. If a lump is then found, that risk of 0.08% would be raised to 5%, using the LR+ of 65 for a mass.

Should the general practitioner attempt to aspirate a breast lump?

No. The sensitivity of fine needle aspiration in expert hands is 88% to 95% and the specificity is between 92% and 99%.[16] This excludes cases where no aspirate was obtained. Aspiration of apparently normal fluid does not therefore exclude carcinoma and aspiration is better left to a specialist as part of the complete assessment of the patient with a lump.

How worrying is a unilateral breast lump in a man?

It is rare but worrying. Refer urgently any man, aged 50 years or older, with a unilateral firm subareolar mass, with or without nipple or skin changes.[5]

● *Could it be gynaecomastia?* Yes. While bilateral breast enlargement (gynaecomastia) does not raise the possibility of breast carcinoma, occasionally gynaecomastia presents unilaterally, with the swelling of the other breast lagging weeks or months behind. A retrospective study of 36 mastectomies in men, median age 63, from Buffalo, New York,[17] found that 83% were found to have gynaecomastia, 11% to have lipomas, while only 1 patient (3%) had breast carcinoma and 1 patient had a melanoma-in-situ. However, the one breast carcinoma could not be distinguished clinically from the other masses. The GP has no alternative but to refer older men, and those with a strong family history of breast cancer, urgently. Men under 50 might be monitored for up to 3 months if the diagnosis of gynaecomastia seems hugely more likely, e.g. at puberty.

● *Does the fact that the patient is taking a drug known to cause gynaecomastia reduce the risk of cancer?* If the patient is taking a drug known to cause gynaecomastia it would be tempting to assume initially that that is the cause. This could be misleading in a man with a unilateral mass. A study from Ireland in which, out of 60 men who underwent a mastectomy, 11 had carcinoma, found that the percentage taking such drugs was the same in those with, and without, carcinoma (27% and 29%).[18]

Nipple discharge

KEY FACTS

- Bilateral discharge does not suggest carcinoma. If it occurs at certain times of life (in association with pregnancy or in the newborn or at puberty), it is likely to be physiological. At other times of life a search for a cause should be made: hypothyroidism, an adverse effect of medication or a prolactin-secreting pituitary tumour.
- Unilateral discharge raises the possibility of carcinoma, papilloma, cyst or duct ectasia. When discharge is unilateral:
  (a) the probability of carcinoma is increased if the discharge is clear or bloodstained rather than opalescent or milky
  (b) the probability of carcinoma is increased if the discharge is from a single duct.

A PRACTICAL APPROACH

- * Refer women with unilateral discharge to a breast surgeon unless they are under 50 years old with discharge from multiple ducts which is not bloodstained.[6]
- * Assess each patient with bilateral discharge individually.

Initial probabilities

Even unilateral persistent discharge is unlikely to be due to cancer, with rates of malignancy of 4% to 21%.[12]

Clinical assessment

Unlike the situation with breast lumps, clinical assessment is useful in deciding whom to refer.
* Ask the following questions:
  ■ *Is it at a time in life when it is expected?* Apart from during lactation, nipple discharge is common in pregnancy, after weaning, in the newborn and sometimes at puberty.
  ■ *Is it bilateral and not at a time of life when it might be expected?* Possibilities are: an unsuspected pregnancy; a prolactin-secreting tumour of the pituitary (usually associated with amenorrhoea); hypothyroidism; or medication (oral contraceptive, spironolactone, chlorpromazine, metoclopramide, methyldopa).
* Check the pregnancy test, serum prolactin level and thyroid function tests (TFTs).
If unilateral:
What colour is it? Bloodstained or serous discharge is more likely to be associated with papilloma and carcinoma, while opalescent discharge is more suggestive of duct ectasia or a cyst (Table 3.8). Milky discharge is likely to be physiological. The commonest type of discharge in carcinoma is watery (45%). In 25% it is bloodstained, in 12% it is serosanguineous and in 6% it is serous.

Table 3.8 Causes of nipple discharge with the type of discharge associated with each[19]

	Bloodstained	Serous	Watery	Opalescent	Milk
Physiological					
Neonatal	0	0	0	0	+
Lactation	0	0	0	0	+
Pregnancy	±	0	0	0	+
Post-lactational	0	0	0	0	+
Mechanical stimulation	0	0	0	0	+
Hyperprolactinaemia	0	0	0	0	+
Ductal pathology					
Duct ectasia	±	±	±	+	0
Cysts	0	0	0	+	0
Papilloma	+	+	±	0	0
Cancer	+	+	±	0	0

Does it arise from multiple ducts or just from one?
Discharge from one duct is more likely to be due
to papilloma or carcinoma. Discharge from
multiple ducts suggests duct ectasia. In a woman
under the age of 50, with a small amount of
discharge from multiple ducts, referral is
unnecessary. Older women should be referred
because of the risk of carcinoma, as should
women whose discharge is bloodstained. Women
with heavier discharge should be referred because
surgery can relieve the symptom even if it is due
to a benign cause, i.e. duct ectasia.[6]

Deciding whether the discharge is from one or from multiple ducts

Each nipple contains about 20 ducts. They can be
seen more easily with a magnifying glass than with
the naked eye.

1. Mop the nipple then look for residual discharge
   lying in the mouth of one or more ducts.
   Bloodstained discharge is easiest to detect.
2. Hold the breast with one hand to tense it, and
   with the tip of a finger of the other hand, stroke
   the subareolar region of the breast towards the
   nipple, one segment at a time. If the discharge is
   localised to one duct, stroking the segment
   which it drains will cause discharge to appear at
   the mouth of that duct.

Points about the nipple and areola[20]

- Nipple inversion occurs in 10% of women,
although self-correcting changes often occur during
pregnancy.
- New nipple retraction is more commonly due to
duct ectasia/periductal mastitis (DE/PDM) than
cancer, although exclusion of the latter is a prime
consideration.
- PDM causes progressive retraction (initially a
transverse slit) in young women; DE is associated
with circular retraction in the perimenopausal
period.
- Erosive adenomatosis of the nipple has a distinct
appearance, which usually allows clinical
differentiation from prolapsing duct papilloma and
Paget's disease. It is not premalignant, but is
associated with an increased cancer risk elsewhere
in the breast.
- Nipple pain associated with breastfeeding may
be associated with candida or staphylococcal
infection.

- Raynaud's phenomenon and complex regional
pain syndrome (CRPS) are rare causes of nipple
pain, sometimes occurring after surgery.
- Secretions from Montgomery's glands, whether
milk-like, serous or bloodstained, are easily
mistaken for nipple discharge, especially in younger
women.

Breast pain

KEY FACTS

- Breast pain in the absence of a mass does
  not suggest the possibility of carcinoma.
- Physiological cyclical mastalgia in a
  menstruating woman is by far the
  commonest type of breast pain. There is no
  difficulty with the diagnosis.
- Non-cyclical pain may be:
  (a) localised, suggesting a specific local
      cause; or
  (b) generalised, suggesting a hormonal
      cause: pregnancy, puberty or
      hyperprolactinaemia.

A PRACTICAL APPROACH

- ✱ In cyclical mastalgia in a menstruating
  woman, explain the physiological nature
  of the condition. Examination is performed
  more for the reassurance of the patient
  than in the expectation of a useful
  finding.
- ✱ In non-cyclical pain that is:
  (a) diffuse, search for a hormonal
      cause
  (b) localised, examine the breast, nipple,
      chest wall and spine for a cause.

Initial probabilities

Breast pain is present in about 50% of patients
presenting to surgical clinics with breast
problems, rising to nearly 70% when women are
interviewed in a screening clinic.[21] A study of
women with breast symptoms in primary care in
the USA[2] found that only 2 out of 169
presentations with pain were due to cancer (1.2%)
and both those patients had a mass. The
combination of pain and a mass gave a
probability of carcinoma of 6.4%. Looked at the

Table 3.9 Frequency of different diagnoses in a specialist mastalgia clinic[22]

Pattern/Diagnosis	Frequency (%)
Pronounced cyclical pain	40
Non-cyclical pain	27
Tietze's syndrome	11
Trauma (post-biopsy)	8
Sclerosing adenosis	4.5
Cancer	0.5
Miscellaneous/non-breast	9

other way round, breast pain is an uncommon symptom in breast cancer (present in <25% of cases) but its presence does not exclude the diagnosis.

Only 10% of women who suffer breast pain present to general practice; 10% of these patients will be referred to a general breast clinic; 10% of these women will require specialist breast pain clinic assessment. Table 3.9 shows the experience of one such clinic.

Clinical assessment

Is there a mass? If so, investigate as for mass.
Is the pain cyclical? In 75% of women who present with breast pain, it is cyclical.[6] If so, there is no need to investigate for underlying pathology. In a postmenopausal woman, check whether the pain is due to HRT.

If not cyclical, is it localised or diffuse?

● *Localised pain* is more likely than diffuse pain to be due to underlying pathology. Examine the breast and, if normal, the chest wall and spine. Pain localised to the nipple may be due to a cracked or inflamed nipple. Localised pain in a lactating woman is usually due to acute mastitis or breast abscess but other signs are usually obvious which confirm these diagnoses.

✳ Refer a patient with localised non-cyclical pain if it is severe enough to bother her.

● *Diffuse pain* may be due to unsuspected pregnancy, the onset of puberty or hyperprolactinaemia. In the latter case, amenorrhoea and galactorrhoea are also likely and the serum prolactin level will confirm the diagnosis. If these are excluded, a therapeutic trial of an NSAID followed by danazol or bromocriptine is justified, with referral if they are ineffective.[6]

Final points

● Cancer, sclerosing adenosis, and post-surgery scars are rare but important causes, while referred pain often presents as mastalgia

● Women with mild to moderate causes of mastalgia are usually satisfied if reassurance can be given, rather than medication or referral.

REFERENCES

1. The BRIDGE Study Group. *The presentation and management of breast symptoms in general practice in South Wales.* Br J Gen Pract 1999;49: 811–812.

2. Barton M, Elmore J, Fletcher S. *Breast symptoms among women enrolled in a Health Maintenance Organization: frequency, evaluation and outcome.* Ann Intern Med 1999;130: 651–657.

3. Dixon J, Mansel R. *ABC of breast diseases: congenital problems and aberrations of normal breast development and involution.* BMJ 1994; 309:797–800.

4. Barton M, Harris R, Fletcher S. *Does this patient have breast cancer?* JAMA 1999;282:1270–1280.

5. NICE. *Referral guidelines for suspected cancer.* London: National Institute for Health and Clinical Excellence, 2005. Online. Available: www.nice.org.uk.

6. Austoker J, Mansel R. *Guidelines for referral of patients with breast problems, 2nd edn.* Sheffield: NHS Breast Screening Programme, 1999.

7. Stone A, Shenker R, McCarthy K. *Adolescent breast masses.* Am J Surg 1977;134:275–277.

8. West K, Rescorda F, Scherer L, et al. *Diagnosis and treatment of symptomatic breast masses in the paediatric population.* J Pediatr Surg 1995;30:182–187.

9. Hughes E, Mansel R, Webster D. *Benign disorders and diseases of the breast: concepts and clinical management.* London: Saunders, 2000.

10. Devitt J. *Benign disorders of the breast in older women.* Br J Surg 1968;55:443–448.

11. Greenall M. *Breast diseases.* In: Morris P, Wood W, eds. Oxford

textbook of surgery, 2nd edn. Oxford: Oxford University Press, 2000:1169–1232.

12. The Steering Committee on Clinical Practice Guidelines for the Care and Treatment of Breast Cancer. 1. *The palpable breast lump: information and recommendations to assist decision-making when a breast lump is detected.* Can Med Assoc J 1998;158 (Suppl 3):S3–8.

13. Van Dam P, Van Goethem M, Kersschot E, et al. *Palpable solid breast masses: retrospective single- and multimodality evaluation of 201 lesions.* Radiology 1988;166:435–439.

14. McIntosh A, Shaw C, Evans G, et al. *Clinical guidelines and evidence review for the classification and care of women at risk of familial breast cancer.* London: National Collaborating Centre for Primary Care/University of Sheffield, 2004. Online.

Available: www.nice.org.uk (search for CG41).

15. Kerlikowske K, Grady D, Barclay J, et al. *Likelihood ratios for modern screening mammography: risk of breast cancer based on age and mammographic interpretation.* JAMA 1996;276:39–43.

16. Kouides R, Mushlin A. *Breast cancer.* In: Black E, Bordley D, Tape T, Panzer R, eds. Diagnostic strategies for common medical problems, 2nd edn. Philadelphia: American College of Physicians, 1999.

17. Volpe C, Raffetto J, Collure D, et al. *Unilateral male breast masses: cancer risk and their evaluation and management.* Am Surg 1999;65: 250–253.

18. O'Hanlon D, Kent P, Kerin M, et al. *Unilateral breast masses in men over 40: a diagnostic dilemma.* Am J Surg 1995;170:24–26.

19. Webster D. *Nipple discharge.* In: Hughes L, Mansel R, Webster D, eds. Benign disorders and diseases of the breast: concepts and clinical management, 2nd edn. London: Saunders, 2000:171–186.

20. Webster D. *Disorders of the nipple and areola.* In: Hughes L, Mansel R, Webster D, eds. Benign disorders and diseases of the breast, 2nd edn. London: Saunders, 2000:199–208.

21. Mansel R, Hughes L. *Breast pain and nodularity.* In: Hughes L, Mansel R, Webster D, eds. Benign disorders and diseases of the breast, 2nd edn. London: Saunders, 2000:95–122.

22. Preece P, Hughes L, Mansel R, et al. *Clinical syndromes of mastalgia.* Lancet 1976;ii:670–673.

4

A cardiac murmur

- Murmurs are common. In young people, as few as 3% with a murmur will have a cardiac lesion. In the old, most with murmurs will have a cardiac lesion and the problem is deciding if it is clinically significant.
- Mitral regurgitation is the commonest lesion in all age groups followed by aortic stenosis in older patients.

- While the clinical examination by cardiologists has been shown to be quite accurate in the diagnosis of cardiac lesions, in the hands of GPs it is much less useful. For this reason, various decision rules have been formulated to assist the GP in the decision whether to refer for further assessment.

A PRACTICAL APPROACH

For clinicians with no confidence in their ability to diagnose cardiac lesions accurately:

* Decide whether the murmur is systolic or diastolic.
* Refer all patients with a diastolic murmur for further assessment.
* If systolic, refer if there is:
  (a) any evidence of cardiac dysfunction, e.g. heart failure, breathlessness without obvious heart failure, syncope, angina
  (b) a murmur that is loud or the patient is 50 or older.

However, two special cautions apply:

1. If deciding not to refer a younger person for the reasons above, check that the murmur meets the criteria for a functional murmur:[1,2]
   (a) it is not loud (i.e. it is <3/6)
   (b) it is mid-systolic, i.e. it does not obscure S_1 or S_2

(c) it is localised to the left sternal border
(d) the patient has no symptoms that could be related to valvular disease
(e) there are no abnormal findings in the rest of the cardiovascular examination.

2. If considering the referral of an older person, make the diagnosis of mild aortic stenosis, or aortic sclerosis, and so avoid referral, if the murmur is an ejection systolic murmur and *none* of the following apply:
   - the murmur is heard over the head of the clavicle
   - there is a thrill
   - S_2 is reduced or absent
   - the carotid pulse is delayed, small and/or slow-rising
   - there is a sustained apical impulse or left ventricular hypertrophy on electrocardiogram (ECG).

This chapter focuses on the murmurs themselves and pays less attention to other, no less essential, aspects of the examination of the cardiovascular system.

Abbreviations used in this chapter

AR: aortic regurgitation
AS: aortic stenosis
ASD: atrial septal defect
MR: mitral regurgitation
MS: mitral stenosis
PR: pulmonary regurgitation
PS: pulmonary stenosis
S_1: first heart sound
S_2: second heart sound
TR: tricuspid regurgitation
TS: tricuspid stenosis
VSD: ventricular septal defect

Prevalence of valvular disease

A US survey found a prevalence of moderate to severe valve disease in 2.5% of the adult population.[3] This varied according to age as follows:

- Age 18–44: 0.7%
- Age 45–64: 2.3%
- Age 65–74: 8.5%
- Age 75 and above: 13.3%.

Prevalence of murmurs and associated cardiac disease

Young adults. Studies report prevalences of systolic murmurs in between 5% and 52%,[4] almost all of whom (86–100%) do not have cardiac disease as judged on echocardiography. The study in which 52% were found to have systolic murmurs was of 509 university students requesting oral contraception.[5] Of the 265 with murmurs, 9 (3%) were found to have cardiac disease (8 valvular and 1 ASD).

Pregnant women. Systolic murmurs are even more common, because of increased blood flow through normal valves. Ninety-seven per cent of pregnant women referred for assessment of a systolic murmur in London were found to be normal on echocardiography.[6] Of the 4 women with cardiac lesions, 3 were immigrants with no previous history of heart disease. The fourth was

known to have had a murmur from childhood. An earlier study had shown that the usual criteria for an innocent murmur (a soft ejection murmur at the left sternal border) was 100% reliable in excluding cardiac disease in 103 pregnant women with a systolic murmur.[7]

The elderly. In a review, between 29% and 60% of elderly people, either screened in general medical clinics or as residents of long-term care facilities, have a systolic murmur.[4] The percentage in whom echocardiography was normal ranged, in different studies, from 44% to 100%. It is clear that the older the patient, the less likely it is that a systolic murmur is functional. In a New Zealand study of patients referred, mainly by cardiologists, for ECGs because of non-specific systolic murmurs, the percentage of abnormal findings in younger adults was fairly constant at 34%.[8] In those aged 50 to 59, it rose to 60% and in those aged over 60 to 89%. Mitral regurgitation was the commonest lesion in these older patients (33%), followed by aortic valve disease (22%).

Patients admitted, for any reason, to hospital. One Copenhagen hospital found that 20% of nearly 3000 unselected admissions were found to have a murmur.[9]

Conclusion

Murmurs are common and are not at all specific for the presence of valvular heart disease. The GP needs to be able to distinguish which patients need referral for echocardiography.

Initial probabilities

No study has been found which gives the prevalence of different cardiac lesions associated with the discovery of a murmur in primary care. The nearest relevant study is one of 203 unselected patients attending an emergency department in Basel, Switzerland who were found to have a systolic murmur.[10] The causes were as follows:

- functional murmur 65%
- MR 21%
- AS 17%
- AR 14%
- TR 7%
- all other causes <2% each.

(The total is >100% because some patients had more than one lesion.)

History

Is the history helpful in deciding whether a murmur indicates cardiac disease?

Yes, hugely.
- The patient with a murmur who describes features of heart failure (e.g. breathlessness or ankle swelling) is more likely to have a cardiac lesion as the cause of the murmur than one who is asymptomatic.
- Conversely, the patient who gives a history suggestive of a high output state (e.g. anaemia, renal failure, pregnancy or thyrotoxicosis) is more likely to have a murmur due to increased flow across a normal valve than one who does not give such a history.
- The history of effort syncope in aortic stenosis suggests that the stenosis is significant. In a study of 106 adults with systolic murmurs suggestive of AS, the 15 with effort syncope all had significant stenosis.[11]
- Finally, the history may reveal that the murmur has been detected before and a diagnosis of cardiac disease, or its absence, made. This history must, however, be treated with caution. A US study of diabetic patients who gave a history of a heart murmur, rheumatic fever or mitral valve prolapse found that 65% had no murmur on two consecutive examinations.[12]

The examination

This is central to the diagnosis of the cause of a murmur. Considering the examination of the cardiovascular system, the questions for the clinician to consider are:
* *Is the patient in heart failure or is there other evidence of impaired cardiac function*, e.g. syncope, angina or breathlessness?
* *Where in the cycle does the murmur occur?*
Systole
  - Holosystolic (or pansystolic) murmur: MR, VSD
  - Mid-systolic (or ejection) murmur: functional murmur, AS, PS, ASD, hypertrophic cardiomyopathy
  - Early systolic murmur: TR, acute MR, VSD
  - Late systolic murmur: mitral valve prolapse, or papillary muscle dysfunction in ischaemic heart disease or left ventricular dilatation.
Diastole
  - Early diastolic murmur: AR, PR
  - Mid-diastolic murmur: TS, MS and sometimes in MR and TR
  - Late diastolic murmur: AR (the Austin Flint murmur), MS, TS.
Continuous murmur
  - Patent ductus arteriosus.

* *What is the character of the sound?* Experience will allow the clinician to identify many murmurs by their frequency and tone even before analysing their other characteristics.
  - A high frequency sustained hissing or 'musical' sound: MR, TR
  - A high frequency blowing sound that decrescendos: AR, PR
  - A low frequency rumble: MS, TS
  - A harsh sound, like someone clearing his throat[2]: AS.
* *Where is the murmur heard best?* If a murmur is heard high in the chest, along the upper sternal border, a site to the left suggests it originates from the pulmonary valve while a site to the right suggests that it is aortic. Aortic lesions are also heard along the left sternal border and at the apex. Mitral lesions are best heard at the apex.
* *Are there other features of the cardiovascular examination which point to the cause of the murmur?* These are discussed under the individual lesions, below.
* *Do any manoeuvres alter the murmur?* Murmurs that become louder during inspiration originate from the right side of the heart. This finding has a sensitivity of 100% and a specificity of 88%.[13] In other words, cardiologists find that all patients with right-sided murmurs show this characteristic; and most who do not have the characteristic do not have a right-sided lesion. The Valsalva manoeuvre, if held for 20 seconds, will make murmurs from the left side of the heart quieter except for the murmur of hypertrophic cardiomyopathy which becomes louder. Other manoeuvres are described[2,13] but are rarely performed in general practice.

How reliable is the examination in the diagnosis of a cardiac murmur?

Two systematic reviews found that cardiologists were good at deciding, on the basis of the clinical examination, whether systolic[4] and diastolic[14] murmurs were innocent, doubtful or an indication of cardiac disorder, although the evidence from some settings was less impressive than from others. Likelihood ratios for the detection or exclusion of each cardiac lesion have been worked out when the examination is undertaken by cardiologists.[2] However, auscultation of the heart is a skill in which the performance of non-specialists is very different. Only a few studies have examined the performance of non-specialists and their performance is much less impressive.

1. In a US study of internal medicine residents in years 1 to 3 of training, using a cardiology patient simulator, the rates of correct identification of three valvular lesions was as follows:[15]
   - MR 52%
   - MS 37%
   - AR 54%.

   Individual residents who repeated the test at the end of that year of training showed no improvement.

2. Another study of physicians in training in the USA, Canada and the UK, mainly in family practice, invited the physicians to identify recordings of 12 sounds from the heart, of which 6 were murmurs, scoring 1 for a correct identification.[16] Corrected scores for the identification of murmurs in the three groups were 12%, 16% and 19% respectively. There was little evidence that the 3 years of training improved performance, with the modest exception of the UK doctors.

However, usually GPs do not need to reach a precise diagnosis. It may be enough:

(a) to distinguish innocent murmurs from those that indicate organic disease. The distinction is important, even in the asymptomatic patient, because of the need for prophylaxis against endocarditis and thromboembolism, as well as in order to allow a decision to be made about future monitoring.

(b) to decide whether an ejection systolic murmur in an older person warrants referral for assessment of aortic stenosis.

The minimum clinical skills a GP needs in the diagnosis of murmurs

1. Distinguishing between innocent murmurs and those that signify organic disease

Two studies found that front-line physicians are not good at making the distinction.

A study of older patients (mean age 64)

A study of emergency department (ED) physicians in Basel, Switzerland, whose clinical expertise might be expected to be similar to that of GPs, found that their clinical examination of patients with systolic murmurs, including chest X-ray (CXR) and ECG, was 82% sensitive and 69% specific for the diagnosis of valvular heart disease (regardless of the exact nature of the lesion).[10] These figures only give their performance a positive likelihood ratio (LR+) of 2.6 and a negative likelihood ratio (LR−) of 0.3. This means that the patient whose probability of valvular heart disease before assessment was, in this study, 35%, has, after assessment, a probability, if judged to have valvular disease, of 59% and, if judged not to have it, of 12%. The assessment therefore neither rules in, nor rules out, valvular disease.

The same study went on to elaborate a simple decision rule for the exclusion of valvular heart disease. This states that the murmur is functional if the patient:

(a) is under 50 years old and

(b) has a murmur that is not loud (i.e. is <3/6).

This rule gave an unimpressive LR+ of 1.5, but a much improved LR− of 0.04 (95% CI 0.01 to 0.3). These figures mean that the probability of valvular heart disease is hardly increased, if the rule is not met, but if the rule is met, the probability falls from 35% to a very useful 2% (Table 4.1).

A study of younger patients (mean age 33)

A study from the general medical clinic of a Boston teaching hospital examined the value of the clinical examination in younger patients. No correlation was found between *systolic* murmurs heard by the physicians (referred to as primary care providers) and the finding of a cardiac lesion on echocardiography.[17] In the assessment of 102

Table 4.1 Value of the Basel rule in the differentiation of valvular heart disease from a functional murmur

Probability of valvular heart disease before the assessment	Basel rule	Likelihood ratio (95% CI)	Probability of valvular heart disease after the assessment (95% CI)
35%	Not met	1.5 (1.3–1.7)	44% (41–47%)
	Met	0.04 (0.01–0.3)	2% (1–14%)

Follow each row from left to right to see how the results of the rule alter the probability of valvular heart disease.

Table 4.2 Value of the Boston rule in the diagnosis of an innocent murmur in younger patients with a systolic murmur

Probability that the murmur is innocent before the assessment	The Boston rule	Likelihood ratio	Probability that the murmur is innocent after application of the rule (95% CI)
65%	Is met	1.7	76% (70–81%)
	Is not met	0.2	28% (16–47%)

Follow each row from left to right to see how the Boston rule alters the probability that the murmur is innocent.

systolic murmurs in adults aged 55 and under, only male sex, older age and a loud murmur (at least 3/6) were significantly associated with pathological findings. In contrast, all four *diastolic* murmurs heard indicated cardiac pathology.

The authors proposed the following decision rule: that murmurs that meet all three of the following criteria can be assumed to be innocent:

1. the murmur is systolic
2. the patient is a woman aged 35 or under
3. the murmur is not loud.

The rule was 90% sensitive and 47% specific for an innocent systolic murmur (LR+ 1.7 (95% CI 1.2 to 2.3); LR– 0.2 (95% CI 0.1 to 0.5)). Using the Basel figure that 65% of murmurs are innocent, the rule would have the following predictive values (Table 4.2):

■ women <35 with soft/moderate murmurs would still have a 24% probability of cardiac pathology
■ all other patients would have a 72% probability of cardiac pathology.

Alone, this decision rule is not sufficient to determine a decision not to refer.

What is the GP to do?

Based on the above studies and those in the sections that follow, only dismiss as innocent a murmur that is:

1. a systolic ejection murmur, i.e. does not obscure S_1 or S_2
2. is only heard at the left sternal border
3. is soft, or, at the most, moderate in intensity
4. does not become louder during a Valsalva manoeuvre (which would indicate hypertrophic cardiomyopathy)
5. is associated with no abnormalities of carotid pulse, blood pressure, jugulovenous pressure or chest palpation
6. in a patient with no symptoms of heart disease.

2. Deciding whether an ejection systolic murmur in an older person warrants referral for assessment of aortic stenosis

● In industrialised countries, aortic stenosis is now largely a degenerative disease of the elderly. It progresses slowly, taking on average 15 years for a stenosis to progress from mild to severe. However, once symptoms occur, the untreated 3-year mortality is 50%.[18] Early diagnosis of severe stenosis is therefore important; but once symptoms begin, their nature and severity are no guide to the severity of the stenosis.[19]

● The problem for the GP is that most older people with an aortic ejection murmur do not need referral; they have a flow murmur without significant stenosis. However, those with stenosis need referral early once symptoms related to the stenosis occur. If the stenosis is severe, referral, even if asymptomatic, would be wise. The GP therefore has to decide clinically whether there is significant stenosis. The ideal would be if the GP could also decide whether the stenosis is severe. However, as shown below, this is less easy. The GP will have to be content with distinguishing moderate or severe stenosis from aortic sclerosis or mild stenosis.[2]

Prevalence of systolic murmurs and AS

Systolic murmurs are common in the elderly, being found in up to half of unselected elderly people.[18] Half of those have been found to have AS.[20] A further 2% have AS without a murmur being audible.

In the Helsinki Ageing Study, 5% of those over 75 years old had moderate or severe AS.[21] In 2.9% of the elderly population it was judged to be critical.

The examination

The murmur: traditionally described as an ejection systolic murmur, with a crescendo in the first half of systole then a diminuendo in the second half. S_1 and S_2 are not obscured. However, the murmur of aortic stenosis may be heard in mid or late systole, or throughout systole, masking S_2. For cardiologists, the characteristic murmur argues modestly for AS (LR+ 3.3) but its absence is more useful in arguing against AS (LR– 0.1).[2] The sound of the murmur may change as the listener moves from the apex (where high frequencies dominate) to the right second intercostal space (where it sounds rougher).

Where to listen for the murmur: apex, left sternal border, upper right second intercostal space, carotid arteries.

Other signs:

- slow rising and delayed carotid pulse
- diminished carotid pulse volume
- left ventricular hypertrophy
- a thrill at the left sternal border
- apical/carotid delay and brachioradial delay.

Calcification of the aortic valve on chest X-ray has been used to increase the probability of AS. Although it is indeed part of the pathological process, it is too common to be useful, being found in half of those aged 55 and over and in 75% of those aged 85.[21]

However, these signs are unreliable as a guide to severity. Furthermore, in heart failure the intensity of the murmur is reduced. *Any* murmur in the presence of heart failure is grounds for an echocardiogram.

A decision rule in the diagnosis of aortic stenosis

Etchells and colleagues from Toronto have suggested and validated a clinical decision rule for non-cardiologists to help the evaluation of a systolic murmur in the older person.[22] Of 123 patients aged >50 referred for an echocardiogram,

13% were found to have moderate to severe AS, 1% mild AS and 46% were classified as having aortic sclerosis. The physicians were instructed to listen for the murmur over the head of the right clavicle (LR+ 2.7; 95% CI 2.2–3.3). If the clavicle was too prominent for the diaphragm to make good contact with skin, it was to be moved down until it did, but always maintaining some contact with the clavicle. If there was no murmur over the clavicle, AS was very unlikely, with an LR– 0.1 (95% CI 0.03 to 0.4) (Table 4.3).

Can a positive clinical diagnosis of AS be made more firmly?

In the Toronto study, the physicians were also instructed to look for four other signs:

1. a reduced S_2
2. a reduced carotid pulse volume
3. a slow rising carotid pulse
4. a murmur that was loudest in the right second intercostal space.

The presence of three or four of these carried an LR+ of 40 (95% CI 7 to 239).

The presence of only one or two of these carried an LR+ of 1.8 (95% CI 0.9 to 2.9), which was clinically and statistically insignificant.

The confidence interval for the LR+ of 40 is too wide to be very useful, although the figure of 40 is supported by an earlier study that examined the reliability of the physical examination and found similar LR+s (around 40) for a long ejection systolic murmur, a late peaking ejection systolic murmur, a decreased or absent aortic second sound and a slow rising carotid pulse.[20] Each carried an LR– of about 0.25. It is interesting that traditionally taught radiation of the murmur to the carotid artery was not found to be useful in the diagnosis of AS.

A Swedish study has confirmed the value of the above signs in the diagnosis of significant AS and adds one feature of the history.[11] A history of

---

Table 4.3 Value of hearing a murmur over the clavicle in the diagnosis of moderate or severe AS

Probability of that condition before the assessment	Murmur over the right clavicle	Likelihood ratio (95% CI)	Probability of that condition after the assessment (95% CI)
5%	Heard	2.7 (2.2–3.3)	12% (11–14%)
	Not heard	0.1 (0.03–0.4)	1% (0–2%)

Follow each row from left to right to see how listening over the clavicle alters the probability of moderate to severe AS. The initial probability of 5% is based on the Helsinki Ageing Study.[21]

effort syncope was present in 15 out of 46 patient with significant AS and absent in all 15 whose AS was mild.

What is the GP to do?

An individual GP cannot know whether his or her clinical skills will give likelihood ratios similar to those above. Faced with a patient aged over 70 with a systolic ejection murmur who is asymptomatic, or whose symptoms are not sufficient to prompt referral unless there is also aortic stenosis, the GP should refer if there are any of the following:

- ■ a history of effort syncope
- ■ an ejection systolic murmur heard over the head of the right clavicle
- ■ a reduced S_2
- ■ a carotid pulse that is slow rising, small in volume or delayed
- ■ a thrill.

Probabilities may be refined further by consideration of the patient's age. In an industrialised country, where rheumatic aortic stenosis is rare, the age cut-off may be set at 70. In the Helsinki Ageing Study, in which 5% of 552 older people were found to have significant AS, none occurred under the age of 72.[21] Increasing age thereafter increases the probability of AS, with 1% of those aged 75 and 6% of those aged 85 judged to have critical AS.

Further details for GPs who aim to go beyond the minimum

Aortic regurgitation

Prevalence

Aortic regurgitation was found on echocardiography in 29% of those aged 55 and over in the Helsinki Ageing Study.[21] However, few of these would have had a murmur. Another study found that only 1% of the elderly had a diastolic murmur.[23]

The examination

The murmur: a high frequency blowing murmur in early diastole, which starts immediately following the second heart sound. For cardiologists it has the following likelihood ratios for the detection of any degree of AR: LR+ 9.9; LR– 0.3.[2]

There may also be:
- ■ a late diastolic murmur (the Austin Flint murmur), thought to be due to the regurgitant jet of blood hitting the wall of the left ventricle
- ■ a mid-systolic murmur due to increased blood flow across the aortic valve. Indeed a study from California[24] found that a systolic murmur was more common than a diastolic murmur, at least when the patient is examined by a non-cardiologist (Table 4.4).

Where to listen for the murmur: right upper sternal border (second and third intercostal spaces); left mid-sternal border (second to fourth intercostal spaces); and between the left sternal border and the apex for the Austin Flint murmur (see below).

Special techniques: sit the patient up, leaning forwards, holding the breath in expiration.

The stethoscope: use the diaphragm, pressing firmly.

Other signs, all of which are due to the ejection of blood from the left ventricle into an aorta in which the pressure is low because of the regurgitation of blood back into the left ventricle during diastole:
- ■ head bobbing in time with the heartbeat
- ■ wide pulse pressure (>50 mmHg)
- ■ a low diastolic pressure (<50 mmHg)
- ■ 'water hammer' or 'collapsing' pulse (a radial pulse which has a rapid upstroke and subsequent collapse when the patient is supine and the arm is raised high in the air)
- ■ brachial-popliteal pulse gradient (Hill's sign), in which the popliteal systolic pressure is ≥20 mmHg higher than the brachial, or the foot systolic pressure is ≥60 mmHg above the brachial

Table 4.4 Detection rates for systolic and diastolic murmur in AR[24]

Degree of regurgitation	Systolic murmur detected	Diastolic murmur detected
Moderate	86%	14%
Mild	50%	4%
None	17%	2%

■ pistol shot sounds (heard over the brachial or femoral artery when the diaphragm is lightly applied)

■ Duroziez murmur (a to-and-fro murmur heard over the brachial or femoral artery when the diaphragm is firmly applied).

However, a study of 34 patients with AR suggests that these signs are only likely to be detected in severe regurgitation.[25] Reliance on them would mean that the majority of patients with AR were missed. The early diastolic murmur remains the most sensitive bedside test, even though, with a sensitivity of 54% to 87% in different studies,[2] it is far from perfect.

Mitral regurgitation

The murmur: pansystolic (LR+ 5.4; LR− 0.2 for moderate or severe MR).[2] There may also be a mid-diastolic murmur because of the increased flow across the mitral valve. The louder the murmur, the more severe the regurgitation. A study from the Mayo Clinic in which murmur loudness, as judged by specialists, was compared to echo findings found that a murmur judged at least 4/6 usefully increased the probability (LR+ 20) of severe regurgitation (regurgitant volume >50 ml) while a murmur judged to be 2/6 or less usefully reduced the probability (LR− 0.08) of severe regurgitation.[26] A murmur judged to be 3/6 was found to have no predictive value about severity. A problem with the study is that no explicit definition of the scoring of murmur intensity was used.

Where to listen for the murmur: apex.

Special techniques: put the patient in the left lateral decubitus position.

Other signs: left ventricular hypertrophy.

Mitral valve prolapse (MVP) is a special case in which the finding of a systolic click and a late systolic murmur defines MVP even if the echocardiogram is normal. Echocardiography shows it to be present in 4% of women and 1% of men in the adult population.

Mitral stenosis

The murmur: a mid to late diastolic murmur. The murmur starts immediately after the opening snap if there is one. The murmur is an indistinct low-frequency rumble, sometimes so indistinct that it is described as 'the absence of silence'. The murmur may crescendo into S_1 (pre-systolic accentuation).

Where to listen for the murmur: apex.

Special techniques: listen with the patient in the left lateral decubitus position.

The stethoscope: use the bell, lightly applied to the chest.

Other signs: the first heart sound may be loud, followed by an opening snap in early diastole if the valves are still mobile. The apex beat may be impalpable or felt as a tap.

Pulmonary regurgitation

The murmur: a low blowing murmur in early diastole, which starts immediately following the second heart sound. In 'normal pressure pulmonary regurgitation' the murmur may be mid diastolic.

Where to listen for the murmur: the left upper sternal border (second intercostal space).

Special techniques: the murmur becomes louder during inspiration. Instruct the patient to breathe quietly. Forced inspiration will obliterate the murmur.

Pulmonary stenosis

The murmur: ejection systolic murmur.

Where to listen for the murmur: left second intercostal space.

Other signs: right ventricular hypertrophy.

Tricuspid regurgitation

The murmur: pansystolic murmur.

Where to listen for the murmur: right sternal border.

Special techniques: the murmur becomes louder during inspiration.

Other signs: a systolic wave in the jugular venous pulse, present in 51% to 83% of patients;[2] a pulsatile enlarged liver.

Hypertrophic cardiomyopathy

Prevalence: between 1 in 1000 and 1 in 5000. It is usually diagnosed before the age of 30.

The murmur: a mid-systolic murmur. It may obscure S_2. There may also be a murmur from associated mitral regurgitation.

Where to listen for the murmur: lower left sternal border to apex.

Special techniques: the murmur becomes louder during a Valsalva manoeuvre (all other systolic murmurs become quieter). Among cardiologists this has a sensitivity of 65% and a specificity of 96%.[13]

ECG: The ECG is likely to show ventricular hypertrophy but is normal in 25% of asymptomatic patients.[27]

Does the loudness of a murmur indicate its severity?

Yes, but only in regurgitant disease.

A US study compared the loudness of the murmur of aortic or mitral regurgitation with echocardiographic findings.[26] Loudness was judged by the patient's physician (mainly cardiologists) and graded from 1 to 6.

■ In AR, all the murmurs found to be inaudible or quiet (0 or 1/6) were associated with mild regurgitation (positive predictive value (PPV) 100%), while 79% of the murmurs graded 3 or above were associated with severe regurgitation. A grading of 2 was unhelpful in the discrimination between mild and severe regurgitation.

■ In MR, a grading of 0 or 1 was associated with mild regurgitation in 88% to 100% according to the echo criterion used, while a grade of 4 or more was associated with severe regurgitation in 91%.

Note that, in the two different lesions, different cut-off points indicate the distinction between mild and severe disease.

In AS, there is no relationship between loudness and the severity of the disease; indeed, the murmur may become quieter as the stenosis becomes more severe and the output of the left ventricle falls. Similarly, in MS, severe disease is associated with a quieter murmur as pulmonary hypertension develops and the cardiac output falls.

Grading the loudness of a murmur

The Levine grading of murmurs is from 1 to 6, in which 1 is so soft it can only be heard after a few seconds' concentration; 2 is intermediate; 3 is loud; 4 is loud and accompanied by a thrill; 5 is so loud it can be heard when only the edge of the stethoscope touches the chest; and 6 when no part of the stethoscope touches the chest.[14]

However, a common error is to score murmur intensity out of 6 less formally, as though on a Likert scale, where 1 is the quietest that can be heard and 6 the loudest that the examiner can imagine. This tends to result in higher scoring than intended by Levine: a moderately loud murmur tends to be scored 3/6 whereas in the Levine scoring it would be scored 2.

Example

An 80-year-old man asks for 'a check-up' because he always feels tired. There are no more specific symptoms. The GP discovers a moderately loud ejection systolic murmur at the apex, left sternal border and second right intercostal space.

She is aware that tiredness may be the presenting symptom of AS and that his age is not necessarily a bar to surgery. She is also aware that other causes of the tiredness are more likely and that, with half the elderly population having been shown to have a systolic murmur, she must exercise some discretion in whom she refers.

Although she has no great confidence in her ability to detect the signs of AS, she decides that the carotid pulse is normal and that there is no thrill, and she assesses S_2 to be normal. However, she can

clearly hear the murmur over the head of the clavicle and she does think that the apex beat is sustained. An ECG confirms left ventricular hypertrophy.

In trying to calculate the probability of significant AS, she starts with a prevalence of 5% at his age, increased to 10% because of his murmur. She adds 15% because of the radiation of the murmur to the clavicle (using McGee's rule, see p. xix) and another 15% because of the left ventricular hypertrophy. This brings him to a probability of significant AS of 40%, but the absence of the other findings reduces it to something like 10% again.

She decides to refer him, given the difficulty of deciding on the cause of fatigue in an 80-year-old, but is able to reassure him that the chance of finding significant heart disease is small.

REFERENCES

1. Bonow R, Carabello B, de Leon AJ, et al. *ACC/AHA guidelines for the management of patients with valvular heart disease: a report of the American College of Cardiology/American Heart Association Task Force on Practice Guidelines.* J Am Coll Cardiol 1998; 32:1486–1588.

2. McGee S. *Evidence-based physical diagnosis.* Philadelphia: Saunders, 2001.

3. Nkomo V, Gardin J, Skelton T, et al. *Burden of valvular heart disease: a population-based study.* Lancet 2006; 368:1005–1011.

4. Etchells E, Bell C, Robb K. *Does this patient have an abnormal systolic murmur?* JAMA 1997;277:564–571.

5. McCracken D, Everett J. *An investigation of the incidence of cardiac murmurs in young healthy women.* Practitioner 1976;216:308–309.

6. Tan J, de Swiet M. *Prevalence of heart disease diagnosed de novo in pregnancy in a West London population.* Br J Obstet Gynaecol 1998;105: 1185–1188.

7. Mishra M, Chambers J, Jackson G. *Murmurs in pregnancy: an audit of echocardiography.* BMJ 1992;304: 1413–1414.

8. Xu M, McHaffie D. *Nonspecific systolic murmurs: an audit of the clinical value of echocardiography.* N Z Med J 1993;106:54–56.

9. Iversen K, Teisner A, Bay M, et al. *Heart murmur and echocardiographic findings in 2907 non-selected patients admitted to hospital.* Ugeskr Laeger 2006;168: 2551–2554.

10. Reichlin S, Dieterle T, Camli C, et al. *Initial clinical evaluation of cardiac systolic murmurs in the ED by noncardiologists.* Am J Emerg Med 2004;22:71–75.

11. Forssell G, Jonasson R, Orinius E. *Identifying severe aortic valvular stenosis by bedside examination.* Acta Med Scand 1985;218:397–400.

12. Guggenheimer J, Orchard T, Moore P, et al. *Reliability of self-reported heart murmur history: possible impact on antibiotic use in dentistry.* J Am Dent Assoc 1998;129:861–866.

13. Lembo N, Dell'Italia L, Crawford M, et al. *Bedside diagnosis of systolic murmurs.* N Engl J Med 1988;318:1572–1578.

14. Choudhry N, Etchells E. *Does this patient have aortic regurgitation?* JAMA 1999;281:2231–2238.

15. St Clair E, Oddone E, Waugh R, et al. *Assessing housestaff diagnostic skills using a cardiology patient simulator.* Ann Intern Med 1992;117: 751–756.

16. Mangione S, Nieman L. *Cardiac auscultatory skills of internal medicine and family practice trainees: a comparison of diagnostic proficiency.* JAMA 1997;278:717–722.

17. Fink J, Schmid C, Selker H. *A decision aid for referring patients with systolic murmurs for echocardiography.* J Gen Intern Med 1994;9:479–484.

18. Das P, Pocock C, Chambers J. *The patient with a systolic murmur: severe aortic stenosis may be missed during cardiovascular examination.* Q J Med 2000;93:685–688.

19. Danielsoen R, Nordrehaug J, Vik-Mo H. *Clinical and haemodynamic features in relation to severity of aortic stenosis in adults.* Eur Heart J 1991;12: 791–795.

20. Aronow W, Kronzon I. *Correlation of prevalence and severity of valvular aortic stenosis determined by continuous-wave Doppler echocardiography with physical signs of aortic stenosis in patients aged 62 to 100 years with aortic ejection systolic murmurs.* Am J Cardiol 1987;60: 399–401.

21. Lindroos M, Kupari M, Heikkila J, et al. *Prevalence of aortic valve abnormalities in the elderly: an echocardiographic study of a random population.* J Am Coll Cardiol 1993; 21:1220–1225.

22. Etchells E, Glenns V, Shadowitz S, et al. *A bedside clinical prediction rule for detecting moderate or severe aortic stenosis.* J Gen Intern Med 1998;13:699–704.

23. Bethel C. *Heart sounds in the aged.* Am J Cardiol 1963;11:763–767.

24. Heidenreich P, Schnittger I, Hancock S, et al. *A systolic murmur is a common presentation of aortic regurgitation detected by echocardiography.* Clin Cardiol 2004; 27:502–506.

25. Frank MJ, Casanegra P, Miglioni AJ, Levinson GE. *The clinical evaluation of aortic regurgitation, with special reference to a neglected sign: the popliteal-brachial pressure gradient.* Arch Intern Med 1965;116:357–365.

26. Desjardins V, Enriquez-Sarano M, Tajik A, et al. *Intensity of murmurs correlates with severity of valvular regurgitation.* Am J Med 1996;100: 149–156.

27. McKenna W. *The cardiomyopathies.* In: Ledingham J, Warrell D, eds. Concise Oxford textbook of medicine. Oxford: OUP, 2000.

5

Chest pain

KEY FACTS

- The complaint of chest pain immediately raises the possibility of serious heart disease and, indeed, 15% of presentations with chest pain are due to ischaemic heart disease. Clinical diagnosis (or at least a suspicion strong enough to justify referral), is usually possible in primary care.
- The majority of complaints of chest pain, however, are due to less serious conditions (e.g. musculoskeletal problems and minor respiratory illness). However, the GP must be alert for two categories of illness:
  1. the serious rarities, e.g. dissecting aneurysm or pulmonary embolus, which it would be tragic to miss, and
  2. the 'hidden' pathologies, e.g. panic disorder, which give rise to major morbidity if not detected.

A PRACTICAL APPROACH

- ★ Ask about factors that help distinguish cardiac from non-cardiac pain: duration, distribution, precipitating factors and type of pain.
- ★ Ask about symptoms that would argue against cardiac pain: the presence of reflux, a respiratory infection, or psychological symptoms (e.g. panic, hypochondriasis, somatisation).
- ★ Tailor the examination to the clues provided by the history.
- ★ Follow up each possibility suggested by the clinical picture (see the appropriate chapter of this book).

Prevalence

In North America in 1985, 1.4% of patient contacts with health care services were for chest pain.[1] Of these, only 7% were admitted to hospital and only 4% presented to the emergency department; 95% of contacts took place in primary care. Figures based on studies in the emergency department and in secondary care must be interpreted with this realisation in mind.

Initial probabilities in general practice

A Belgian study found the following final diagnoses in 320 patients who presented with chest pain, either at home or in a GP clinic:[2]
- musculoskeletal pain 21%
- tracheitis or bronchitis 16%
- heart neurosis 10%
- intercostal neuralgia 8%
- psychopathology 7%
- peptic ulcer or gastritis 5%
- oesophagitis 5%
- serious cardiovascular disorders (includes myocardial infarction) 5%
- angina or arrhythmia 10%
- serious lung disease 3%
- unstable angina 0%
- others 10%
- unknown 1%.

Other studies from primary care show some variation in these figures but the principles remain the same.[3]

These prevalences are very different from those reported from emergency departments. The same Belgian study found that, among 580 patients who presented with chest pain to an emergency department, 28% had a serious cardiovascular disorder and a further 13% had unstable angina. Non-cardiac causes of chest pain were correspondingly less common. Similar results in primary care and emergency department populations have been found in the USA.[1,4–6]

Other points

• Certain features of the patient will alter these probabilities. Angina and myocardial infarction are more common in older patients, while trauma, pleurisy and costochondritis are more common in younger adults. Costochondritis is more common in blacks than in other races and in women than in men.

• The above diagnoses may coexist. In a group of Spanish patients with proven coronary artery disease and continuing chest pain at rest, 50% were also found to have panic disorder, 33% were found to have gastro-oesophageal reflux disease (GORD), 11% had oesophageal dysmotility and 6% had biliary colic.[7]

• While it is obviously important not to miss the diagnosis of coronary heart disease (CHD), it is also important not to over-refer patients in whom the probability of CHD is low. Only 11% to 44% of patients referred to cardiac outpatient clinics have cardiac disease.[8] Once the possibility of cardiac disease is raised in a patient with chest pain, it can be hard to shake off. Investigation, even if negative, can entrench the idea that cardiac disease is present.

• In those in whom the probability of cardiac disease is low, it is still important to make a precise diagnosis of the cause of the chest pain. A study from Oxford[9] found that half of those with non-cardiac chest pain continue to suffer from pain, that they consult as often as those with cardiac pain and that they suffer from significantly more anxiety and depression. Over 2 years of follow-up, about half (whether cardiac or non-cardiac) continued to suffer from frequent distressing chest pain, emotional distress and impaired quality of life.

Diagnosis

Make an initial diagnosis as outlined below, then check it out in more detail as is shown in the appropriate chapter in Part 2.

The history will permit a correct diagnosis to be made in the majority of cases.

■ *A history of central chest pain or pressure*, brought on by exertion and relieved by rest, will lead to further assessment (see *Stable angina*, p. 488). Three more sophisticated questions have been found useful in patients referred for angiography in the discrimination of cardiac from non-cardiac pain:[10]

(a) *Regularity.* If you go uphill (or do whatever causes the pain) on 10 separate occasions, on how many do you get the pain? 'Cardiac' answer = 10.

(b) *Pain at rest.* Of 10 pains in a row how many occur at rest? 'Cardiac' answer = < 2.

(c) *Duration.* How many minutes does the pain usually last? 'Cardiac' answer = <5 minutes.

If none of the answers suggest cardiac disease, the probability that the chest pain is cardiac falls to 2% in a person aged <55, even in a hospital setting, although in a person aged 55 and over it only falls to 12%. In primary care, those post-test probabilities would be considerably lower.

■ *If the chest pain is new and continues for more than 15 minutes*, especially if the pain is severe and the patient is unwell with sweating or nausea or vomiting, the assessment should be made urgently along the lines of *Acute coronary syndrome*, see page 289.

■ *A patient who complains of chest tightness* may not be describing pain at all but dyspnoea, and further questions are needed to be clear which of the two is being felt. If dyspnoea is the problem, see *Dyspnoea*, page 83.

■ *Pain that is confined to one side of the chest* is unlikely to be cardiac. A history of worsening with movement or posture should lead to an assessment of *chest wall pain* (see 'Musculoskeletal pain' in *Pleuritic chest pain*, p. 222). Pain that was brought on by a violent movement suggests muscular or joint strain. Trauma raises the possibility of rib fracture. Pain and tenderness over one or more costochondral junctions is diagnostic of costochondritis.

■ *A feeling of a lump in the throat and chest*, an acid taste, reflux of acid or feeling bloated after meals, point to a GI cause, see *Dyspepsia* (p. 75) and *Heartburn* (p. 154). However, the fact that the patient refers to the pain as 'heartburn' or 'indigestion' should not lead the physician down the path of GI investigations unless other aspects of the history point there too. Patients can find it very difficult to distinguish cardiac from oesophageal pain. A study from Boston showed that the fact that a patient presenting to the emergency department with chest pain described it as 'indigestion' had no effect on the probability of a coronary event either way.[4]

Roughly half of patients with non-cardiac chest pain have abnormally low oesophageal pH and presumed GORD.[11] A trial of a proton pump inhibitor (PPI) may be helpful (see below) but an apparent response may be due to chance or to a placebo effect. Dysphagia is the only symptom that specifically points to the upper GI tract.

The value of the PPI test in non-cardiac chest pain

A meta-analysis of 8 small trials of a PPI in non-cardiac chest pain found that the PPI was useful in the diagnosis of reflux disease. When compared to the gold standard of endoscopy and 24-hour pH monitoring, the PPI test was 80% sensitive and 74% specific for the diagnosis of GORD. That gave useful likelihood ratios: LR+ 3.1, LR– 0.3.[12]

■ *Patients with evidence of respiratory infection* and chest pain should be examined with the diagnosis of pleurisy in mind.

■ *Pleuritic pain*: see *Pleuritic chest pain* (p. 222).

■ *Psychological disorders*. Patients in whom no physical cause for the pain is found do not necessarily have a psychosomatic problem, but it is this group in whom more detailed psychological assessment should be made in order to see whether a positive psychological diagnosis can be made. The main possibilities are:

(a) panic

(b) somatisation

(c) hypochondriasis.

Several studies have found that at least 30% of patients with otherwise unexplained chest pain suffer from panic disorder.[13] Ask whether the pain tends to occur in certain situations (supermarkets, lifts) and whether, during an attack, the patient feels short of breath, dizzy, shaky, with a racing heart and trembling limbs. If the answer is 'yes', see 'Is this panic disorder' (p. 333). The pain that is felt as part of somatisation and hypochondriasis usually shows none of the characteristics of angina; however, real problems arise in patients who suffer both angina and one of the psychological disorders that can mimic it.

■ Other pointers will prompt other lines of investigation.

One diagnostic possibility that is not discussed elsewhere will be discussed here.

Is this a dissecting aneurysm?

Fewer than 1% of patients presenting with acute chest or back pain to an emergency department in Hamburg were found to have a dissection.[14] In primary care, the incidence becomes vanishingly small. Most cases are not diagnosed when first seen in secondary care and 39% remain undiagnosed after 24 hours in hospital.[15] In primary care, the diagnosis is even harder to make, although most will be admitted because the GP recognises that the patient is severely ill.

The following *clinical features* suggest dissection:[15]

■ severe (90%), tearing (39%) pain of sudden onset (84%), radiating to the upper back (32%), lower back (32%) or abdomen (23%)

■ one or more predisposing features: male sex, late middle age, hypertension, Marfan's syndrome, bicuspid aortic valve, previous aortic valve replacement, cocaine use, giant cell arteritis, late pregnancy

■ diminution or loss of carotid, brachial or femoral pulses

■ the murmur of aortic regurgitation

■ hemiplegia or paraplegia

■ haematuria.

Where percentages are quoted above they represent the proportion of patients with that symptom; i.e. they are sensitivities for that symptom in making the diagnosis of dissection. Positive likelihood ratios are disappointingly low, being rarely above 2, but negative likelihood ratios are more useful, i.e. the absence of the symptom argues against the patient having a dissection. For instance, suddenness of onset carries an LR+ of 1.6 (95% CI 1.0 to 2.4) and an LR– of 0.3 (95% CI 0.2 to 0.5). However, studies vary so much in patient selection and methodology that meta-analysis to produce pooled statistics is rarely possible.[15] Pooling of the sensitivities of different aspects of the examination found similar heterogeneity. None of the pooled figures reached a sensitivity of even 50%.[15]

Combinations of symptoms and signs are more helpful. The Hamburg study found that if the patient had a history suggestive of dissection (sudden, tearing pain radiating to the back) plus a pulse or blood pressure deficit, the combination gave an LR+ of 10 (95% CI 1.4 to 80), and an LR– of 0.9 (95% CI 0.9 to 1.0).[14] However, as with all studies of dissections, the numbers are so small that the wide confidence intervals make the results almost useless.

Finally, the ECG has no characteristic pattern in dissection. In 7%, the ECG suggests myocardial infarction with new Q waves or ST elevation.[15] Such an ECG should not deter the GP from suggesting dissection to the admitting medical team if the clinical picture suggests it: it may save the patient from disastrous thrombolysis.

Example

A 60-year-old man consults his GP because of upper right-sided chest and shoulder pain that had been present since the previous day. The GP, knowing that the man is waiting for an angioplasty because of a stenosis of the right anterior descending coronary artery, is tempted to reach immediately for the phone to call an ambulance. But the patient looks well and she takes further details of the history.

The pain came on while sawing wood. He is right-handed. Movements of the arm bring on the pain. There is tenderness over the upper pectoralis major.

The GP is clear that this is musculoskeletal pain. Despite the fact that the pre-test probability of the pain being cardiac was high, the detailed clinical assessment argued too strongly against it. To further convince herself, and the patient, she checks the ECG, which is unchanged.

She sends him home and he has his angioplasty 3 weeks later as planned.

REFERENCES

1. Rosser W, Henderson R, Wood M, et al. *An exploratory report of chest pain in primary care.* J Am Board Fam Pract 1990;3:143–150.

2. Buntinx F, Knockaert D, Bruyninckx R, et al. *Chest pain in general practice or in the hospital emergency department: is it the same?* Fam Pract 2001;18:586–589.

3. Nilsson S, Scheike M, Engblom D, et al. *Chest pain and ischaemic heart disease in primary care.* Br J Gen Pract 2003;53:378–382.

4. Lee T, Cook E, Weisberg M, et al. *Acute chest pain in the emergency room. Identification and management of low-risk patients.* Arch Intern Med 1985; 145:65–69.

5. Klinkman M, Stevens D, Gorenflo D. *Episodes of care for chest pain: a preliminary report from MIRNET.* J Fam Pract 1994;38:345–352.

6. Pope J, Ruthazer R, Beshansky J, et al. *Clinical features of emergency department patients presenting with symptoms suggestive of acute cardiac ischemia: a multicenter study.* J Thrombos Thrombol 1998;6:63–74.

7. Ros E, Armengol X, Grande L, et al. *Chest pain at rest in patients with coronary artery disease. Myocardial ischemia, esophageal dysfunction, or panic disorder?* Dig Dis Sci 1997;42:1344–1353.

8. Chambers J, Bass C. *Atypical chest pain: looking beyond the heart.* Q J Med 1998;91:239–244.

9. Gill D, Mayou R, Dawes M, Mant D. *Presentation, management and course of angina and suspected angina in primary care.* J Psychosom Res 1999;46:349–358.

10. Cooke R, Smeeton N, Chambers J. *Comparative study of chest pain characteristics in patients with normal and abnormal coronary angiograms.* Heart 1997;78:142–146.

11. Castell D, Katz P. *The acid suppression test for unexplained chest pain.* Gastroenterology 1998;115:222–224.

12. Cremonini F, Wise J, Moayyedi P, et al. *Diagnostic and therapeutic use of proton pump inhibitors in non-cardiac chest pain: a metaanalysis.* Am J Gastroenterol 2005;100:1226–1232.

13. Fleet R, Dupuis G, Marchand A, et al. *Detecting panic disorder in emergency department chest pain patients: a validated model to improve recognition.* Ann Behav Med 1997;19:124–131.

14. von Kodolitsch Y, Schwartz A, Nienaber C. *Clinical prediction of acute aortic dissection.* Arch Intern Med 2000;160:2977–2982.

15. Klompas M. *Does this patient have an acute thoracic aortic dissection?* JAMA 2002;287:2262–2272.

6

Constipation

KEY FACTS

The referral of all patients who present in primary care with constipation would overload any gastroenterology service. Referral, therefore, has to be based on an assessment of the probability of serious or treatable disease.

A PRACTICAL APPROACH

* Do not accept the patient's complaint of constipation; check that the problem really is the infrequent passage of hard stools.
* Consider whether the symptoms suggest true constipation or irritable bowel syndrome, by applying the Rome II criteria for each (see pp. 39 and 424).
* In those with true constipation, search for a precipitating cause: medication, an anal condition, a lifestyle change.
* Ask about pointers towards organic disease: bleeding, anal pain, abdominal pain, recent onset, weight loss, tiredness.
* Check formally whether the patient meets the criteria for a diagnosis of functional constipation or of irritable bowel syndrome.
* Check whether pelvic floor dysfunction is present; in this condition, the difficulty passing stool is out of proportion to the hardness of the stool.
* Examine the abdomen and rectum.
* Refer those who have some pointer towards the presence of serious pathology or who might benefit from a retraining programme.

Prevalence

In the USA, 21% of adult women and 8% of men report constipation and 9% of women and 3% of men report infrequent defecation (<3 times a week).[1] A systematic review of constipation in North America found an average prevalence of 15% (range 1.9% to 27%). Self-reports by patients gave the highest estimates, but two studies using face-to-face interviews gave prevalences below 4%.[2] One of the face-to-face studies found that the prevalence in those less than 40 years old was 2%, rising after the age of 60 to reach 10% in those aged 80 and over.

Is the patient really describing constipation?

Constipation is the infrequent passage, with difficulty, of hard or lumpy stools. In a survey in Canadian family practice, almost half of patients complaining of constipation met the criteria for irritable bowel syndrome and not constipation.[3] A study from Israel found that half of patients used the word in a way that their doctors did not regard as signifying constipation.[4]

Initial probabilities

No studies have assessed the initial probabilities in patients presenting with constipation in primary care. The possibilities are as follows:

■ *Functional constipation*, to which any of the following may contribute: constitutional tendency, inactivity, inadequate diet and fluid intake, and a lack of a regular defecatory habit

■ *Drug use*. In the Canadian survey described above, one-fifth of patients complaining of constipation were taking an antidepressant and almost half were taking an analgesic. Other preparations that cause it are verapamil, NSAIDs, anticholinergics, and those containing iron, aluminium or calcium

- Painful anal conditions
- Crohn's disease
- Acquired megacolon (as seen in neurological disorders or scleroderma)
- Neurological disorders, e.g. spinal cord lesions, Parkinson's disease
- Diverticular disease
- Pregnancy
- Depression
- Colorectal carcinoma (see below)
- Hypothyroidism
- Hypercalcaemia
- In patients under the age of 25, consider the possibility of a late presentation of Hirschsprung's disease.

The history and examination

* Ask about pointers towards organic disease: bleeding, anal pain, abdominal pain, recent onset, weight loss, tiredness.
* If pain is a feature, check for other clues to the diagnosis of irritable bowel syndrome (IBS) (see p. 424). The single most useful question is likely to be whether pain is felt between bowel movements, as in IBS, or only when the patient feels the need to defecate.
* Ask about the factors mentioned above (diet, activity, defecatory habits) which might strengthen the conclusion that the constipation is not due to organic disease.
* Assess for pelvic floor dysfunction. Try to differentiate from the history between slow colonic transit and difficulty evacuating stool, although often both are present.[5] In slow transit, stool presents itself to the rectum for evacuation infrequently, and may therefore be harder to evacuate than normal. In pelvic floor dysfunction, stool arrives at the rectum with normal frequency but is evacuated with difficulty. The importance of making the diagnosis of pelvic floor dysfunction is that it responds well to retraining and poorly to dietary change, exercise and laxatives. Clues in the history are:
  - straining to pass stool is excessive and prolonged, even when the stool that is eventually passed is not hard
  - pressure on the perineum or in the vagina seems to help
  - digital evacuation is used.

* Ask what medication is taken.
* Check the abdomen for a mass, either tumour or a loaded colon.
* Examine the rectum for an anal cause and for evidence of hard stool. Look, in women, for a rectocele. Assess the anal tone and the ability of the patient to expel the examining finger: say 'try to push my finger out'. A poor expulsive effort is evidence of pelvic floor dysfunction.[5]

Investigations

In the absence of pointers towards organic disease, manage without investigation. The diagnosis is very likely to be 'functional constipation' (see box below). This diagnosis is more secure the longer the constipation has been present and the older the patient.

Does a new complaint of constipation warrant investigation for colorectal cancer?

Not necessarily, unless there are other pointers. A UK study examined 2268 patients with distal colonic symptoms referred by GPs, of whom 95 were found to have colorectal cancer.[6] Altered bowel habit in the direction of constipation argued *against* a finding of cancer *in this group of patients* (LR+ 0.3; 95% CI 0.1 to 0.8. LR– 1.1; 95% CI 1.0 to 1.2). Constipation reduced the chance of finding cancer from a baseline of 4.2%, among those with colonic symptoms of any sort, to 1%. Note, however, that this is still higher than in the asymptomatic population: a new complaint of constipation still increases the risk of colorectal cancer above that in the general population (annual incidence 0.05%).[7] A case-control study from Exeter found that the probability of colorectal carcinoma in a patient with constipation was even lower than this, at 0.42%[8] (see *Colorectal carcinoma*, p. 366).

Referral

* Refer all with constipation under age 25 unless it is transient. Contrary to the situation in older adults, the possibility of organic pathology is greater in this age group if the constipation is longstanding.
* Investigate or refer other patients if there are pointers towards organic disease.

The Rome II criteria for functional constipation[9]

It is present if, in the preceding 12 months, two or more of the following have been present for at least 12 weeks, which need not be consecutive:

1. straining in >1/4 defecations
2. lumpy or hard stools in >1/4 defecations
3. a sensation of incomplete evacuation in >1/4 defecations

4. a sensation of anorectal obstruction/blockage in >1/4 defecations
5. manual manoeuvres to facilitate >1/4 defecations (e.g. digital evacuation, support of the pelvic floor)
6. <3 defecations per week.

Patients should have no pointers to organic disease from the history, examination and, if appropriate, laboratory tests.

Example

A GP is making his regular visit to patients in a residential care home. The nurse in charge asks for a supply of enemas for a female patient aged 82 who is chronically constipated. The GP ascertains that there are many likely causes: inactivity, a low fibre diet, no regular toilet habit. He examines her and confirms the presence of hard stool in the rectum. Anal tone is normal but she is unable to make any expulsive effort when asked.

The GP diagnoses pelvic floor dysfunction (in addition to probably functional constipation) and calls in the nurse specialist who has an interest in faecal continence and pelvic floor function.

REFERENCES

1. Everhart J, Go V, Johannes R, et al. *A longitudinal survey of self-reported bowel habits in the United States.* Dig Dis Sci 1989;34:1153–1162.

2. Higgins P, Johanson J. *Epidemiology of constipation in North America: a systematic review.* Am J Gastroenterol 2004;99:750–759.

3. Ferrazzi S, Thompson G, Irvine E, et al. *Diagnosis of constipation in family practice.* Can J Gastroenterol 2002;16:159–164.

4. Herz M, Kahan E, Zalevski S, et al. *Constipation: a different entity for patients and doctors.* Fam Pract 1996; 13:156–159.

5. Locke G, Pemberton J, Phillips S. *American Gastroenterological Association medical position statement: guidelines on constipation.* Gastroenterology 2000;119: 1761–1766.

6. Selvachandran S, Hodder R, Ballal M, et al. *Prediction of colorectal cancer by a patient consultation questionnaire and scoring system: a prospective study.* Lancet 2002;360: 278–283.

7. Hamilton W, Sharp D. *Diagnosis of colorectal cancer in primary care: the evidence base for guidelines.* Fam Pract 2004;21:99–106.

8. Hamilton W, Round A, Sharp D, et al. *Clinical features of colorectal cancer before diagnosis: a population-based case-control study.* Br J Cancer 2005;93:399–405.

9. Thompson W, Longstreth G, Drossman D, et al. *Functional bowel disorders and functional abdominal pain.* Gut 1999;45 (Suppl II):43–47.

Convulsions in adults

7

KEY FACTS

- The diagnosis of epilepsy is easy in a patient who has several tonic-clonic convulsions spread out over time with complete recovery between attacks.
- Difficulties arise:
  - in patients who have a single attack; or
  - where there are convulsive movements other than a tonic-clonic convulsion; or
  - where the manifestations of epilepsy occur without convulsions.

A PRACTICAL APPROACH IN A PATIENT NOT KNOWN TO HAVE EPILEPSY

- ★ Take a detailed history of the fit from any available witness. Explore the possibility that drugs or alcohol are the cause.
- ★ Examine for fever, neck stiffness, evidence of head injury and for focal neurological signs.
- ★ If the history is of loss of consciousness with convulsive movements, but not of a true tonic-clonic convulsion, consider the possibility of cerebral anoxia, e.g. from a vasovagal attack or from cardiac syncope.
- ★ Admit for urgent investigation the patient who has not recovered when seen. Refer urgently a patient who has made a full recovery and no cause for the fit has been found.
- ★ Be alert to the possibility that bizarre sensations, feelings or behaviour may (rarely) have an epileptic cause.

Misdiagnosis of convulsive disorders is common. One estimate is that 20–30% with a diagnosis of epilepsy may have been misdiagnosed.[1]

Prevalence in the community

A study from Rochester, Minnesota, over a 50-year period, found an incidence of all convulsive disorders of 130 per 100 000 person years.[2] This gave a prevalence in 1980 of epilepsy of 0.68% of the population.

Initial probabilities

Initial probabilities from the Rochester study were as follows:
- *Epilepsy*: 44 per 100 000 population:
  (a) generalised:
  - tonic-clonic 23%
  - myoclonic 6%
  - absence 3%
  - other 8%
  (b) partial:
  - complex 36%
  - simple 14%
  - other 7%
  (c) unclassified 3%.
- A single unprovoked seizure: 61 per 100 000.
- *Acute symptomatic seizures*: 25 per 100 000 (although the figure was assessed as 39 in an earlier study):[3]
  - trauma 17%
  - withdrawal 16%
  - stroke 16%
  - central nervous system (CNS) infection 14%
  - metabolic 9%
  - neoplastic 7%
  - toxic 6%
  - encephalopathy 5%

initial acute respiratory infection should be assessed as for chronic cough.

Chronic cough

Initial probabilities

Comprehensive figures are only available for patients referred to specialist clinics with cough. In a *meta-analysis*, the following were consistently found to be the *commonest causes*:[3]
- *rhinitis* (upper airway cough syndrome, previously called post-nasal drip syndrome) 34%
- *asthma* 25%
- *reflux oesophagitis* 20%.

In a US study of non-smokers with a normal or stable chest X-ray, who were not taking an ACE inhibitor, one or more of the above three were the cause of cough in 99.4% of patients.[6]

Individual studies found the following prevalences:
- chronic bronchitis 12–16%
- post-infectious cough 13–27%
- bronchiectasis 4–18%
- eosinophilic bronchitis 13%.[7]

Less common causes include:
- carcinoma of the bronchus
- tuberculosis (TB)
- occupational bronchitis
- heart failure
- interstitial lung disease
- chronic aspiration
- tonsillar enlargement[8]
- psychological cough[9]
- pertussis[10]
- tropical pulmonary eosinophilia.[11]

Finally, *no cause* may be found. Even pulmonary specialists may be unable to find a cause for chronic cough in 12% of referrals.[12] Alternatively, more than one cause may be found in a fifth[13] to over half[6] of cases.

Prevalences in primary care may be very different. However, the one study that has reported on patients with cough for more than 2 weeks found prevalences not unlike those in specialist clinics for asthma (39%) and chronic obstructive pulmonary disease (COPD) (7%).[4]

An approach to the clinical assessment

The *history* should include questions about:
- smoking
- nasal symptoms
- phlegm
- wheeze
- dyspnoea
- heartburn and reflux
- use of an ACE inhibitor
- exposure to dust or to known allergens
- whether the cough began with an acute respiratory infection
- whether the patient is ill, with fever or weight loss, or has other symptoms
- risk factors for TB or AIDS, foreign travel and other relevant conditions.

The *examination* should include
- the nose, which may reveal the boggy appearance of rhinitis, or nasal polyps
- the throat, where post-nasal catarrh or enlarged tonsils may be visible
- the lungs, for wheeze or focal signs.

A pattern of symptoms and signs may suggest a diagnosis which can then be confirmed by further tests: see *Asthma*, page 337, *Rhinorrhoea*, page 233, *Oesophagitis*, page 76.

Less common physical signs. Occasionally a positive finding will point towards one of the less common diagnoses, for instance clubbing or a left supraclavicular node in carcinoma of the bronchus.

Pertussis. There is a clinical impression that pertussis has a distinct clinical picture.[10] The cough is worse at night and on exercise, and may cause vomiting. A whoop may be heard but is less common in adults than in small children. The cough may last 3 months and the same cough may return with the next few upper respiratory tract infections. The fact that the patient was immunised as a child does not rule out the diagnosis.

When the diagnosis is not obviously clinically

A problem arises when none of the usual symptoms or signs of the underlying cause of the cough is present. The most common syndromes are known respectively as *cough-variant asthma*, *upper airway cough syndrome* (post-nasal drip) and *silent reflux oesophagitis*.

Even when the usual pointers to these diagnoses are absent, the *pattern* of the cough may suggest the diagnosis:
- *In cough-variant asthma*, the cough is rarely constant but, like wheeze in overt asthma, will vary within the day and from day to day. The patient may have noticed triggers such as exercise, cold or excitement.

■ *In upper airway cough syndrome*, the cough may show the pattern of allergic rhinitis (triggered by exposure to allergens), or of vasomotor rhinitis (triggered by cold or emotion).

■ *In silent reflux*, the cough may be worse after meals, on stooping or lying down.

Does the evidence support the above approach in the diagnosis of the cause of chronic cough?

Studies from secondary care do not; they have failed to show that the history is a useful predictor of the diagnosis, except for specific situations such as ACE inhibitor use, smoking-related disease, or exposure to TB.

■ A review of studies that looked at the predictive value of different aspects of the cough (timing or character of the cough, whether or not there is sputum and, if so, how much) found that the history was of no value in making the diagnosis.[14]

■ A study from a Belfast chest clinic found little difficulty in assigning most patients with dry cough into one of three categories:[13]

 (a) cough-variant asthma (worse at night or on exercise or in cold, and precipitated by aerosols or sprays)

 (b) post-nasal drip (dripping sensation at the back of the throat, need to keep clearing the throat)

 (c) reflux (dyspepsia, cough worse after meals, on stooping or when supine).

However, these histories barely increased the probability of each condition, with no LR+ greater than 2. The negative likelihood ratios were 0.2 or less, but based on so few patients that they were not statistically significant.

■ A study from specialist clinics shows how difficult it is to diagnose carcinoma of the bronchus because of cough. In a large study from Philadelphia, the presence of cough for 6 weeks or over had a sensitivity of 48% and a specificity of 71% for the diagnosis of cancer (LR+ 1.7; LR– 0.7).[15] Even in this specialist setting, that gave a positive predictive value for cancer of only 3% and a negative predictive value of 99%.[16] In other words, it was fairly useless if cough was present, and the risk of cancer was only slightly reduced if cough was absent.

However, this does not mean that the history is not useful in primary care. It seems more likely that those cases in which clinical assessment permits a diagnosis are managed in primary care without referral. Only cases which present diagnostic difficulty are referred, so it is not surprising that their diagnosis depends on investigations. The idea that the history can assist the diagnosis in primary care is supported by a primary care study from the Netherlands, which examined the value of the clinical assessment in the diagnosis of airways obstruction (asthma or COPD) as the cause of a complaint of cough for 2 weeks or more in people not known to have respiratory disease.[4]

The study found that certain features permitted a diagnosis of airways obstruction to be made with increasing certainty the more features were present:

■ a current or past history of breathlessness or wheeze, or both

■ cough that is provoked by allergens (e.g. pets, hay, mould or house dust)

■ cough that is triggered by various non-allergic stimuli (fog, smoke, exercise or cold air).

The study found no predictive value from a past history of atopy in childhood, a family history of asthma or a history of nocturnal cough.[4]

Investigations

Chest X-ray is the first-line investigation in any patient with chronic cough when the diagnosis is not clear from the history and examination. It is likely to be the only way that some of the less common diagnoses (cancer, TB) are discovered (see p. 429).

Spirometry may detect unsuspected asthma or COPD (see pp. 340 and 357) but there is no evidence about how useful this is in the absence of clinical pointers towards those diagnoses. If spirometry is found to be abnormal in a patient whose cough is not suggestive of either of those diagnoses, there remains the problem of deciding whether the spirometry findings are coincidental. A therapeutic trial, as outlined below, would be needed.

More specific investigations may be dictated by specific clinical suspicions. In acute cough, where pertussis is suspected, send a pernasal swab for culture. If seen later in the illness, send serum for serology.

What to do when the clinical assessment and investigations provide no clues?

An empirical approach to these cases has been suggested as follows:[1]

* *Treat as for rhinitis.* Give an oral antihistamine, with or without a decongestant (although a response may indicate rhinitis or it may be due to the antitussive action of the antihistamine). If there is no response but there are some pointers towards rhinitis from the clinical assessment, persevere with nasal steroids, anticholinergics or antihistamines.

If still no response:

* *Treat as for asthma* with an inhaled steroid. Be prepared to wait 8 weeks for a full response.

If still no response:

* *Treat as for reflux* with a proton pump inhibitor.

Other points

* The empirical treatment for eosinophilic bronchitis is inhaled steroids; but a response may be due to asthma and spirometry would be needed to distinguish these two. A difference in the history is that symptoms in asthma are variable, whereas in eosinophilic bronchitis they are not.

* Stop an ACE inhibitor if the cough is sufficiently troublesome, and it began shortly after starting the drug. Cough occurs in 5–10% of those who take an ACE inhibitor. However, patience is needed in assessing the response to discontinuing the drug. The median time from stopping the drug to the cessation of cough is 26 days.[1]

Eosinophilic bronchitis

First described in 1989, this condition is probably underdiagnosed as a cause of chronic cough.[7] The diagnosis depends on the finding of sputum eosinophilia >3%, but many patients have no sputum and many laboratories are not experienced in the complex handling of the sputum sample necessary to produce a reliable result. This author suggests that, in primary care, the diagnosis can be made tentatively in a patient with chronic cough for which no other cause has been found, who has normal spirometry and no peak flow variability, and who responds to a 4-week course of inhaled steroids.

Referral

Further investigations in the hands of specialists are very likely to find a cause for a chronic cough even if that cause is not apparent in primary care. As well as chest X-ray and spirometry, the patient is likely to undergo a methacholine challenge test, induced sputum analysis, endoscopy of the upper and possibly lower respiratory tract, and investigations for reflux. High resolution CT scan of the chest may detect bronchiectasis in patients in whom the chest X-ray is normal. In a study from Hull, of patients with a mean duration of cough of 6 years, a cause was found in 93% of cases;[17] 26% were diagnosed solely on clinical assessment plus chest X-ray and spirometry.

Referral is justified in a patient sufficiently distressed by cough in whom assessment and therapeutic trials in primary care have failed to reveal a cause. However, the possibility of finding a sinister cause of longstanding non-progressive dry cough is remote and referral need not be made for the exclusion of serious disease.

Chronic cough in children

A study from tertiary care in Brisbane has shown that the aetiology of chronic cough in children is very different from that in adults.[18] The authors examined 108 patients under 18 who had cough for >3 weeks. The mean age was 2.6 years and the mean duration of cough was 6 months. They found that the most common cause was protracted bacterial bronchitis due to the common respiratory pathogens: *Haemophilus influenzae*, *Moraxella catarrhalis* and *Streptococcus pneumoniae*. The figures were as follows:

- protracted bacterial bronchitis 40%
- bronchiectasis 6%
- aspiration 5%
- asthma 4%
- eosinophilic disorders 4%
- gastro-oesophageal reflux disease 3%
- upper airway cough syndrome 3%
- *Mycoplasma pneumoniae* infection 2%
- pertussis 1%
- tuberculosis 1%
- bronchiolitis obliterans 1%.

The rest resolved spontaneously (22%) or remained undiagnosed (6%).

Note two points:

• These aetiologies are markedly different from those in the adult. The most common cause, protracted bacterial bronchitis, was characterised by a moist cough which resolved within 2 weeks of a course of antibiotics.

• The figure of 1% with pertussis is in marked contrast to the finding from primary care in Oxford that 37% (95% CI 30% to 44%) of children aged 5–16 with cough for at least 2 weeks had serological evidence of pertussis.[19] The difference is likely to be due to the younger mean age of the Brisbane group and the much longer mean duration of cough.

Example

A 23-year-old woman presents with a dry cough for the last 3 years. It tends to be worse in spring and summer and easier in the autumn and winter. She used to play tennis on the local grass court but found her cough made her unable to play. There is no other relevant history. Her nose and throat look normal and the chest moves normally with no wheeze.

The GP feels he has too many clues. The cause could be cough-variant asthma triggered by exercise or grass pollen from the fields around the court; or it could be upper airway cough syndrome, also triggered by spring and summer allergens.

He checks her spirometry but is not surprised to find it normal since she is symptom free at the time. He decides on a therapeutic trial, stating with nasal steroids for 4 weeks, followed by inhaled steroids for 4 weeks.

She reports modest improvement with the nasal steroids followed by much greater improvement with the inhaled steroids. He concludes that asthma is the main cause but with the possibility that allergic rhinitis is also contributing.

REFERENCES

1. Pratter M, Brightling C, Boulet L, et al. *An empiric integrative approach to the management of cough.* Chest 2006;129(1 (Suppl)):S222–S231.

2. Pratter M, Bartter T, Akers S, et al. *An algorithmic approach to chronic cough.* Ann Intern Med 1993; 119:977–983.

3. Morice A. *The diagnosis and management of chronic cough.* Eur Respir J 2004;24:481–492.

4. Thiadens H, de Bock G, Dekker F, et al. *Identifying asthma and chronic obstructive pulmonary disease in patients with persistent cough presenting to general practitioners: descriptive study.* BMJ 1998;316:1286–1290.

5. Holmes W, Macfarlane J, Macfarlane R, et al. *Symptoms, signs, and prescribing for acute lower respiratory tract illness.* Br J Gen Pract 2001;51:177–181.

6. Mello C, Irwin R, Curley F. *Predictive values of the character, timing, and complications of chronic cough in diagnosing its cause.* Arch Intern Med 1996;156:997–1003.

7. Brightling C, Ward R, Goh K, et al. *Eosinophilic bronchitis is an important cause of chronic cough.* Am J Respir Crit Care Med 1999;160: 406–410.

8. Birring S, Passant C, Patel R, et al. *Chronic tonsillar enlargement and cough: preliminary evidence of a novel and treatable cause of chronic cough.* Eur Respir J 2004;23:199–201.

9. Currie G, Gray R, McKay J. *Chronic cough.* BMJ 2003;326: 261.

10. Ross A, Fleming D. *Don't forget pertussis . . . (letter).* BMJ 2003;326: 1036–1037.

11. Malavige G. *. . . and tropical pulmonary eosinophilia.* BMJ 2003;326: 1037.

12. Poe R, Harder R, Israel R, et al. *Chronic persistent cough. Experience in diagnosis and outcome using an anatomic diagnostic protocol.* Chest 1989;95:723–728.

13. McGarvey L, Heaney L, Lawson J, et al. *Evaluation and outcome of patients with chronic non-productive cough using a comprehensive diagnostic protocol.* Thorax 1998;53:738–743.

14. Pratter M. *Overview of common causes of chronic cough.* Chest 2006; 129 (Suppl 1):S59–S62.

15. Boucot K, Seidman H, Weiss W. *The Philadelphia pulmonary neoplasm research project. The risk of lung cancer in relation to symptoms and roentgenographic abnormalities.* Envir Res 1977;13:451–469.

16. Liederkerken B, Hoogendam A, Buntinx F, et al. *Prolonged cough and lung cancer: the need for more general practice research to inform clinical decision-making.* Br J Gen Pract 1997; 47:505.

17. Kastelik J, Aziz I, Ojoo J, et al. *Investigation and management of chronic cough using a probability-based algorithm.* Eur Respir J 2005;25: 235–243.

18. Marchant J, Masters I, Taylor S, et al. Evaluation and outcome of young children with chronic cough. Chest 2006;129:1132–1141.

19. Harnden A, Grant C, Harrison T, et al. *Whooping cough in school age children with persistent cough: prospective cohort study in primary care.* BMJ 2006;333:174–177.

9

Deafness

- Chronic bilateral deafness is common and serious. It is associated with social isolation, functional disability and depression.
- Early diagnosis allows the patient to learn to use a hearing aid before too disabled to do so. Occasionally it reveals a treatable underlying disease.
- Deafness that is sudden in onset, or that affects a younger person, or is conductive or unilateral, raises the possibility of treatable cause, e.g. trauma, cerebello-pontine angle tumour or middle or inner ear infection.

A PRACTICAL APPROACH

- * *Is the onset of deafness sudden?*
  - If seen in the first 3 weeks, refer urgently unless there is a clear cause which can be managed in primary care, e.g. wax or acute otitis media.
- * *If not sudden in onset*
  - Confirm the deafness bilaterally with a whisper test.
  - Ask about the effect of the deafness on the patient's life.
  - Examine the ears for wax or abnormalities of the drum.
  - Use the Rinne test to decide if the deafness is perceptive or conductive.

- * *In unilateral deafness or bilateral conductive deafness.* Refer for further assessment.
- * *In chronic bilateral perceptive deafness.* Manage in primary care, with referral to an audiology clinic for assessment for an aid, provided none of the above warning features is present.

Definitions

These are based on formal audiological testing. A common definition is that a hearing loss in the better ear of >25 dB is considered mild, >40 dB is considered moderate and >60 dB is considered severe deafness.[1]

For the GP, these definitions have two limitations:

1. The necessary soundproof room, equipment and trained staff are not available.
2. Deafness measured formally does not necessarily equate to disability due to deafness. Disability is the result of the interaction between the patient's deafness and a number of other psychological, physical and environmental factors.

Prevalence

Older people. The prevalence is 25% to 40% of the population over 65 years old increasing to >80% of those over 85.[2] In many of these, the hearing loss will be mild. The Blue Mountains Hearing Study in Australia found the following breakdown according to severity of deafness in a population aged 55 to 99:[1]

- mild deafness 39%
- moderate deafness 13%
- severe deafness 2%.

Younger people. Surveys less often include young people, but those that do include them find appreciable disability. A Danish study of 31- to 50-year-olds found that 2.7% reported problems which restricted their daily activities and a further 11.6% reported some problem with their hearing.[3]

Importance of early diagnosis

- Deafness is associated with social isolation, low self-esteem, depression, functional disability and even dementia.[4] Provision of an aid alleviates these problems, although benefit in dementia has not been demonstrated.[5]
- Deafness is underdiagnosed and undertreated.[4] Not only does this lower the quality of life for the time that the deaf person is without an aid, but it also appears that some people pass the point at which they can learn to use an aid.
- The extent of underprovision and underuse of hearing aids in the UK has been shown by an MRC survey.[6] Half of those who failed the whisper test did not have an aid. Of those who had an aid, 40% did not use it regularly. There is thus a 'rule of halves' which applies to deafness.

There appear to be three main reasons for the failure to use an aid:

1. Using an aid is technically demanding, requiring manual dexterity to insert and operate. Learning these skills for the first time is hard for the very old.
2. A deaf person loses the ability to discriminate speech from background noise. It is a skill which may take a year to relearn. At first, patients complain that the aid magnifies everything and doesn't make it easier to hear. Provision of an aid at an early stage of deafness will preserve this skill.
3. Many devices in use need adjustment or replacement.[7]

Early diagnosis, early referral and re-referral should alleviate these problems.

Types of deafness and their causes

Conductive (<10%)

- Wax
- Foreign body
- Perforation of the tympanic membrane
- Otitis media
- Otosclerosis
- Cholesteatoma
- Tumour
- Traumatic damage to the ossicular chain or the foramen ovale.

Sensorineural (>90%)

- Presbyacusis
- Noise-induced
- Toxic
- Inner ear infection
- Genetic
- Ménière's disease.

Some disorders are so common (e.g. presbyacusis and wax) that a mixed deafness frequently occurs.

Deafness of sudden onset

Refer urgently if seen in the first 3 weeks (preferably in the first 72 hours) unless there is an obvious cause, e.g. wax or acute otitis media, which can be treated in primary care. Urgent treatment may lead to improved outcomes in barotrauma, acute viral infection and presumed vascular disease.

Deafness of gradual onset

Diagnosing deafness, and the type of deafness, from the history

* *Ask the patient whether he or she is aware of any difficulty hearing.* In mild deafness, the question is only modestly helpful. In alleged moderate and severe deafness, it is not much more helpful if positive but it is very helpful in ruling out deafness if the answer is negative (Table 9.1). There is a clinical impression that the same question, posed to other family members, would prove more useful. If the patient says he or she has no difficulty hearing, then moderate or severe deafness is unlikely to be present.
* *Ask if the problem is unilateral or bilateral.*
* *Ask what impact the deafness has on the patient's life.* This can be done formally with the Hearing Handicap Inventory for the Elderly (Screening Version) (HHIE-S) or informally by asking whether the deafness interferes with the person's social life, or the ability to enjoy theatre, church, the radio or television.

The HHIE-S has been used as a screening tool for the presence of deafness. Using a score of >8 (out of a possible maximum of 40) as

Table 9.1 Likelihood ratios for a single question about deafness in the detection of deafness

Severity of deafness	Probability of deafness before you ask the question*	Patient's reply	Likelihood ratio (95% CI)	Probability of deafness according to the patient's reply
Mild[2]	50%	Yes	2.2 (1.8–2.8)	70%
		No	0.5 (0.4–0.6)	33%
Moderate[2]	50%	Yes	2.5 (1.7–3.6)	71%
		No	0.1 (0.1–0.2)	9%
Severe[1]	50%	Yes	2.0 (1.9–2.1)	67%
		No	0.0 (0.0–0.3)	0%

Follow each row from left to right to see how the patient's reply alters the probability that they are deaf.
*For the sake of this illustration, imagine that you are completely without an opinion about whether the patient is deaf or not (for instance because the family reports deafness but so far in the consultation the patient has been able to understand you perfectly).

positive for hearing loss, the HHIE-S has an LR+ of 4.5 (95% CI 3.1 to 6.6) and an LR− of 0.5 (0.4 to 0.7).[2] Setting the threshold for a positive score higher does not seem to improve the likelihood ratios. Note that this use of the inventory was not the purpose for which it was introduced, which was to measure the *handicap* due to deafness. As a screening test for deafness, it is less sensitive, and so less useful, than the single question: 'do you have any difficulty hearing?'[1]

* *Ask about possible causes*: noise exposure, drug exposure, a history of infection and note the patient's age. Relevant drugs are furosemide, gentamicin, high-dose erythromycin and NSAIDs.
* *Ask about other aural symptoms*: tinnitus (see p. 262), vertigo (see p. 63), earache, as well as headache and the patient's general health.
* *In the younger person ask about a family history* of genetic sensorineural deafness or otosclerosis.

Subtleties

There is a clinical impression that certain types of hearing loss suggest certain aetiologies:
■ paracusis (words are clearer in a noisy environment) suggests a conductive disorder
■ a feeling of fullness in the ear suggests middle ear disease or Ménière's disease
■ hyperacusis (sound is uncomfortable) and diplacusis (the same sound has a different pitch in different ears) suggest inner ear disease.

The Hearing Handicap Inventory for the Elderly (Screening Version) (HHIE-S)

1. Does a hearing problem cause you to feel embarrassed when meeting new people?
2. Does a hearing problem cause you to feel frustrated when talking to members of your family?
3. Do you have difficulty hearing when someone speaks in a whisper?
4. Do you feel handicapped by a hearing problem?
5. Does a hearing problem cause you difficulty when visiting friends, relatives or neighbours?
6. Does a hearing problem cause you to attend religious services less often than you would like?
7. Does a hearing problem cause you to have arguments with family members?
8. Does a hearing problem cause you difficulty when listening to television or radio?
9. Do you feel that any difficulty with your hearing limits or hampers your personal or social life?
10. Does a hearing problem cause you difficulty when in a restaurant with relatives or friends?

Score 4 for 'yes'; 2 for 'sometimes'; 0 for 'no'. A positive result is >8 out of a possible maximum score of 40.[1]

The examination

1. *Look in the ear.* Wax, if found, will not necessarily be the cause of the deafness but it will be necessary to remove it in order to examine the drum as well as to see if hearing does improve. A study of people aged at least 75 in the UK found that wax was present in 38% of those who failed the whisper test. Of those who agreed to be syringed, nearly half (48%) then passed the whisper test on retrial.[6] Once the drum can be seen, look for perforation, dullness, inflammation or scarring.

2. *Test for deafness* on both sides. The whisper test has been validated for use in primary care (see box opposite).

3. *If deafness is found,* determine whether it is conductive or perceptive (see box below).

The whisper test

This is a good screening test and is easily performed. A meta-analysis found likelihood ratios of LR+ 6.1 (95% CI 4.5 to 8.4) and LR– 0.03 (95% CI 0.0 to 0.24).[2] This means that if the chance of the patient being deaf before the test is 50%, the probability changes to 86% if positive and 3% if negative.

1. Stand behind the patient at arm's-length with your head behind the ear to be tested.

2. Cover the patient's other ear with a finger in the meatus. Move it gently to and fro to mask the whisper in that ear.

3. Whisper, and ask the patient to repeat what he or she has heard: for children under 6 years old use a phrase, e.g. 'bread and butter' or 'Father Christmas'; for children over 6 years old, multisyllabic numbers, e.g. '362436'. Correctly hearing 3 out of 6 numbers is a 'pass'.

Tests to distinguish conductive from perceptive deafness

The Rinne test

A 512 cps tuning fork is struck and its base pressed firmly against the mastoid process. The tines of the fork are then held adjacent to the external auditory meatus and the patient is asked which is louder (*the loudness comparison method*).

If louder by the meatus this is a normal or *positive* Rinne test, i.e. if deafness is present, it is *perceptive*. Because doctors easily become confused about which test result is called positive, it is better to report the result in terms of whether bone conduction (BC) or air conduction (AC) is better, i.e. AC > BC.

If louder when pressed to the mastoid, this is a *negative* Rinne test, i.e. if deafness is present, it is *conductive*, BC > AC.

False negatives can occur in severe unilateral perceptive deafness. Bone conduction appears better than air conduction, but the sound is in fact being heard by the good ear.

Note that there is another way of conducting this test. The fork can be held pressed to the mastoid until the patient signals that it can no longer be heard. It is then moved to the meatus and the patient says whether it can be heard (*the threshold method*). This takes longer than the comparison method and has been found to be inferior in one study.[8]

The Weber test

Once the side of the deafness has been discovered, apply the tuning fork to the top of the head. Note that the test is of no use in a patient whose ears are equally deaf.

(a) If the sound is heard on the *deaf side*, then the deafness is *conductive*.

(b) If the sound is heard on the *good side*, the deafness is *perceptive*.

Is the distinction between conductive and perceptive deafness reliable?

In a recent meta-analysis, Bagai and colleagues suggested that the Rinne and Weber tests should no longer be used as screening methods for deafness because they are too inaccurate.[2] However, that is different from their role in distinguishing between conductive and perceptive deafness in a patient in whom it has been established that deafness is present. Further problems arise from three factors:

1. some studies use the inferior *threshold method*
2. some studies include patients with mild deafness, in whom the tests are less reliable
3. some studies do not specify that the tuning fork was pressed *firmly* on the mastoid.

The second of these issues was examined in a study of patients with conductive deafness from New York. If the deafness was <15 dB then a positive Rinne (AC > BC) was always a false positive. All positives only became true positives in hearing losses of 30 dB and above. The Rinne test should not be used for those with very mild deafness.

The third issue was examined in a study from Guy's Hospital London. Light pressure on the mastoid produced a sensitivity of 27% and a specificity of 100% while, with firm pressure, the figures were 73% and 93%.[9] Again, the more severe the deafness, the better the performance of the test.

A study from Glasgow that explicitly avoided these three problems found that the Rinne was 87% sensitive and 95% specific for conductive deafness when the deafness due to the conductive element (the air–bone gap) was 25 dB.[8] The sensitivity rose to 95% with an air–bone gap of 30 dB without loss of specificity. A study from Ohio, in which the *mean* hearing loss was 23 dB, found figures that were almost as good (sensitivity for the detection of a conductive loss 73%, specificity 97%; LR+ 22 (95% CI 17 to 28), LR– 0.3 (95% CI 0.2 to 0.4).[10] In other words, if the test suggests the deafness is conductive, it almost always is. Table 9.2 shows how this affects the probability of conductive deafness using the Glasgow results.

The audioscope

This handheld instrument is a combined audiometer and auriscope. It allows the clinician to test the patient with pure tones of different loudness at different frequencies. It is recommended for screening for deafness in primary care settings by some authorities in Canada, the USA and the UK, but a meta-analysis of six studies found that its likelihood ratios are no better than the whisper test (LR+ 2.4 (95% CI 1.4–4.1); LR– 0.07 (95% CI 0.03–0.17)).[2]

When is further investigation necessary?

Referral for investigation

Refer all with obstructive deafness or sensorineural deafness in the younger person (e.g. under 50) and all with sensorineural deafness of sudden onset, or unilateral sensorineural deafness. Refer the latter two urgently.

A study from Columbus, Ohio found that, in a series of patients referred with unilateral sensorineural deafness, 5% had acoustic neuromas and another 6% had significant retrocochlear lesions.[11] However, on a population basis such findings are rare, with an annual incidence of acoustic neuroma of 0.001%.

Referral for a hearing aid

Refer older people with bilateral sensorineural deafness of gradual onset, with normal tympanic membranes, without further investigation. The one exception, where a specific diagnosis is needed, is noise-induced hearing loss where the diagnosis would affect employment or entitlement to compensation.

The timing of referral for a hearing aid can be difficult. If the patient is having any difficulty with an aspect of life because of deafness and requests referral for an aid, there is no problem. However, if the patient asks to defer referral, there are two points to consider:
1. It is easier to learn to use an aid before manual and intellectual dexterity are lost.
2. Provision of an aid while deafness is mild to moderate avoids losing the ability to discriminate between speech and background noise.

Table 9.2 Probability that a mild (25 dB) hearing loss is conductive when the Rinne test is performed

Probability of conductive deafness before the test	Rinne test result	Likelihood ratio (95% CI)	Probability of conductive deafness after the test (95% CI)
50%	Negative BC > AC	17 (6–50)	94% (86–96%)
	Positive AC > BC	0.14 (0.07–0.3)	12% (7–21%)

Follow each row from left to right to see how the Rinne test alters the probability that the deafness is conductive.

The pre-test probability of 50% might arise in an older patient with some scarring of both drums from old otitis media. The patient's age increases the probability of perceptive deafness but this is balanced by the appearance of the drums, which increases the probability that it is conductive.

What if the patient complains of deafness but the whisper test (and audiometer) is normal?

Tests for deafness in primary care are crude compared to the complexity of the auditory system. The hearing loss may be in different frequencies from those tested, or it may be due to an inability to distinguish a sound above background noise.

The King–Kopetzky syndrome (auditory processing disorder) is hearing handicap in the presence of normal hearing on auditory testing. It is thought to be due to a failure of central processing and is not psychogenic. It may be present to some degree in 10% of children but its prevalence in adults is not known. It has been found in 5% to 37% of patients who attend audiology clinics with hearing problems.[12] Often the diagnosis is used as a 'basket' term for patients with a complaint of hearing loss in whom the audiogram is normal. Many of these will turn out to have another cause when followed up.

* Believe the patient who reports a hearing difficulty.

* Refer for more sophisticated testing:

  (a) those with a family history of perceptive deafness

  (b) those whose difficulty seems to be progressive

  (c) those with other audio-vestibular symptoms (tinnitus, vertigo or imbalance)

  (d) those with other conditions that could affect hearing, e.g. multiple sclerosis or cerebrovascular disease

  (e) those whose symptoms are unilateral, in case it represents an early cerebello-pontine angle tumour

  (f) those disabled by their symptoms.

REFERENCES

1. Sindhusake D, Mitchell P, Smith W, et al. *Validation of self-reported hearing loss. The Blue Mountains Hearing Study.* Int J Epidemiol 2001; 30:1372–1378.

2. Bagai A, Thavendiranathan P, Detsky A. *Does this patient have hearing impairment?* JAMA 2006;295: 416–428.

3. Karlsmose B, Lauritzen T, Parving A. *Prevalence of hearing impairment and subjective hearing problems in a rural Danish population aged 31–50 years.* Br J Audiol 1999;33: 395–402.

4. Yueh B, Shapiro N, MacLean C, et al. *Screening and management of adult hearing loss in primary care.* JAMA 2003;289:1976–1985.

5. Mulrow C, Aguilar C, Endicott J, et al. *Quality-of-life changes and hearing impairment: a randomized trial.* Ann Intern Med 1990;113:188–194.

6. Smeeth L, Fletcher A, Ng E, et al. *Reduced hearing, ownership, and use of hearing aids in elderly people in the UK – the MRC Trial of the Assessment and Management of Older People in the Community: a cross-sectional survey.* Lancet 2002;359:1466–1470.

7. Sangster J, Gerace T, Seewald R. *Hearing loss in elderly patients in a family practice.* Can Med Assoc J 1991;144:981–984.

8. Browning G, Swan I, Chew K. *Clinical role of informal hearing tests.* J Laryngol Otol 1989;103:7–11.

9. Johnston D. *A new modification of the Rinne test.* Clin Otolaryngol 1992;17:322–326.

10. Burkey J, Lippy W, Schuring A, et al. *Clinical utility of the 512-Hz Rinne tuning fork test.* Am J Otol 1998;19:59–62.

11. Daniels R, Swallow C, Shelton C, et al. *Causes of unilateral sensorineural hearing loss screened by high-resolution fast spin echo magnetic resonance imaging: review of 1070 consecutive cases.* Am J Otol 2000;21: 173–180.

12. Kennedy V, Wilson C, Stephens D. *When a normal hearing test is just the beginning.* J R Soc Med 2006;99: 417–420.

Delirium (acute confusional state)

10

KEY FACTS

- Delirium is common in severely ill patients and is often undetected.
- Suspect it in any ill person whose cognitive function has changed, even when the changes seem minor and even 'understandable' given the severity of the illness. Difficulty concentrating or fluctuation between restlessness and sleepiness may be the only signs.
- While any delirious person is likely to need admission, assessment of the cause by the GP can often lead to appropriate referral. For instance, a patient with an acute myocardial infarction can be directed immediately to the cardiological team rather than sent to the emergency department as 'delirium ?cause'.

A PRACTICAL APPROACH TO THE CONFUSED PATIENT

- ★ Make an initial judgement whether the patient is acutely confused or demented, or both, based on whether the symptoms are acute, or chronic, or chronic with an acute exacerbation.
- ★ Confirm the diagnosis of delirium with the three questions of the Confusion Assessment Method (CAM).
- ★ Decide from the history and clinical presentation whether the patient is suffering from acute intoxication or from substance withdrawal.
- ★ Look for evidence of acute medical illness including acute constipation or retention of urine.
- ★ Admit, without sedation, a patient with delirium if no cause that is manageable in primary care is found.

Prevalence and diagnostic difficulty

- The point prevalence in adults in the population is 0.4%, rising to 1.1% of those aged 55 and older.[1]
- 10% of patients aged 65 and older presenting at an emergency department (ED) and requiring a stretcher have delirium. In most of them, the diagnosis of delirium is missed by the ED physician (a Montreal study showed the physician's assessment was 35% sensitive and 98% specific for the diagnosis of delirium; LR+ 17, LR– 0.66).[2]
- 55% of patients, not known to have dementia, who are admitted with delirium are diagnosed as suffering from dementia in the following 2 years. In most, the diagnosis can be made as soon as the delirium subsides.[3]

The World Health Organization (WHO) diagnosis of delirium: the ICD-10 definition[4] (reproduced with permission of WHO)

A. There is clouding of consciousness, i.e. reduced clarity of awareness of the environment, with reduced ability to focus, sustain or shift attention.

B. Disturbance of cognition is manifest by both:

  (1) impairment of immediate recall and recent memory, with relatively intact remote memory

  (2) disorientation in time, place or person.

C. At least one of the following psychomotor disturbances is present:

  (1) rapid, unpredictable shifts from hypoactivity to hyperactivity

  (2) increased reaction time

  (3) increased or decreased flow of speech

  (4) enhanced startle reaction.

D. There is disturbance of sleep or of the sleep–wake cycle, manifest by at least one of the following:

  (1) insomnia, which in severe cases may involve total sleep loss, with or without daytime drowsiness, or reversal of the sleep–wake cycle

  (2) nocturnal worsening of symptoms

  (3) disturbing dreams and nightmares, which may continue as hallucinations or illusions after awakening.

E. Symptoms have rapid onset and show fluctuations over the course of the day.

F. There is objective evidence from history, physical and neurological examination or laboratory tests of an underlying cerebral or systemic disease (other than psychoactive substance-related) that can be presumed to be responsible for the clinical manifestations in criteria A–D.

Suspect it in those at risk

These are those with multiple risk factors:
- old age
- cognitive impairment
- acute illness
- dehydration
- disturbed serum biochemistry
- drugs prone to cause sedation or confusion.

Diagnosis

* Check whether the *ICD-10 criteria* (above) are met. Very similar is the *Confusion Assessment Method (CAM)*, which states that the patient has delirium if:

- there was an acute onset with a fluctuating course;
- there is inattention; and
- there is either disorganised thinking or an altered level of consciousness. Consciousness may be depressed or the patient may be hyperalert.

The CAM has a sensitivity of at least 94% and a specificity of at least 90% (LR+ 9.4; LR– 0.07) for the diagnosis of delirium, when used by non-psychiatrists and compared to psychiatrists as the gold standard.[5]

Differential diagnosis

- *Dementia*. The time course should differentiate the two. Underlying dementia in a patient with delirium can usually be diagnosed only once the delirium clears.

- *Intoxication*. The patient behaves in a way that is characteristic of intoxication with the responsible substance. If the characteristic features of delirium supervene, the diagnosis is of substance intoxication delirium.

- *Substance withdrawal*. The patient behaves in a way that is characteristic of withdrawal from the responsible substance. If the characteristic features of delirium supervene, the diagnosis is of substance withdrawal delirium.

- *Epilepsy*. Confusion may last for minutes or, rarely, up to an hour after a tonic-clonic or a complex partial seizure. However, prolonged epileptic confusional states, without convulsions, do occur but their diagnosis is not a matter for the GP who will admit anyone with prolonged confusion to hospital.[6]

- *Acute psychosis*. The hallucinations and delusions are more organised, without the fluctuations in conscious level and cognition seen in delirium.

- *Severe acute stress disorder*. Again, the fluctuations in conscious level and cognition seen in delirium are absent.

- *Transient global amnesia*. Patients may perform complex actions but have no recollection of them afterwards. There is no drowsiness and no other neurological features.

What is the cause of the delirium?

The diagnosis of delirium is only the start of the diagnostic process. The commonest causes of delirium are:

■ *A medical condition*: for instance, infection, hepatic or renal failure, cancer, head injury, myocardial infarction, stroke, major surgery, or diabetic ketoacidosis or other metabolic disturbance.

■ *Intoxication*. Alcohol, cannabis, cocaine, opioids, hallucinogens and benzodiazepines are common causes.

■ *Substance withdrawal*. The list of substances is similar to those causing intoxication.

■ *Medication*: especially sedatives, opioids, anticholinergics, antiparkinsonian drugs, corticosteroids.

■ *Urinary retention, constipation or pain*: which may precipitate delirium in someone with underlying cognitive impairment, or with another serious illness.

A proposal for the assessment of the patient with altered mental state can be found in the Clinical Policy document of the American College of Emergency Physicians.[7]

Example

A GP is telephoned by a residential care home about a male patient who is aged 72 and suffering from mild to moderate dementia of Alzheimer type. The previous evening he had become 'difficult' and the on-call doctor had prescribed sedation. This had been only partially successful.

When the GP visits she learns that he had become restless and begun to shout, having been his normal self earlier in the day. He kept trying to get out of bed and took no notice of the nurses' attempts to calm him down.

The sudden onset of disturbed behaviour alerts the GP to the likelihood of an underlying cause. She finds no cardiac abnormality nor evidence of chest infection but abdominal examination reveals that the bladder is distended halfway to the umbilicus. She arranges immediate admission for urinary retention and within 48 hours he has recovered his normal calm.

REFERENCES

1. American Psychiatric Association. *Diagnostic and statistical manual of mental disorders, 4th edn, text revision.* Washington DC: American Psychiatric Association, 2000.

2. Elie M, Rousseau F, Cole M, et al. *Prevalence and detection of delirium in elderly emergency department patients.* Can Med Assoc J 2000;163:977–981.

3. Rahkonen T, Luukkainen-Markkula R, Paanil S, et al. *Delirium episode as a sign of undetected dementia among community dwelling elderly subjects: a 2 year follow up study.* J Neurol Neurosurg Psychiatry 2000;69:519–521.

4. WHO. *The ICD-10 classification of mental and behavioural disorders: diagnostic criteria for research.* Geneva: World Health Organization, 1993.

5. Inouye S, van Dyck C, Alessi C, et al. *Clarifying confusion: the confusion assessment method. A new method for detection of delirium.* Ann Intern Med 1990;113:941–948.

6. Duncan J. *Diagnosis and management of epilepsy in adults: Scottish Intercollegiate Guidelines Network, 2003: Appendix A.* Online. Available: www.sign.ac.uk.

7. American College of Emergency Physicians. *Clinical policy for the initial approach to patients presenting with altered mental status.* Ann Emerg Med 1999;33: 251–281. Online. Available: www.acep.org.

11

Diarrhoea

Acute diarrhoea (less than 4 weeks)

KEY FACTS

- Most cases are due to infection and are self-limiting.
- A few will represent the onset of more serious disease, e.g. inflammatory bowel disease.

A PRACTICAL APPROACH

- * Send stool for examination in only a few specific situations:
  (a) suspected food poisoning, or
  (b) the patient is systemically unwell, or
  (c) there is rectal bleeding, or
  (d) the patient is immunocompromised, or
  (e) the diarrhoea is related to a hospital stay or to antibiotic use.

Background

In the UK, the incidence of acute diarrhoea is almost 1 episode per adult per year.[1] No reliable information exists about the pre-test probabilities in primary care. In secondary care in the USA, only 8.4% of stools examined are found to contain pathogens.[2] In primary care, almost all patients recover without a specific diagnosis being made.

Common causes

■ Gastroenteritis: 19% of the population develop an acute intestinal infection per year, although only 1 in 6 of those presents in primary care.[3] *Campylobacter* is the commonest organism isolated in symptomatic adults (12.2%), with rotavirus second (7.7%)[4]

■ Drug-induced diarrhoea, especially laxatives and antibiotics

■ Alcohol misuse

■ Anxiety

■ Surgical emergencies

■ An acute onset of inflammatory bowel disease (IBD).

Assessment

- * *Ask especially*:
  (a) whether other people have been affected
  (b) what drugs have been taken
  (c) whether there has been blood in the stool
  (d) the patient's occupation and whether the episode relates to foreign travel.
- * *Examine*:
  (a) the mouth for evidence of dehydration
  (b) the abdomen, for a surgical cause, or in the elderly, for evidence of severe constipation
  (c) the rectum in those at risk of severe constipation, to exclude the possibility of impaction with overflow diarrhoea.
- * *Send stool for laboratory examination if any of the following apply*:
  (a) The patient is sufficiently ill to need antibiotic treatment if a pathogen is found.
  (b) There is blood in the stools. This increases the probability of *Shigella*, *Salmonella*, *Yersinia*, *Campylobacter* or pathogenic *Escherichia coli*, although a positive result will still only be found in 20%.[2]
  (c) Two or more people are affected who have had the same food or drink and in whom the onset is within a few hours of each other. In the UK, suspected food poisoning should be notified to the public health authorities even

before the results of the stool culture are known.

(d) The patient has recently returned from a country where parasitic infections are endemic. Stool examination for ova and parasites has a sensitivity and a specificity of 80% to 90%, LR+ 4 to 5, LR– 0.1 to 0.2.[5]

(e) The patient is HIV positive or is immunocompromised for any other reason. Opportunistic organisms can be found in 85% of patients with AIDS who have diarrhoea.[6]

(f) The patient was recently in hospital or has recently had broad-spectrum antibiotics. Request examination for *Clostridium difficile*.

* *If the stool test is negative do not send further specimens.* In a US study of 107 patients, there was complete agreement between the first and subsequent stool examinations in 106 of them.[7] In the one patient in whom the first sample missed the diagnosis (of *Shigella*), that first sample was a rectal swab, not a specimen in a pot.

* *Refer as suspected inflammatory bowel disease (IBD)* if the diarrhoea continues for 2 weeks, the history as outlined above provides no alternative diagnoses, and the stool culture is negative. Refer more urgently if the diarrhoea is heavily bloodstained, the patient is dehydrated or systemically unwell, or abdominal pain is prominent. With a prevalence of 0.2%,[8] a practice of 2000 patients will have 4 patients with IBD at any one time.

Chronic diarrhoea

KEY FACTS

* Chronic diarrhoea is common and, in the large majority of cases, the aetiology is functional.
* In a small but significant number of cases, an important treatable cause will be found.

A PRACTICAL APPROACH

* In the clinical assessment, look for clues as to the cause:
  (a) foreign travel, the fatty stool of malabsorption
  (b) an infectious onset
  (c) an association with dairy foods
  (d) drug or laxative use
  (e) alarm features (e.g. weight loss, rectal bleeding, and abdominal or rectal mass) which increase the probability of colorectal carcinoma or inflammatory bowel disease.

* Follow up any clues with appropriate investigations.

* In the absence of a diagnosis, consider the need for referral.
  ■ This will be necessary in the older patient, in those with alarm symptoms and in those whose diarrhoea is of recent onset.
  ■ It may not be necessary for the younger patient with no alarm symptoms whose diarrhoea is longstanding and who meets the criteria for irritable bowel syndrome or functional diarrhoea.

Definition

Diarrhoea for >4 weeks. The cut-off of 4 weeks is arbitrary, as is the definition of diarrhoea recommended by the British Society of Gastroenterology: the abnormal passage of three or more loose or liquid stools per day and/or a daily stool weight of >200 g.[9]

Prevalence

Prevalences of 4% to 5% are found in Western populations,[9] increasing to 14% in the elderly.[10]

Initial probabilities

■ *Functional bowel disorders* comprise up to 40% of referrals to gastroenterologists[11]
■ Malabsorption
■ *Infection.* This may be:
  (a) active chronic infection, e.g. giardiasis, or due to *Cryptosporidium*, or *Entamoeba histolytica*, or
  (b) it may be a functional disorder following acute infection. A study from UK general practice shows that 17% of patients with irritable bowel syndrome (IBS) attribute the onset to a bout of acute gastroenteritis.[12] The chance of developing IBS seems to be higher with more severe illness: a rate of IBS following infection with *Campylobacter* and *Shigella* of 1 in 10 has been reported.[12] In the 3 months after gastroenteritis, patients are 6

times more likely to consult their GP with gastrointestinal symptoms, mainly diarrhoea, than are controls[13]

■ *Lactose intolerance*, whether primary or following gastroenteritis, or as part of coeliac disease or NSAID use[9]

■ *Inflammatory bowel disease* (prevalence 0.2% in most European populations, see above)

■ *Colorectal carcinoma*. A change of bowel habit in the direction of diarrhoea increases the probability of colorectal carcinoma to 8% among patients referred to secondary care because of distal colonic symptoms.[14] A case-control study from Exeter suggests that much of this apparent risk is due to selection bias and that the probability of colorectal carcinoma in a patient with diarrhoea in primary care is only 0.94%[15] (see *Altered bowel habit*, p. 3, and *Colorectal carcinoma*, p. 365)

■ *Coeliac disease* (prevalence 0.5% in European populations) (see *Coeliac disease in adults*, p. 361)

■ *Endocrine disorders*: e.g. hyperthyroidism or diabetes (when it is usually due to metformin)[16]

■ Previous GI surgery

■ Alcohol

■ Drugs

■ Autonomic neuropathy

■ *Factitious diarrhoea* (present in 4% of those referred to a district gastroenterology service but 20% of those attending tertiary referral centres).[9] Patients may use laxatives or just add water to their stools. Laxative users often suffer from an eating disorder (see *Eating disorders*, p. 383).

History

Check, from the history:

■ *Other symptoms*, e.g. abdominal pain, rectal bleeding, weight loss.

■ *The patient's description of the stool*: pale, bulky, foul-smelling stool suggests malabsorption; loose stool containing blood and mucus suggests IBD or carcinoma.

■ *Timing*: whether the diarrhoea is intermittent or continuous and whether it happens at night. Intermittent symptoms that do not disturb the patient from sleep point towards functional diarrhoea.

■ *A history of overseas travel*: 3% of travellers overseas develop diarrhoea that lasts for >4 weeks.[17]

■ *A history of eating disorders* (a pointer to laxative abuse).

■ *A family history* of neoplastic or inflammatory bowel disease, or coeliac disease.

■ *Drug use*: alcohol, drugs (e.g. laxatives, magnesium-containing antacids, antihypertensives, NSAIDs, theophyllines, antibiotics), or food additives such as sorbitol and fructose.

■ *Previous surgery*. There are various mechanisms:

(a) resection of ileum or right side of colon leading to diarrhoea due to lack of absorptive surface, decreased transit time or malabsorption of bile acid

(b) gastric surgery or jejunoileal bypass surgery leading to bacterial overgrowth

(c) resection of the terminal ileum leading to bile acid diarrhoea typically occurring after meals and responding to cholestyramine

(d) cholecystectomy, which may result in chronic diarrhoea in up to 10% of patients by causing increased gut transit, bile acid malabsorption and increased enterohepatic cycling of bile acids.

■ A history of pancreatic disease.

■ *Systemic disease*, e.g. thyrotoxicosis, diabetes mellitus (autonomic dysfunction), scleroderma (bacterial overgrowth).

■ *A history of intolerance to dairy products*, which might suggest lactase deficiency (although only half the patients with the condition will have noticed the connection).

Red flags for organic disease[9]

1. Duration <3 months
2. Continuous or nocturnal symptoms
3. Significant weight loss
4. Rectal bleeding.

Examination

Examine the abdomen and rectum. No figures exist for the value of this in the diagnosis of diarrhoea in primary care.

Investigations

(a) *Blood tests* for malabsorption: full blood count (FBC), liver function tests (LFTs), calcium, B_{12}, folate, ferritin, coeliac serology (antiendomysial antibody). In addition, check the erythrocyte sedimentation rate (ESR) as a pointer towards organic disease and the thyroid function tests (TFTs) in case the diarrhoea is due to hyperthyroidism.

(b) *Stool tests, and other tests, for malabsorption*. If blood tests suggest that malabsorption is present, and there will be a delay before the patient can be seen by a gastroenterologist, discuss with the laboratory the most appropriate next step. Analysis of fat concentration in a single stool sample has largely replaced the 3-day collection. Some laboratories will offer analysis of radiolabelled by-products of fat hydrolysis on breath testing.[9] Pancreatic function can be assessed by analysis of stool elastase.

(c) *Stool tests*: three fresh stools for ova, cysts and parasites (sensitivity 60–90% for the detection of protozoan infections);[9] three stools at at least 48-hour intervals are needed because of the intermittent nature of egg and larvae excretion. Also request stool culture plus stool enzyme-linked immunosorbent assay (ELISA) for *Giardia*. The latter is 92% sensitive and 98% specific for giardiasis.[9] Inform the laboratory where the patient has been, if foreign travel is implicated.

(d) *Trial of a lactose-free diet* appears to be more effective in the diagnosis of lactose intolerance than is blood or stool testing following lactose ingestion. The patient should avoid all diary products for 3 weeks while recording bowel symptoms. If objective confirmation is needed, the hydrogen breath test is probably the most reliable.[18]

(e) *Tests for the presence of laxatives* in urine or stool can be conducted in specialist laboratories.[9]

No studies have examined the effectiveness of these investigations in primary care.

Rome II criteria for functional bowel disorders[19]

Irritable bowel syndrome:
Abdominal discomfort or pain for 12 weeks or more in the last year with at least two of the following features:

1. relieved by defecation
2. onset associated with a change in the frequency of the stool
3. onset associated with a change in the form of the stool, especially if any of the following are present:
   (a) abnormal stool frequency (>3 a day or <3 a week)
   (b) abnormal stool form
   (c) abnormal passage of stool (straining, urgency or a feeling of incomplete defecation)
   (d) mucus
   (e) a feeling of abdominal distension.

Functional diarrhoea:
At least 12 weeks, which need not be consecutive, in the preceding 12 months of:

1. liquid (mushy) or watery stools
2. present >¾ of the time, and
3. no abdominal pain.

REFERENCES

1. Feldman R, Banatvala N. *The frequency of culturing stools from adults with diarrhoea in Great Britain.* Epidemiol Infect 1994;113:41–44.

2. Slutsker L, Ries A, Greene K, et al. *Escherichia coli 0157:H7 diarrhea in the United States: clinical and epidemiological features.* Ann Intern Med 1997;126:505–513.

3. Wheeler J, Sethi D, Cowden J, et al. *Study of infectious intestinal disease in England: rates in the community, presenting to general practice, and reported to national surveillance.* BMJ 1999;318:1046–1050.

4. Tompkins D, Hudson M, Smith H, et al. *A study of infectious intestinal disease in England: microbiological findings in cases and controls.* Commun Dis Public Health 1999;2: 108–113.

5. Massey B. *Acute diarrhea.* In: Black E, Bordley D, Tape T, Panzer R, eds. Diagnostic strategies for common medical problems, 2nd edn. Philadelphia: American College of Physicians, 1999.

6. Smith P, Lane H, Gill V, et al. *Intestinal infections in patients with the acquired immunodeficiency syndrome (AIDS). Etiology and response to therapy.* Ann Intern Med 1988;108: 328–333.

7. Chitkara Y, McCasland K, Kenefic L. *Development and implementation of cost-effective guidelines in the laboratory investigation of diarrhea in a community hospital.* Arch Intern Med 1996;156: 1445–1448.

8. MeReC. *Inflammatory bowel disease.* MeReC Bulletin 1999;10, No. 12. Online. Available: www.npc.co.uk (choose MeReC).

9. Thomas P, Forbes A, Green J, et al. *Guidelines for the investigation of chronic diarrhoea.* Gut 2003;52 (Suppl v):v1–v15.

10. Talley N, O'Keefe E, Zinsmeister A, et al. *Prevalence of gastrointestinal symptoms in the elderly: a population-based study.* Gastroenterology 1992; 102:895–901.

11. Talley N, Weaver A, Zinsmeister A, et al. *Onset and disappearance of*

gastrointestinal symptoms and functional gastrointestinal disorders. Am J Epidemiol 1992;136:165–177.

12. Spiller R. *Postinfectious irritable bowel syndrome.* Gastroenterology 2003;124:1662–1671.

13. Cumberland P, Sethi D, Roderick P, et al. *The infectious intestinal disease study of England: a prospective evaluation of symptoms and health care use after an acute episode.* Epidemiol Infect 2003;130:453–460.

14. Selvachandran S, Hodder R, Ballal M, et al. *Prediction of colorectal cancer by a patient consultation questionnaire and scoring system: a prospective study.* Lancet 2002;360: 278–283.

15. Hamilton W, Round A, Sharp D, et al. *Clinical features of colorectal cancer before diagnosis: a population-based case-control study.* British Journal of Cancer 2005;93:399–405.

16. Lysy J, Israeli E, Goldin E. *The prevalence of chronic diarrhea among diabetic patients.* Am J Gastroenterol 1999;94:2165–2170.

17. Kolars J, Fischer P. *Evaluation of diarrhea in the returned traveler.* Prim Care 2002;29:931–945.

18. Shaw A, Davies G. *Lactose intolerance: problems in diagnosis and treatment.* J Clin Gastroenterol 1999; 28:208–216.

19. Thompson W, Longstreth G, Drossman D, et al. *Functional bowel disorders and functional abdominal pain.* Gut 1999;45 (Suppl II):43–47.

Dizziness

- Patients with vertigo are usually suffering from benign positional vertigo (BPV), vestibular neuronitis or Ménière's disease; and the first two of these can be diagnosed with confidence in primary care.
- Older patients more often suffer from non-vertiginous dizziness, for a variety of cardiovascular, neurological and psychiatric reasons.
- Among those presenting with dizziness will be a few with serious underlying disorders (e.g. cardiac arrhythmias, stroke disease) in whom a precise diagnosis must be made.

A PRACTICAL APPROACH

- * Ascertain if possible whether the patient is describing vertigo (which must include a sensation of spinning), unsteadiness, presyncope or some other vaguer type of light-headedness.
- * Ask about the duration of the attack and of the condition as a whole, whether the onset was sudden, whether there is deafness or tinnitus, and whether the patient has nausea or vomiting at the time of the attack.
- * Examine the ear, check the blood pressure sitting and standing and look for nystagmus.
- * Form an initial diagnosis on the basis of the above, then examine the patient further to verify it. The initial possibilities will depend on the age of the patient. Older patients are

most likely to suffer from unsteadiness due to multiple cerebrovascular and neurological problems. Younger patients are more likely to suffer from a specific vestibular condition, or from the light-headedness of an anxiety disorder.
- * In a patient with a clinical picture that does not fit into one of the organic causes of dizziness, or in whom there are pointers towards a psychological cause, ask specific questions directed at diagnosing hyperventilation.

There can be few physicians so dedicated to their art that they do not experience a slight decline in spirits on learning that their patient's complaint is of giddiness. (Matthews WB. *Practical Neurology*, 2nd edn. Blackwell, Oxford, 1970.)

The GP's spirits need not sink in the way Professor Matthews describes. In primary care, the management of giddiness includes the drama of the acute first episode of vertigo, the confident clinical diagnosis of benign positional vertigo (BPV) and other characteristic syndromes, and the referral for assessment and rehabilitation of older people who are unsteady because of a combination of neurological and cardiovascular problems.

Prevalence

Between 2.2%[1] and 4%[2] of all patients registered with a GP in the UK present to their GP each year with dizziness, comprising 0.7% of all consultations. In the USA, dizziness accounts for 8 million clinic visits/year.[3] Of people aged over 65 years, 30% report dizziness at some stage, whereas only 1.8% of young adults report it.[3] In

* *Ask* what precipitates it, how long it lasts, whether there is nausea, vomiting or a feeling of fullness in the ears, whether the patient has ever fallen or gone unconscious, how many attacks there have been over what period of time.
* *Ask* about the patient's health and past history especially if there is any deafness, tinnitus, visual difficulty, heart disease, neck pain, psychiatric disorders, and what medication is taken or was being taken at the onset of the condition.
* *Ask*, in those with vertigo, about a family history. It is present in 25% of those with otosclerosis and in 7% of those with Ménière's disease.[7]

From the answers to these questions it is usually possible to make an *initial diagnosis* as follows, which can then be tested in more detail (see below).

Vertigo

* If the history is of episodes of vertigo, brought on by lying down or turning over in bed, which last only seconds, consider benign positional vertigo (BPV).
* If the history is of episodes of severe vertigo with vomiting, lasting for hours or days and with a background of tinnitus and deafness, consider Ménière's disease.
* If the history is of a single episode of vertigo settling over days to a feeling of unsteadiness, with normal hearing and no tinnitus, consider vestibular neuronitis.
* If the history is of unilateral deafness and tinnitus as well as vertigo or even with a vague unsteadiness, consider acoustic neuroma or another cerebello-pontine angle lesion.

Disequilibrium

* If the dizziness is associated with an unsteady gait, or a focal neurological lesion, consider cerebrovascular disease or another central neurological problem.
* If the complaint is of disequilibrium with a past history of vertigo, the cause may be a vestibular lesion with compensation.

Presyncope

* If the dizziness occurs when standing up quickly and resolves on sitting down, consider postural hypotension.
* If the dizziness occurs in specific situations (e.g. relaxing in the theatre or when tense about having blood taken), consider a vasovagal attack.

Light-headedness

* If the dizziness occurs in situations where the patient feels frightened, check for hyperventilation.

The older the patient the harder it will be to make a single diagnosis on the basis of the history.

The examination

In all patients, check the blood pressure seated, examine the ear drum and test for spontaneous nystagmus by having the patient follow your finger to each side and upwards. More detailed examination will be necessary once it has been decided which diagnoses need further investigation.

Step 2. Refining the possibilities suggested by the initial assessment

Is this benign paroxysmal positional vertigo?

* Check that the history is suggestive: episodes of vertigo, lasting only seconds, triggered by a change of posture (lying down, turning over in bed, sitting up from lying, but not looking up or standing up from sitting). The patient is likely to be aged >50. Symptoms may be variable with remissions of weeks, months or years between episodes. Any deafness or tinnitus will be coincidental.
* Check that there are no pointers towards other causes of dizziness (which may coexist).
* Perform the Hallpike manoeuvre. In a study from general practice in Ireland of patients with vertigo, in which the Hallpike manoeuvre was performed by GPs, it had a sensitivity of 56% and a specificity of 81% for the diagnosis of BPV, giving an LR+ of 3.0 (95% CI 1.0 to 8.7) and an LR− of 0.5 (95% CI 0.3 to 0.9).[8] In this study, when the GPs suspected the diagnosis of BPV enough to perform the test, the final diagnosis of BPV was made in 63%. If the Hallpike manoeuvre was positive, the probability of BPV rose to 83%.

The Hallpike manoeuvre (Fig. 12.1)

* Obtain the patient's consent to the manoeuvre and ask her to keep her eyes open when feeling dizzy.
* Sit her on the couch so that, if she lies down, her head will be off the end of the couch.
* Stand in front of the patient and hold her head in both hands, turning it 45° towards the test ear.
* Keeping the head turned, lie the patient down rapidly with the head at 30–45° below the horizontal (or, if not possible, at least 10°) (the head hanging position).
* Maintain the head hanging position for 30–60 seconds and observe the patient's eyes. Note whether nystagmus occurs. Maintain that position for about 1 minute after the onset of nystagmus to check that it stops.
* Return the patient to the upright position while maintaining 45° neck rotation. The nystagmus and vertigo should recommence.
* Repeat on the opposite side if no nystagmus is seen on the first side. The affected ear is the one that is underneath when the nystagmus occurs.

Note that the nystagmus may only last a few seconds and will not occur at all in some patients, in whom the diagnosis must be made on the history alone. Note also that the patient will experience vertigo at the same time as the nystagmus.

* If the history and the Hallpike manoeuvre are positive, accept the diagnosis of BPV. Further history and examination are only needed if there is a suspicion that the patient suffers from another cause of dizziness as well, because, for instance, of episodes of syncope or symptoms suggesting postural hypotension or hyperventilation.

* If the history is suggestive but the test is negative, believe the history. In the Irish study (above), a negative test only reduced the probability from 63% to 48%. Alternatively, repeat the test. This can raise the sensitivity to 78%.[17]

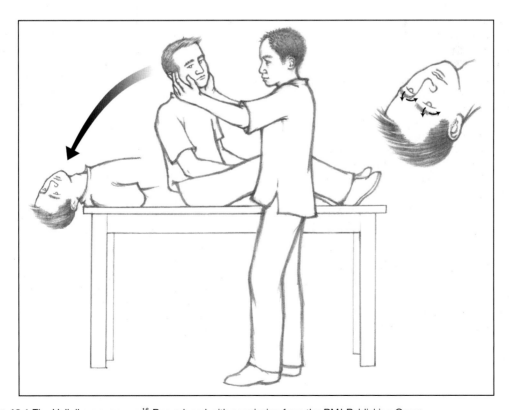

Figure 12.1 The Hallpike manoeuvre.[16] Reproduced with permission from the BMJ Publishing Group.

Is this Ménière's disease?

The diagnosis is made on the presence of all three of the following:[18]
1. at least two attacks of vertigo lasting at least 20 minutes each; and
2. hearing loss; and
3. tinnitus or fullness in the ear.

However, most come to the notice of the GP before the triad is present, as episodic vertigo, unilateral deafness and/or tinnitus. The overall clinical picture often points to the correct diagnosis. Attacks usually last for a mean of 20 minutes but may last hours. Most patients have between one and four attacks a month. Nausea, and sometimes vomiting, is usually present and many patients have to retire to bed. Vertigo is usually the first symptom to appear followed by a unilateral sensorineural deafness. Even if deafness is not apparent when seen between attacks, the patient may report deafness, or at least fullness in the ear, during the attack.

The onset is usually between the ages of 20 and 50. It is unilateral in the early stages but bilateral in 40% of those with longstanding disease. There is a family history in 7.7%.

The implications of the diagnosis are sufficiently worrying for all patients to be referred to a specialist for confirmation. This will allow the detection of rarer causes of vertigo with deafness, such as otosclerosis.

Is this vestibular neuronitis?

The diagnosis is made on the triad of:[12]
1. vertigo that is usually sudden in onset, although the patient may report several days of increasing symptoms
2. absence of cochlear symptoms (deafness and tinnitus)
3. no central neurological symptoms or signs.

It is a single episode which lasts 1 to 5 days and is the most intense of all causes of vertigo, with nausea (in 94%) and vomiting (in 54%). Movements of the head worsen the symptoms and the gait is unsteady; 68% have nystagmus during the attack. As the brain compensates for the vestibular nerve damage, the vertigo ceases but the patient may feel unsteady for months with apparent mild relapses as central compensation fluctuates. Like Ménière's disease,

it mainly affects the young and middle-aged. A study of 60 cases found a range of ages from 13 to 69.[12]

Retrospectively the clinical picture permits a diagnosis. If symptoms persist, an audiogram and a caloric test will confirm the diagnosis. But the dilemma for the GP is in distinguishing the initial attack from a more sinister, acute peripheral (e.g. pyogenic infection of the inner ear) or central lesion (e.g. cerebellar infarction).
* Check that the patient has no tinnitus.
* Check that hearing is normal.
* Check the drums and external auditory canal. Middle ear disease with extension inwards does not occur without drum abnormality. Ramsay Hunt syndrome may manifest itself as vesicles in the external auditory canal and on the pinna. Look for evidence of mumps.[7]
* Perform the head impulse test (see box below and Fig. 12.2). It is said always to be positive in acute vestibular neuronitis and negative in a central lesion.[19] Limitations of the test are that the patient who is distressed by vertigo and vomiting will find it hard to cooperate; and an inexperienced clinician might miss the flick of the eyes after the head has been moved (see box).

The head impulse test[19]

* Hold the patient's head with both hands. Ask the patient to fix his gaze on a distant object.
* In a quick movement, rotate the patient's head about 15°, watching his eyes.

In vestibular disease, the patient loses fixation momentarily and the eyes then flick back to fix on the object again.

The above examination will fail to distinguish the patient who is in the first few hours of an episode of vestibular neuronitis from one with a first attack of Ménière's disease or of basilar migraine. The longer time course of the first and the recurrent attacks of the last two will make the diagnosis; but the treatment of all three in the first attack is symptomatic and the patient will come to no harm from the confusion.

Is this acoustic neuroma?

Half of patients with an acoustic neuroma experience true vertigo at some stage, and more experience postural instability. The vertigo comes

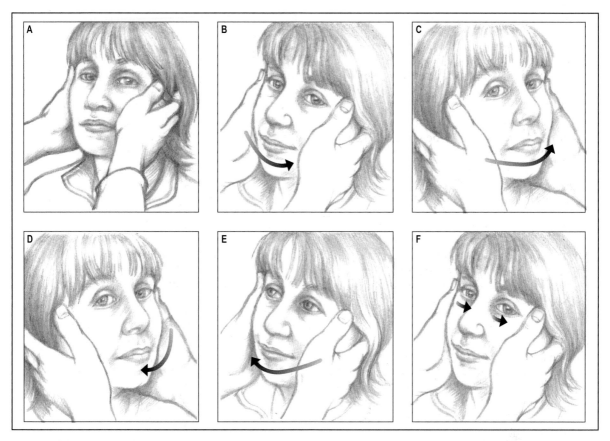

Figure 12.2 The head impulse test. A–C show the patient able to fixate while her head is turned to her left. D–F show that she loses fixation when her head is turned to her right, then regains it. Diagnosis: right peripheral vestibular lesion. After Halmagyi,[19] with permission of the Royal College of Physicians of London.

in attacks lasting from a few minutes to several hours and comes usually no more frequently than monthly. By the time the attacks start, the patient will already have hearing loss (in 95% of cases) and tinnitus (in 83% of cases).[12] See *Deafness* (p. 53) and *Tinnitus* (p. 262).

Is this sudden deafness?

A review of 21 cases of sudden deafness from Finland[12] found that 18 had vertigo and 18 had tinnitus. The vertigo either came as short episodes or as a long episode accompanying the deafness. The deafness and tinnitus distinguish it from vestibular neuronitis but, at first presentation, it cannot be distinguished from Ménière's disease or acoustic neuroma. Referral for investigation is required.

Is there a central cause for this vertigo?

The following suggest a central cause for vertigo:[7,15]
- vertigo that is persistent and worsening
- atypical vertigo, e.g. where the rotation experienced is vertical
- severe headache
- altered consciousness
- other symptoms: diplopia, visual disturbance
- other signs: cranial nerve and long tract signs, dysarthria and ataxia, papilloedema
- nystagmus which is vertical or purely torsional and not horizontal.
- The aetiology of vertigo of central origin will be suggested by the time course and the extent of the lesion. A cerebrovascular

pathology is suggested by acute onset with resolution in 24 hours (transient ischaemic attack – TIA) or over months or years (stroke). A tumour will have an onset that is slower but then worsening progressively. Multiple sclerosis will be suggested by the younger age of the patient, the evidence of plaques elsewhere and by the sequence of remissions and relapses.

• Once vertigo of central onset is identified, specialist referral is needed.

• Less well-defined episodes of dizziness, without vertigo, are associated with a risk of falling but not with stroke and do not need referral as a TIA. A large study of people aged 65 and over in Newcastle found no increase in the risk of stroke, over almost 4 years of follow-up, in those with faints, black-outs and non-rotational dizziness.[20] The stroke risk ratio for those with vertigo, however, was 2.48 (95% CI 1.48 to 4.15). These patients were also more likely to have abnormal T wave changes on ECG and possibly more likely to have atrial fibrillation. In this unselected aged population, the presence of vertigo was 25% sensitive and 88% specific for subsequent stroke within 4 years, giving a positive predictive value of 10.4% and a negative predictive value of 96%. In other words, an older patient who reported vertigo had a risk of a stroke in the next 4 years of 10%. One whose dizziness had no element of vertigo had a stroke risk of only 4%.

Is this migraine?

A study of 200 unselected patients with migraine seen in a specialist clinic[21] found vestibular or cochlear symptoms in 59% of migraine sufferers, either as a prodrome, or during the headache, or in between attacks. In 5% they were disabling. The diagnosis is usually clear because the patient has recognised the association with the headaches, but until a pattern becomes established, the diagnosis may only be made in retrospect. The vestibular symptoms were either a feeling of giddiness or a true vertigo; the cochlear symptoms were hearing loss, distortion of pitch or tinnitus. Migraineurs are also more likely to report giddiness between attacks of headache than controls; the aetiology of this is not clear.

Is this postural hypotension?

Check the blood pressure sitting then standing, and again after standing for 3 minutes. Several definitions of postural hypotension exist. One is that a fall in systolic pressure alone is not significant but a fall in mean pressure of at least 20 mmHg is.[10] Another is that the condition exists if there is a fall in systolic pressure of ≥20 mmHg or in diastolic of ≥10 mmHg on changing from supine to standing.[22]

Even then, a significant fall does not mean this is the cause of the patient's symptoms and a negative test does not rule it out. A study of frail, elderly nursing home residents[23] found that 51% had demonstrable orthostatic hypotension on at least one reading, but only 13% had it on all readings. Measurements were most likely to be positive before breakfast and least likely to be positive after lunch. The diagnosis is made on the history of feeling faint on standing from a sitting or lying position, confirmed by the finding of a significant fall on at least one occasion.

Is this hyperventilation?

Hyperventilation causes light-headedness and may complicate other forms of dizziness or exist in its own right, as part of an anxiety or panic disorder. It may occur in acute attacks or take a chronic form. The diagnosis is made from a history in which other somatic symptoms (e.g. tightness in the chest, tingling in the fingers and round the mouth, blurred vision) are prominent. A formal questionnaire, the Nijmegen questionnaire, has been shown to be 91% sensitive and 95% specific for hyperventilation (LR+ 18, LR− 0.1).[24] This means that, if the initial probability of a psychological cause for dizziness is 21%, as shown in the two studies quoted above, a positive response to the Nijmegen questionnaire raises that probability to 83% while a negative response lowers it to 2%.

A study from Cambridge, England found that 74% of patients referred to a vestibular clinic in whom the diagnosis of hyperventilation was made would have been missed had the questionnaire not been used.[25]

- *Do you have any of the following and, if so, how often?* Feeling tense, chest pain, blurred vision, dizzy spells, feeling confused or out of touch, tight feelings in chest, bloated feeling in stomach, faster/deeper breathing, short of breath, tingling in fingers, unable to breathe deeply, stiff fingers/arms, tight feelings around mouth, cold hands/feet, heart racing (palpitations), feelings of anxiety.
- The patient is asked to score how often each symptom is experienced on a scale of 1 (never) to 5 (very frequently).
- A GP may not wish to score the questionnaire formally but the questions it contains are a useful guide to the sort of questions to ask. The questions may be divided into three components: difficulty with breathing; peripheral tetany; and central effects. A patient may have symptoms predominantly from one group only, so at least three questions should be asked; for instance:
    - 'Do you ever feel you can't take a deep enough breath?'
    - 'Do you ever get tingling in the fingers or round the mouth?'
    - 'Do you ever feel out of touch with, or distant from, your surroundings?'

---

* Look for other features that suggest psychogenic dizziness:
    - a vague and imprecise history such as a sensation of motion (rocking, tilting, levitating, etc.) that does not suggest vertigo
    - brief attacks that can occur several times per day; however, other patients will show a more chronic pattern
    - normal or inconsistent clinical examination and investigations
    - multiple other complaints that raise the suspicion of a somatisation disorder.
* *Perform the hyperventilation test.* Ask the patient to breathe deeply and rapidly for 3 minutes and to signal if doing so brings on the exact symptoms of the dizziness. A study from Utah[26] found that most patients with a positive test had other causes for their dizziness. In their hands, the test was 100% sensitive but only 79% specific for hyperventilation as the cause of their dizziness (LR+ 4.8 (95% CI 2.8 to 6.8); LR− 0.0 (95% CI 0.0 to 1.5)). In their study, the initial probability that hyperventilation was the cause of the dizziness was 5%. A positive test only raised that to 19% but a negative test excluded it. In other words, a

negative result helps to rule out the diagnosis but, even if the test is positive, the patient's dizziness is probably not due to hyperventilation, unless suspicion of the diagnosis is already very strong.

* Do not diagnose dizziness of psychological origin as a diagnosis of exclusion; specific pointers to a psychological diagnosis must be present.
* Do not assume that if you have made a positive diagnosis of psychogenic dizziness, the patient does not also have an organic cause. A study of patients with psychogenic dizziness in a tertiary balance centre in Philadelphia found that only a third had purely psychogenic dizziness. In the other two-thirds, the neurological disorder had either caused the psychological disorder or triggered it in a patient with a pre-existing psychiatric disorder.[27]

Is this due to cardiovascular disease?

A study of 50 consecutive patients aged 60 and over who presented in primary care with dizziness, plus a further 50 referred to a geriatric clinic because of dizziness, found certain aspects of the history useful in establishing that cardiovascular disease (CVD) was the cause of the dizziness (Table 12.1).[9] For instance, if the dizzy patient gave a history of pallor during an episode of dizziness, the probability of it being due to CVD rose from 45% (the prevalence of dizziness due to CVD in that group) to 95%. If there was no history of pallor, the probability of CVD as the cause of the dizziness fell to 33%. In general, the questions are useful in ruling in the diagnosis and less useful in ruling it out. No analysis was performed to see whether the questions were independent of each other. They cannot therefore be applied one after the other, though clearly a combination of positive answers raises the probability of CVD still further.

The difficulty of diagnosing carotid sinus sensitivity in general practice

The above study found carotid sinus sensitivity to be the most common cardiovascular abnormality causing or contributing to dizziness in 26% of all dizzy patients in the study. It was diagnosed when carotid sinus massage reproduced the dizziness with either asystole for at least 3 seconds, or a fall of systolic BP of at least 50 mmHg, whether lying or standing. However, it is not a test to be conducted in primary care. European guidelines require the use of continuous ECG and blood pressure monitoring

Table 12.1 Questions in patients over 60 and how they alter the probability that cardiovascular disease is the cause of dizziness where the prevalence of CVD as the cause was 45%[9]

Question	Answer	LR+ (95% CI)	Probability according to the answers
Syncope	Present	13 (4.1–39)	91%
	Absent	0.3 (0.2–0.5)	21%
Dizziness described as 'light-headedness'	Present	8.6 (3.2–23)	88%
	Absent	0.4 (0.3–0.6)	25%
Pallor when symptoms felt	Present	22 (3.1–159)	95%
	Absent	0.6 (0.5–0.8)	33%
Need to sit or lie down when symptoms felt	Present	5.9 (2.7–13)	83%
	Absent	0.4 (0.3–0.6)	25%
Symptoms triggered by prolonged standing	Present	5.3 (1.3–22)	81%
	Absent	0.7 (0.5–0.9)	35%
Other CVD diagnoses already made	Yes	1.9 (1.2–3.0)	60%
	No	0.6 (0.4–0.9)	33%

Follow each row from left to right to see how each answer alters the probability of CVD being the cause of the dizziness.

as well as warning of the 0.45% risk of serious neurological complications.[28]

Dizziness as a geriatric syndrome

The suggestion has been made that dizziness in the older patient should be managed like 'confusion' or 'taking to bed', as a non-specific manifestation of impairment in a number of areas.[10] A population-based study from New Haven, Connecticut found seven characteristics that were associated with a complaint of dizziness:[10]

- anxiety trait
- depressive symptoms
- impaired balance
- past myocardial infarction
- postural hypotension
- five or more medications
- impaired hearing.

These characteristics illustrate how psychological, cardiovascular, neurological, sensory and iatrogenic factors can contribute to a complaint of dizziness. Alone, each characteristic carried a modest relative risk of dizziness of about 1.5. None of the elderly people with none of the seven characteristics complained of dizziness. Half of those with four factors complained of it.[29]

However, specific causes of dizziness still occur in the older person, and some occur more

commonly than in younger people. A study from the USA of elderly city residents aged at least 72 years, found that 9% of those with dizziness or unsteadiness had unrecognised BPV. It was associated with a description of 'spinning' rather than 'light-headedness'. Those with unrecognised BPV were more likely to be depressed and more likely to have fallen in the previous 3 months.[30]

A test which may be helpful in patients in whom the diagnosis is not clear is Romberg's test (see box). It can distinguish organic problems from psychological ones though it cannot distinguish peripheral vestibular problems from central causes of vertigo or unsteadiness.[9]

Romberg's test

* Ask the patient to stand still. If she is unsteady there is no point in proceeding.
* Ask her to close her eyes. If she loses her balance the test is positive. This suggests that she has impaired sensory input (vestibular and/or proprioceptive), but that she normally compensates for this lack by using visual clues.

Other causes of dizziness

These may be obvious from the situation or may defy diagnosis:

written with the intention that they should be over-ridden when clinical judgement suggests a different approach to diagnosis and management. For instance, the UK guidelines make strong use of the cut-off of age 55 in the assessment of the need for initial endoscopy. Yet a retrospective study from the University of Wisconsin found that, of 341 upper GI malignancies diagnosed, 65 were in patients under 55 and 21 in patients under 45.[22] Of the 65 malignancies in those <55, 5 presented with uncomplicated dyspepsia. A prospective study from Poland, where the incidence of gastric cancer is double that in the UK, found that 24% of those diagnosed with

gastric cancer were aged under 45.[23] Twenty-seven per cent of the patients with cancer had no alarm features at presentation (although the study did not report on the percentage without alarm features in the under 45s). The GP who suspects carcinoma for a reason not included in the guidelines should not be deterred from referral.

One caution should be stated on this topic. The GP may be tempted to use endoscopy to reassure the patient, even when it is not recommended by the guidelines. Such reassurance does not seem to work. A Dutch study of patients with functional dyspepsia found no such benefit from endoscopy.[24]

Example

A 42-year-old chief executive from the local primary health care trust presents, at a time of stress, with a 4-week history of 'indigestion' felt in the centre of the epigastrium. Sometimes food seems to ease it but at other times it sets it off. There is no reflux but she has been woken by it at night. The GP asks about weight loss, black stool, vomiting and dysphagia. The patient has had none of them. She has been taking antacids over the last 4 weeks which help for a few hours at a time. She doesn't take any other medication.

Examination of the abdomen is normal. The GP orders a haemoglobin test.

The GP explains that he thinks she has a problem with acid irritating the stomach. Whether there is an

ulcer or an inflamed oesophagus it is impossible to say, and he doesn't recommend endoscopy, which would not affect the treatment anyway. He wants to give a proton pump inhibitor for 4 weeks and then see her again. He asks her whether there is any help he can give with the stress she is under but she waves the offer away.

She does, however, ask about the possibility of serious disease. He gives the probabilities as follows, modifying them for this patient with her short history and response to antacid: a 1 in 3 chance of an ulcer or oesophagitis; a 1 in 2 chance that the acid is irritating the stomach but without ulceration; and the rest a collection of diagnoses, with cancer <1%.

REFERENCES

1. Scottish Intercollegiate Guidelines Network. *Dyspepsia.* Edinburgh: SIGN, 2003. Online. Available: www.sign.ac.uk (choose 'guidelines').

2. Logan R, Delaney B. *Implications of dyspepsia for the NHS.* BMJ 2001; 323:675–677.

3. Heikkinen M, Pikkarainen P, Takala J, et al. *Etiology of dyspepsia: four hundred unselected consecutive patients in general practice.* Scand J Gastroenterol 1995;30:516–523.

4. Voutilainen M, Mantynen T, Kunnamo I, et al. *Impact of clinical symptoms and referral volume on endoscopy for detecting peptic ulcer and gastric neoplasms.* Scand J Gastroenterol 2003;38:109–113.

5. Rudmann A. *Peptic ulcer disease.* In: Black E, Bordley D, Tape T, et al, eds. Diagnostic strategies for common medical problems, 2nd edn. Philadelphia: American College of Physicians, 1998:127–139.

6. Colin-Jones D. *Management of dyspepsia: report of a working party.* Lancet 1988;1:576–579.

7. Agreus L, Talley N. *Challenges in managing dyspepsia in general practice.* BMJ 1997;315:1284–1288.

8. Moayyedi P, Talley N, Fennerty M, et al. *Can the clinical history distinguish between organic and functional dyspepsia?* JAMA 2006;295:1566–1576.

9. Bytzer P, Moller Hanson J, Schaffalitzky de Muckadell O. *Predicting endoscopic diagnosis in the dyspeptic patient. The value of predictive score models.* Scand J Gastroenterol 1997;32:118–125.

10. Lydeard S, Jones R. *Factors affecting the decision to consult with dyspepsia: comparison of consulters and non-consulters.* J R Coll Gen Pract 1989;39:495–498.

- upper respiratory infection (head cold) 7%
- COPD/emphysema/bronchiectasis 4%
- acute laryngitis/tracheitis 3%
- pneumonia 3%
- ischaemic heart disease 2%
- anxiety/stress 1%
- sinusitis 1%
- atrial fibrillation 1%.

These probabilities were found to vary with the age of the patient. For instance, the probability of asthma fell to 5% in those aged 65 to 74 and to 3% in those aged >74. Heart failure, on the other hand, did not occur in patients under the age of 45. Age 45 to 64 it was 4%, age 65 to 74 it was 13% and >74 years old it was 21%.

Other possibilities are:
- pulmonary embolus
- pneumothorax
- pericardial effusion – found in 14% of patients presenting to the emergency department with dyspnoea in whom the initial work-up revealed no cause[5]; the signs of cardiac tamponade (hypotension, raised jugular venous pressure and quiet heart sounds) are late and none of the patients in this series had them
- pleural effusion
- diabetic ketoacidosis
- stridor
- neuromuscular weakness
- acute blood loss.

The initial assessment

An initial diagnosis will be made rapidly in most patients because the symptoms and signs present a typical pattern. In many patients, the underlying disorder will already have been diagnosed on a previous occasion. However, even specialists cannot rely on their clinical impression. In a US pulmonary clinic,[6] the initial diagnosis based on history, examination and chest X-ray in patients with dyspnoea for at least 3 weeks was only correct in 66% of cases. The specialists were best at diagnosing common causes (e.g. asthma or COPD) and most likely to miss the less common causes.

Typical patterns

Asthma: a history of acute episodes of wheezing with cough in a patient with clinically obvious airways obstruction during an attack (wheezing and possibly intercostal indrawing). There is often an obvious pattern to the attacks (night-time, or after exercise, or on exposure to an allergen). See *Asthma*, page 337.

Respiratory infection: no history of previous episodes (unless there is underlying respiratory disease); fever, purulent sputum, and localised chest signs in an unwell patient. See *Acute respiratory infections*, page 299.

Heart failure: either the picture of acute left ventricular failure (pallor, sweating, tachycardia, raised blood pressure, bilateral crackles at the bases) or congestive cardiac failure (without the pallor and sweating but with swollen ankles, a raised jugular venous pressure and an enlarged tender liver). See *Heart failure*, page 398.

COPD: a long history of productive cough, usually in a smoker or one at risk of occupational respiratory disease, with signs of airways obstruction. A barrel chest may be present if there is emphysema. See *Chronic obstructive pulmonary disease*, page 354.

Less common causes

If the typical history and clinical signs of these conditions do not suggest a diagnosis, more detailed examination may suggest the cause: the crackles of interstitial lung disease; the hyper-resonance, reduced breath sounds and tracheal deviation of a pneumothorax; the dullness of a pleural effusion; the pallor of anaemia. Patients with panic disorder are usually more troubled by dizziness, paraesthesiae or nausea than by dyspnoea, even when the hyperventilation is apparent to an observer. In stridor, the characteristic noise is as loud in inspiration as in expiration.

One particular problem that may occur is the older patient with severe dyspnoea, in whom the diagnosis lies between acute left ventricular failure (LVF) and asthma and who is too dyspnoeic to perform a lung function test. Wheezing may occur in both conditions, or be absent in both, but crackles make the diagnosis of LVF a little more likely.

Diagnosis

Confirm the diagnosis with a test of respiratory function. This becomes more important the older the patient and the more likely it is that two or more conditions coexist.

Table 14.1 Value of the peak flow in the diagnosis of a pulmonary cause in the patient with acute dyspnoea in primary care. Based on a probability before the assessment of 40%[4]

Peak flow result (L/min)	Likelihood ratio (95% CI)	Probability of a pulmonary cause after the peak flow measurement
≤150[7]	3.9 (1.6–9.4)	72%
>150	0.2 (0.1–0.5)	12%
≤200[8]	2.5 (1.4–4.3)	62%
>200	0.4 (0.2–0.8)	21%

Follow each row from left to right to see how each peak flow result alters the probability of a pulmonary cause.
Note that these studies cannot be compared to show that the cut-off of 150 L/min is better than that of 200 L/min. The first study only admitted patients whose lung disease was asthma or COPD; the second study included patients with pneumonia. This may explain the poorer performance of the peak flow in the second study.

■ *Peak expiratory flow rate (PEFR).* In cases of difficulty, a single peak flow rate may be useful in distinguishing heart failure from airways obstruction in patients with moderate or severe dyspnoea. In a US emergency department,[7] using a cut-off of 150 L/min, a PEFR ≤150 was 87% sensitive and 78% specific for airways obstruction (LR+ 3.9 (95% CI 1.6 to 9.4); LR– 0.2 (95% CI 0.1 to 0.5)) and a PEFR >150 L/min was 78% sensitive and 87% specific for heart failure (LR+ 6.0 (95% CI 2.0 to 18); LR– 0.3 (95% CI 0.1 to 0.6)). Another study, in a different US emergency department,[8] using a cut-off of 200 L/min, found that the PEFR was slightly more reliable than the clinical judgement of the emergency department physician in distinguishing cardiac from pulmonary disease (72% of diagnoses correct versus 69% correct) but also noted that ill patients may perform the test poorly and give falsely low readings. These studies are summarised in Table 14.1.

■ *Spirometry.* Using spirometry rather than a peak flow may increase specificity. In a study of 200 adults referred to a pulmonary function laboratory,[9] forced expiratory volume in 1 second/forced vital capacity (FEV_1/FVC), using a cut-off of 70%, was 82% sensitive and 98% specific for airways obstruction measured against a composite standard of clinical judgement and body plethysmography. It was most sensitive (92%) in those with moderate or severe disease and least sensitive (64%) in those with mild airways obstruction.

Chest X-ray (CXR) is rarely used to make an unsuspected diagnosis. Rather, it is used to confirm or refute a diagnosis made clinically. Occasionally, however, it may reveal a cause of dyspnoea that could not be suspected clinically: for instance, a small pneumothorax or the shadowing of fibrosing alveolitis or sarcoidosis.

Blood tests (haemoglobin (Hb), blood sugar, thyroid function tests (TFTs) and urea and electrolytes (U&Es) are likely to reveal the diagnosis in 2% of those in whom the diagnosis is not suspected clinically.[1]

Example

A smoker aged 55 presents with moderate dyspnoea for 2 weeks and a history of some recent loss of exercise tolerance over months which he describes as 'wheezing'. He is wheezing but also has some bilateral basal crackles. The history of deterioration over some months makes acute respiratory infection unlikely and the GP judges the initial probabilities as follows: airways obstruction (whether asthma or COPD) 50%, heart failure 30%, and other causes, especially infection, still a possibility.

The peak flow is 140 L/min. This increases the probability of airways obstruction to 80% (Fig. 14.1). It reduces the probability of heart failure to 11% (Fig. 14.2). These changes are not enough to clinch the diagnosis and CXR, ECG and the response to an inhaled beta$_2$-agonist are needed, as set out in the relevant sections.

In primary care

A Swedish study found an annual incidence of UTI in primary care of 45 per 10 000 males of all ages.[6]

Initial probabilities

A German study of 79 men presenting in primary care with acute urinary symptoms found that 60% had a UTI.[2] Of these, half had a positive culture on MSU of $>10^5$ colony forming units (CFU)/ml. The other half had counts between 10^3 and 10^5 CFU/ml. Diagnoses made in the 40% who were culture negative were not reported. Those with a clinical diagnosis of acute prostatitis were excluded from the study.

Possible diagnoses, therefore, in a man with acute urinary symptoms are:
- UTI
- acute urethritis
- acute prostatitis
- urethral syndrome
- benign prostatic hypertrophy with an acute presentation
- an overactive bladder with an acute presentation
- an exacerbation of chronic prostatitis.

The probabilities of these diagnoses vary with age and with other risk factors for UTI.

Infection is more likely in those with:[2]
- older age: the annual incidence in men >80 years old is >10 times that in those <60[7]
- diabetes
- indwelling catheter
- history of urinary surgery
- bladder or prostate cancer
- renal failure
- antibiotics in the last 2 weeks
- chronic prostatitis
- a history of anal sexual intercourse.

Features of the clinical assessment that help the diagnosis

The symptoms of frequency, urgency, hesitancy and poor stream are common to many disorders. In the German study above, only dysuria was independently associated with a diagnosis of UTI.[2]

In the absence of further studies giving information about the accuracy of the clinical assessment, we have to fall back on traditional descriptions:

- *Acute urethritis* is suggested by the presence of discharge. Investigation is by urethral swab and first pass urine examination. Urethral swabs should include swabs for *Gonococcus* and *Chlamydia*.
- *Acute prostatitis* is suggested by fever, and acute urinary symptoms in the presence of pain in the perineum, genitals, back or lower abdomen. The patient may notice that the urine stream is diminished. The prostate will be tender and possibly enlarged. There may or may not be urethral discharge and abnormal findings in the urine. The four-glass test is the traditional investigation (see below).
- *Urethral syndrome* is a diagnosis that will only be made once the chronic nature of symptoms becomes apparent and the MSU is repeatedly negative.
- *Benign prostatic hypertrophy* occasionally presents acutely. 'Filling' symptoms include frequency, urgency and nocturia, but not dysuria. 'Voiding' symptoms include hesitancy, poor stream and terminal dribbling. More detailed questioning will almost always reveal a longer history of difficulty.
- *An overactive bladder* is found in 19% of men >60 years old.[8] Again, detailed history taking is likely to reveal a longer history.
- *An acute exacerbation of chronic prostatitis*. There is likely to be a long history, although the patient may be asymptomatic for much of the time. Ten per cent will have bacteriuria but in 90% the prostatitis is abacterial. It is suggested by the presence of urinary symptoms (dysuria, frequency, hesitancy, poor stream and, possibly, malaise and fever) with genital, perineal or pelvic pain (see *Lower urinary tract symptoms in men*, p. 171).

The frail elderly present a special problem. Significant bacteriuria is common, as are symptoms of dysuria, frequency and urgency.[9] The diagnosis of UTI should be based on the existence of new urinary symptoms, combined with bacteriuria and pyuria. A Canadian study of elderly people in long-term care facilities found that bacteriuria was so common that the combination of bacteriuria and fever was only predictive of UTI in 10% of patients with this combination.[10]

Examination

Examination in a man with suspected UTI is more likely to be useful than in a woman.
- Discharge from the meatus may indicate urethritis.
- Genital and rectal examination may reveal epididymo-orchitis, prostatitis or carcinoma of the

prostate. A recent systematic review concluded that a finding of prostatic cancer on rectal examination in a man with lower urinary tract symptoms (LUTS) was likely to be coincidental.[11] However, the finding of a prostate that is irregular, with hard nodules, or enlarged with loss of the midline sulcus, cannot be ignored. The sensitivity of rectal examination for carcinoma of the prostate in screening studies is 64% (95% CI 47% to 80%) and the specificity 97% (95% CI 95% to 99%).[11]

● Loin tenderness, especially if combined with high fever, suggests pyelonephritis.

Investigations

● *Dipstick.* The accuracy of the dipstick is similar to that in women (see *Dysuria in women*, p. 96). A positive test for nitrites and/or leucocyte esterase has a positive likelihood ratio of 2.6 for infection and a negative likelihood ratio of 0.1.

● *MSU.* Microscopy and culture of the midstream specimen of urine is the gold standard for infection. However, the conditions for the transport of the test (see box) are often not met in general practice and a negative test may be less powerful in ruling out infection than if performed in a setting closer to the laboratory.

● *What is a positive MSU?* In men, a threshold of $>10^2$ CFU/ml appears to distinguish significant infection most effectively.[12] Significant pyuria exists when more than 5 white cells are seen per high power field. Both organisms and cells are needed to diagnose a UTI.

● *How should the MSU be performed?* Despite its name, the MSU need not be midstream, at least in men. A US study compared 308 paired (initial and midstream) urines and found no significant difference in terms of significant bacteriuria. In addition, they found that cleansing the meatus, and whether the patient was circumcised, made no difference.[13]

● *Prostatitis is a diagnostic problem.* The predictive values of investigations for prostatitis have not been worked out. The diagnosis is suggested by finding white cells in ejaculate, in prostatic secretions produced by prostatic massage or in glasses 3 or 4 of the four-glass test. In the non-inflammatory form of chronic prostatitis (also called chronic pelvic pain

syndrome) there is no excess of white cells and the diagnosis is made on the clinical picture and the exclusion of other disorders.[14] The diagnosis is not easy: the clinical picture is rarely diagnostic and interpretation and, indeed, performance of the tests can be hard. A prospective study of patients attending urology clinics in Italy found that prostatic massage produced enough secretion for examination in only 44%.[15]

● *Prostate specific antigen (PSA).* Dysuria has not been shown to be associated with the presence of carcinoma of the prostate and so performing a PSA in a man complaining only of dysuria is screening, not diagnosis. However, studies suggest that *other* lower urinary symptoms are associated with carcinoma. A case-control study from Exeter, UK found that retention, impotence, frequency, hesitancy, nocturia and haematuria were associated with carcinoma with odds ratios of 2.4 to 11.[16] However, none of these symptoms proved to be independently useful once a PSA test was performed. A PSA >4 ng/ml was found to have a positive likelihood ratio of 29 (95% CI 19 to 43) for prostatic cancer. Even a rectal examination lost its independent value when the PSA was included in the multivariate analysis. The authors of the study argue that a PSA is therefore needed in all men complaining of lower urinary symptoms other than dysuria. The difficulty with this advice is that a case-control study cannot avoid the problem of verification bias: controls were not subjected to prostatic biopsy and so it is not known whether they had the same degree of prostatic cancer which remained undetected. See page 471 for a fuller discussion. The question remains undecided.

Transport of the midstream urine sample

The urine should be passed into a sterile bottle and examined within 2 hours, in order to minimise bacterial overgrowth and cell destruction. Four hours is considered the outside limit unless the sample is refrigerated at 4°C.

Dip-inoculum cultures are more robust when these conditions cannot be met but they give no information on cell counts.

The four-glass test for prostatic infection

- The patient passes urine into three separate glasses then voluntarily stops his stream. The physician massages the prostate per rectum and the patient then passes urine into the fourth glass. All four are sent for microscopy and culture. If specimen 3 or 4 has a substantially greater colony count than specimen 1 (e.g. >10-fold) the infection is likely to be prostatic.
- The absence of a gold standard test for prostatitis means that the predictive power of this test has not been assessed.[17] Urologists do not perform the four-glass test[18] and there are insufficient grounds to encourage GPs to do so.
- The test should not be confused with the two-glass test, in which a colony count in the first sample that is higher than that in the second indicates urethral infection.

Are further investigations needed in a man with a proven UTI?

Traditional advice has been that investigation is needed in men with UTI because of the high frequency of clinically significant abnormalities. In older men, investigation was thought to be less useful, because as men approach the age of 80 the prevalence of UTI comes to equal that of women.

In fact the reverse seems to be the case. An Israeli study of 29 men with UTI under the age of 45 found that only one had an abnormality, which was bladder outflow obstruction. The authors concluded that investigation after a single episode of infection in younger men was not justified.[19]

In contrast, a Swedish study[20] of 85 men aged 18–86 with a mean age of 63 found that 19 had upper urinary tract abnormalities, of whom one

needed surgery for calyceal stones, and 35 had lower urinary tract abnormalities, of which 20 were surgically correctable. However, crucially, the authors found that all those who required surgery had one of the following:

- a history of voiding difficulty
- acute retention at the time of the infection
- microscopic haematuria at follow-up
- an early recurrence of symptomatic UTI.

It seems that the older the patient, the more rewarding investigation will be, but that at no age is investigation needed for a single uncomplicated infection.

What urinary tract abnormalities are likely?

A study of 100 men referred to a UK district general hospital for investigation of UTI found the following abnormalities on intravenous urography (IVU):[21]

Upper urinary tract:
- hydronephrosis 7
- kidney stone 3
- ureteric stone 2
- small/scarred kidney 3
- pelvic kidney 1
- ureteric dilatation 3.

Lower urinary tract:
- residual urine 26
- bladder diverticulum 7
- bladder stone 1.

If investigations are undertaken, the combination of abdominal X-ray (AXR) and ultrasound scan (USS) is 100% sensitive and 93% specific compared to IVU as well as being safer.[21] The AXR is needed because of the tendency of the USS to miss urinary stones.

Example

A man aged 75 presents with a 1-week history of dysuria, frequency and urgency. He has no fever. He laughs off a question about lower urinary tract symptoms (LUTS), saying 'doesn't everyone at my age?', but it appears that there is a history of increasing difficulties over several years.

Examination reveals no bladder enlargement or testicular swelling. The prostate is possibly enlarged. The GP cannot decide if it is tender; the patient is too distressed by the rectal examination in general.

The dipstick is positive for nitrites but negative for leucocyte esterase. The GP reasons that the clinical picture suggests a probability of UTI of 70%, increased to 88% by the dipstick result. She gives a course of antibiotics. An MSU subsequently shows a growth of *Escherichia coli* >10^5/ml and 5 cells per high power field (i.e. showing significant bacteriuria but just falling short of proving a UTI).

A week later the patient's symptoms have returned to their previous level.

The GP feels that the diagnosis lies between a UTI and an exacerbation of chronic prostatitis. She decides that the presence of dysuria sways her in favour of the former. The presence of LUTS means that this is a complicated UTI and she refers him for investigation. A significant residual urine, secondary to bladder outflow obstruction, is found.

REFERENCES

1. Zackrisson B, Ulleryd P, Aus G, et al. *Evolution of free, complexed, and total serum prostate-specific antigen and their ratios during 1 year of follow-up of men with febrile urinary tract infection.* Urology 2003;62:278–281.

2. Hummers-Pradier E, Ohse A, Koch M, et al. *Urinary tract infection in men.* Int J Clin Pharmacol Ther 2004;42:360–366.

3. Krieger J, Ross S, Simonsen J. *Urinary tract infections in healthy university men.* J Urol 1993;149:1046–1048.

4. Clemens J, Meenan R, O'Keeffe Rosetti M, et al. *Incidence and clinical characteristics of National Institutes of Health type III prostatitis in the community.* J Urol 2005;174: 2319–2322.

5. Luzzi G. *Chronic prostatitis and chronic pelvic pain in men: aetiology, diagnosis and management.* Eur Acad Dermatol Venereol 2002;16:253–256.

6. Ferry S, Burman L, Mattsson B. *Urinary tract infection in primary health care in northern Sweden.* I. Epidemiology. Scand J Prim Health Care 1987;5:123–128.

7. PRODIGY. *Urinary tract infection (lower) – men: Sowerby Centre for Health Informatics at Newcastle, 2006.* Online. Available: www.prodigy.nhs. uk/guidance March 2006.

8. Adey G, Steele G. *The overactive bladder.* In: Kirby R, O'Leary M, eds. Hot topics in urology. Edinburgh: Saunders, 2004.

9. McMurdo M, Gillespie N. *Urinary tract infection in old age: over-diagnosed and over-treated.* Age Ageing 2000;29:297–298.

10. Orr P, Nicolle L, Duckworth H, et al. *Febrile urinary tract infection in the institutionalized elderly.* Am J Med 1996;100:71–77.

11. Hamilton W, Sharp D. *Symptomatic diagnosis of prostate cancer in primary care: a structured review.* Br J Gen Pract 2004;54:617–621.

12. Orenstein R, Wong E. *Urinary tract infection in adults.* Am Fam Physician 1999;59:1225–1234, 1237.

13. Lipsky B, Inui T, Plorde J, et al. *Is the clean-catch midstream void procedure necessary for obtaining urine culture specimens from men.* Am J Med 1984;76:257–262.

14. Krieger J, Nyberg LJ, Nickel J. *NIH consensus definition and classification of prostatitis.* JAMA 1999;282:236–237.

15. Rizzo M, Marchetti F, Travaglini F, et al. *Prevalence, diagnosis and treatment of prostatitis in Italy: a prospective urology outpatient practice study.* BJU Int 2003;92:955–959.

16. Hamilton W, Sharp D, Peters T, et al. *Clinical features of prostate cancer before diagnosis: a population-based, case-control study.* Br J Gen Pract 2006;56:756–762.

17. Lipsky B. *Urinary tract infections in men.* Ann Intern Med 1989;110:138–150.

18. McNaughton Collins M, Fowler FJ, Elliott D, et al. *Diagnosing and treating chronic prostatitis: do urologists use the four-glass test?* Urology 2000;55:403–407.

19. Abarbanel J, Engelstein D, Lask D, et al. *Urinary tract infection in men younger than 45 years of age: is there a need for urologic investigation?* Urology 2003;62:27–29.

20. Ulleryd P, Zackrisson B, Aus G, et al. *Selective urological evaluation in men with febrile urinary tract infection.* BJU Int 2001;88:15–20.

21. Andrews S, Brooks P, Hanbury D, et al. *Ultrasonography and abdominal radiography versus intravenous urography in investigation of urinary tract infection in men: prospective incident cohort study.* BMJ 2002;324:454–456.

Dysuria, nocturia, frequency and urgency in women

16

KEY FACTS

- Acute urinary symptoms in women in primary care are due to urinary tract infection (UTI) in half of cases; which means that the other half have another disorder, usually a genital infection or the urethral syndrome.
- The typical symptoms of lower urinary infection plus the absence of vaginal discharge or irritation (or any other pointer to another disorder) make the diagnosis of UTI very likely. Empirical treatment without confirmation is justified.

- The diagnosis of UTI is more likely if the urine is cloudy and smelly; and less likely if it is clear.
- Dipstick tests will further refine the probabilities, the test for nitrites being more useful than those for leucocyte esterase or for blood.
- Patients whose diagnosis remains in doubt need a midstream urine (MSU), as do patients with recurrent symptoms, with systemic disturbance or with 'complicated' infections.

A PRACTICAL APPROACH

- ★ Ask about symptoms that would point to a diagnosis of UTI (e.g. dysuria, nocturia, frequency, urgency) and about symptoms that would point towards an alternative diagnosis (e.g. discharge, vulval irritation or dyspareunia).
- ★ Assess risk factors for UTI and any complications (e.g. diabetes, pregnancy, incontinence) which would make the diagnosis more serious.
- ★ Omit examination unless there are suggestions in the history that it might be worthwhile (e.g. loin pain or vaginal discharge or irritation).

- ★ Note the clarity and smell of the urine and perform a dipstick test.
- ★ If the probability of a UTI is now strong, treat as such. Otherwise, send an MSU.
- ★ If the probability of vaginitis or a sexually transmitted disease (STD) fits the clinical picture better, investigate as appropriate (see p. 274).
- ★ If the patient has neither a UTI nor a vaginitis, urethritis or pelvic infection, consider the possibility of urethral syndrome.
- ★ Only investigate women with recurrent UTIs if there is persistent haematuria or infection of the upper urinary tract.

Background

- Urinary tract infection (UTI) in women is common, but only half of those with symptoms suggestive of UTI (acute dysuria/frequency/urgency) have one.

- The clinical assessment is a poor guide in the assessment of which women have a UTI.
- Symptoms will resolve in half of those with proven UTI, without treatment, falsely suggesting to doctor and patient that the aetiology was not bacterial infection.[1]

- GPs have two tests at their disposal but use them inappropriately; they are more likely to send a urine sample to the laboratory if the dipstick test is positive,[2] whereas the opposite approach makes more sense.
- Factors other than the clinical presentation seem to influence GPs in their decision about antibiotic treatment. London GPs were found to be 4.5 times more likely to prescribe antibiotics if they did not know the patient well.[3]

Prevalence

Five per cent of women of reproductive age have significant bacteriuria.[4] Three per cent of the female population present annually with acute urinary symptoms.[5]

Initial probabilities

The initial probabilities when a woman presents in primary care with acute urinary symptoms are:

- urinary tract infection 48%[4] or 62% if the diagnosis is based on a cut-off of $\geq 10^3$ colony forming units (CFU)/ml.[6]
- urethral syndrome (estimates suggest 25%[7] but, being a diagnosis by exclusion, the rate depends on the intensiveness of the search for another cause)
- vaginitis due to *Gardnerella, Candida, Trichomonas* or to bacterial vaginosis (no estimate of prevalence found)
- *Chlamydia* urethritis 3.7% (in a Scandinavian study of women aged 15 to 35)[8]
- genital herpes simplex
- interstitial cystitis (rare and by definition only diagnosed after symptoms have persisted for 6 months without the discovery of another cause).

Do risk factors for infection alter these probabilities?

The following all increase the probability that the symptoms are due to bacterial infection:[1]

- *Sexual intercourse* in the previous 48 hours (risk increased 60-fold).[7] Different authors suggest that the use of a diaphragm does[9] or does not[7] increase the risk.
- *Previous proven UTI.* A recurrence of the same symptoms raises the probability of a UTI to 84%, at least in intelligent women (LR+ 4.0 (95% CI 2.9 to 5.5); LR– 0.0 (95% CI 0.0 to 0.1)).[10] In other words, if a patient who had had a previous UTI said she didn't think that was another one, she was always right.

- *Pregnancy.*
- *Diabetes.*
- *The elderly.*
- *Indwelling catheter* or incontinence requiring aids of some sort. In one survey, this accounted for 9% of UTIs in primary care.[5]

Other factors often quoted (e.g. type of clothing, volume of fluid consumed) do not appear to be risk factors.[9]

The probability of a sexually transmitted disease (STD) is increased by a history of:

- multiple partners
- sexual intercourse without using condoms
- a new complaint of vaginal discharge, genital discomfort or pain.

However, note that a diagnosis of UTI does not necessarily reduce the probability of an STD. A study from New York found a 17% prevalence of STD in women aged 18–55 with frequency, urgency, dysuria and no new vaginal discharge.[11] The prevalence of STD was the same in those with and without bacteriuria (using a cut-off of 10^2 CFU/ml). A check for STD should be made in those at risk even if a UTI is found.

How does the clinical assessment assist the diagnosis?

Symptoms that point to a UTI. A cross-sectional study in primary care in the Balearic Islands of unselected women with urinary symptoms found that specific symptoms were associated with an increased probability of UTI, but not by much (Table 16.1).

A meta-analysis,[4] performed before publication of the Balearic Islands study, has added the further symptoms of haematuria and fever as useful (Table 16.2) but found that flank pain and lower abdominal pain did not shift the diagnosis in either direction.

Symptoms that make the diagnosis of UTI less likely. See Table 16.3.

Do combinations of symptoms help to refine the diagnosis?

A study from Boston of 821 young women presenting in primary care with acute urinary or vaginal symptoms found that certain combinations of symptoms were useful in directing the examination and investigation (Table 16.4).[13] The prevalence of UTI in the group was 12%.

Table 16.1 Symptoms in the prediction of UTI in women with urinary symptoms in primary care.[12] The pre-test probability of UTI in this study was 48%

Symptom	Presence	Likelihood ratio (95% CI)	Probability of UTI according to presence or absence of the symptom
Painful voiding	Present	1.3 (1.1–1.5)	55%
	Absent	0.7 (0.6–0.8)	39%
Urgency	Present	1.3 (1.1–1.5)	55%
	Absent	0.6 (0.5–0.7)	36%
Frequency	Present	1.2 (1.1–1.3)	53%
	Absent	0.4 (0.4–0.5)	27%
Tenesmus	Present	1.2 (1.0–1.3)	53%
	Absent	0.7 (0.6–0.8)	39%
Burning	Present	1.1 (0.97–1.2)	50%
	Absent	0.8 (0.7–0.9)	42%

Follow each row from left to right to see how each symptom alters the probability of a UTI.
Combinations of these symptoms do not usefully increase the probability of UTI.

Table 16.2 Symptoms in the prediction of UTI in women with urinary symptoms in primary care,[4] based on a pre-test probability of UTI of 48%

Symptom	Presence	Likelihood ratio (95% CI)	Probability of UTI according to presence or absence of the symptom
Fever	Present	1.6 (1.0–2.6)	60%
	Absent	0.9 (0.9–1.0)	45%
Haematuria	Present	2.0 (1.3–2.9)	65%
	Absent	0.9 (0.9–1.0)	45%

Follow each row from left to right to see how each symptom alters the probability of a UTI.

Table 16.3 Symptoms that reduce the probability of UTI in women with urinary symptoms in primary care.[12] The pre-test probability of UTI in this study was 48%

Symptom	Presence	Likelihood ratio (95% CI)	Probability of UTI according to presence or absence of the symptom
Lower abdominal discomfort	Present	0.7 (0.6–0.8)	39%
	Absent	1.6 (1.4–1.8)	60%
Genital discomfort	Present	0.7 (0.5–0.9)	39%
	Absent	1.1 (0.9–1.4)	50%
Dyspareunia	Present	0.6 (0.4–0.8)	36%
	Absent	1.1 (0.8–1.5)	50%
Increased vaginal discharge	Present	0.6 (0.4–0.8)	36%
	Absent	1.1 (0.8–1.5)	50%
Perineal discomfort	Present	0.5 (0.3–0.8)	32%
	Absent	1.1 (0.9–1.4)	50%

Follow each row from left to right to see how each symptom alters the probability of a UTI.
However, none of these likelihood ratios are far enough removed from 1 to alter hugely the probability of UTI.

Table 16.4 Combinations of symptoms in the prediction of UTI in women with urinary symptoms in primary care,[4,13] based on a pre-test probability of UTI of 48%

Combination of symptoms	Likelihood ratio	Probability of UTI according to presence or absence of the symptoms
Dysuria and frequency without vaginal discharge or irritation	25	96%
Dysuria or frequency present but vaginal discharge or irritation present as well	0.7	39%
Vaginal discharge or irritation present without dysuria	0.3	22%

Follow each row from left to right to see how each combination of symptoms alters the probability of a UTI.

Table 16.5 Signs in the prediction of UTI in women with urinary symptoms in primary care,[4] based on a pre-test probability of UTI of 48%

Sign	Presence	Likelihood ratio (95% CI)	Probability of UTI according to presence or absence of the sign
Vaginal discharge on examination	Present	0.7 (0.5–0.9)	39%
	Absent	1.1 (1.0–1.2)	50%
Loin tenderness	Present	1.7 (1.1–2.5)	61%
	Absent	0.9 (0.8–1.0)	45%

Follow each row from left to right to see how each sign alters the probability of a UTI.

■ If the patient had 'internal' dysuria and frequency but no vaginal discharge or irritation, a pelvic examination was unlikely to reveal vaginal, urethral or cervical infection (positive predictive value (PPV) for vaginitis 1% in this group). Indeed, a UTI was so likely that urinalysis could be avoided (PPV for UTI 77% in this group, or 96% in women in whom the pre-test probability was a more typical 48%).

■ When the opposite was the case (the patient had vaginal discharge or irritation but no 'internal' dysuria or frequency), urinalysis was unnecessary because the probability of UTI was so low (PPV for UTI 4% in this group although it would be 22% in women in whom the pre-test probability was a more typical 48%).

■ When both 'internal' dysuria ± frequency *and* vaginal discharge ± irritation were present it was not possible to distinguish vaginitis from a UTI; pelvic examination and urinalysis were needed.

Note the importance of asking whether the dysuria was deep inside the body ('internal') or felt in the labia as the urine was passed.

Is examination helpful?

Not much. The Journal of the American Medical Association meta-analysis found only two features of the examination that were significant and they are usually not present.[4] Even if they are, they do not alter the probabilities enough to be useful (Table 16.5).

Is it possible to distinguish an upper from a lower UTI?

Clinical features of an upper UTI are, by consensus, high fever, possibly with rigors, vomiting, loin pain and tenderness.[7] The likelihood ratios for these features are unknown.

Does naked eye (and nose) examination of the urine help in the diagnosis of UTI?

■ *A cloudy urine* suggests a UTI (sensitivity 85%, specificity 60%; LR+ 2.1(95% CI 1.7 to 2.6), LR– 0.25 (95% CI 0.1 to 0.4)).[14] Most of the false positives are due to the presence of phosphate crystals. A study in which these were dissolved with acetic acid solution found the test was considerably more accurate (sensitivity 94%, specificity 79%; LR+ 4.5 (95% CI 3.2 to 6.3), LR– 0.07 (95% CI 0.02 to 0.3)).[15]

■ *A smelly urine* suggests a UTI (sensitivity 22%, specificity 96%; LR+ 5.1 (95% CI 2.3 to 12), LR– 0.8 (95% CI 0.7 to 0.9)).[14] This does not seem to hold for parents' assessment of the smell of their children's urine.[16]

A UK primary care study, from Southampton, has combined four clinical features into a clinical decision rule:[6]
■ cloudy urine
■ offensive smell
■ moderately severe dysuria
■ moderately severe nocturia.

They found no other clinical variables that had independent predictive power; and they noted that mild symptoms were much less useful. The likelihood ratios and probabilities for the rule are shown in Table 16.6.

What tests are useful?

Dipstick for nitrites and leucocyte esterase

● Bacteria convert nitrates to nitrites in the urine. The conversion takes several hours, and so the test should only be performed on urine that has been in the bladder for several hours (e.g. an early morning sample or a sample from a woman who has not passed urine for at least 4 hours).

● The leucocyte esterase test detects pyuria.[17]

● Studies of the accuracy of the dipstick test show enormous variation, with sensitivities ranging from 18% to 71% and specificities from 82% to 99%.[17] These variations depend on the type of patient studied, the setting in which the study is performed, the person who performs it and the gold standard used for the diagnosis. Only studies of patients with suspected UTI in primary care, tested by the doctor or nurse, are relevant here.

● The Southampton study mentioned above is unique in that it uses the currently recommended European standard for the diagnosis of UTI ($\geq 10^3$ CFU/ml for a positive MSU), and it combines testing for blood with nitrites and leucocyte esterase (Table 16.7).[6]

In common with a previous meta-analysis, testing for protein was found to have no independent value.[17]

The leucocyte esterase test

The poor performance of the leucocyte esterase test is disappointing. The meta-analysis mentioned above found that, alone, it had a useless positive likelihood ratio of 1 and an almost useless negative likelihood ratio of 0.8.[17] This poor performance seems to be due in part to overgenerous interpretation of the test by the doctor. When performed by a nurse, the test gives the figures in Table 16.8.

Table 16.6 The probability of UTI according to the Southampton clinical decision rule, based on a pre-test probability of UTI of 62%

Number of features	Likelihood ratio	Probability of UTI
None	0.25	29%
At least 2	2.1	77%
All 4	12	95%

The study used a cut-off of $\geq 10^3$ CFU/ml for a positive MSU, hence the high pre-test probability.

Table 16.7 Performance of the dipstick test (where the pre-test probability of UTI is 62%)[6]

Result	Likelihood ratio	Probability of UTI according to the dipstick result
All three negative	0.2	27%
N or L+B positive	2.6	81%
N+B or N+L positive	7.2	92%
All three positive	9.1	94%

Follow each row from left to right to see how each result alters the probability of a UTI.
N = nitrites, L = leucocyte esterase, B = blood.

Table 16.8 Performance of the dipstick test by a nurse (where the pre-test probability of UTI is 50%)[17]

Test	Result	Likelihood ratio	Probability of UTI according to the dipstick result
Leucocyte esterase only	Positive	1.9	66%
	Negative	0.5	34%

Follow each row from left to right to see how each result alters the probability of a UTI.

The nurse is less easily persuaded that the test is positive, so the probability of a UTI, when it is judged positive, is higher. Laboratory workers are even harder to convince that the dipstick is positive, giving them an LR+ of 3.1 without any decrease in value of the LR−.[17]

The question of spectrum bias (bias introduced by the nature of the population tested) was assessed by a study from Yale. When the clinician thought the patient had a UTI (because of a classical clinical picture), the sensitivity of the dipstick was good (92%). When the clinician thought the patient probably did not have a UTI (because of less characteristic symptoms), the sensitivity of the test was poor (56%).[18] So the test is least helpful when it is most needed.

In conclusion, a dipstick that is negative to nitrites and leucocyte esterase is useful in reducing the probability of a UTI. A dipstick that is positive to nitrites shifts the probability usefully in the direction of a UTI. A GP who finds the result to be a negative nitrite and a positive leucocyte esterase might do well to have the urine retested by a nurse, or ignore the result.

Microscopy and culture of a clean catch MSU

Compared to the dipstick, microscopy and culture is costly and takes at least 24 hours to give a result. It is necessary:

(a) as the 'gold standard' test in cases which, after clinical assessment and dipstick test, are still in doubt; or

(b) where it is important to know the sensitivity of the organism.

However, transport conditions in primary care may not be ideal (see box) and false negatives may occur.

Transport of the MSU

The urine should be passed into a sterile bottle and examined within 2 hours, in order to minimise bacterial overgrowth and cell destruction. Four hours is considered the outside limit unless the sample is refrigerated at 4°C.

Dip-inoculum cultures are more robust when these conditions cannot be met but they give no information on cell counts.

What constitutes a positive MSU?

For decades, the cut-off for significant bacteriuria has been a pure growth of 10^5 colony forming units (CFU) per ml. However, counts of 10^2 to 10^4 CFU/ml may be significant, especially in Gram-positive infections or with atypical organisms, e.g. *Proteus*.[19] The use of counts lower than 10^5 increases the sensitivity of the test but reduces its specificity. European guidelines recommend using a cut-off of 10^3 for pure growths of *Escherichia coli* and a higher cut-off for more unusual organisms or mixed growths.[20]

The finding of >5 white cells per high power field increases the likelihood that the bacterial count is significant.

Complicated cases

An MSU is needed in complicated cases. Treatment failure and recurrent infection are more likely. They are:

- known abnormality of the urinary tract
- diabetes
- immunosuppression
- pregnancy
- indwelling catheter
- recent instrumentation.

Further investigations

- *Women with multiple proven UTIs.* A search for an underlying anatomical or neurological abnormality has traditionally been recommended in women with recurrent infections.[19] Investigation is important in children, where 12–20% of those with a UTI will be found to have an abnormality,[21] and in men, where half will have an abnormality[22] (but see p. 90). However, more recent evidence in women suggests that further investigation, initially an ultrasound scan of the urinary tract, is only needed in women with persistent haematuria or an upper UTI.[7]

- *Women in whom a UTI, vaginitis and STD have been excluded and whose symptoms recur.* The urethral syndrome is the likely diagnosis but the fact that it is diagnosed by exclusion and is of unknown aetiology makes it unsatisfactory for doctor and patient. Whether to refer a patient for a urological opinion will depend on the severity of the symptoms and the patient's distress.

Example

A 30-year-old woman presents with severe dysuria and some frequency. She has just started a new sexual relationship. She has not noticed any vaginal discharge. She is well in herself and there are no other pointers from the history.

The GP decides that this is simple cystitis and decides to treat her empirically without examination or further testing. She, however, has brought a urine sample with her and he examines it in order not to seem over-hasty. It is clear to the naked eye, which, he knows, carries a likelihood ratio of 0.25. Still, he reasons, that only reduces the probability of UTI from, say 80% (because of the severe dysuria and no vaginal discharge) to 50% (Fig. 16.1). He tests for nitrites and leucocyte esterase with a dipstick. Both are negative. The negative likelihood ratio of 0.2 reduces her probability of UTI to 17% (Fig. 16.2).

The GP backtracks and examines her. There is nothing to find, but he takes swabs from the cervix and urethra as well as asking her to send an MSU. He's disappointed (for her sake) when both swabs grow *Gonococcus* while the MSU is sterile.

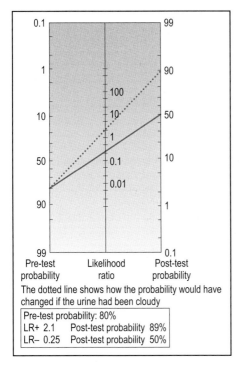

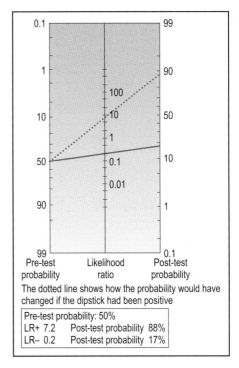

Figure 16.1 The probability of UTI before and after the visual examination of the urine in the example on p. 98.

Figure 16.2 The probability of UTI before and after the dipstick test in the example on p. 98.

REFERENCES

1. MeReC. *Urinary tract infection.* MeReC Bulletin 1995;6(8):1–6.

2. Fahey T, Webb E, Montgomery A, et al. *Clinical management of urinary tract infection in women: a prospective cohort study.* Fam Pract 2003;20:1–6.

3. Nazareth I, King M. *Decision making by general practitioners in diagnosis and management of lower urinary tract symptoms in women.* BMJ 1993;306:1103–1106.

4. Bent S, Nallamothu B, Simel D, et al. *Does this woman have an acute uncomplicated urinary tract infection?* JAMA 2002;287:2701–2710.

5. Ferry S, Burman L, Mattsson B. *Urinary tract infection in primary health care in northern Sweden.* I. Epidemiology. Scand J Prim Health Care 1987;5:123–128.

6. Little P, Turner S, Rumsby K, et al. *Developing clinical rules to predict urinary tract infection in primary care settings: sensitivity and specificity of near patient tests (dipsticks) and clinical scores.* Br J Gen Pract 2006;56: 606–612.

7. Car J. *Urinary tract infection in women: diagnosis and management in primary care.* BMJ 2006;332:94–97.

8. Osterberg E, Aspevall O, Grillner L, et al. *Young women with symptoms of urinary tract infection. Prevalence and diagnosis of chlamydial infection and evaluation of rapid screening of bacteriuria.* Scand J Prim Health Care 1996;14:43–49.

9. Remis R, Gurwith M, Gurwith D, et al. *Risk factors for urinary tract infection.* Am J Epidemiol 1987;126: 685–694.

10. Gupta K, Hooton T, Roberts P, et al. *Patient-initiated treatment of uncomplicated recurrent urinary tract infections in young women.* Ann Intern Med 2001;135:9–16.

11. Shapiro T, Dalton M, Hammock J, et al. *The prevalence of urinary tract infections and sexually transmitted disease in women with symptoms of a simple urinary tract infection stratified by low colony count.* Acad Emerg Med 2005;12:38–44.

12. Medina-Bombardo D, Segui-Diaz M, Roca-Fusalba C, et al. *What is the predictive value of urinary symptoms for diagnosing urinary tract infection in women?* Fam Pract 2003; 20:103–107.

13. Komaroff AL, Pass T, McCue J, et al. *Management strategies for urinary and vaginal infections.* Arch

Intern Med 1978;138:1069–1073.

14. Ditchburn R, Ditchburn J. *A study of microscopical and chemical tests for the rapid diagnosis of urinary tract infections in general practice.* Br J Gen Pract 1990;40:406–408.

15. Bulloch B, Bausher J, Pomerantz W, et al. *Can urine clarity exclude the diagnosis of urinary tract infection?* Pediatrics 2000;106:E60.

16. Struthers S, Scanlon J, Parker K, et al. *Parental reporting of smelly urine and urinary tract infection.* Arch Dis Child 2003;88:250–252.

17. Deville L, Yzermans J, van Duijn N, et al. *The urine dipstick test useful to rule out infections. A meta-analysis of the accuracy.* BMC Urol 2004;4:4.

18. Lachs M, Nachamkin I, Edelstein P, et al. *Spectrum bias in the evaluation of diagnostic tests: lessons from the rapid dipstick test for urinary tract infection.* Ann Intern Med 1992;117:135–140.

19. DTB. *Managing urinary tract infection in women.* Drug Ther Bull 1998;36:30–32.

20. European Confederation of Laboratory Medicine. *European urinalysis guidelines: summary.* Scand J Clin Lab Invest 2000;60:1–96.

21. DTB. *The management of urinary tract infection in children.* Drug Ther Bull 1997;35:65–69.

22. Andrews S, Brooks P, Hanbury D, et al. *Ultrasonography and abdominal radiography versus intravenous urography in investigation of urinary tract infection in men: prospective incident cohort study.* BMJ 2002;324:454–456.

Erectile dysfunction

17

KEY FACTS

Diagnosis of the cause of erectile dysfunction (ED) is usually possible after a history and brief examination.

- A psychogenic cause is suggested by a rapid onset, intermittent loss of erection and preservation of nocturnal erections. Refer for specific sexual psychotherapy without investigation.
- An underlying mental disorder is suggested by low mood or symptoms of anxiety or disturbance in the ability to function outside the area of sexual activity.
- An underlying physical disorder will usually already have manifested itself. Erectile dysfunction may be caused by the disorder or the medication taken for it.
- If the history suggests an organic cause but the patient is not known to have a relevant physical disorder, restrict the search to the two causes for which there is specific treatment: hypogonadism and vascular disease.

A PRACTICAL APPROACH

- * Ask about timing, whether there have been other sexual problems and whether nocturnal erections occur.
- * Ask about other medical disorders and their medication.
- * Ask about any penile deformity when erect.
- * Check the patient's mental state.
- * Only examine if the history suggests an organic cause or you sense that the patient has physical concerns about his genitalia which examination may elucidate and perhaps relieve.
- * If genital examination reveals a local cause, refer to a urologist.
- * If the patient is taking a drug know to cause ED, consider stopping it once an alternative has been found but with the understanding that most patients on such drugs do not experience ED and that in this patient it may be coincidental.
- * If an organic cause has been identified, for which there is no specific treatment, offer a trial of an oral phosphodiesterase type-5 inhibitor.
- * In other patients: check serum testosterone at 9.00 am.
  - (a) If two specimens are low, refer for endocrinological assessment.
  - (b) If normal, give a trial of an oral phosphodiesterase type-5 inhibitor.
  - (c) If successful, continue it as treatment. However, in addition, investigate further those patients with abnormalities on examination. For instance, patients with diminished arterial pulses need an assessment of their risk of cardiovascular disease. Patients with abnormal neurological findings need further assessment.
  - (d) If no response to the phosphodiesterase type-5 inhibitor, refer, if the patient wishes, for further investigation, especially if vascular or neurological abnormalities have been detected.

Definition

'The inability of the male to attain and maintain erection of the penis sufficient to permit satisfactory sexual intercourse' (US National Institutes of Health).[1] It may be divided into categories according to severity: mild, moderate and complete. Assessment of severity may be left to the patient or defined by the patient's score on a questionnaire, e.g. the International Index of Erectile Function Questionnaire.[1]

Prevalence

In the population

Estimates vary according to the population studied, the definition of ED used, and the interview method.

A relatively low estimate comes from Germany (19% of men aged 30 to 80)[2] and a relatively high one from Finland (76% of men aged 50 to 75).[3] The largest study comes somewhere between those extremes: 31 000 men in the USA, aged 53 to 90, gave a prevalence of 33%.[4] All studies show a marked increase with age, with figures of 2% at the age of 30 to over 50% at age 80.[2] This does not mean that ED is an inevitable part of ageing; there is always a cause, and with the advent of oral therapy, there is treatment that is effective regardless of age.

Those studies with high prevalences include patients whose impotence was minimal. The Massachusetts Male Aging Study reports a prevalence of 52% in men aged 40 to 70, but one-third of those described it as minimal and in only 9.6% was it complete.[5]

In primary care

A study of 1512 primary care attenders in London aged 18 to 75 gave a prevalence of ED of 8.8%.[6] Of the sample, 22% had sexual dysfunction sufficient to merit an ICD-10 diagnosis of sexual dysfunction, of which ED was the most common. Yet only 4% had a record of sexual dysfunction in their notes in the previous 2 years. Only a small minority of patients with sexual dysfunction, therefore, consult their GP with it in a way that leads the GP to record it, although 21% said they had sought sexual advice from a doctor at some time in their life.

The problem

Only a small proportion of those who could be helped present to their general practitioner. Reasons for this include a poor understanding of what services are available, an idea that ED is unimportant or part of normal ageing, embarrassment and also issues relating to the general practitioner's gender, class and attitude towards later life sexuality.[7]

Initial probabilities

The following figures are derived from the prevalences in *secondary* care. In primary care, more patients will be seen whose ED is due to medication or to alcohol abuse, but it appears that the proportions with ED of psychological and organic aetiology are similar to those in secondary care.[8]

A. Probabilities in a patient presenting with ED without known concurrent disease

■ *Vascular causes*: 42%, of which two-thirds are arterial and one-third are due to a venous leak.[9]

■ *Psychological causes*: These are more common in the younger patient, with a prevalence of 39% in patients <40 years old in a Spanish clinic, with another 20% of mixed organic and psychological aetiology.[10] A US clinic found similar figures: 40% psychogenic and 25% mixed.[11] The patient may have a specific sexual problem of which performance anxiety in young men is the commonest, or the ED may be part of a more general disorder, usually depression or anxiety. Once a man experiences ED, anxiety about his performance may complicate the picture, whatever the original cause.

■ *Medication*: 25%.[12]

■ *Hypogonadism*: 8% of referred patients in a French study were found to have a low serum testosterone with most cases occurring in older patients.[9] In this study, it was low in 4% of those aged <50 and in 9% of those aged >50. Other studies range from 2%[13] to 16%.[14]

■ *Hyperprolactinaemia*: 0.2% in the French study, of whom 1 patient had a pituitary tumour (0.1%).[9]

■ *Diabetes*: However, diabetes is rarely the cause of ED in patients not known to have diabetes.[1]

■ *Hypo- and hyperthyroidism*: A very small number of patients with previously undetected thyroid disease are found in cross-sectional studies of men with ED. It is not clear whether the prevalence is higher than in the general population.

■ *Alcohol*: 75% of patients in alcohol rehabilitation programmes have ED.[12] However, only very heavy drinking seems to put patients at risk. The US survey of 31 000 men found that drinking >30 g/day was no more associated with ED than abstinence, although more moderate drinkers had a *reduction* in ED risk.[4]

■ *Illicit drugs* (amfetamines, cocaine, heroin, marijuana, morphine, steroids) are all potential causes of ED but are only occasionally the cause of ED in patients not already in treatment for the misuse.

B. Probabilities in a patient presenting with ED with known concurrent disease

See below under 'Does the patient have a relevant medical or surgical condition?'

The history

The detailed history of the problem

In a New York study of men referred for ED, the history had a sensitivity of 96.5% and a specificity of 50% in diagnosing organic ED; LR+ 1.9 (1.2 to 3.2); LR– 0.07 (0.01 to 0.50).[15] In other words, if the history suggests that it is psychological, it probably is. It is less good at confirming an organic diagnosis.

＊ Ask:

■ Was the onset sudden or had the patient noticed a gradual loss of rigidity over months or years?
■ Is it constant or intermittent?
■ Are there any other sexual problems?
■ Does it only occur when attempting intercourse or is masturbation affected?
■ Do nocturnal erections occur?

A sudden onset, concurrent premature ejaculation, normal erection with masturbation, ED with one partner and not another, and the continuation of nocturnal erections all point to a psychological cause. Not all studies have found sudden onset useful.[16,17] For a more detailed analysis of the discriminatory power of different aspects of the history see Appendix 1 on page 107.

Attention to detail in interpreting the history is needed. For instance, an apparent sudden onset may in fact be gradual but the man may not realise it if he has not attempted intercourse in the preceding months or years. A Turkish study of young men with 'honeymoon impotence' of sudden onset found that 28% had penile vascular abnormalities and 4% had neurological abnormalities.[18] The apparent sudden onset was the result of a lack of previous attempts at intercourse.

More detail about the history

Do nocturnal erections occur? This is the single most useful question in the distinction of organic from psychogenic ED. The value of the patient's report has been tested in a small study.[19] The presence of nocturnal erections was 86% sensitive and 100% specific for the diagnosis of psychogenic ED (LR+ infinitely high; LR– 0.1). In other words, if nocturnal erections occur the impotence is psychological. It is essential to ask the question as follows: 'Do you experience erections on waking at least twice a week that would be sufficient for vaginal penetration?' The same question, but asking about '100% full erection', has no discriminatory power.[19]

Formal testing, using equipment of various designs, has confirmed the value of morning erections in larger studies. They achieve sensitivities and specificities of between 80% and 95%.[20] The report by the patient of nocturnal or early morning erections gives results very similar to these objective findings.[16,21]

In conclusion, erections on waking, if present, are a powerful pointer away from organic disease. A report of a lack of nocturnal erections is useful but does not rule out a psychological cause; severe depression is commonly associated with lack of nocturnal erections. Alternatively, erections may be occurring unnoticed by the patient.

Is libido reduced? This question is often asked but with little reason to think that it will prove useful. Libido is reduced in hypogonadism, but also in depression so it is not a useful test in distinguishing endocrine from psychological causes.[22] It is not even useful in the identification of hypogonadism (Table 17.1).[9] Note that some men find it hard to distinguish between loss of libido and ED.[23]

Does the patient have a relevant medical or surgical condition?

The finding of a condition known to be associated with ED poses the problem of whether the condition has caused ED in this patient. A short cut is to look for the three causes of impotence that need specific treatment: endocrine, psychogenic and certain types of reversible vascular impotence. If these are not present, the cause is academic and the patient, if he wishes to have treatment, can be treated with oral therapy.[24] Oral therapy is effective regardless of the severity, aetiology (psychogenic,

Table 17.1 Usefulness of reduced libido in the diagnosis of hypogonadism from a study of French men referred because of ED[9]

Prevalence of hypogonadism	Libido	LR (95% CI)	Probability of hypogonadism according to libido status
7%	Low	1.4 (1.03–1.8)	10%
	Normal	0.8 (0.6–1.03)	6%

Follow each row from left to right to see how little the status of the patient's libido alters the probability of hypogonadism.

diabetes, depression, ischaemic heart disease, hypertension, peripheral vascular disease, spinal cord injury or radical prostatectomy) or the age and ethnicity of the patient.[25]

The conditions in more detail:

■ *Chronic medical conditions.* A study of US male medical outpatients found that 34% had ED.[26] The single commonest cause was not the illness for which they were attending the hospital but the medication (25%), and the second commonest was psychogenic (14%).[26] The US survey of 31 000 men found that chronic diseases were significantly associated with ED, after correction for age, other diseases and risk factors, and the effect of medication. The adjusted relative risks and their 95% confidence intervals were as follows:

(a) hypertension 1.2 (1.1 to 1.3)

(b) heart disease 1.4 (1.1 to 1.6)

(c) diabetes 1.5 (1.2 to 1.9)

(d) stroke 1.4 (1.0 to 1.9)

(e) cancer (other than prostatic cancer) 1.4 (1.1 to 1.6).[4]

■ *Cardiovascular disease.* Complete ED is found in 39% of those with treated heart disease and in 15% of those on antihypertensives.[12] How many of these are due to atheroma of the pelvic arteries is not clear. The presence of intermittent claudication, diminished lower limb pulses, with or without bruits, wasting of the buttock muscles and ED (Leriche's syndrome) suggests it. However, normal peripheral pulses do not rule out the diagnosis of an arterial cause, which may be localised to the pelvic vessels. When detected, arterial stenosis is potentially amenable to surgery, as is a venous leak when discovered by duplex ultrasonography.

■ *Diabetes.* Complete ED is found in 28% of diabetics[12] and increases with age and with duration of the disease. It may be due to autonomic neuropathy, or, more commonly, to microvascular or macrovascular disease. It is, however, rarely the presenting symptom of diabetes. A blood sugar is not recommended as part of the work-up unless the

patient has risk factors for diabetes that would warrant screening anyway (e.g. obesity, strong family history, previous glucose intolerance).[1] Diabetic patients with ED of neuropathic origin often report that dry orgasm occurred in the year or so prior to the development of ED.[8] A small Italian study found that no patients had autonomic neuropathy and ED without evidence of peripheral neuropathy as well. They also noted the importance of psychogenic factors even in those with physical abnormalities.[27]

■ *Penile disease.* Peyronie's disease may cause pain on erection and deviation of the penis. It may also cause disruption of the veno-occlusive mechanism, causing ED. So can congenital malformations, trauma or surgery.[12] Note that diseases of the penis can cause marked deviation of the erect penis with virtually nothing to find when it is flaccid. The patient's description is the best guide to the presence of an anatomical abnormality which may have triggered the ED.

■ *Other urological disease.*

(a) Prostatic cancer may cause ED as it invades the parasympathetic fibres on the posterolateral aspect of the prostate.[8] Both simple and radical prostatectomy and external beam irradiation carry a high risk of ED because of damage to the autonomic fibres that encircle the prostate. One large study found ED in >80% of men treated for prostatic cancer regardless of method of treatment.[28]

(b) Lower urinary tract symptoms are significantly associated with ED (odds ratio 2.1) independent of age,[2] but the reason for this is not clear. Benign prostatic hypertrophy does not cause ED.[8]

■ *Spinal cord injury, peripheral neuropathy.* Erectile dysfunction will almost never be the presenting symptom of spinal cord injury or disease. Furthermore, most patients with spinal cord lesions retain reflex erections. Complete impotence is only to be expected in total destruction of the spinal segments S2–S4 or their roots. Patients with peripheral neuropathy are likely to have other symptoms and signs.

Does the patient have a relevant psychiatric condition?

■ *Depression.* Complete ED is found in 90% of men with severe depression.[12] Nocturnal erections are often lost. However, in less severe depression, the presence of depression and ED may be linked or, since both are common, coincidental. Furthermore, any ED may be due to an antidepressant: rates of 7–30% have been reported according to the drug used.[29] Assess the patient for depression (see *Depression*, p. 373).

■ *Anxiety.* Generalised anxiety and social phobia are commonly associated with ED. Check for them (see *Anxiety*, p. 328)

■ *Specific psychological sexual dysfunction*, of which performance anxiety in young men is the commonest. Erectile dysfunction due to performance anxiety is usually of sudden onset. There may have been a trigger that the patient can recall. Masturbation and nocturnal erections will be preserved. Other specific causes are guilt, fear of hurting a partner who has dyspareunia, an underlying relationship problem or the patient's partner may have a sexual problem. Secondary psychological problems may complicate a physical primary cause.

Is the patient taking medication known to cause ED?

If so, and the patient is sufficiently troubled, stop it once a suitable alternative has been found. If the drug cannot be stopped, changing to a lower dose may be enough.

The commonest drugs responsible are as follows:
■ antihypertensives especially high-dose thiazides and beta-blockers
■ antidepressants, whether tricyclic antidepressants, selective serotonin reuptake inhibitors (SSRIs) or monoamine oxidase inhibitors (MAOIs)
■ other psychotropics, e.g. benzodiazepines and phenothiazines
■ others: cimetidine, digoxin, metoclopramide and anabolic steroids.

However, since psychiatric disorders and cardiovascular disease are themselves causes of ED, it is hard to decide, from cross-sectional studies, whether the disease or the medication is the cause of the problem.

The US survey of 31 000 men found that drugs were sometimes a more powerful predictor of ED than the diseases for which they were being given. The main classes of drugs, corrected for age, other risk factors and morbidity, gave the following relative risks (95% CI) for ED:

■ antidepressants 1.7 (1.2 to 2.2)
■ beta-blockers 1.2 (1.1 to 1.5)
■ alpha-blockers 1.3 (1.0 to 1.7).

Thiazides were not found to be associated with an increased risk. The study was performed in 2000 and so it is likely that patients were on low thiazide doses.[4]

Caution: Do not attribute ED to a drug just because the drug is known to cause it. The problem may be due to the underlying disorder or it may be coincidental. In the Treatment of Mild Hypertension Study, chlorthalidone was significantly associated with ED but acebutolol, amlodipine and enalapril were not and doxazosin showed a tendency towards benefit.[30] In principle, only accept that the drug was the cause of the ED if erections return to their previous state when the drug is stopped. However, in practice, the experience of ED may have so damaged the patient's confidence that ED continues for psychological reasons even when the causative drug has been stopped.[31] One pointer towards a true drug effect is if orgasm and ejaculation are also affected. A study of patients on imipramine, phenelzine and placebo found that orgasm and ejaculation were affected more than erection.[32]

Is the patient misusing a substance known to cause ED?

Erectile dysfunction is described in those who misuse alcohol and illicit drugs (see above).[12] Between 50% and 80% of alcoholics have ED.[33] There is less evidence of an effect with lower intake (see above).

Chronic marijuana use may decrease testosterone levels and precipitate ED. This comes as a surprise to users who recall the enhanced sexual function associated with the testosterone surge of acute intermittent use. Erectile dysfunction is more regularly associated with opiate misuse. Cigarette smoking can cause ED both by causing atherosclerosis and by its direct action in causing vasoconstriction of the internal pudendal artery.[33]

The examination

This is the least useful assessment tool. A small study from a New York sexual dysfunction centre found marginal use from the physical examination in the detection of organic disease which did not reach statistical significance: LR+ 1.3 (1.03 to 2.3); LR– 0.7 (0.3 to 1.4).[15] False positives occur when organic disease is found and is assumed to be the cause of ED. False negatives occur because many organic causes of ED cannot be detected on examination. A larger study might still show a significant contribution from the examination.

* Check blood pressure, peripheral pulses, penis, testes, secondary sexual characteristics and a brief test for peripheral neuropathy and sensation in the saddle area.

* If there is reason to suspect neurological disease, test anal sphincter tone. An intact bulbocavernosus reflex makes neurological disease less likely as the cause of the impotence. Insert a gloved finger into the anus and squeeze the glans penis. A positive test occurs when there is reflex contraction of the anal sphincter. No studies have assessed its value as part of the physical examination. When it has been assessed formally, using measurement of latency, it achieved a sensitivity of 55–70% and a specificity of 95% (LR+ 11–14, LR– 0.3–0.5) for neurological disease.[20]

Combining history, examination and the presence or absence of nocturnal erections, in the small New York study, detected all the cases of organic ED and only attributed 1 case to an organic cause when it was found by more detailed investigation to be psychogenic; sensitivity 100%, specificity 83%; LR+ 5.9 (1.9 to 14) LR– 0 (0.0 to 0.3).[15]

Blood tests

Check total serum testosterone at 9.00 am. Younger men, especially, have a diurnal cycle with a morning peak. Repeat the test if it is low. If there has been recent illness, wait 3 months before repeating the test. One study found that 40% with low levels on the first test were normal when repeated.[9] Order follicle stimulating hormone (FSH) and luteinising hormone (LH) with the repeat testosterone. Low or low-normal levels of these hormones raise the possibility of hypopituitarism. High levels suggest primary hypogonadism. Serum prolactin is unlikely to be raised if the serum testosterone is normal and so may be omitted from the initial screen.

Interpreting a low serum testosterone

* Refer any patient with a level <7 nm/L (<2 ng/ml). Referral for a level 7–10.5 nm/L (2–3 ng/ml) is justified if there is a clinical suspicion of hypogonadism or if the laboratory gives the higher figure as the upper limit of normal for the method used.

* When referring, warn the patient that the interpretation of serum testosterone results is complex and the question of whether the decline seen with age is pathological is not resolved.[34] Lack of sexual activity can itself cause a low testosterone level. In Buvat's study, of those with low testosterone only 10% had organic hypogonadism as the cause of their ED. Of these, half had Leydig cell failure and half had a pituitary tumour.[9] In the others, the low testosterone was judged to be incidental. However, those with low levels sometimes benefited from androgen therapy regardless of whether the low testosterone was judged to indicate organic hypogonadism: 36% improved.[9]

* Do not dismiss the idea of hypogonadism if the free testosterone is normal and the total testosterone is low. Some argue that testosterone bound to albumin is bio-available and should be included.

Example

A man aged 45 consults because he has developed complete impotence with his wife since being made redundant from work. The problem had been coming on over 6 months and he attributes it to worry over his employment. He does not masturbate for religious reasons and has not noticed nocturnal erections. His self-esteem has taken a blow from the loss of his job but he does not have a depressive illness. He wants to recover his potency because his wife is distressed by its loss.

He has no other illnesses and does not misuse drugs or alcohol.

The GP's examination is more thorough than usual because of the lack of nocturnal erections. It includes the genitals, secondary sexual characteristics, femoral pulses and sensation in the saddle area. It is normal.

The GP cannot decide whether the impotence is organic, psychological or a mixture of the two. Her experience tells her to believe a patient who thinks his impotence is psychological; but the gradual onset and apparent lack of nocturnal erections is more suggestive of an organic cause. Then again, the absence of an obvious physical condition makes organic disease less likely.

Because of this uncertainty she checks the serum testosterone, which is normal. A trial of a phosphodiesterase type-5 inhibitor is successful. The patient is happy to continue this and to accept that referral for further investigations is unlikely to yield useful information.

Appendix 1
Discriminatory power of different questions in the separation of psychogenic and organic erectile dysfunction

A study of 176 men referred with erectile dysfunction (ED) to Leiden University Hospital found that the following questions contributed independently to the differentiation between a psychogenic and an organic cause (Tables 17.2–17.4).[17] The prevalence of a psychological cause in the sample was 38%.

None of these questions shifts the probabilities very much. However, using all 10 questions gave much more useful figures for the diagnosis of a psychogenic cause (Table 17.4).

There are two problems with this study for GPs:
1. These patients were referred, mainly to a urology clinic. It is likely that they represent only the more difficult cases seen in primary care. The questions may be even more useful in unselected patients in primary care.

2. The study excluded 22 patients judged to have a mixture of causes (psychogenic and organic), which is the most difficult group to assess. Had the questions been applied to those excluded patients, 11 would have been classified as organic and 7 as psychogenic. Only the clinical judgement of the GP can reconcile pointers in different directions and decide on a diagnosis that includes different concurrent causes.

Table 17.2 Seven questions made a psychogenic cause more likely if the answer was positive. Prevalence of psychogenic ED 38%

Questions	Likelihood ratio (95% CI)	Probability of a psychological cause
Question 1	**Do you find you have erections on waking?**	
Yes	1.3 (1.1–1.5)	44%
No	0.3 (0.1–0.7)	17%
Question 2	**Is it at least 50% of the rigidity of your previous normal erections?**	
Yes	1.4 (1.1–1.8)	52%
No	0.5 (0.3–0.9)	30%
Question 3	**If you masturbate is your normal erection at least 50% of the rigidity of your previous erections?**	
Yes	1.8 (1.3–2.5)	53%
No	0.5 (0.3–0.8)	23%
Question 4	**Do you think your ED is associated with psychological problems?**	
Yes	1.9 (1.4–2.6)	54%
No	0.5 (0.3–0.7)	24%
Question 5	**When you used to have intercourse did you experience premature ejaculation?**	
Yes	1.5 (1.1–2.1)	52%
No	0.6 (0.4–0.9)	28%
Question 6	**Was the onset of ED sudden?**	
Yes	1.3 (0.9–2.0)	47%
No	0.8 (0.7–1.1)	36%
Question 7	**Is there tension in your relationship with your partner?**	
Yes	1.6 (1.1–2.3)	47%
No	0.7 (0.5–0.97)	29%

Follow each row from left to right to see how each symptom alters the probability of psychogenic erectile dysfunction.

Table 17.3 Three questions made a psychogenic cause *less* likely if the answer was positive. Prevalence of psychogenic ED 38%

Questions	Likelihood ratio (95% CI)	Probability of a psychological cause
Question 8	**Has there been a decline in your sexual interest?**	
Yes	0.8 (0.7–0.97)	34%
No	2.6 (1.3–5.3)	62%
Question 9	**Has your penis reduced in size?**	
Yes	0.7 (0.5–0.9)	30%
No	1.5 (1.1–2.2)	49%
Question 10	**Before the onset of ED did you have intercourse more than once a month?**	
Yes	0.8 (0.7–0.97)	34%
No	2.6 (1.2–5.3)	62%

Follow each row from left to right to see how each symptom alters the probability of psychogenic erectile dysfunction.

Table 17.4 Ten questions made a psychogenic cause much more likely if the majority of answers pointed in that direction. Prevalence of psychogenic ED 38%

Majority of answers	Likelihood ratio (95% CI)	Probability of a psychological cause
Pointing to a psychological cause	15 (4.8–44)	93%
Pointing to an organic cause	0.25 (0.2–0.4)	18%

Follow each row from left to right to see how each combination of symptoms alters the probability of psychogenic erectile dysfunction.

REFERENCES

1. Pharmacy Benefits Management – Medical Advisory Panel. *The primary care management of erectile dysfunction: VHA PBM-SHG Publication No. 99-0014, 1999.* Online. Available: www.vapbm.org (choose 'treatment guidelines').

2. Braun M, Sommer F, Haupt G, et al. *Lower urinary tract symptoms and erectile dysfunction: co-morbidity or typical 'aging male' symptoms?* Eur Urol 2003;44:588–594.

3. Shiri R, Koskimaki J, Hakama M, et al. *Prevalence and severity of erectile dysfunction in 50- to 75-year-old Finnish men.* J Urol 2003;170: 2342–2344.

4. Bacon C, Mittlemen M, Kawachi I, et al. *Sexual function in men older than 50 years of age: results from the health professionals follow-up study.* Ann Intern Med 2003;139:161–168.

5. Feldman H, Goldstein I, Hatzichristou D, et al. *Impotence and its medical and psychosocial correlates: results of the Massachusetts Male Aging Study.* J Urol 1994;151:54–61.

6. Nazareth I, Boynton P, King M. *Problems with sexual function in people attending London general practitioners: cross sectional study.* BMJ 2003;327: 423–426.

7. Gott M, Hinchliff S. *Barriers to seeking treatment for sexual problems in primary care: a qualitative study with older people.* Fam Pract 2003;20: 690–695.

8. Mulley A, Goroll A. *Medical evaluation and management of erectile dysfunction.* In: Gorroll A, Mulley AJ, eds. Primary care medicine. Baltimore: Lippincott Williams & Wilkins, 2000.

9. Buvat J, Lemaire A. *Endocrine screening in 1022 men with erectile dysfunction: clinical significance and cost-effective strategy.* J Urol 1997; 158:1764–1767.

10. Sanchez de la Vega L, Amaya Gutierrez J, Alonso Flores J, Garcia Perez M. *Erectile dysfunction in those under 40. Etiological and contributing factors.* Arch Esp Urol 2003;56: 161–164.

11. Melman A, Tiefer L, Pedersen R. *Evaluation of first 406 patients in urology department based Center for Male Sexual Dysfunction.* Urology 1988;32:6–10.

12. Wagner G, Saenz de Tejada I. *Update on male erectile dysfunction.* BMJ 1998;316:678–682.

13. Maatman T, Montague D. *Routine endocrine screening in impotence.* Urology 1986;27:499–502.

14. Govier F, McClure R, Kramer-Levien D. *Endocrine screening for sexual dysfunction using free testosterone determinations.* J Urol 1996;156: 405–408.

15. Davis-Joseph B, Tiefer L, Melman A. *Accuracy of the initial history and physical examination to establish the etiology of erectile dysfunction.* Urology 1995;45:498–502.

16. Ackermann M, D'Attilio J, Antoni M, et al. *The predictive significance of patient-reported sexual functioning in Rigiscan sleep evaluations.* J Urol 1991;146: 1559–1563.

17. Speckens A, Hengeveld M, Lycklama G, et al. *Discrimination between psychogenic and organic erectile dysfunction.* J Psychosom Res 1993; 37:135–145.

18. Usta M, Erdogru T, Tefekli A, et al. *Honeymoon impotence: psychogenic or organic in origin?* Urology 2001; 57:758–762.

19. Segraves K, Segraves R, Schoenberg H. *Use of sexual history to differentiate organic from psychogenic impotence.* Arch Sex Behav 1987;16: 125–137.

20. Black E. *Impotence.* In: Black E, Bordley D, Tape T, Panzer R, eds. Diagnostic strategies for common medical problems. Philadelphia: American College of Physicians, 1999.

21. Ackerman M, D'Attilio J, Antoni M, Campbell B. *Assessment of erectile dysfunction in diabetic men: the clinical relevance of self-reported sexual functioning.* J Sex Marital Ther 1991; 17:191–202.

22. Shabsigh R, Klein L, Seidman S, et al. *Increased incidence of depressive symptoms in men with erectile dysfunction.* Urology 1998;52: 848–852.

23. Arduca P. *Erectile dysfunction. A guide to diagnosis and treatment.* Aust Fam Physician 2003;32:414–420.

24. Sharlip I. *Diagnostic evaluation of erectile dysfunction in the era of oral therapy.* Int J Impot Res 2000;12 (Suppl 4):S12–S14.

25. Fink H, Mac Donald R, Rutks I, et al. *Sildenafil for male erectile dysfunction.* Arch Intern Med 2002; 162:1349–1360.

26. Slag M, Morley J, Elson M, et al. *Impotence in medical clinic outpatients.* JAMA 1983;249:1736–1740.

27. Benvenuti F, Boncinelli L, Vignoli G. *Male sexual impotence in diabetes mellitus: vasculogenic versus neurogenic factors.* Neurourol Urodyn 1993;12:145–151.

28. Siegel T, Moul J, Spevak M, et al. *The development of erectile dysfunction in men treated for prostate cancer.* J Urol 2001;165:430–435.

29. Nurnberg H. *Erectile dysfunction and comorbid depression: prevalence, treatment strategies, and associated medical conditions.* J Clin Psychiatry 2003;64 (Suppl 10):3–4.

30. Grimm RJ, Grandits G, Prineas R, et al. *Long-term effects on sexual function of five antihypertensive drugs and nutritional hygienic treatment in hypertensive men and women.* Hypertension 1997;29:8–14.

31. Morse W, Morse J. *Erectile impotence precipitated by organic factors and perpetuated by performance anxiety.* Can Med Assoc J 1982;127: 599–601.

32. Harrison W, Rabkin J, Ehrhardt A, et al. *Effects of antidepressant medication on sexual function: a controlled study.* J Clin Psychopharmacol 1986;6:144–149.

33. Keene L. *Drug-related erectile dysfunction.* Adverse Drug React Toxicol 1999;18:5–24.

34. Plymate S. *Which testosterone assay should be used in older men?* J Clin Endocrinol Metab 1998;83: 3436–3438.

18

Fatigue

When the history is of fatigue for more than 2 weeks the approximate probabilities are:
- depression in a quarter
- a physical disease in a quarter
- no cause found in a quarter
- the final quarter contains many possibilities, with chronic fatigue syndrome (CFS) accounting for 2% of the total.

When the history is of fatigue for more than 6 months without a diagnosis the approximate probabilities are:
- depression in half
- somatisation disorder and other psychiatric disorders in a quarter
- chronic fatigue syndrome in 10%
- prolonged fatigue syndromes and chronic physical disorders in the remainder.

Tailor your approach according to how long the symptoms have been present. The longer the duration the more intensive the search for a psychiatric cause, or for chronic fatigue syndrome, should be.
- Ask about mood, about current or recent infections, about use of alcohol and other drugs, about sleep, sleepiness and snoring.
- Ask specifically whether there is muscle fatigue after exertion and whether there are mental changes other than tiredness.
- Ask about muscle pain unrelated to exertion.

- Examine the patient, looking for anaemia, hypo- or hyperthyroidism, and the lymphadenopathy and hepatosplenomegaly of chronic infection or of widespread malignancy.
- Check the FBC, ESR, fasting blood sugar and endomysial antibodies ($\pm$ tTGA).

If you reach the point when all reasonable avenues have been explored without reaching a diagnosis, seek to obtain the patient's agreement to a policy of 'watchful waiting'. Make a single referral to a physician interested in the problem if the patient is unable to accept that approach.

Prevalence

In the general population

In response to a questionnaire, 38% of adults living in southern England reported substantial fatigue and 18% had had it for >6 months.[1] In another study, 9% of British adults under the age of 65 reported unexplained fatigue of >6 months' duration.[2]

In primary care

Around 5% to 10% of patients in primary care present with fatigue as their main complaint[3-5] with another 5% to 10% having it as a subsidiary complaint.[6] Doctors classify far fewer as presenting with fatigue (1.2% in the UK).[7] Women are three to four times more likely to complain of fatigue than are men.[8]

Initial probabilities

What are the initial probabilities when fatigue is recorded by the GP as the presenting complaint, regardless of duration?

In a large Dutch study, 58 family doctors coded the presenting symptoms and final diagnoses in over half a million episodes of care.[9] The most common diagnoses were as follows:

- 'tiredness' as final diagnosis 43%
- viral disease 6%
- iron deficiency anaemia 3%
- depressive disorder 2%
- mental disorder (NOS) 1%
- infectious mononucleosis 0.7%
- anaemia (NOS) 0.3%
- infectious disease (NOS) 0.3%.

NOS = not otherwise stated, i.e. for which there was no more precise diagnosis.

It seems that, in primary care, a specific diagnosis in a patient with short-term tiredness is uncommon.

Note: The doctors' work-up in this study was less rigorous than in those studies (below) that were specifically aimed at elucidating the cause of the patients' fatigue.

What are the pre-test probabilities when it is the main complaint and present for at least 2 weeks?

- *Depression.* Studies vary from 17%[4] to 40%[10] with a summary of five studies giving 25%.[11]
- *Other psychiatric diagnoses* (mainly anxiety and dysthymia) 25%.[11]
- *Boredom, overwork, other types of unhappiness* short of psychiatric illness.[12]
- *Alcohol misuse.* Screening of unselected patients aged 18–64 will find that 16% drink excessively and that 2.6% have evidence of dependency.[13] The probability that alcohol is the cause of a complaint of fatigue is unknown (see *Alcohol misuse*, p. 312).
- *Insomnia.* The complaint is common but the degree to which it is the cause of fatigue is unknown (see *Insomnia*, p. 160).
- *Obstructive sleep apnoea* 2.4% (1 out of 42 patients).[10]
- *Chronic fatigue syndrome (CFS)* 0.2% to 2.6%.[14] It is impossible to make a final diagnosis at this stage since, by definition, it must have been present for 6 months (see below). However, the SOFA screening test can be used after 4 weeks to screen for prolonged fatigue syndromes (see p. 113) and at 6 weeks a working definition of CFS is possible.[15]
- *Fibromyalgia* 2.4%.[10]

- *Other physical disorders* 15%[11] to 17%[10]:
  - (a) *Anaemia* 4% (8 out of 210 patients in England and Wales).[16]
  - (b) *Hypothyroidism* 1.5% (3 out of 210).[16] However, this is not significantly more than the baseline rate of overt hypothyroidism in the UK (1.4% for women; <0.1% for men).[17] The overall rate of biochemical thyroid disorder in older women is higher (5% in a Swedish study).[18] The highest rate will be found in women >50 years old, in whom another study showed that 1 in 71 unselected women have undiagnosed symptomatic hypothyroidism.[19]
  - (c) *All types of infection* (e.g. cytomegalovirus, hepatitis, mononucleosis) 3%[16] to 15%.[11] However, a UK cohort study of 1199 people with infections has shown that, overall, past infection is not associated with chronic fatigue.[20] This does not, however, mean that specific fatigue syndromes that can follow uncommon infections, such as infectious mononucleosis, encephalitis, meningitis and Lyme disease do not exist, just that they are rare.[21]
  - (d) *Diabetes* 0.5% (1 out of 210).[16] This frequency might be expected by chance since 1–2% of the population have unsuspected diabetes.[22]
  - (e) *Gluten intolerance.* One in 300 of the UK population has gluten intolerance, 2 out of 3 of them undetected. In a group of 29 adults with unsuspected coeliac disease, the main complaint in 6 was fatigue. Most did not complain of gastrointestinal symptoms.[23]
  - (f) *Carcinomatosis* 0.5% (1 out of 210).[16]
  - (g) *Autoimmune disease.*
  - (h) *Low cardiac output.*
  - (i) *Chronic neurological disorders*, e.g. multiple sclerosis, motor neurone disease.
  - (j) *Chronic lung disease.*
- *Drugs*, e.g. beta-blockers, hypnotics, anxiolytics, diuretics, antihistamines, anti-epileptics, anticonvulsants, antipsychotics, antidepressants or opioids. A drug that is being taken is, however, not necessarily the cause. A meta-analysis found that beta-blockers only caused fatigue in 1 in 57 patients treated for a year.[24]
- *Low systolic blood pressure.* It is associated with fatigue but the association is not independent of psychological dysfunction. Low blood pressure is therefore not a cause in its own right[25] (see box on p. 112).
- *No cause found* in 20%[11] to 28%.[26]

How do the pre-test probabilities change when it is the main complaint and present for at least 6 months?

■ *Current psychiatric disorder* is more likely: 60%[27] to 67%.[28] Referrals from primary care gave the frequencies below.[29] However, the figures must be interpreted with caution. Only 2% of patients with fatigue are referred, so referrals to a secondary care clinic give little insight into the situation in primary care.[16]

    (a)   Depression 47%

    (b)   Somatisation disorder 15%

    (c)   Anxiety 9%, but beware; it may be coincidental – all anxiety disorders combined have a lifetime prevalence of 25%.[30]

■ *Chronic fatigue syndrome* 4%[28] to 11%[31] to 31%.[32] The lower figures apply to uninvestigated patients. The highest figure applies to patients in whom the diagnosis is reached by excluding other diagnoses. By definition, CFS is present if the patient has severe disabling fatigue affecting both mental and physical functioning which has not always been present but which has been present for at least 6 months.[33] There should be no known physical cause; and psychosis, bipolar affective disorder, eating disorder and organic brain disease must have been excluded. Stricter definitions are now preferred (see p. 351).[15]

■ *Non-specific chronic fatigue:* 69% of patients in whom other diagnoses, other than CFS, have been excluded.[32]

Note: The diagnosis of depression or anxiety does not exclude the diagnosis of CFS, nor vice versa. Patients with CFS are twice as likely to be depressed as those with non-specific fatigue.[32]

Rarities

■ *Myasthenia gravis.* The patient has fluctuating muscular weakness and muscles are easily fatigued. The patient may not have noticed ptosis but it may be obvious if the patient is asked to look up for 1 minute. Refer if this test is positive.

■ *Addison's disease.* Pigmentation of skin and buccal mucosa are late signs, as is hypotension. Suspect it in someone with anorexia, weight loss, fatigue and weakness, especially if there is a history, or family history, of thyroid disease, type 1 diabetes or premature ovarian failure. The short synacthen test is needed (a 9.00 am cortisol is often normal in early Addison's disease). In the test, the plasma cortisol is measured before, and at 30 and 60 minutes after, 250 μg synacthen intramuscular (IM).

■ *Chronic infections: Lyme disease, brucellosis.* Look for evidence of multisystem involvement, especially migratory polyarthritis.

Hypotension

Hypotension (systolic <110 in men or <100 mmHg in women) has been considered to be a cause of chronic fatigue in German-speaking countries for decades but not in English-speaking countries.[34] Cross-sectional studies have shown an association between constitutional hypotension and chronic fatigue and one prospective study has found an association between constitutional hypotension and the subsequent development of 'easy fatigability', with a relative risk (RR) for women of 5.0 (95% CI 1.4 to 17.4) and an RR for men of 1.7 (95% CI 0.8 to 3.5).[35] Whether the hypotension causes the tiredness is still unproven.

The history

1. *Depression.* Look for depression by asking two questions:[36]

    ■ 'In the last month have you often been bothered by feeling down, depressed or hopeless?'

    ■ 'In the last month have you often been bothered by little interest or pleasure in doing things?'

    If the patient answers yes to either of these, the test is positive. A positive response has a sensitivity of 96% (95% CI 90% to 99%) and a specificity of 57% (95% CI 53% to 62%); LR+ = 2.2; LR− = 0.08. The positive predictive value was 33% and the negative predictive value 98% in a primary care adult population in the USA where the prevalence of major depression was 18%.[36] This means that, in a similar population, the test is very good at ruling out depression if negative (a negative test reduced the probability of depression to 2%); but if the test is positive the patient still has probably not got a major depressive illness. If positive, check in more detail (see *Depressive illness*, p. 373).

2. *Anxiety.* Look for anxiety by asking 'Do you find yourself worrying a lot or on edge?' If the answer is yes, check in more detail (see *Anxiety disorders*, p. 328).

3. *Dissatisfaction.* Look for dissatisfaction with life, short of psychiatric disorder. Ask 'Do you usually get out of bed in the morning looking forward to the day ahead?'

4. *Ask about sleep.* There are three parts to this:

  (a) *Check that the patient is getting enough good quality sleep.* Insomnia may reflect an underlying psychiatric disorder, the result of shift work, or be due to a lifestyle that is too demanding for that individual. Daytime fatigue may result.

  (b) *Check that the patient is not getting an excessive amount of sleep.* Hypersomnia may be due to depression, drugs, hypothyroidism or physical illness, and further questions will be needed.

  (c) *Check whether the problem is daytime sleepiness rather than fatigue.* If so, see *Sleepiness*, page 243. However, be aware that most of the causes of fatigue in this list can also present with daytime sleepiness.

5. *Ask about snoring*, though 20% of adults snore – more if they are male, obese or elderly.[37] While sensitive for sleep apnoea, it is therefore not specific. Ask about episodes of apnoea while asleep and a tendency to fall asleep unintentionally.[38] If any of these is present, see *Sleep apnoea* (p. 439).

6. *Ask about alcohol use.* Ask 'How often do you have an alcoholic drink?' If the answer is on 4 or more days a week, ask the full Audit-C questionnaire (see *Alcohol misuse*, p. 313).

7. *Prolonged fatigue syndromes* (i.e. chronic fatigue syndrome and idiopathic chronic fatigue). Screen for these with the SOFA Scale (see below). If positive, see *Chronic fatigue syndrome* (p. 350).

8. *Infectious mononucleosis.* Ask about sore throat, fever and swollen glands at the start of the illness; 40% of patients with infectious mononucleosis admit to fatigue 6 months later.[39]

9. *Concomitant illness.* Ask about other illnesses already diagnosed.

10. *Drugs.* Ask about drugs, whether prescribed, over the counter or illicit.

SOFA (Schedule of Fatigue and Anergia)[40] (with kind permission of Springer Science and Business Media)

Ask the patient to comment on the following statements in relation to how they have been over the last few weeks:

1. I feel tired for a long time after physical activity.
2. My concentration is poor.
3. My muscles feel very tired after physical activity.
4. I get headaches.
5. I need to sleep for long periods.
6. I get muscle pain after physical activity.
7. I sleep poorly.
8. I have problems with my speech (e.g. feeling 'lost for the word').
9. My memory is poor.
10. I get muscle pain even at rest.

  * Score 1 for each question if the patient says the statement is true 'a good part of the time' or 'most of the time'. Score 0 if the statement is only true 'some of the time' or less. The screen is positive for prolonged fatigue syndrome if the patient scores 3 or more.

Tested in 1513 Australian GP attenders, this gave a sensitivity of 81% and a specificity of 100% for the diagnosis of prolonged fatigue syndrome. This gives an LR+ that is infinitely high (lower limit of 95% CI 163) and an LR– of 0.2 (0.1 to 0.3).

  * If positive, use the same test to test for the more specific diagnosis of chronic fatigue syndrome. Score 1 if the patient has had symptoms which have been at least moderate or frequent for the last month and which cause major disruption to their usual daily activities. Score 0 if the symptom is less severe than that. The test is positive for chronic fatigue syndrome if the patient scores 2 or more. Tested in 368 Australians with a clinical diagnosis of CFS and 430 controls, this gave a sensitivity of 93% and a specificity of 95%; LR+ 19 (95% CI 13 to 26); LR– 0.07 (0.02 to 0.3).

The examination

A routine physical examination is unlikely to be helpful if the history has not provided any clues. The yield in one study of fatigue was 2%.[11,41] If the decision is made to examine the patient, look for:

1. *Pallor.*[42] Pallor at one site, e.g. conjunctiva (LR+ 2.2), raises the probability of anaemia from the baseline of 4% to only 10%. If pallor at multiple sites is present (LR+ 4.5), the probability rises to 15%. Overall, examination can detect about half of anaemic patients, but the absence of pallor cannot be used to rule out anaemia;[43] no LR– is

below 0.5. If anaemia is suspected, see *Anaemia*, page 318.

2. *Hypotension* (systolic <110 in men or <100 in women) (see box on p. 112).

3. *Signs of hypothyroidism.*[42] Take the patient's hand, feel the pulse and listen to the voice. The finding of coarse skin (LR+ 5.6) increases the probability of hypothyroidism from a baseline of 1.5% to 8%. If the patient also has hypothyroid speech (LR+ 5.4), it increases to 32%. Further LR+s are: bradycardia below 70/min, 4.1; wrist puffiness, 2.9; periorbital puffiness, 2.8; goitre, 2.8. The absence of any signs virtually rules the diagnosis out (LR– 0.01). If hypothyroidism is suspected, see *Hypothyroidism*, page 416.

4. *Signs of hyperthyroidism.*[42] The finding of lid retraction (LR+ 31.5) means that the probability that this is hyperthyroidism rises from a baseline of 1.5% to 34%. Lid lag is also useful (LR+ 17.6), but if lag and retraction are both positive, the LR of only one of them can be used, because the two signs share the same pathophysiology. Other useful signs are fine tremor (LR+ 11.4), moist warm skin (LR+ 6.7), and tachycardia 90 or above (LR+ 4.4). The absence of any signs virtually rules the diagnosis out (LR– 0.01). If hyperthyroidism is suspected see *Hyperthyroidism*, page 412.

5. *The lymphadenopathy and hepatosplenomegaly* of chronic infection or of widespread malignancy.

Investigations

The yield is unlikely to be high: 5%,[11] 8%,[26] or 9%.[16] A study from New York State found that a battery of tests revealed no useful clues as to the cause of the fatigue in 22 patients who had had fatigue for at least a year.[44]

Check:

■ *The full blood count (FBC)* for:

(a) anaemia: it may be the cause of the fatigue or a marker for chronic disease; 2–5% of the UK population are anaemic, with a higher prevalence in premenopausal women and a much higher prevalence in older people[45] (see *Anaemia*, p. 318).

(b) macrocytosis of alcohol misuse or hypothyroidism.

■ *The erythrocyte sedimentation rate (ESR)* for chronic disease.

■ *For* diabetes, check either the *random* or the *fasting sugar*. If either is >6 mmol/L, more tests are needed; see *Diabetes* (p. 379).

■ *The thyroid stimulating hormone (TSH)* for thyroid disease, unless a thorough history and examination have ruled out thyroid disease (see above). The sensitivity and specificity of the TSH are both >99% for hyperthyroidism and 99% for hypothyroidism.[46] This means that in a patient complaining of fatigue who has no other signs or symptoms of hypothyroidism, a raised TSH raises the probability that the fatigue is due to hypothyroidism from 1.5% to 60% while a normal TSH reduces it to 0.02%. Note that an abnormal TSH will be found in a further 32%, because of the high baseline rate of asymptomatic thyroid disease. It may reflect an abnormality of thyroid function but does not explain the fatigue in those patients. If abnormal,[47] see *Hypothyroidism* (p. 416) or *Hyperthyroidism* (p. 412).

■ *Endomysial antibodies (EMA)* for coeliac disease. Estimates of sensitivity range from 64%[48] to 95%[49] and of specificity from 64%[49] to 100%.[50] One reason for a false negative test is that it measures IgA and will be falsely negative in the 2% of the UK population who are IgA deficient. An alternative test, the tissue transglutaminase antibody (tTGA) test, can be performed on IgA and IgG. Although overall it is no more sensitive or specific than the EMA, the combination of tTGA and EMA can reduce the number of false negatives. However, the range of different sensitivities in different studies makes it impossible to estimate likelihood ratios. If positive, see *Coeliac disease* (p. 361)

In addition, the UK Royal Colleges recommend that the following be checked in any patient with a history >6 months:[51]

■ liver function tests
■ urea and electrolytes
■ creatine kinase.

Additional points

● Most patients with fatigue do not present. Those who present are more likely to have poor social support, and be vulnerable to social or work stress.

● A patient may have both a physical and a psychiatric reason for fatigue. Psychiatric complications are especially common in chronic physical illness.

tubal damage, endometriosis and polycystic ovary syndrome.

Factors that will alter these probabilities

■ *Age*. A woman aged 35–39 has a chance of conceiving that is half that of a woman aged 19–26.[6] This decline with age means that a woman aged 35 has a 94% chance of conceiving during 3 years of trying and a woman aged 38 a 77% chance.[2] Male fertility also declines with age but less dramatically and is only detectable when the woman is also older. A woman aged 35 with a partner aged 40 seems to have a chance of conception on the day of peak fertility that is about two-thirds that of a woman of 35 with a partner who is also 35.[6]

■ *Whether either partner has had a previous pregnancy*. A previous conception almost doubles the chance that a couple will conceive spontaneously.[1]

■ *The timing of intercourse*. The woman's most fertile time is from 6 days before ovulation until ovulation itself. Couples who wait for evidence of ovulation before having intercourse are missing the window of opportunity.[6] The peak of fertility is 2 days before ovulation.

■ *The frequency and success of intercourse*. Couples who are anxious about conceiving may find that their ability to achieve successful intercourse is affected.

■ *Over- or underweight*. A body mass index (BMI) <20, if associated with irregular menstruation or amenorrhoea, decreases a woman's fertility. A BMI >30 in a man or woman is associated with subfertility.[2]

■ *Lifestyle*. Smoking by either partner, and excess alcohol or caffeine intake by the woman, are associated with subfertility. Studies have difficulty eliminating possible confounders but the evidence is strongest for smoking, which shows that female smokers are 3.4 times more likely to take over a year to conceive than non-smokers.[1] Anabolic steroids, cannabis and cocaine have all been shown to interfere with male fertility.

■ *Medication*. Sulfasalazine, tetracyclines and allopurinol are all associated with reduced male fertility.

■ *Occupation*. Exposure to metal fumes (as in welding), solvents and pesticides can lower male fertility.[7]

■ *Menstrual history*. Oligo- or amenorrhoea increases the probability of fertility problems.

■ *Past medical history*. A history of pelvic inflammatory disease, past chemotherapy for malignancy, or an undescended testicle will increase the probability of fertility problems.

Assessment in primary care

∗ Start investigations as soon as the couple voice anxiety about conceiving.

∗ Aim to consider referral after 1 year, or sooner if there is good reason to predict difficulties, e.g. oligo- or amenorrhoea, abnormal sperm count or woman's age over 35.

∗ Refer the couple directly to a specialist centre holding the contract for the treatment of subfertility, not to a general gynaecology clinic.

Assessment of the woman

∗ Take a history, including details of menstrual cycle, previous pregnancies, pelvic infections or operations. Regular periods are a reliable guide to the fact that the woman is ovulating. Check that they are having intercourse at the woman's most fertile time (as well as throughout the cycle). Do not recommend temperature charts or luteinising hormone (LH) detection kits. They have not been shown to increase the chance of conception.[8]

∗ Examine for evidence of pelvic pathology.

∗ Assess whether the woman is ovulating:

(a) *Progesterone level*. Take blood 7 days before menstruation is due. A level of >16 nmol/L suggests ovulation, and a level of >30 nmol/L confirms it. Borderline levels may be due to a deficient luteal phase, or to mistimed sampling. Levels <16 nmol/L confirm that the cycle was anovulatory.

(b) *Measure follicle stimulating hormone (FSH) and LH* in a woman with irregular cycles in whom it is impossible to predict when to check the blood progesterone. Take blood between day 2 and 6 of the cycle. High levels (FSH >10 IU/L or LH >10 IU/L) suggest an ovarian problem.

Note: There is no value in measuring thyroid function tests (TFTs) or prolactin in women with regular menses in the absence of galactorrhoea or symptoms of thyroid disease.

Assessment of the man

∗ Take a history covering the points listed above.

∗ Examine the genitalia, noting the secondary sex characteristics while doing so.

∗ Arrange for semen analysis. Attention to detail is important.

1. Semen should be produced by masturbation 3 days after the last ejaculation, and examined within an hour. A condom should not be used. Keep the sample warm on the way to the laboratory.

2. If the count is low, repeat after 3 months and refer to a specialist fertility clinic if still low. Explain to the patient who has had a recent illness that that may have temporarily depressed the count and that 3 months is needed for it to recover. However, if the count is severely low, refer after a single count.

3. Warn the patient that even a 'normal' sperm count does not mean that there is not some sperm dysfunction which can only be detected by more sophisticated tests.

Normal values for semen (WHO)

(a) volume: ≥2 ml

(b) pH 7.2 or higher

(c) concentration: ≥20 million per ml

(d) total sperm number ≥40 million per ejaculate

(e) motility: ≥50% with ≥25% showing progressive motility

(f) vitality: ≥75% live

(g) morphology (strict criteria): >15% normal forms

(h) white blood cells: <1 million per ml

Refer, armed with the above results, if the tests are abnormal or if the history shows a likely cause, or if the couple have been trying for a year, or if the woman is over age 35.

Two investigations are needed in the assessment of the patient who is trying to conceive, not in order to discover a cause for the subfertility but in order to assist a healthy pregnancy should conception occur:

• rubella status

• cervical smear, unless up to date.

Example

A very serious-minded couple in their late 30s consult their GP because the woman has failed to become pregnant after trying to do so since they married 9 months before. There have been no previous pregnancies for either partner; indeed this is the woman's first sexual relationship. Her periods have been irregular since the marriage, usually coming 1 or 2 weeks late. They are only having intercourse from 2 weeks after the start of each period, so as not to 'waste his sperm', as she puts it.

The GP detects no other clues from their histories. She examines them both and finds the women very tense, almost amounting to vaginismus. The man, too, is shy and she wonders about the success of intercourse.

She organises blood tests for the woman (FSH and LH on day 4 of the cycle) and a semen analysis (giving him written instructions).

She decides that at this stage the urgent thing is to try to defuse their anxiety. She points out that a 9-month delay is something they share with about 20% of all couples; that their ages only reduce their fertility to half what it would have been 15 years earlier, and that she notices how tense they are about the whole business. She asks gently if that anxiety is getting in the way of their having sex in an easy, spontaneous manner. They exchange glances but cannot bring themselves to answer. The GP doesn't press the point but makes a note to invite them to talk about the issue when they return for their test results.

REFERENCES

1. Taylor A. *ABC of subfertility: extent of the problem.* BMJ 2003;327:434–436.

2. NICE. *Fertility: assessment and treatment for people with fertility problems.* London: National Institute for Clinical Excellence, Clinical Guideline 11, 2004. Online. Available: www.nice.org.uk.

3. Martin T. *Infertility in a large Royal Air Force general practice.* J R Army Med Corps 1989;135:68–75.

4. Weiss T, Meffin E, Jones R, et al. *Trends in causes and treatment of infertility at Flinders Medical Centre, Adelaide, 1976–1989.* Med J Aust 1992;156:308–311.

5. Wiswedel K, Allen D. *Infertility factors at the Groote Schuur Hospital Fertility Clinic.* S Afr Med J 1989; 76:65–66.

6. Dunson D, Colombo B, Baird D. *Changes with age in the level and duration of fertility in the menstrual cycle.* Hum Reprod 2002;17: 1399–1403.

7. Figa-Talamanca I, Traina M, Urbani E. *Occupational exposures to metals, solvents and pesticides: recent evidence on male reproductive effects and biological markers.* Occup Med 2001;51:174–188.

8. RCOG Guideline Development Group. *The initial investigation and management of the infertile couple.* London: Royal College of Obstetricians and Gynaecologists, 1998. Online. Available: www.rcog. org.uk.

20

Haematuria

- The management of macroscopic haematuria is dominated by the search for urological cancer, which is the cause in over 20% of men aged >60 with the condition.

- Microscopic haematuria, in contrast, carries a risk of malignancy <1% and management involves considering a host of possible conditions.

A PRACTICAL APPROACH

Macroscopic haematuria
* Refer all to a urologist urgently unless there is a proven symptomatic urinary tract infection (UTI) at the time and the haematuria resolves completely with one course of treatment.
* Refer urgently to a urologist patients aged 40 and over if they have persistent or recurrent UTIs associated with haematuria.
* Refer to a nephrologist those with negative urological investigations.
* Consider referring young patients with a glomerular filtration rate (GFR) <60 to a nephrologist in the first instance.

Microscopic haematuria
* Check the midstream urine (MSU), urinary protein and serum creatinine and calculate the GFR.

* If there is evidence of glomerular disease (GFR <60, urinary albumin:creatinine ratio >30 mg/mmol, or protein:creatinine ratio >45 mg/mmol), refer to a renal physician.
* If the urinary protein and GFR are normal, refer the patient who is aged <50 to the urologist, but not urgently. This is a NICE recommendation even though the evidence for it is not strong.
* Refer patients aged 50 or over with normal renal function to a urologist urgently.
* If investigations in secondary care are normal, monitor the patient with repeat tests of urine and serum creatinine, with assessment of GFR, after 6 months then annually,
* If the haematuria was associated with unilateral abdominal or loin pain, consider the possibility of a urinary calculus.

Definitions

- *Macroscopic haematuria* is visible blood in the urine originating from the urinary tract.
- *False haematuria* is blood in the urine which originates from outside the urinary tract (most commonly from the menses).
- *Pseudo-haematuria* is a reddening of the urine due to something other than blood. These may be foods (beetroot, berries), drugs (rifampicin, nitrofurantoin, chloroquine, hydroxychloroquine, furazolidone, phenazopyridine or phenolphthalein) or breakdown products (myoglobinuria in conditions involving muscle breakdown, haemoglobinuria in in-vivo haemolysis).
- *Microscopic haematuria* is an abnormal number of red blood cells in the urine invisible to the naked eye. Normal urine contains occasional red cells. The

arbitrary definitions of microscopic haematuria are >12 500 red cells per ml of urine or >3 red cells per high power field of urinary sediment.[1] Urine dipsticks become positive at a level of 15 000 to 20 000 red cells per ml.[2]

Prevalence

In the general population

Macroscopic haematuria: 1%.[2]

Microscopic haematuria: between 0.19% and 16.1% in different population studies.[3] The differences probably reflect populations of different ages, different methods of testing, different diagnostic thresholds and different numbers of tests per patient. The study which found the highest prevalence used a threshold of 1 red cell per high power field.[4] The prevalence varies markedly with age, from 1.2% in men aged 18 to 33,[5,6] to about 20% in men aged 60 and over,[7] or over 50.[8]

In primary care

Macroscopic haematuria. A Belgian study found a prevalence in primary care of 0.49% per year.[9]

Microscopic haematuria is by definition an opportunistic finding:

(a) during opportunistic dipstick testing of urine in those who are asymptomatic (e.g. for insurance medicals, or in pregnancy)

(b) when the urine is being tested due to the presence of certain symptoms, e.g. a suspected UTI, or ankle or facial swelling

(c) as part of the investigation of other findings, e.g. a raised creatinine, a reduced GFR or a raised blood pressure (assessing for target organ damage).

In general medical patients, estimates of prevalence vary from 5% to 13%.[10] In primary care, the prevalence will depend on the screening activity of the practice. Routine screening for microscopic haematuria is not recommended by UK guidelines.

Initial probabilities

Macroscopic haematuria

■ *Urological cancer*: 10.3%. This figure is divided into bladder cancer 8.3% (95% CI 5.9% to 11.5%) and other cancers (mainly renal and prostatic) 2.0% (95% CI 0.9% to 4.0%).These probabilities are highly dependent on the age and sex of the patient (Table 20.1).

■ *Non-malignant conditions.* No figures exist for their probabilities in patients with macroscopic haematuria in primary care. In a UK study of referrals for macroscopic or microscopic haematuria to an open access haematuria clinic,[11] the following percentages were found:

(a) benign prostatic hypertrophy (BPH): 12%

(b) urological cancer: 10%

(c) calculi: 4%

(d) strictures or stenosis: 3%

(e) no cause found: 72%.

The absence of patients with UTIs shows that this was a selected group, some of whom had been managed in primary care without referral.

Microscopic haematuria

No figures exist for the probabilities of the different conditions that are possible in the patient found to have microscopic haematuria in primary care. A recent overview cast doubt on the value of testing for microscopic haematuria because of its poor sensitivity and specificity in urological cancer as well as in benign urological

Table 20.1 Probability of urological cancer in a patient presenting in primary care with macroscopic haematuria according to age and sex[9]

Men	Probability of urological cancer (95% CI)	Women	Probability of urological cancer (95% CI)
Age <40	0% (0–12.0%)	Age <40	0% (CI not given)
Age 40–59	3.6% (0.6–13.4%)	Age 40–59	6.4% (1.7–18.6%)
Age >59	22.1% (15.8–30.1%)	Age >59	8.3% (3.4–17.9%)

Follow each row from left to right to see how age and sex alter the probability of urological cancer.

conditions.[12] A US review supports this idea, pointing out that the positive predictive value of microscopic haematuria for cancer in screening studies is often no higher than the prevalence in the general population.[3]

Patients who come to cystoscopy give the following figures:[4,13–15]

(a) urological and prostatic malignancy 0.5%

(b) BPH 8–24%

(c) urethral lesions 13–25%

(d) non-malignant bladder lesions 3–5%

(e) bladder calculi 1–2%.

(f) UTI 2–4%.

However, again, these are a selected group. Some, especially those who are asymptomatic or who have a UTI, will have been treated in primary care and not referred.

Other conditions which may give rise to microscopic haematuria are:

■ *glomerulonephritis* and other causes of glomerular disease

■ *interstitial nephritis* (due to various drugs including penicillins, cefalosporins, ciprofloxacin, NSAIDs, furosemide)

■ *acute haemorrhagic cystitis* due to cyclophosphamide (and certain other drugs)

■ *trauma* to the kidneys (such as by a blunt blow) or perineum (such as by falling astride a motorbike, or onto a fence from a height)

■ *renal cysts*/polycystic kidney disease

■ *appendicitis or diverticulitis*, which may cause haematuria by contact inflammation

■ *anticoagulant therapy*: in the past, haematuria in a patient on an anticoagulant has been ascribed to the medication. However, it appears that the anticoagulant may rather cause a significant urological tumour to present earlier; figures from 13% to 45% have been found for significant urological causes underlying bleeding in such patients[16]

■ *NSAIDs*

■ *exercise-induced haematuria*: up to 20% of long-distance runners may develop a temporary microscopic haematuria afterwards for up to a few days

■ *renal infarction* (may be due to an embolism, e.g. after myocardial infarction, or occur in sickle-cell disease) or renal vein thrombosis (in severe dehydration, related to the combined oral contraceptive pill, nephrotic syndrome, pregnancy or trauma)

■ *tuberculosis*

■ *schistosomiasis* (directly or indirectly, it is a risk factor for urological malignancy)

■ *angiomyolipoma*

■ *medullary sponge kidney*

■ *arteriovenous malformations* (look for an abdominal bruit)

■ *papillary necrosis* (in sickle-cell disease, diabetes, and in aspirin and NSAID use, especially in analgesic abusers)

■ *infective endocarditis*. Urine was tested for blood in 106 patients in Denmark with suspected infective endocarditis. The LR+ for the diagnosis of infective endocarditis was 4.5 and the LR− 0.35. In this study, a positive test raised the probability from 59% to 86%, and a negative test lowered it to 33%.[17] A positive test therefore adds a further piece of the jigsaw that may prompt admission, but neither rules it in nor excludes it effectively

■ *sickle-cell disease*.

Details of the clinical examination are discussed under the different possible diagnoses (below).

What investigations are useful in primary care?

* *Confirm that macroscopic haematuria is present with a dipstick.* It has a sensitivity of 86% and a specificity of 85% when compared to microscopy as the gold standard.[18] If negative, but the patient reports blood in the urine, repeat the test at least three times; bleeding may be intermittent. However, if the patient's history of haematuria is clear, believe it despite subsequent negative tests.

* *Send a midstream urine for microscopy and culture.* This is to look for infection, not to confirm the dipstick result. If the dipstick is positive for blood but the MSU is negative, trust the dipstick. Red cells may have lysed in the urine while being transported to the laboratory.

Other tests are only necessary in primary care in microscopic haematuria, since all patients with macroscopic haematuria and no UTI should be referred to a urologist. They are urine protein, urine protein : creatinine ratio (or albumin : creatinine ratio) and serum creatinine, and are discussed under the different possible diagnoses (below).

Causes of a falsely positive urine dipstick test for microscopic haematuria
- Myoglobinuria, e.g. from strenuous exercise. If this is a possibility, repeat after a week, and consider a second repeat after one month, as microscopic haematuria may itself be intermittent.
- Iodine-containing solutions or dressings.
- Hypochlorite contamination.

Causes of a falsely negative urine dipstick test for microscopic haematuria
- Excess vitamin C.
- Rifampicin.
- Phenolphthalein.
- Acidic urine.
- Air-exposed or expired dipsticks.

Who should be referred?

The UK Guidelines of the National Institute for Health and Clinical Excellence (NICE)[19] make the following recommendations:

1. Urgent referral is advised for patients with:
   - painless macroscopic haematuria at any age
   - haematuria and recurrent or persistent urinary infection if aged 40 or above
   - unexplained microscopic haematuria if aged 50 and above
   - an abdominal mass which appears to be arising from the urinary tract.

2. Patients with macroscopic haematuria and symptoms suggestive of urinary infection should be investigated for urinary infection. Urgent referral should follow if investigation does not confirm the suspicion of infection and should be considered if haematuria continues despite effective treatment.

3. Microscopic haematuria in patients aged 50 and under should be investigated with urinary protein, serum creatinine and assessment of GFR. If abnormal, the patient should be referred to a renal physician; if normal, to a urologist.

Note: The NICE Guideline also gives recommendations for the referral of patients with manifestations of urological cancer other than haematuria which are not relevant here.

The Guidelines of the Renal Association, available on www.renal.org (choose UK CKD guide), support most of these recommendations but suggest that a presentation, at any age, of microscopic haematuria and a urine protein:creatinine ratio >45 mg/mmol should prompt referral directly to a nephrologist. They also stress the need to refer to a nephrologist a patient who has macroscopic haematuria and negative urological investigations.

Is this urological malignancy?

What factors in the history influence the diagnosis?

Age and sex. Urological malignancy is more common in men than in women and in older rather than in younger patients. In a Belgian primary care study which yielded 126 patients with urological cancer, not one was aged under 40 and only 12 were in patients under 60.[9]

The presence of other symptoms. The evidence is contradictory. The Belgian study (above) found that other symptoms did not significantly alter the initial probabilities. Contrary to expectations, complaints of dysuria and frequency did not significantly reduce the probability of cancer.[9] However, a UK study, in which patients were entered into the study if they were referred to a haematuria clinic, found that a number of clinical features altered the probability of cancer. Macroscopic haematuria was a far greater indicator of cancer (positive predictive value (PPV) 25%) than microscopic haematuria (PPV 2%).[11] After adjusting by logistic regression, the features that independently predicted the presence of cancer (apart from age and sex) were:
- macroscopic rather than microscopic haematuria
- a history of no more than one UTI, and
- hesitancy.

What examination should be performed?

* Examine the abdomen and loins. Tenderness shifts the probability towards renal colic as the cause of haematuria.[20]
* Examine the prostate digitally. Two out of 36 urological cancers presenting with haematuria in the Hull study were prostatic.[11]

Is this renal/glomerular disease?

Definitions

Chronic kidney disease (CKD) is classified as follows:[21]

Stage 1: Normal GFR; GFR >90 ml/min/1.73 m^2 but with other evidence of chronic kidney damage

Stage 2: Mild impairment; GFR 60–89 ml/min/1.73 m^2 with other evidence of chronic kidney damage (see below)

Stage 3: Moderate impairment; GFR 30–59 ml/min/1.73 m^2

Stage 4: Severe impairment; GFR 15–29 ml/min/ 1.73 m^2

Stage 5: Established renal failure (ERF); GFR <15 ml/ min/1.73 m^2 or on dialysis

'Other evidence of chronic kidney damage' may be one of the following:

■ persistent microalbuminuria

■ persistent proteinuria

■ persistent haematuria (after exclusion of other causes, e.g. urological disease)

■ structural abnormalities of the kidneys demonstrated on ultrasound scanning or other radiological tests, e.g. polycystic kidney disease, reflux nephropathy

■ biopsy-proven chronic glomerulonephritis (most of these patients will have microalbuminuria or proteinuria, and/or haematuria).

Patients found to have a GFR of 60–89 ml/ min/1.73 m^2 without one of these markers should not be considered to have CKD and should not be subjected to further investigation unless there are additional reasons to do so.

Proteinuria

One '+' or greater on a dipstick is significant. If random, repeat it on an early morning sample to avoid orthostatic proteinuria.

If positive, send urine for protein:creatinine ratio or albumin:creatinine ratio, according to local practice.

The following are considered to constitute significant proteinuria:

■ protein:creatinine ratio >45 mg/mmol

■ albumin:creatinine ratio >30 mg/mmol.

Microalbuminuria

One '+' or greater on a dipstick is significant. If random, repeat it on an early morning sample to avoid orthostatic proteinuria.

If positive, send urine for albumin:creatinine ratio. A ratio ≥2.5 mg/mmol (male) or ≥3.5 mg/ mmol (female) is significant. Two repeat samples over the subsequent 1 to 3 months are needed. At least two positives are needed to confirm the diagnosis.

How is the GFR calculated?

● The serum creatinine alone is an insensitive measurement of renal function, which only becomes abnormal after considerable renal function has been lost. A study in primary care showed that calculating the GFR increased the detection of patients with CKD from 22% to 85%.[22]

● Laboratories nationally should be starting to report GFR results based on age, sex, creatinine and race. An on-line calculator version of the 4-variable

equation can be found at: http://www.renal.org/ eGFR/eguide.html.

Steps to be taken if a GFR <60 is discovered for the first time.

* Assume it is due to acute renal failure until proved otherwise (although most cases will turn out to be due to chronic renal disease). Admit if the clinical condition is sufficiently severe. Otherwise repeat the serum creatinine within 5 days. Suspect acute renal failure if there has been a >1.5-fold rise; or a fall in GFR of >25%; or oliguria (urine output <0.5 ml/kg/hour), in the context of an acute illness.

* Review medication for drugs that can impair renal function: e.g. diuretics, NSAIDs.

* Examine for bladder distension.

* Check for haematuria and proteinuria; if found, they increase the probability of glomerulonephritis, which may be rapidly progressive.

* Look for a clinical condition which may be causing renal failure, e.g. sepsis, heart failure, hypovolaemia.

A decision about the cause of renal impairment is beyond the province of the GP, whose role is to ascertain that impairment is present and decide whether to refer to a urologist or renal physician and how urgently. The NICE guidelines (above) set out the criteria for referral. However, the GP may note the features of glomerulonephritis (below) which would assist the decision to refer to a renal physician urgently.

Glomerulonephritis

Glomerulonephritis is more likely to be the cause of haematuria when associated with any of the following:[2]

■ *proteinuria*, usually less than 3 g in 24 hours

■ a *raised serum creatinine* or *reduced GFR*, especially where there is a trend in the change away from normal, and particularly where the change is occurring relatively quickly

■ *red blood cell dysmorphism, red blood cell casts* and/ or *acanthocytes* in an MSU result (sensitivity 88% and specificity 95% for glomerular disease)[23]

■ *systemic malaise, arthralgia, weight loss* and evidence of *an acute phase response (C-reactive protein/ erythrocyte sedimentation rate/plasma viscosity raised)*

■ patients with *new, worsening or refractory hypertension* (although urinary obstruction from a urological cancer can also cause this)

■ *a positive family clinical history of renal/glomerular disease*

- a recent or ongoing *sore throat, respiratory tract infection* or an episode of *tonsillitis* or *gastroenteritis*.

Is this renal colic?

Prevalence

The point prevalence of urinary calculi is 2–3%[24] with a lifetime prevalence of 10–20% for men and 3–5% for women. The annual incidence of renal colic in the general population is 1 to 2 per 1000.[25]

Clinical features

- Abdominal pain of <12 hours' duration
- Loss of appetite
- Loin or renal tenderness
- Haematuria (macroscopic or microscopic).

In a Finnish study of 1333 patients with abdominal pain, the presence of all four of the above features was 84% sensitive and 99% specific for renal colic, giving an LR+ of 84 and an LR– of 0.16.[20] Microscopic haematuria was the most useful of these, with a sensitivity of 75% and specificity 99% (LR+ 73, LR– 0.3).

However, a later, smaller US study suggests that if the patient has acute flank pain, examining the urine for red cells adds little to the diagnosis. In a study of 267 patients with acute flank pain, the finding of more than 5 red cells per high power field was only 37% sensitive and 76% specific for a calculus, giving likelihood ratios that are almost useless clinically (LR+ 1.54; LR– 0.83).[26] Reducing the threshold for a positive test to more than 1 red cell per high power field improved the sensitivity to 70% but reduced the specificity to 49% and so has little effect on the likelihood ratios (LR+ 1.37; LR– 0.61).

Investigations

Most patients with renal colic will be admitted and investigated in secondary care. However, sometimes the patient presents after the crisis has passed.
- *An abdominal X-ray* to show the urinary tract (kidneys, ureters and bladder; KUB) may be helpful, but its sensitivity and specificity are poor. Studies are bedevilled by the problem of what constitutes the gold standard investigation. The most pessimistic figures come from an overview from the University of Washington,[24] which found that the KUB had a sensitivity of 45% to 59% and a specificity of 71% to 77% (LR+ 2.57; LR– 0.53). The

sensitivity of the KUB is limited by the fact that 15% of stones are not radio-opaque and that smaller radio-opaque stones are not detected. The specificity is limited by the fact that calcification in blood vessels and elsewhere can mimic calculi.
- *Ultrasound scan (USS).* The same study found that USS has a sensitivity of 19% and a specificity of 97%, (LR+ 6.33; LR– 0.84). Ultrasound scan is especially poor at visualising ureteric stones.
- If there is doubt, the definitive investigation is currently the helical computed tomography (CT) scan (sensitivity 95% to 100%; specificity 94% to 96%) or, if CT is unavailable, the intravenous urogram (sensitivity 64% to 87%; specificity 92% to 94%).[24]

These unimpressive figures for KUB and USS mean that, even using the higher estimates, if a patient presents with a clinical picture that gives a 50% probability of renal colic, a positive KUB only increases that likelihood to 72% overall (although, of course, certain X-ray appearances will be diagnostic of a calculus) and a negative KUB only reduces it to 35%. A positive USS is more useful. It would increase the probability of calculus to 86%. However, a negative USS would make no significant impact on the probability.

Thinking through the implications of these figures reveals that there is only a small place for these investigations in primary care. A patient with reasonable suspicion of a calculus would need to be referred for definitive investigations even if the tests are negative. A patient with a positive test would need to be referred for a decision about management. Only in the patient in whom there is real doubt about the need for referral might they be helpful. For instance, if the probability based on the clinical picture is low, at 10%:
(a) a positive KUB will raise that to 22% and a negative KUB will lower it still further to 6%
(b) a positive USS following a positive KUB would then raise the probability to 64% (while a negative USS would leave it unchanged.)
(c) A positive USS following a negative KUB would raise the probability to 29% and so would trigger referral for further investigation.

Using the likelihood ratios above and the nomogram on page xxiv will show how these figures are arrived at.

In conclusion, if the clinical picture suggests renal colic, KUB and USS add little to the assessment in primary care. However, if the GP is undecided about the need for further investigation, a positive result from either will help the decision; a negative result from the KUB will sway the decision against referral but only slightly, while a negative USS will make no difference.

In brief, the GP should ignore negative imaging results but act, cautiously, on positives.

For a discussion of the diagnosis of urinary tract infection see pages 92 (women) and 87 (men).

Example

A 52-year-old company director presents with a letter from her new firm. A pre-employment medical has detected microscopic haematuria. She comes with a fresh sample which is normal for protein and blood.

The GP ascertains that the original sample was not taken during menstruation. The patient says she is far too busy to take any exercise. She has never seen blood in the urine. There is no personal or family history of renal problems and she is well in herself.

The blood pressure is normal and no renal mass is palpable.

The GP tests for microalbuminuria, orders an MSU and serum creatinine. All are normal with a GFR >90 ml/min/1.73 m^2.

The GP is tempted to dismiss the report of microscopic haematuria as an artefact but knows that he should not: blood loss into the urine can be intermittent. He discusses with the patient the slim chance that there is urological pathology and says that current guidelines recommend urological investigation. He has to admit that there is a possibility of cancer even if it is only 1 in 200. The patient requests referral.

Ultrasound scan and cystoscopy are normal and the patient is discharged. However, the dipstick at the urology unit was again positive. The GP and patient agree to a review of blood pressure, urine for protein and blood and serum creatinine in 6 months, then annually if stable.

REFERENCES

1. Grossfeld G, Wolf JJ, Litwan M, et al. *Asymptomatic microscopic hematuria in adults: summary of the AUA best practice policy recommendations.* Am Fam Physician 2001;63:1145–1154.

2. EdREN. *How to manage microscopic haematuria.* The Renal Unit, Royal Infirmary of Edinburgh (EdREN), 2006. Online. Available: http://renux.dmed.ed.ac.uk/EdREN/Unitbits/HaematGuide.html.

3. Grossfeld G, Carroll P. *Evaluation of asymptomatic microscopic haematuria.* Urol Clin North Am 1998;25:661–676.

4. Mohr D, Offord K, Owen R, et al. *Asymptomatic microhematuria and urologic disease: a population-based study.* JAMA 1986;256:224–229.

5. Froom P, Ribak J, Benbassat J. *Significance of microhaematuria in young adults.* BMJ 1984;288:20–22.

6. Froom P, Gross M, Ribak J, et al. *The effect of age on the prevalence of*

asymptomatic microscopic haematuria. Am J Clin Pathol 1986;86:656–657.

7. Britton J, Dowell A, Whelan P, et al. *A community study of bladder cancer screening by the detection of occult urinary bleeding.* J Urol 1992;148:788–790.

8. Messing E, Young T, Hunt V, et al. *Home screening for haematuria: results of a multiclinic study.* J Urol 1992;148:289–292.

9. Bruyninckx R, Buntinx F, Aertgeerts B, et al. *The diagnostic value of macroscopic haematuria for the diagnosis of urological cancer in general practice.* Br J Gen Pract 2003;53:31–35.

10. Connelly J. *Microscopic hematuria.* In: Black ER, Bordley DR, Tape TG, Panzer RJ, eds. Diagnostic strategies for common medical problems. Philadelphia: American College of Physicians, 1999:518–526.

11. Summerton N, Mann S, Rigby A, et al. *Patients with new onset haematuria: assessing the discriminant*

value of clinical information in relation to urological malignancies. Br J Gen Pract 2002;52:284–289.

12. Malmstrom P-U. *Time to abandon testing for microscopic haematuria in adults?* BMJ 2003;326:813–815.

13. Greene L, O'Shaughnessy E, Hendricks E. *Study of five hundred patients with asymptomatic microscopic haematuria.* JAMA 1956;161:610–613.

14. Carson C, Segura J, Greene L. *Clinical importance of microhaematuria.* JAMA 1979;241:149–150.

15. Golin A, Howard R. *Asymptomatic microscopic haematuria.* J Urol 1980;124:389–391.

16. Schuster G, Lewis G. *Clinical significance of haematuria in patients on anticoagulant therapy.* J Urol 1987;137:923–925.

17. Benn M, Hagelskjaer L, Tvede M. *Infective endocarditis, 1984 through 1993: a clinical and microbiological survey.* J Intern Med 1997;242:15–22.

18. Gleeson M, Connolly J, Grainger R, et al. *Comparison of reagent strip (dipstick) and microscopic haematuria in urological out-patients.* Br J Urol 1993; 72:594–596.

19. NICE. *Referral guidelines for suspected cancer.* London: National Institute for Health and Clinical Excellence, 2005. Online. Available: www.nice.org.uk. Reproduced with permission.

20. Eskelinen M. *Usefulness of history-taking, physical examination and diagnostic scoring in acute renal colic.* Eur J Urol 1998;34:467–473.

21. The Renal Association, The Royal College of Physicians, The Royal College of General Practitioners. *Chronic kidney disease in adults: UK guidelines for identification, management and referral, 2006.* Online. Available: http://www.renal.org (search on 'CKD guide').

22. Akbari A, Swedko P, Clark H, et al. *Detection of chronic kidney disease with laboratory reporting of estimated glomerular filtration rate and an educational program.* Arch Intern Med 2004;164:1788–1792.

23. Offringa M, Benbassat J. *The value of urinary red cell shape in the diagnosis of glomerular and post-glomerular haematuria. A meta-analysis.* Postgrad Med J 1992;68: 648–654.

24. Portis A, Sundaram C. *Diagnosis and initial management of kidney stones.* Am Fam Physician 2001;63: 1329–1338.

25. Lloyd J, Jugool S, Mclain D. *Renal colic or just a pain in the side for the surgeon? A comparison study of general practitioner referrals suggestive of renal colic under a cross cover system.* Internet J Urol 2005;2(2).

26. Bove P, Kaplan D, Dalrymple N, et al. *Reexamining the value of haematuria testing in patients with acute flank pain.* J Urol 1999;162: 685–687.

21

Haemoptysis

KEY FACTS

- The commonest causes of haemoptysis are lung cancer, bronchiectasis and chest infections (including pneumonia). The incidence of tuberculosis varies according to the population surveyed.
- Initial evaluation of patients with haemoptysis should include a chest X-ray (CXR).

- The computed tomography (CT) scan and bronchoscopy are complementary investigations. High resolution CT scan is the investigation of choice for demonstrating bronchiectasis; bronchoscopy will reveal endobronchial lesions and is required for biopsies.

A PRACTICAL APPROACH

- ★ Admit those with massive haemoptysis, severe pneumonia or a clinical picture that raises the possibility of pulmonary embolus.
- ★ Refer those whose CXR raises the suspicion of carcinoma of the bronchus urgently. They will require further investigation: CT scan followed by bronchoscopy if indicated.
- ★ Assess those with localised shadowing and a clinical picture suggestive of acute infection. If they have fewer than two risk factors for carcinoma (male, over 40 years, smoking >40 pack years) and symptoms resolve, order a CXR at 6 weeks. If normal, they can be reassured without further investigation.

- ★ Manage those with an initially normal CXR as follows:
  - ■ Patients with two or more risk factors for cancer (male, over 40 years, smoking >40 pack years), or persistent haemoptysis, or other symptoms (e.g. weight loss): refer for a CT scan.
  - ■ Patients with a normal CXR, small, non-recurrent haemoptysis, fewer than two risk factors for malignancy and no clinical pointers for other pathology (e.g. bronchiectasis, tuberculosis, pulmonary embolus) may be observed.

Background

The incidence of haemoptysis as a presenting symptom in primary care is unclear.

- Haemoptysis is the symptom of coughing blood from the lower respiratory tract.
- In one survey of people over the age of 40 registered with a UK general practice, 4.3% of responders had experienced an episode of haemoptysis lasting 3 days or more; 1.7% reported haemoptysis in the previous year.[1] This is equivalent to 17 patients/1000 of the population over the age of 40 years/year. This survey did not attempt to distinguish blood originating from the mouth, nasopharnyx or stomach so probably overestimates the incidence of haemoptysis.
- Only 71% of the patients reported seeking medical advice. Of these, 74% reported having had a chest X-ray (all but one of the smokers, but less than half of the non-smokers) and 37% were referred to hospital for further investigation.
- Haemoptysis in children is rare, with even specialist centres only reporting about 4 cases per year.[2,3]

Prevalence of the main causes of haemoptysis in the population

Pulmonary malignancy

Pulmonary malignancy may be primary or metastatic. Primary lung cancer is the most common cause of cancer deaths for men, with a rising incidence in women. Smoking is by far the greatest risk factor. The incidence rises sharply with age, is rare under the age of 40, with the most common age group at diagnosis being 70–74.[4] With an incidence of 80/100000/year in men and 38/100000/year in women,[5] a general practitioner is likely to diagnose at least one new case of lung cancer each year.

Bronchiectasis

The prevalence of bronchiectasis is not known.[6,7] Overlap with the symptoms of chronic obstructive pulmonary disease results in significant underdiagnosis: nearly a third of patients presenting to their general practitioner with an acute exacerbation of chronic obstructive pulmonary disease had evidence of bronchiectasis on a high resolution computed tomographic (HRCT) scan.[8]

Tuberculosis

The incidence of respiratory tuberculosis is rising, with a rate in the UK of 9.5/100000 in year 2000.[5] This increase is greatest in urban areas, with half of notifications occurring in patients from ethnic minorities.[9] Other high-risk groups include patients with impaired immunity, e.g. human immunodeficiency virus (HIV), patients on steroids, the homeless and those dependent on alcohol or drugs.

Chest infections

The annual incidence of lower respiratory tract infections treated in the UK has been estimated at between 4400 and 8400/100000.[10] Primary care studies suggest that 6% of people presenting with 'chest infections' have radiological evidence of pneumonia.[11]

Pulmonary embolus

A hospital survey estimated the incidence of admissions with a pulmonary embolus at about 25/100000 population/year, though this is likely to be an underestimate as many cases are first diagnosed at postmortem.[12]

Initial probabilities

There are no studies analysing the prevalence of the causes of haemoptysis in the undifferentiated population presenting to primary care or emergency departments. The following data are from secondary care practice and, if the survey cited above is representative,[1] relate to about a third of the cases of haemoptysis seen in general practice.[13–20] In addition, some of the studies selectively focused on those patients admitted with haemoptysis, potentially the group with the greatest morbidity.[21–26] Table 21.1 details the diagnostic yield of these studies.

The commonest identified causes of haemoptysis are:

- *Pulmonary malignancy.* There was a reported prevalence of all pulmonary malignancy ranging from 10% to 44%, about 90% of which were primary lung cancers.[14,16–20]
- *Bronchiectasis.* The reported prevalence of bronchiectasis in the surveys varied considerably, from 0 to 25%. Computed tomography scan is the investigation of choice for detecting bronchiectasis: studies only including bronchoscopy identified less than 1%.[15–17,21]
- *Tuberculosis.* Respiratory tuberculosis has a marked geographical variation, with rates as high as 33% in Kuwait attributed to a high expatriate population from endemic countries,[25] or as low as 0% in some UK and US groups.[14,21,23]
- *Chest infections.* Most studies attributed between 4% and 16% of cases of haemoptysis to pneumonia, though three series reported no cases. The variation in reported prevalence of bronchitis as a cause of

Table 21.1 Final diagnosis in all adults presenting to secondary care with haemoptysis

Author	Population	Investigations	Pulmonary malignancy	Bronchiectasis	Pneumonia	Bronchitis	TB	Pulmonary embolus	Cardiovascular	Bleeding disorders	Other	No diagnosis
Hirshberg et al[13]	Israeli tertiary centre (n = 208)	CXR, CT scan, VQ scan, bronchoscopy	39 (19%)	41 (20%)	33 (16%)	37 (18%)	3 (1%)	5 (2%)	8 (4%)	8 (4%)	25 (12%)	17 (8%)
Set et al[14]	Cambridge, UK (n = 91)	CXR, CT scan, bronchoscopy	34 (37%)	14 (15%)	4 (4%)	13 (14%)	0	0	1 (1%)	0	3 (3%)	22 (24%)
Santiago et al[15]	Los Angeles, USA (n = 264)	CXR, bronchoscopy	78 (29%)	2 (1%)	15 (6%)	62 (23%)	15 (6%)	0	1 (1%)	0	35 (13%)	57 (22%)
Johnston and Reisz[16]	Kansas City, USA (n = 148)	CXR, bronchoscopy	29 (19%)	1 (1%)	8 (5%)	55 (37%)	10 (7%)	2 (1%)	2 (1%)	2 (1%)	30 (20%)	5 (3%)
Reisz et al[17]	Missouri, USA (n = 288)	CXR, bronchoscopy	73 (25%)	2 (1%)	29 (10%)	76 (26%)	23 (8%)	4 (1%)	2 (1%)	4 (1%)	54 (19%)	21 (7%)
Wong et al[18]	Kuala Lumpur, Malaysia (n = 160)	CXR, CT scan, bronchoscopy	55 (34%)	16 (10%)	23 (14%)	1 (1%)	27 (17%)	0	2 (1%)	1 (1%)	15 (9%)	18 (11%)
Gong and Salvatierra[19]	Los Angeles, USA (n = 129)	CXR, bronchoscopy	31 (24%)	Combined infective causes 56 (43%)			4 (3%)	2 (2%)	5 (4%)	4 (3%)	13 (10%)	14 (11%)
Herth et al[20]	Boston, USA (n = 722)	CXR, bronchoscopy, ±CT scan	232 (40%)	0	33 (6%)	'COPD' 184 (31%)	73 (12%)	24 (4%)	0	0	41 (6%)	135 (19%)
Weaver et al[21]	Chicago, USA (n = 70 inpatients)	CXR, + bronchoscopy	28 (40%)	0	6 (9%)	(22 (32%)	0	0	2 (3%)	0	7 (10%)	1 (1%)
McGuiness et al[22]	New York, USA (n = 57 inpatients)	CXR, CT scan, bronchoscopy	7 (12%)	14 (25%)	0	4 (7%)	9 (16%)	0	0	0	10 (17%)	11 (19%)
Haponik et al[23]	Baltimore, USA (n = 32 inpatients)	CXR, CT scan	14 (44%)	0	0	3 (9%)	0	0	0	0	3 (9%)	12 (38%)
Fidan et al[24]	Istanbul, Turkey (n = 108 inpatients)	CXR, ± bronchoscopy and HRCT	37 (34%)	27 (25%)	11 (10%)	0	19 (18%)	5 (5%)	1 (1%)	0	3 (3%)	0
Abal et al[25]	Kuwait (n = 52 inpatients)	CXR, ± bronchoscopy and HRCT	5 (10%)	11 (21%)	0	3 (6%)	17 (33%)	0	1 (2%)	0	2 (4%)	13 (25%)
Bouley et al[26]	France (n = 6349 inpatients)	Not stated	949 (15%)	558 (9%)	427 (7%)	543 (9%)	Not stated	Not stated	848 (13%)	141 (2)	206 (3%)	2677 (42%)

COPD, chronic obstructive pulmonary disease; CT, computed tomography; CXR, chest X-ray; HRCT, high resolution CT; VQ, ventilation–perfusion.

haemoptysis (0% to 32%) may be partly methodological. Many studies reporting a high incidence assumed that if bronchitis were present and no other cause was identified, it was the source of bleeding.[15–17,20,21] Other studies only implicated bronchitis if an active bleeding point had been visualised.[22,19] The observed seasonal variation in hospital admissions for haemoptysis is consistent with an infective trigger for a significant proportion of episodes.[26]

■ *Pulmonary embolism*. Most studies attributed up to 2% of cases of haemoptysis to pulmonary emboli, though a higher proportion was reported in one series of inpatients.[24] Some studies may have included embolic disease in the category of 'cardiovascular cause'.[26]

■ *Other causes*. Many studies listed a substantial number of 'other causes'. Among the commonest were cardiovascular conditions (e.g. left ventricular failure) implicated in up to 4% of cases in most series. One large survey of over 6000 hospital admissions categorised 13% as 'cardiovascular', probably reflecting the bias resulting from selectively surveying inpatients.[26] Bleeding disorders, including anticoagulation, accounted for a similar number of cases.

■ *Cryptogenic haemoptysis*. There was wide variation in the proportion of cases for which no cause was identified (0% to 42%). This may be methodological, as some studies rigorously noted areas of active bleeding and others accepted the existence of pathology as a likely source of bleeding.

■ *Co-morbidity* may significantly influence the causes, e.g. pneumonia accounted for 28 (56%) cases of haemoptysis in a series of HIV-positive patients from New York: Kaposi sarcoma was diagnosed in 5 (10%).[27]

Children

In a large survey of children admitted to a hospital in Texas over a decade, the commonest cause of haemoptysis was cystic fibrosis (149/228 (65%)), 93% occurring in children over the age of 10 years. Congenital heart disease accounted for 37/228 (16%) of cases, predominantly in infants or teenagers. Acute pneumonia caused 13/228 (6%) of cases.[28]

Clinical assessment

Does this patient have a lung cancer?

The most common presenting symptoms of bronchial carcinoma are cough, weight loss, dyspnoea, chest pain, haemoptysis, bone pain and clubbing.[4] Haemoptysis occurs in 6% to 35%

of presentations,[29] often triggering an early presentation,[30] and is the symptom that most strongly predicts lung cancer, with a likelihood ratio of approximately 13.[31]

Investigations

■ *Chest X-ray.* Consider making an urgent referral to the lung cancer multidisciplinary team while awaiting the chest X-ray results if the patient is a smoker or ex-smoker older than 40 years with persistent haemoptysis, or in the presence of signs of sinister signs such as superior vena cava obstruction or stridor.[4]

■ *Contrast-enhanced chest CT scan* should be offered to further the diagnosis and stage the disease in patients with known or suspected lung cancer.[4]

■ *Bronchoscopy* should be performed on patients with central lesions who are able and willing to undergo the procedure.[4]

Does this patient have bronchiectasis?

The most common presenting symptoms of bronchiectasis are chronic cough and sputum production, often with wheeze.[7] Haemoptysis is common, occurring in 51% of patients in one survey, often recurrent and may be copious.[32]

Investigations

■ HRCT scan is the investigation of choice for detecting bronchiectasis.[33]

Does this patient have pneumonia?

Common presenting symptoms of pneumonia include cough and sputum production, wheeze, chest pains or aches, sweating and sore throat.[10,11]

Investigations

■ Although investigations are rarely needed in primary care for the management of uncomplicated chest infections,[10,11,34] the occurrence of haemoptysis should prompt urgent referral for a chest X-ray. Failure of the acute respiratory symptoms or signs to resolve should also prompt investigation.

Does this patient have tuberculosis?

Presenting symptoms of pulmonary tuberculosis include fever and night sweats, cough, weight loss and haemoptysis.

Investigations

■ A chest X-ray should be arranged.

■ In addition, three early morning sputum samples should be sent for microscopy, culture and sensitivity for acid-fast bacilli, prior to prompt referral for specialist care.

Does this patient have a pulmonary embolus?

The classical presentation of a pulmonary embolus is of an acute onset of dyspnoea, pleuritic pain, cough and haemoptysis in a patient with known risk factors (immobility, recent surgery, obstetric, lower limb problems, or malignancy).[12] The diagnosis may be refined using validated scores to assess the probability of embolus (see *Pulmonary embolism*, p. 477).

■ A negative D-dimer test excludes the diagnosis in patients with low or moderate clinical probability of pulmonary embolus. If the prior clinical probability is high, further investigations are indicated regardless of the results of the D-dimer test.[12]

■ Inpatient investigations include isotope lung scanning, pulmonary angiography and, more recently, computed tomographic pulmonary angiography.[12]

What does the GP do?

■ *Massive haemoptysis* (defined as >600 ml in 48 hours) is a life-threatening emergency. It is a recognised complication of tuberculosis, carcinoma of the bronchus and of chronic lung suppuration due to bronchiectasis.[17,33] It may be a terminal event in young adults with cystic fibrosis.[28] From the perspective of primary care, the only decision is to admit urgently.

■ *Patients with haemoptysis and a localised abnormality on their chest X-ray* will require urgent referral according to the clinical picture and the X-ray appearance: i.e. to the lung cancer services if cancer is the most likely diagnosis or to the pulmonary clinic if the picture is that of bronchiectasis or tuberculosis. High resolution CT scan is the initial investigation of choice.[33,35,36] A patient with haemoptysis and clinical and radiological evidence of pneumonia should be assessed for urgent admission, though those with a small haemoptysis, no markers of severity and no co-morbidity may be managed at home. A CXR should be arranged at 4–6 weeks, and the patient followed up to establish complete resolution and exclude underlying malignancy. Referral for further investigation should be considered in those at high risk (male, smokers >40 pack years, >50 years of age).

■ *Patients with a clinical picture of pulmonary embolus* need immediate admission (see p. 477).

■ *Patients with haemoptysis, a normal chest X-ray and a clinical diagnosis of a 'chest infection'.* Those whose respiratory symptoms do not resolve within 6 weeks, and those at high risk of malignancy, should be considered for further investigation.

■ *Patients with haemoptysis, no clear clinical diagnosis and a chest X-ray that is reported as normal or with no localised suspicious abnormalities* pose a diagnostic problem. Table 21.2 details the outcome of studies on patients with haemoptysis who have a normal, or non-localising, chest X-ray.[14,37–42] The incidence of sinister pathology is relatively low in this group of patients, with up to 90% having a normal bronchoscopy, and two-thirds having a normal CT scan. However, a pulmonary malignancy was identified in up to 7% of patients. The main risk factors for the identification of malignancy are male gender, age over 50 years and a smoking history >40 pack years,[37] leading to recommendations that patients with two or more of these risk factors should be considered for further investigation (normally a CT scan).[33,35] Younger (e.g. under 40 years), non-smoking patients are at low risk and may simply be observed,[35] unless the haemoptysis is heavy or persistent (>30 ml in 24 hours).[35]

Outcome in patients for whom no cause for haemoptysis is identified

Table 21.3 details the findings of four studies that have followed patients for 1 to 3 years after negative investigations. The respiratory prognosis is generally good, and although up to one in five will have recurrent haemoptysis,[42] most will have resolved within 6 months.[43] There is a small, but increased, risk of developing a lung cancer, though it is not clear whether the diagnosis was 'missed' at the time of the original investigations, or had developed subsequently.[20,38,43]

22

Headache

KEY FACTS

- In primary care, chronic headache has the following causes:
  - tension-type headache 78%
  - migraine 16%
  - other causes, none of which has a prevalence >2%.

- In acute headache, most cases are due to acute infectious disease, while some represent the onset of one or other type of chronic headache. However, a few will be due to serious urgent neurological disease (e.g. subarachnoid haemorrhage or cerebral tumour).

A PRACTICAL APPROACH

In chronic recurrent headache:
* Take a brief history, decide on the likely headache type, then focus down on that diagnosis with more detailed questions.
* Then consider whether any other type of headache is also present, especially tension-type headache in a migraine sufferer and analgesic headache in anyone who takes analgesics for headache.
* Decide whether examination is likely to be useful. It will clearly be needed if you are considering diagnoses in which physical findings may be present: giant cell arteritis or cluster headache during an attack. There are benefits from measuring the blood pressure and examining the fundus, including demonstrating to the patient that they are being taken seriously, but they are unlikely to reveal a cause if the history has not already suggested it.

In acute or subacute headache:
* Take a history as above but also look for red flags for serious pathology.
* Examine the patient briefly if the history suggests a primary headache but in more detail if there are pointers to a secondary headache.
* Stress to the patient that most headache diagnoses are made over time. A diagnosis at first presentation is often tentative and open to review.

In all cases:
* Check why the patient presented at this moment. The full diagnosis may include issues only marginally related to the headache.

The causes of headache are legion; not all the rarer causes can be considered here.

Prevalence in the population and in primary care

- In Denmark, 63% of males and 86% of females have tension headache in any one year and 6% of males and 15% of females have migraine.[1] In 5% of sufferers, the headache is daily or nearly daily.
- Despite this, the consultation rate for headaches, including migraine, in the UK is only 2.4 per hundred person years.[2] The proportion of those with migraine who *ever* consult varies according to the country. In Canada it is 81%, in the UK 58%, in Japan 31%.[3]

The problem with diagnosis

Studies from the USA and France show that only about half of those who present with headache that is subsequently judged to be migraine receive a correct diagnosis from their physicians.[3] Missed diagnosis of migraine is most likely in those without aura, in men, in those who are also depressed and in those with headache that is not severe.

Initial probabilities

In patients presenting in primary care with a new headache, these are:[4,5]
- tension headache alone 24%
- migraine alone 13%
- other (including viral infections, upper respiratory tract infections (URTIs) and trauma) 47%
- undiagnosed or mixed 15%
- serious intracranial pathology 0.95% (this figure only represents tumours, subarachnoid haemorrhages and subdural haemorrhages, of which, in this study, at a rate of 12 per 100 000 patients per year, there were 25, 17 and 8 respectively; 60% of these patients had symptoms other than headache and/or had neurological signs).

Of these new headaches, 45% were judged to be severe or disabling.

CHRONIC RECURRENT HEADACHE

(For new acute headache, see below.)

Initial probabilities in the population

- Tension-type headache 78%[1]
- Migraine 16%[1]
- Medication overuse headache 2%, though this accounts for half of all daily headaches in a headache clinic
- Cluster headache 0.4%[6]
- Giant cell arteritis 0.2% of patients aged 50 and older.[7]

Diagnostic problems

- *A patient may have two or more types of headache.* Tension-type headaches are as common in migraineurs as in those without migraine.[8] Three-quarters of migraine sufferers therefore also get tension-type headaches. By the time a patient is referred to a headache clinic, the majority have more than two diagnoses.[9] The physician will tend to diagnose the headache that is most frequent and stop there.[10] This leads to an apparent incomplete response to treatment.
- *Is it worth separating migraine from tension-type headache?* There is controversy about the possibility and the value of separating tension-type headache from migraine in the majority of patients who present in primary care. At one end of the spectrum is the convergence view that both are part of the same pathophysiological process.[11] At the other is the view that the treatment of each headache type is different and every patient has the right to a specific diagnosis.[12] In between are the views that, in mild to moderate cases, the treatment (analgesics and NSAIDs) is the same[2] and so differentiation does not matter; and that symptoms often overlap and that extra care needs to taken to separate the syndromes where possible.[10] In more severe cases, where it does matter, differentiation is easier. Indeed, disabling symptoms are hardly ever due to tension-type headache.[13]

The history

In making the diagnosis, the history is supreme. It is a rare patient in whom the examination, or imaging, reveals a relevant abnormality which was not suspected from the history.

* Ask the following questions:
  1. *How many different types of headache does the patient experience*? Separate histories are necessary for each type of headache. It is reasonable to concentrate on the one that is most bothersome to the patient but other headaches should always be reviewed in case they are clinically important.
  2. *Questions about timing*
     (a) Why consulting now?
     (b) How recent in onset?
     (c) How frequent, and what temporal pattern (especially distinguishing between episodic and daily or unremitting)?
     (d) How long lasting?
  3. *Questions about character*
     (a) Intensity of pain
     (b) Nature and quality of pain
     (c) Site and spread of pain
     (d) Associated symptoms
  4. *Questions about cause*
     (a) Predisposing and/or trigger factors
     (b) Aggravating and/or relieving factors
     (c) Family history of similar headache

5. *Questions about response*
   (a) What does the patient do during the headache?
   (b) How much is activity (function) limited or prevented?
   (c) What medication has been used and is being used, and in what manner?

6. *State of health between attacks*
   (a) Completely well, or residual or persisting symptoms?
   (b) Concerns, anxieties, fears about recurrent attacks and/or their cause.

(Questions reproduced by permission of the British Association for the Study of Headache.[14])

* Where the diagnosis is not clear from the history, ask the patient to keep a headache diary. This often resolves the issue.[13]

What follows illustrates how to interpret the answers to the above questions.

Initial screening of a patient with recurrent headache

1. Checking for migraine

Is there an aura before at least some of the headaches? Typical features are homonymous visual loss and/or fortification spectra (a flickering jagged crescent), dysphasia and unilateral paraesthesiae in the face, arm or hand. Vaguer symptoms ('blurred vision', 'spots before the eyes' that do not flicker) do not suggest migrainous aura. If the patient describes an aura, check the diagnosis of migraine with aura (see below).

If there is no aura, is it still migraine? There is evidence for two sets of questions.

1. For a screening test, combining three questions gives good results and adding further questions

is no more helpful. In a study in primary care in the USA,[15] Lipton and colleagues found that the most useful questions were about the presence of:
   (a) *nausea*
   (b) *photophobia*
   (c) *disability due to headache* (on at least 1 day in the last 3 months).

The presence of at least 2 out of 3 gave a sensitivity of 81% (95% CI 77% to 85%), and a specificity of 75% (95% CI 64% to 84%) for migraine using the diagnosis by a migraine specialist as the gold standard. This gives the likelihood ratios and post-test probabilities in Table 22.1.

If the screening test is positive, check out the diagnosis of migraine in more detail (see below). If negative, screen for other conditions before returning to the possibility that this is migraine.

2. Another study, from Canada, found that three questions, two of them different from Lipton's, were equally reliable:
   (a) if the headache was *not* daily, *and*
   (b) either it was unilateral *or*
   (c) it was severe enough to stop the patient from doing things.

A positive response had a sensitivity of 86% and a specificity of 73% for migraine (LR+ 3.2; LR− 0.2).[16]

Further details: Lipton's study[15] found that a positive answer to any of nine questions was significantly associated with the presence of migraine in patients presenting with headache in primary care in the USA (Table 22.2):

• These questions are not necessarily independent of each other, and each likelihood ratio cannot be applied in turn. Instead a total score of positive answers can be calculated. A total of 6 positive answers was found to have a sensitivity of 77% (95%

Table 22.1 The probability of migraine after asking Lipton's three questions, based on a pre-test probability of migraine of 16% in a patient with chronic recurrent headache in primary care

Score	LR (95% CI)	Probability of migraine after asking the questions
≥2 out of 3	3.2 (2.7–3.9)	38%
≤1 out of 3	0.2 (0.2–0.2)	5%

Follow each row from left to right to see how the score alters the probability of migraine.

Table 22.2 Useful features in the history for the diagnosis of migraine[15] based on a pre-test probability of migraine of 16% in a patient with chronic recurrent headache in primary care

Item	Presence	LR (95% CI)	Probability of migraine according to the answer
Pain is worse on one side	Present	1.5	22%
	Absent	0.5	9%
Pain is pulsing, pounding or throbbing	Present	1.1	17%
	Absent	0.6	10%
Pain is moderate or severe	Present	1.1	17%
	Absent	0.4	7%
Pain is made worse by activities like walking or climbing stairs	Present	1.6	23%
	Absent	0.6	10%
Nausea is present	Present	3.2	38%
	Absent	0.5	9%
Spots, stars, zigzags, lines or grey areas for several minutes or more before or during the headaches (aura symptoms)	Present	1.7	24%
	Absent	0.8	13%
Light bothers you (a lot more than when you don't have headaches)	Present	2.9	36%
	Absent	0.3	5%
Sound bothers you (a lot more than when you don't have headaches)	Present	1.9	27%
	Absent	0.3	5%
Functional impairment due to headache on at least 1 day in last 3 months	Present	1.8	26%
	Absent	0.2	4%

Follow each row from left to right to see how the response to the question alters the probability of migraine.

CI 72 to 81%), and a specificity of 74% (95% CI 62 to 84%) for migraine using the diagnosis by a migraine specialist as the gold standard. This is no better than using just the three screening questions above.

- Note that some questions are more useful in arguing *against* the diagnosis if negative, than they are useful in arguing *in favour of* it if positive; e.g. 'throbbing pain' or 'pain that is moderate or severe'. The most useful negative response that argues against migraine is if there is virtually no functional impairment as a result of the headache. Nausea is the symptom that argues most strongly for the diagnosis.

- These figures are less impressive than those of an earlier systematic review[17] in which the following were found: nausea LR+ 19.2, LR– 0.2, photophobia LR+ 5.8, LR– 0.25; but the order of usefulness of symptoms is strikingly similar.

If a patient passes the screening test, more specific questions are needed to confirm or refute the diagnosis (see below) to discover the 16% to 19% who screen positive but who do not have migraine.

2. Checking for tension-type headache

If the initial screen does not suggest migraine, is the headache consistent with tension-type headache? That is, is it a mild to moderate generalised headache without the features of migraine and without specific pointers to one of the conditions below? If so, see the more detailed work-up below.

3. Checking for headache related to neck pathology (cervicogenic headache)

The once-accepted clinical picture was of pain in the neck radiating to the back of the head aggravated by neck movements. However, there is no acceptance that this entity exists and much stricter criteria for the diagnosis have been agreed (see below).

4. Checking for headache related to trauma

Did the headache start within 7 days of significant trauma to the head or neck? If so, see below.

5. Checking for medication overuse headache

Is the patient using analgesics, ergotamine or triptans on at least 10 to 15 days each month? Is the headache associated with any other substance use? See below.

6. Checking for cluster headaches

Are the headaches focused around one eye, do they come in bouts at least once a day? If so, check out the possibility further (see below).

7. Checking for giant cell arteritis

Is the patient white and aged 50 or over? Check for the possibility of giant cell arteritis (see below). While continuous headache is more common, a low grade onset could present as chronic episodic headache.

8. Checking for serious intracranial pathology[18]

Are any of the following present:

  (a) sudden onset (either instantaneous or reaching its peak within 5 minutes of onset)

  (b) occipitonuchal location of symptoms

  (c) the presence of other symptoms (drowsiness, confusion, motor difficulties, etc.)

  (d) age >55

  (e) focal or general neurological signs?

Chronic daily headache

This is a description, not a diagnosis. It is said to be present when a patient has headache daily for weeks or months and when the headache is present for at least half the time.[14] It may be due to any or all of the following: tension-type headache, medication overuse, depression or cervicogenic headache. It is not a feature of migraine.

Examination

Check the patient's blood pressure and check for papilloedema.[19] In the absence of pointers from the history, a general neurological examination and investigations are very unlikely to be useful.[20] A study of 100800 patients in a health maintenance organisation in the USA examined the 89 CT scans performed on patients with chronic isolated headache. No useful abnormalities were found.[21] Even in the young, no investigations are routinely recommended.[22]

More detailed work-up

Does this patient have migraine?

* Check the history against the International Headache Society (IHS) criteria for migraine with, and without, aura.

IHS diagnostic criteria for migraine with aura[23] (reproduced with permission of Blackwell Publishing)

A. At least 2 attacks which meet the criteria B and C:

B. Aura, consisting of at least one of the following, is present, is not accompanied by motor weakness and is fully reversible:

  1. visual symptoms, including positive features (e.g. flickering lights, spots or lines) and/or negative features (i.e. loss of vision); or

  2. sensory symptoms, paraesthesia or numbness; or

  3. dysphasia.

C. At least 2 of the following are present:

  1. homonymous visual symptoms and/or unilateral sensory symptoms

  2. at least one aura symptom develops gradually over at least 5 minutes and/or different aura symptoms occur in succession over at least 5 minutes

  3. each symptom lasts between 5 and 60 minutes.

D. Headache typical of migraine without aura begins during the aura or within 60 minutes.

Variations on this pattern occur. The aura may not be followed by headache, in which case the diagnosis is of migrainous aura without headache. The aura may include motor weakness, in which case the diagnosis is hemiplegic migraine.

Note that patients often report the visual symptoms as affecting one eye only, not realising that flickering lights seen on one side are homonymous, not uniocular.

IHS diagnostic criteria for migraine without aura[23] (reproduced with permission of Blackwell Publishing)

A. At least 5 attacks fulfilling criteria B to D.

B. Headache attacks lasting 4–72 hours (untreated or unsuccessfully treated).

C. Headache has at least two of the following characteristics:
   1. unilateral location
   2. pulsating quality
   3. moderate or severe pain intensity

   4. aggravation by, or causing avoidance of, routine physical activity (e.g. walking or climbing stairs).

D. During headache, at least one of the following:
   1. nausea and/or vomiting
   2. photophobia and phonophobia.

E. Not attributed to another disorder.

Comment on the use of the IHS diagnostic criteria

● The criteria are intended for clinical, as well as research, use and have been shown to be useful in the diagnosis of headache disorders. A Venezuelan study found that the criteria had sensitivities and specificities of between 84% and 96% for the diagnoses of migraine, tension-type headache, and migraine and tension-type headache combined, compared to a neurological consultation as the gold standard.[24] These figures give positive likelihood ratios of 5 to 24 and negative likelihood ratios of 0.2 to 0.04. Furthermore, when doctors use the criteria independently to diagnose patients, the correlation between their results is strong.[25]

● The criteria inevitably have a rigidity that does not mirror the infinite variety of human experience. Clearly, a patient with symptoms typical of migraine without aura who has only had four attacks, and who then goes on to have a fifth attack, had migraine all along, even though the criteria were not met until that fifth attack. Furthermore, other types of migraine are specified in the IHS classification but are too lengthy to be included here.

● A study from primary care in France suggests that five questions are as useful as the full IHS criteria in the diagnosis of migraine.[26] They are:

   ■ Is the headache pulsatile?
   ■ Does it last between 4 and 72 hours (untreated)?
   ■ Is it unilateral?
   ■ Is there nausea?
   ■ Is the headache disabling?

These questions have the predictive values shown in Table 22.3.

Trigger factors in migraine

The systematic review mentioned above found that the literature confirmed certain triggers for migraine which may be helpful in making the diagnosis in cases of doubt.[17] A relationship with some foods (especially chocolate and cheese), alcohol, stress, weather change and menses is significantly associated with an increased probability that a headache is migraine rather than tension-type headache. Positive likelihood ratios range from 7.1 (95% CI 4.5 to 11.2) for chocolate, to 1.3 (95% CI 1.1 to 1.5) for alcohol. Only the LR+ for chocolate and cheese (4.9 (95% CI 1.9 to 12.5)) are usefully high. In none is the LR− usefully low, i.e. the absence of such a trigger does not usefully argue against the diagnosis. Strange to report is that an apparent trigger of smells, e.g. perfume, argues *against* the diagnosis of migraine (LR+ 0.6 (95% CI 0.4 to 0.8)).

Family and past history in the diagnosis of migraine

The same systematic review[17] found that a family history of migraine argued strongly in favour of the diagnosis (LR+ 7.1 (95% CI 4.5 to 11.2)) and a personal history of childhood vomiting attacks (LR+ 2.4) and motion sickness (LR+ 2.2) were also useful. A negative family history argues against migraine (LR− 0.5 (95% CI 0.5 to 0.5)); a negative personal history of childhood vomiting or motion sickness is not useful either way.

Is this a tension-type headache?

* Check the history against the IHS criteria for tension-type headache.

Table 22.3 Value of Michel's five questions in the diagnosis of migraine,[26,27] based on a pre-test probability of 16%

Number of questions positive	Likelihood ratio (95% CI)	Probability of migraine
1 or 2	0.4 (0.3–0.5)	7%
3	3.5 (1.3–9.2)	40%
4 or 5	24 (1.5–388)	82%

Note how wide the confidence intervals are for the positive likelihood ratios.

IHS diagnostic criteria for tension-type headache[23] (reproduced with permission of Blackwell Publishing)

The IHS recognises two types:

Episodic

A. At least 10 episodes occurring on <15 days a month for at least 3 months with the following characteristics:

B. Headache lasting from 30 minutes to 7 days.

C. Headache has at least 2 of the following characteristics:

   (a) bilateral location

   (b) pressing/tightening (non-pulsating) quality

   (c) mild or moderate intensity

   (d) not aggravated by routine physical activity such as walking or climbing stairs.

D. Both of the following negatives apply:

   (a) no nausea or vomiting (although anorexia may occur)

   (b) no more than one of photophobia or phonophobia.

E. Not attributed to another disorder.

Chronic

which is similar except that the headache is present for most days of the year, lasts hours each time or is continuous, and mild nausea may occur.

Are these cluster headaches?

* Check the history against the IHS criteria for cluster headaches.

The IHS diagnostic criteria for cluster headaches[23] (reproduced with permission of Blackwell Publishing)

A. At least 5 attacks fulfilling the following criteria:

B. Severe or very severe unilateral orbital, supraorbital and/or temporal pain lasting 15 to 180 minutes if untreated.

C. Headache is accompanied by at least one of the following:

   (a) ipsilateral conjunctival injection and/or lacrimation

   (b) ipsilateral nasal congestion and/or rhinorrhoea

   (c) ipsilateral eyelid oedema

   (d) ipsilateral forehead and facial sweating

   (e) ipsilateral miosis and/or ptosis

   (f) a sense of restlessness or agitation.

D. Attacks have a frequency of from one every other day to 8 a day.

E. Not attributed to another disorder.

They are six times more common in men than in women,[17] with an age of onset between 20 and 40 years. About 5% show autosomal dominant inheritance, so a strong family history helps to confirm the diagnosis, although its absence does not weaken it. Attacks are usually so severe that the patient is restless and wants to move around, in marked contrast to migraine. The short duration of each attack and the tendency of attacks to cluster, coming often daily, or more often, for 1 to 2 months (the cluster period), further helps make the distinction. Finally, cluster periods tend to recur at about the same time every year.

However, note that cluster-type headaches are also associated with increased risk of intracranial pathology (see p. 150).

Is this cervicogenic headache?

* Check the history against the IHS criteria for cervicogenic headache.

The IHS diagnostic criteria for cervicogenic headache[23] (reproduced with permission of Blackwell Publishing)

A. Pain referred from a source in the neck and perceived in one or more regions of the head and/or face, fulfilling criteria C and D.

B. Clinical, laboratory and/or imaging evidence of a disorder or lesion within the cervical spine or soft tissues of the neck known to be, or generally accepted as, a valid cause of headache.

C. Evidence that pain can be attributed to the neck disorder or lesion based on at least one of the following:
   1. demonstration of clinical signs that implicate a source of pain in the neck
   2. abolition of headache following diagnostic blockade of a cervical structure or its nerve supply using placebo or other adequate controls.

D. Pain resolves within 3 months after successful treatment of the causative disorder or lesion.

- Note that the IHS 1988 definition, which described the then commonly accepted picture of pain in the neck or occiput, aggravated by neck movements, has been completely replaced.
- There are good reasons for imposing these strict criteria. Almost everyone over 40 has evidence of cervical spondylosis on X-ray; its finding in a patient with headache has no effect on the diagnosis, even in those with limitation of neck movements.
- In practice, it would hardly ever be possible to make a diagnosis of cervicogenic headache in primary care using these new criteria, for four reasons:
  1. The cervical disorders accepted under criterion B are tumours, infections and rheumatoid arthritis but not cervical spondylosis, osteochondritis or myofascial tender spots.
  2. There is no evidence that any clinical signs reliably indicate a source of pain in the neck, so criterion C1 is theoretical at the moment.
  3. Criterion C2 is not practicable in primary care.
  4. It is rarely possible to treat a cervical disorder so successfully that the pain resolves, so criterion D is of little use either.

Is this giant cell arteritis (GCA)?

Meta-analysis has examined which factors allow the diagnosis of GCA to be made or excluded (Tables 22.4 and 22.5). The problem for the GP is that these likelihood ratios were worked out from patients referred for temporal artery biopsy. The referring physician had already made a decision that GCA was a strong

Table 22.4 Most useful symptoms in the diagnosis of giant cell arteritis, based on a prevalence of 39% in referred patients

Symptom	Positive likelihood ratio (95% CI)	Probability of giant cell arteritis if the symptom is present
Jaw claudication[28]*	4.2 (2.8–6.2)	73%
Neck pain (mainly in the back of the neck)[29]	3.7 (1.8–7.7)	70%
Diplopia[28]	3.4 (1.3–8.6)	68%
Weight loss/anorexia[29]	1.6 (1.2–2.0)	51%
Fever[29]	1.6 (1.1–2.5)	51%

Follow each row from left to right to see how the symptom, if present, increases the probability of giant cell arteritis.
*Check that it really is claudication (pain coming on after starting to chew) and not a temporomandibular joint disorder (pain from the start of chewing).

Table 22.5 Most useful signs in the diagnosis of giant cell arteritis,[28] based on a prevalence of 39% in referred patients

Sign	Positive likelihood ratio (95% CI)	Probability of giant cell arteritis if the sign is present
Prominent or enlarged temporal artery	4.3 (2.1–8.9)	73%
Absent temporal artery	2.7 (0.6–13)	63%
Temporal artery tenderness	2.6 (1.9–3.7)	62%

Follow each row from left to right to see how the sign, if present, increases the probability of giant cell arteritis. Again, the negative likelihood ratios of these signs are clinically unhelpful. In other words, if the sign is negative, the probability of arteritis is hardly reduced.

enough possibility to make that referral. No study has captured the value of symptoms in primary care in this field. They are likely to be higher than in referred patients. For instance, headache has an LR+ of 1.2 for the diagnosis of GCA in secondary care. This must be because almost all patients referred have headache; its value will therefore have been used up in primary care.

Because of this, the baseline probability of giant cell arteritis used in Tables 22.4 and 22.5 is 39% – the prevalence of arteritis in referred patients. The GP who performs a full history and examination and decides to refer is likely to achieve the post-test probabilities in these tables, not the much lower probabilities that would come from applying these likelihood ratios to the pre-test probability of GCA in a patient with headache in primary care (0.2%).

Factors which increase the probability of the diagnosis

The negative likelihood ratios for almost all these symptoms are close to 1 and so useless in excluding the diagnosis. The exception is headache, which has an LR– of 0.7 (95% CI 0.6 to 0.8).[28] In other words, the absence of headache argues against the diagnosis (although only modestly in a patient referred for temporal artery biopsy).

Two other features of the history strongly support the diagnosis in a patient with headache in primary care, although likelihood ratios for them are not available:
■ *loss of vision*, especially if ophthalmoscopy shows the changes of ischaemic optic neuritis
■ *Polymyalgia rheumatica* (PMR).

Combining these likelihood ratios for symptoms and signs, using the nomogram on page xxiv in a patient with several positive findings can produce a post-test probability that is strongly in favour of the diagnosis. For instance, take a patient with a pre-test probability of, say, 20% because of an age of 70, and a history of the recent onset of headache combined with weight loss and malaise. The presence of jaw claudication raises the probability of GCA to 51%. If there is also neck pain, it rises to 80% and, if there is also an enlarged temporal artery, to 95%. However, beware of combining likelihood ratios that are not independent of each other. The meta-analysis used above did not attempt to assess the independence of the different factors and therefore a common sense approach is needed. For instance, only one abnormality of the temporal artery can be used: if the artery is enlarged, it is unlikely that the finding of tenderness adds much to the diagnosis.

A raised erythrocyte sedimentation rate (ESR) is disappointingly unhelpful both in screening and in the confirmation of the diagnosis:
■ A raised ESR regardless of the level: LR+ 1.1 (0.82 to 2.9)
■ ESR >50: LR+ 1.2 (1.0 to 1.4)
■ ESR >100: LR+ 1.9 (1.1 to 3.3).

The only factors that usefully reduce the probability of the diagnosis are:[28]
■ temporal artery clinically normal: LR– 0.53 (0.38 to 0.75)
■ Normal ESR (LR– 0.2 (0.08 to 0.51)
■ Age under 50 (in a review of 8 studies, only 2 of 1435 positive biopsies were from patients aged <50).

As an example, in a patient in whom the initial probability of GCA is thought to be 20%, but whose temporal artery is found to be clinically normal, the probability of GCA falls to 12%. If the ESR is also normal, it falls to 3%. In the absence of any positive pointers towards the diagnosis, a trial of steroids would not be justified and most physicians would judge that watchful waiting rather than biopsy was justified.

The problem with temporal artery biopsy

The sensitivity and specificity of a positive temporal artery biopsy, once considered the gold standard for the diagnosis of giant cell arteritis, is now uncertain. The two main causes for concern are:

1. It is clear that some patients with a negative biopsy would have been positive if longer, bilateral segments of artery had been examined.
2. One-third of patients with clinical evidence of the disease have negative biopsies.[30] How many of them have the disease is not clear.

An estimate of the value of temporal artery biopsy in the diagnosis of GCA gives it a sensitivity of 80% and a specificity of 95% (LR+ 16; LR− 0.21).[31]

A new gold standard for the diagnosis of GCA, of a persistent clinical diagnosis at 1 year, has been suggested.[32]

Who should have a trial of steroids and who should be biopsied?

The sensitivity and specificity of a trial of steroids is unknown. The present consensus is that a patient with a clear clinical picture should be treated with steroids regardless of the biopsy result. If there is a dramatic response to steroids within 48 hours, the diagnosis is confirmed. Biopsy is therefore only really useful in patients whose clinical picture is not sufficiently clear for a trial of steroids to be justified.

Does the patient have headache induced by a substance or by its withdrawal?

Analgesic overuse headache

* Check the history against the IHS criteria for analgesic overuse headache.

> **The IHS diagnostic criteria for analgesic overuse headache[23] (reproduced with the permission of Blackwell Publishing Ltd)**
>
> A. Headache is present on >15 days per month with at least one of the following characteristics, and fulfils criteria C and D:
>   1. the headache is bilateral; and/or
>   2. pressing/tightening in nature and/or
>   3. mild to moderate in intensity.
> B. The patient uses simple analgesics on ≥15 days per month for at least 3 months.
> C. The headache has developed or worsened during analgesic use.
> D. The headache resolves within 2 months of stopping.

- The diagnostic criteria for *ergotamine-induced headache* and *opioid-overuse headache* are similar but may occur after use of the drug on only 10 days per month.
- Since the criteria include the need to withdraw medication for 2 months before the diagnosis can definitely be established, the diagnosis is of 'probable medication-overuse headache' until the drug has been withdrawn.
- Headache may worsen initially when the drugs are withdrawn, making patient and doctor think, erroneously, that the diagnosis of medication overuse is wrong. In fact, worsening of headache, with nausea, vomiting, insomnia and anxiety in the first 10 days after withdrawing the drug *strengthens* the diagnosis of medication overuse.[33]

Caffeine withdrawal headache

It is characterised by bilateral and/or pulsating headache after a high caffeine dose is taken for at least 2 weeks and then stopped. Headache starts within 24 hours of the last caffeine intake, is relieved completely within 1 hour of taking caffeine and resolves within 7 days of total caffeine withdrawal.

Oestrogen withdrawal headache

This occurs in someone using exogenous oestrogen for at least 3 weeks which is then stopped. It develops within 5 days of stopping and resolves within 3 days.

Acute substance-induced headaches

They are typically bilateral fronto-temporal headaches, pulsating and aggravated by physical activity. Their timing is important in making the diagnosis:

Oral or inhaled nitrates – onset within 10 minutes and resolving within 1 hour.

Monosodium glutamate – onset within 1 hour resolving within 72 hours.

Cocaine – onset within 1 hour resolving within 72 hours.

Cannabis – onset within 12 hours resolving within 72 hours.

Alcohol – onset within 3 hours resolving within 72 hours.

Delayed substance-induced headache (hangover)

This occurs with alcohol. It develops as the alcohol level declines and resolves within 72 hours. In migraine sufferers, the amount of alcohol may be modest.

Is the headache one of a group of benign paroxysmal headaches?

Certain severe transient headaches of sudden onset may mimic subarachnoid haemorrhage (SAH) and, until a pattern is established, can only be distinguished from SAH by negative investigations. In the first attack, the patient will need to be referred urgently, even if the headache is short-lived and improving when seen by the physician.

Paroxysmal hemicrania

This is similar to cluster headache with the following differences:[23,34]

(a) at least 20 attacks are required for the diagnosis (not >5)

(b) the attacks are shorter (2–30 minutes not 15–180 minutes)

(c) attacks are more frequent (>5 a day for at least half the time instead of at least every other day)

(d) attacks do not centre on the eye

(e) attacks are completely prevented by indometacin.

Ice-pick headache

This is characterised by transient head pain occurring as a single stab or a series of stabs. It is exclusively or predominantly felt in the distribution of the first division of the trigeminal nerve (orbit, temple or parietal area). Stabs last for up to a few seconds. There may be one or many each day. There are no accompanying symptoms.

Cough headache

This is characterised by a sudden onset, lasts from 1 second to 30 minutes, and is brought on by and occurs only in association with coughing, straining and/or Valsalva manoeuvre; 40% are secondary to intracranial disease, mainly Arnold–Chiari malformation type 1. Cerebral aneurysms may give rise to cough headache. Refer all.

Exertional headache

This is characterised by pulsating headache, lasting from 5 minutes to 48 hours, brought on by and only occurring during or after physical exertion. The symptoms cannot be attributed to another disorder. Again if the patient presents with the first attack, it is essential to refer as possible SAH.

Coital headaches

Pre-orgasmic headache is a dull ache in the head and neck occurring during sexual activity and increasing with increasing excitement. Orgasmic headache is characterised by sudden severe headache occurring at orgasm and not attributable to another disorder. When the first attack is sudden and severe, the patient will need referral for suspected SAH.

Thunderclap headache

A severe headache whose onset is instantaneous, it may last hours or days. It can only be distinguished from a SAH by negative investigations. It may recur. In a Dutch study, 36% of patients presenting in primary care with sudden severe headache fell into this category.[35]

Is this headache related to trauma?

Acute post-traumatic headache (adapted from the IHS classification)[23]

This is headache, without any typical characteristics, which meets the following requirements:

(a) a history of head trauma severe enough to cause concussion or unconsciousness

(b) the headache developed within 7 days of the trauma or after regaining consciousness

(c) either the headache resolved within 3 months or 3 months have not yet passed.

Chronic post-traumatic headache

This is as for acute, but headache lasts more than 3 months. It may be associated with poor balance, loss of concentration, irritability, depression and insomnia.

Acute headache attributed to whiplash injury (adapted from the IHS classification)[23]

This is headache which meets the following requirements:

(a) a history of whiplash (sudden acceleration/deceleration movement of the neck) associated at the time with neck pain

(b) headache develops within 7 days of the injury

(c) either the headache resolves within 3 months or 3 months have not yet passed.

Chronic headache attributed to whiplash injury

This is as for acute, but headache lasts more than 3 months.

Note: Both migraine and tension-type headache may be triggered by trauma to the head or neck. They may exist alone or together with a post-traumatic headache.

The patient's perspective

Most people with headaches never consult a physician about them.[36] Those who do consult tend to have more severe symptoms, but not necessarily so; the decision to consult is the result of a number of factors: the patient's psychological state, social situation and illness beliefs, as well as factors that the GP is more likely to attend to, such as concern about serious disease and about relieving symptoms. Studies of hospital referrals for headache show that satisfaction with the consultation was associated with subsequent improvement, and this improvement seems to relate not to the use of specific treatments but to whether the doctor had met their personal concerns.[37,38] At the risk of stating the obvious, the GP needs to check what has brought the patient to that consultation, rather than concentrating exclusively on accurate diagnosis and medical treatment.

NEW ACUTE OR SUBACUTE HEADACHE

● Most patients will be suffering from an acute illness (e.g. generalised viral infection or upper respiratory tract infection) and the symptoms of this will make the diagnosis obvious. Others will be suffering from the onset of one of the chronic types of primary headache. However, a new acute headache raises the possibility of other conditions, some of which need urgent treatment.

● The problem for the GP is that serious conditions are uncommon. The Ambulatory Sentinel Practice Network (ASPN), based in Denver, Colorado, found that 58 practices, over a 19-month period, had only 25 patients with an intracranial tumour, 15 with subarachnoid haemorrhage and 8 with a subdural haemorrhage; a rate of 12 per 100 000 patients per year.[5] Furthermore, only half of these patients presented with headache. In that time, using data from a previous ASPN report,[4] about 4500 patients would have presented with a new headache, giving a prevalence of one of those three serious pathologies in 1 in 180 patients with new headache. Despite that, only four of those diagnoses were missed, and two of those were because of undue reliance on a negative CT scan.

Check for the following red flags

* Are there new-onset seizures, papilloedema, cranial nerve palsy or other *progressive neurological deficit*?[39] Refer urgently for suspected cerebral tumour. One study of patients presenting to the emergency department with headache who had an abnormality on neurological examination found that 39% of them had intracranial pathology.[18]

* Does the spouse or partner give a history of *mental changes* (memory loss, fatigue or personality change) in addition to the headache? These were present in the majority of patients with malignant glioma in a Swedish study, and only discovered by interviewing someone other than the patient.[40] They are grounds for urgent referral.[39]

* Does the headache raise the possibility of *raised intracranial pressure* (woken by headache, worse on straining or bending down, vomiting, drowsiness)? Refer urgently.

* *Is the headache associated with aura*, other than the visual aura typical of migraine? A meta-analysis has found an association with intracranial pathology (LR+ 3.2 (95% CI 1.6 to 6.6)).[27]

* *Is the headache 'cluster' in type*, i.e. severe pain in or around the eye, occurring in frequent bouts, followed by a pain-free interval? A meta-analysis has found an association with intracranial pathology (LR+ 11 (95% CI 2.2 to 52)), even though this is also the pattern of true cluster headaches, which are not associated with intracranial pathology.[27]

* Is the patient *over 50 years old* with a new continuous headache? Consider the possibility of giant cell arteritis (see above). Older patients are also more likely to have intracranial pathology.[18]

* Is this the *worst headache* the patient has ever had? A US study found that 20 out of 107 patients presenting to an emergency department in Houston, Texas with their worst ever headache were suffering from a subarachnoid haemorrhage (SAH).[41] However, this may only apply to those who attend an emergency department. In one study, 9.1% *of the population* reported at least one 'almost unbearable' headache in the previous year.[42]

* *Was the onset sudden and severe?* The probability of SAH is 25%.[43] Even if there are no other symptoms or signs, the probability of SAH is 12%.
* Was there *loss of consciousness?* This raises the possibility of SAH even if the patient seems to be recovering well.
* Was the *onset gradual but progressively worsening?* Consider an intracranial lesion.
* Is there *systemic disturbance* (e.g. fever, vomiting) with no systemic illness to explain it? Consider meningitis, or, if there is no neck stiffness, cerebral abscess.
* Is *one eye inflamed* with a fixed pupil? A patient with acute glaucoma may not have noticed the unilateral loss of vision. Less acute attacks may cause headache and coloured haloes round lights without rendering the patient prostrate.
* Are there *focal neurological signs, disturbed cognition and a stiff neck?* Consider the possibility of SAH and admit. However, most patients with SAH seen in primary care will not have a stiff neck. Even by the time they reach the emergency department, Lambert found that

64% of patients with SAH did not have neck stiffness.[44]

* Does the history suggest *carbon monoxide poisoning* (i.e. more than one person in the household affected, headache relieved by leaving the house, gas appliance burns with a yellow or orange flame)? There were 21 deaths in 1996/7 in the UK from this cause with many more affected without fatality.[45]
* *A pattern which does not fit any of the primary headache entities.*
* New-onset headache in a patient with *cancer or who is HIV positive.* One study of HIV-positive patients with a chief complaint of headache found that 82% had an identifiable serious cause of headache. Cryptococcal meningitis (39%) and CNS toxoplasmosis (16%) were the leading causes.[46]

Note: Beware being falsely reassured by the fact that the patient's headache appears to improve with analgesics. Several case studies have reported apparent response to treatment in patients with intracranial haemorrhage, viral meningitis and meningeal carcinomatosis.[47]

Example

A 20-year-old refuse collector presents with headaches that have bothered him for 6 months, although he has been prone to headaches for longer than that. They often last all day. He describes them as being 'all over' the head but there are no other pointers, specifically no aura, no nausea, no photophobia. They are present when he wakes up. They tend to occur on a Saturday but occasionally they happen in the week. If so, he is able to work the next day but will prefer not to go out that night.

The GP is not getting a clear picture of any characteristic headache. The Saturday occurrence makes her think of migraine, but the lack of any of Lipton's criteria (nausea, photophobia, disability) or of more than one of the Canadian criteria (not daily, and unilateral or disabling) reduce the probability of that from 13% to 3% (Fig. 22.1).

A few more questions suggest that tension-type headache fits better (it is bilateral, not pulsating and only moderate) but the regularity is unlike a tension-type headache, as is the fact that movement makes the headache worse.

Finally the GP hits the bullseye with the question: 'What do you do on a Friday night?', getting the answer 'I get slaughtered, don't I?'. To the question 'Do you think alcohol could be playing a part?' he says that that's what his girlfriend thinks but he's dismissed the idea because he doesn't vomit, in contrast to his friends who do, when hung over. Also,

the headache goes on all day whereas his friends are drinking again by Saturday lunchtime.

The GP feels she is getting to understand her patient better as the consultation proceeds and asks what he does on the night before he gets a headache in the week. To her surprise they are not related to drinking. Putting together the fact that his post-alcohol headache is not typical of a hangover, except in timing of the onset, and that some headaches are not alcohol related, she decides that he probably has migraine without aura, mainly alcohol-induced, even though the headaches do not meet the IHS criteria for migraine without aura. She is aware that there is evidence that a history of alcohol triggering the headache argues in favour of migraine but that the LR+, at 1.3, hardly affects the probability. However, she is sophisticated enough to understand that such an LR is a composite figure for a large population. Within that population will be some patients in whom the link between alcohol and migraine is strong, but they are almost swamped, statistically, by the majority in whom there is no link.

The patient then volunteers that his father had migraine. This usefully increases the probability of migraine to 13% (Fig. 22.2), although this is still no more than the population average.

The patient finds migraine, triggered by alcohol, a more acceptable diagnosis than hangovers and is prepared to talk about cutting down.

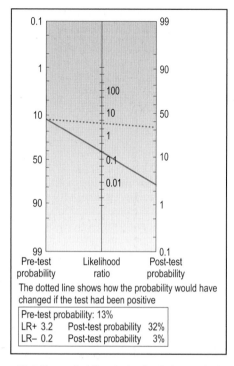

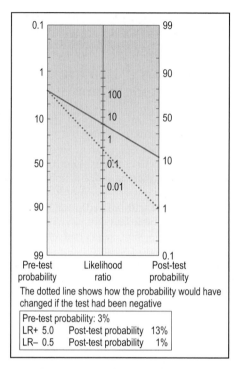

Figure 22.1 The probability of migraine before and after asking the three questions in the example on p. 151.

Figure 22.2 The probability of migraine before and after the emergence of the fact that there is a family history in the example on p. 151.

REFERENCES

1. Rasmussen B, Jensen R, Olesen J. *A population-based analysis of the diagnostic criteria of the International Headache Society.* Cephalalgia 1991; 11:129–134.

2. Ridsdale L. *'I saw a great star, most splendid and beautiful': headache in primary care.* Br J Gen Pract 2003;53: 182–184.

3. Edmeads J, Lainez J, Brandes J, et al. *Potential of the Migraine Disability Assessment (MIDAS) Questionnaire as a public health initiative and in clinical practice.* Neurology 2001;56 (Suppl 1): S29–S34.

4. Becker LA, Iverson DC, Reed FM, et al. *Patients with new headache in primary care: a report from ASPN.* J Fam Pract 1988;27:41–47.

5. Becker LA, Green LA, Beaufait D, et al. *Detection of intracranial tumors,* subarachnoid hemorrhages, and subdural hematomas in primary care patients: a report from ASPN, Part 2. *J Fam Pract 1993;37:135–141.*

6. Sjaastad O, Bakketeig L. *Cluster headache prevalence. Vaga study of headache epidemiology.* Cephalalgia 2003;23:528–533.

7. Lawrence R, Helmick C, Arnett F, et al. *Estimates of the prevalence of arthritis and selected musculoskeletal disorders in the United States.* Arthritis Rheum 1998;41: 778–799.

8. Ulrich V, Russell M, Jensen R, Olesen J. *A comparison of tension-type headache in migraineurs and in non-migraineurs: a population based study.* Pain 1996;67:501–506.

9. Sanin L, Mathew N, Bellmeyer L, Ali S. *The International Headache Society (IHS) headache classification* as applied to a headache clinic population. Cephalalgia 1994;14: 443–446.

10. Kaniecki R. *Migraine and tension-type headache: an assessment of challenges in diagnosis.* Neurology 2002;58(9 (Suppl 6)):S15–20.

11. Cady R, Schreiber C, Farmer K, Sheftell F. *Primary headaches: a convergence hypothesis.* Headache 2002;42:204–216.

12. Task Force of the International Headache Society. *Organisation and delivery of services to headache patients.* Cephalalgia 1997;17:702–710.

13. Lipton R, Cady R, Stewart W, et al. *Diagnostic lessons from the Spectrum Study.* Neurology 2002; 58(9 (Suppl 6)):S27–31.

14. British Association for the Study of Headache. *Guidelines for all doctors*

in the diagnosis and management of migraine and tension-type headache, 2004. Online. Available: www.bash. org.uk.

15. Lipton R, Dodick D, Sadovsky R. *A self-administered screener for migraine in primary care.* Neurology 2003;61:375–382.

16. Pryse-Phillips W, Aube M, Gawal M, et al. *A Headache Diagnosis Project.* Headache 2002;42:728–737.

17. Smetana G. *The diagnostic value of historical features in primary headache syndromes.* Arch Intern Med 2000;160:2729–2737.

18. Ramirez-Lassepas M, Espinosa C, Cicero J. *Predictors of intracranial pathologic findings in patients who seek emergency care because of headache.* Arch Neurol 1997;54:1506–1509.

19. Steiner T, Fontebasso M. *Headache.* BMJ 2002;325:881–886.

20. Quality Standards Subcommittee of the American Academy of Neurology. *Practice parameter: the utility of neuroimaging in the evaluation of headache in patients with normal neurologic examinations.* Neurology 1994;44:1353–1354.

21. Weingarten S, Kleinman M, Elperin L, et al. *The effectiveness of cerebral imaging in the diagnosis of chronic headache.* Arch Intern Med 1992;152:2457–2462.

22. Lewis D, Ashwal S, Dahl G, et al. *Practice parameter: evaluation of children and adolescents with recurrent headaches.* Neurology 2002;59: 490–498.

23. Headache Classification Subcommittee of the International Headache Society. *The international classification of headache disorders.* Cephalalgia 2004;24 (Suppl 1).

24. Colina-Garcia R, Carrasquero-Arias S. *Diagnostic value of the criteria of the International Headache Society in the differential diagnosis of primary headaches.* Rev Neurol 2003;36: 903–906.

25. Granella F, D'Alessandro R, Manzoni G, et al. *International Headache Society classification:*

interobserver reliability in the diagnosis of primary headaches. Cephalalgia 1994;14:16–20.

26. Michel P, Henry P, Letenneur L, et al. *Diagnostic screen for assessment of the IHS criteria for migraine by general practitioners.* Cephalalgia 1993;13 (Suppl 12):54–59.

27. Detsky M, McDonald D, Baerlocher M, et al. *Does this patient with headache have a migraine or need neuroimaging?* JAMA 2006;296: 1274–1283.

28. Smetana G, Shmerling R. *Does this patient have temporal arteritis?* JAMA 2002;287:92–101.

29. Hayreh S, Podhajsky P, Raman R, Zimmerman B. *Giant cell arteritis: validity and reliability of various diagnostic criteria.* Am J Ophthalmol 1997;123:285–296.

30. Pountain G, Hazleman B. *Polymyalgia rheumatica and giant cell arteritis.* BMJ 1995;310:1057–1059.

31. Kantor S. *Temporal arteritis.* In: Black E, Bordley D, Tape T, Panzer R, eds. Diagnostic strategies for common medical problems, 2nd edn. Philadelphia: American College of Physicians, 1999:429–437.

32. Sudlow C. *Diagnosing and managing polymyalgia rheumatica and temporal arteritis.* BMJ 1997;315:549.

33. DTB. *Management of tension-type headache.* Drug Ther Bull 1999;37: 41–44.

34. Zidverc-Trajkovic J, Pavlovic A, Mijajlovic M, et al. *Cluster headache and paroxysmal hemicrania: differential diagnosis.* Cephalalgia 2005;25: 241–243.

35. Linn FHH, Wijdicks EFM, van der Graaf Y, et al. *Prospective study of sentinel headache in aneurysmal subarachnoid haemorrhage.* Lancet 1994;344:590–593.

36. O'Flynn N, Ridsdale L. *Headache in primary care: how important is diagnosis to management?* Br J Gen Pract 2002;52:569–573.

37. Fitzpatrick R, Hopkins A, Harvard-Watts O. *Social dimensions of*

healing: a longitudinal study of outcomes of medical management of headaches. Soc Sci Med 1983;17: 501–510.

38. Fitzpatrick R, Hopkins A. *Referrals to neurologists for headache not due to structural disease.* J Neurol Neurosurg Psychiatry 1981;44: 1061–1067.

39. NICE. *Referral guidelines for suspected cancer.* London: National Institute for Health and Clinical Excellence, 2005. Online. Available: www.nice.org.uk.

40. Salander P, Bergenheim A, Hamberg K, et al. *Pathways from symptoms to medical care: a descriptive study of symptom development and obstacles to early diagnosis in brain tumour patients.* Fam Pract 1999;16: 143–148.

41. Morgenstern LB, Luna-Gonzales H, Huber JC, et al. *Worst headache and subarachnoid hemorrhage: prospective, modern computed tomography and spinal fluid analysis.* Ann Emerg Med 1998;32: 297–304.

42. Newland C, Illis L, Robinson P, et al. *A survey of headache in an English city.* Res Clin Stud Headache 1978;5:1–20.

43. Linn FHH, Wijdicks EFM, van der Graaf Y, et al. *Prospective study of sentinel headache in aneurysmal subarachnoid haemorrhage.* Lancet 1994;344:590–593.

44. Lambert K. *Sudden onset headache in the A&E Department (unpublished).* Durham: University of Durham, 1999.

45. CMO's update: DOH, 1997:2.

46. Lipton R, Feraru E, Weiss G, et al. *Headache in HIV-1 related disorders.* Headache 1991;31:518–522.

47. American College of Emergency Physicians. *Clinical policy: critical issues in the evaluation and management of patients presenting to the emergency department with acute headache.* Ann Emerg Med 2002;39:108–122.

23

Heartburn

KEY FACTS

The complaint of heartburn poses several problems:
(a) it can be difficult to be sure what the patient means by it
(b) even if the patient means what the doctor means by it, it correlates poorly with objective evidence of acid reflux or oesophagitis
(c) symptoms are only modestly useful in the diagnosis of gastro-oesophageal reflux disease
(d) objective tests (endoscopy, pH monitoring) are useful if positive but negative results do not exclude gastro-oesophageal reflux disease (GORD)
(e) a positive response to a trial of a proton pump inhibitor confirms acid-related disease but only slightly increases the probability of GORD.

A PRACTICAL APPROACH

* If the patient reports heartburn and/or reflux, remember that the diagnosis at this stage is of dyspepsia; the probability that it is GORD is less than 50%.
* Ask about the severity of symptoms. The patient's judgement that they are troublesome is more useful than an arbitrary count of hours or days in which symptoms are felt.[1]
* Ask about alarm symptoms that might indicate serious upper gastrointestinal disease: dysphagia, weight loss, vomiting, haematemesis or melaena.
* Examine the abdomen.
* Check the haemoglobin in patients who are older, who smoke, take NSAIDs or have a past history of peptic ulcer or gastrointestinal bleeding.
* In those who do not require referral because of any findings in the points above, institute a trial of a proton pump inhibitor.

Definitions

● The dyspepsia guideline of the Scottish Intercollegiate Guidelines Network (SIGN)[2] defines dyspepsia as a 'pain or discomfort centred in the epigastrium' and excludes from the guideline patients with heartburn. It also excludes patients with heartburn and dyspepsia where heartburn is the dominant symptom. This is because of an assumption that gastro-oesophageal reflux disease (GORD, or GERD in American usage) can be diagnosed clinically.

● The dyspepsia guideline of the National Institute for Health and Clinical Excellence (NICE)[3] takes the opposite stance, including those with heartburn and/or regurgitation in their definition of dyspepsia on the grounds that GORD cannot be reliably distinguished clinically from other types of dyspepsia in primary care.

● The Global Consensus Group has published the Montreal definition of GORD: 'a condition which develops when the reflux of stomach contents causes troublesome symptoms and/or complications'.[1] This avoids the problems raised by trying to define GORD by the imperfect methods by which it is diagnosed (endoscopy, oesophageal pH monitoring, and response to a proton pump inhibitor).

- The distinction between GORD and other causes of dyspepsia is important because of the different treatments that are needed, both in the lifestyle advice that is appropriate and the fact that *Helicobacter pylori* eradication is not useful in the treatment of GORD. Indeed, eradication may worsen symptoms. A Hong Kong study found that eradication, in Chinese patients with GORD, doubled the probability of treatment failure at 12 months: from 21% to 43%; an adjusted hazard ratio of 2.47 (95% CI 1.05 to 5.85).[4]

Several problems exist with any discussion of the diagnosis of GORD:

- *GORD can exist when the endoscopy is normal.* Of patients with a final diagnosis of GORD, only 60% have endoscopic evidence of oesophageal inflammation.[5] In primary care, it is likely that even fewer will have such evidence since only those with more severe symptoms tend to be entered into studies. Options to detect those with GORD but with normal endoscopy include 24-hour oesophageal pH monitoring and 'the omeprazole test' but, in the absence of a gold standard, their accuracy is not clear.
- *Oesophagitis on endoscopy can exist with normal oesophageal pH.* A Swedish study[6] found that 25% of patients with oesophageal erosions had normal oesophageal pH, as did 47% of those with inflammation of the distal oesophagus. There is therefore no clear 'gold standard'.
- *Endoscopists do not agree* on the finding of low-grade oesophagitis. A Danish study found that, while agreement between three endoscopists on the diagnosis of erosive oesophagitis (grades 2–4) was good (kappa 0.68–0.79), agreement on grade 1 was only 0.34–0.47.[7] This latter is only fair to moderate agreement, although better than the agreement you would expect from chance (which gives a kappa of 0).

- *The finding of hiatus hernia* is often erroneously thought to mean that symptoms are due to reflux. In fact, any association is often incidental.[5] It does appear, however, that if oesophagitis is present, it is likely to be more severe if hiatus hernia is also present, and more severe the larger the hiatus hernia.[8]
- *There is a large overlap between heartburn and dyspepsia.* One estimate is that over half the patients in the community with dyspepsia also have heartburn.[9] Furthermore, the reliable diagnosis of one condition does not exclude the existence of the other; 10% of patients with GORD also have peptic ulcers and over half of patients with peptic ulcers report heartburn.[10]

Prevalence in the community

Studies from Minnesota[11] and Finland[12] have given similar results: 20% of adults who responded to a questionnaire reported heartburn and/or regurgitation at least weekly. In Finland, only 16% used medication and only 5.5% had sought medical advice in the last year.

Incidence in primary care

Two to four per cent of all consultations in primary care are for dyspepsia, of which about a quarter are for GORD.[13]

Can the GP diagnose GORD clinically?

The chapter on dyspepsia (see p. 75) gives the value of GPs' clinical diagnosis of GORD in three studies of unselected patients with dyspepsia in primary care. The figures for a GP diagnosis of GORD are shown in Table 23.1.

In other words, the GP can make, and exclude, the diagnosis better than by chance, but only just. If the GP diagnoses GORD, the patient probably still does not have it.

Table 23.1 Value of the clinical assessment in the diagnosis of GORD, where the initial probability of GORD in a patient with dyspepsia is 25%[14–16]

GP's diagnosis	Likelihood ratio	Probability of GORD if diagnosed by the GP (95% CI)
GORD	2.4	37% (33–41%)
Not GORD	0.7	14% (13–16%)

Follow each row from left to right to see how the GP's diagnosis alters the probability of GORD.

What aspects of the history are important?

- Several studies have examined the accuracy of symptoms in the diagnosis of GORD.[17–19] They show that only heartburn and regurgitation are predictive.
- Another study confirmed that belching, traditionally associated with GORD, occurred as frequently in those with functional dyspepsia.[20]
- An attempt has been made to improve on this poor performance by using a formal questionnaire. The initial study by the authors of the questionnaire was positive,[21] but a subsequent larger study on primary care patients found it was no better than GPs' clinical judgement and neither was particularly

useful in the diagnosis of GORD in this group of patients, in a situation designed, as closely as possible, to represent normal practice.[22] Gastroscopy and the response to a proton pump inhibitor were the gold standard for the diagnosis of GORD. The details are as follows: a score >7 on the questionnaire had an LR+ of 1.5 (95% CI 1.2 to 1.7) and an LR– of 0.6 (95% CI 0.5 to 0.8) against the gold standard of oesophagitis on endoscopy. When the diagnosis was made on a positive endoscopy or a positive omeprazole test, the likelihood ratios were not significantly different.

The questionnaire is included here, not in order to encourage its formal use, but to see what questions the GP might ask in an informal way:

The Carlsson–Dent reflux disease questionnaire

(Reprinted from 'The usefulness of a structured questionnaire in the assessment of symptomatic gastroesophageal reflux disease' by Carlsson R, Dent J, Bolling-Sternevald E et al. *Scandinavian Journal of Gastroenterology*, www.tandf.no/gastro, 1998;33:1023–1029, by permission of Taylor & Francis AS.)

Please answer the following questions by ticking 1 box only, except for question 3, where you must tick one box for each statement.

1. Which one of these four statements BEST DESCRIBES the main discomfort you get in your stomach or chest?
   - A burning feeling rising from your stomach or lower chest up towards your neck (5)
   - Feelings of sickness or nausea (0)
   - Pain in the middle of your chest when you swallow (2)
   - None of the above (0)

2. Having chosen one of the above, please now choose which one of the next three statements BEST DESCRIBES the timing of your main discomfort?
   - Any time, not made better or worse by taking food (–2)
   - Most often within 2 hours of taking food (3)
   - Always at a particular time of day or night without any relationship to food (0)

3. How do the following affect your main discomfort?
   - Larger than usual meals
   - Food rich in fat
   - Strongly flavoured or spicy food

   For each, score (1) if worsened, (–1) if improved or (0) if no effect/unsure.

4. Which one of the following BEST DESCRIBES the effect of indigestion medicines on your main discomfort?
   - No benefit (0)
   - Definite relief within 15 minutes (3)
   - Definite relief after 15 minutes (0)
   - Not taken (0)

5. Which one of the following BEST DESCRIBES the effect of lying flat, stooping or bending on your main discomfort?
   - No effect (0)
   - Brings it on or makes it worse (1)
   - Gives relief (–1)
   - Don't know/doesn't apply (0)

6. Which one of the following BEST DESCRIBES the effect of lifting or straining (or any other activity that makes you breath heavily) on your main discomfort?
   - No effect (0)
   - Brings it on or makes it worse (1)
   - Gives relief (–1)
   - Don't know/doesn't apply (0)

7. If food or acid tasting liquid returns to your throat or mouth, what effect does it have on your main discomfort?
   - No effect (0)
   - Brings it on or makes it worse (2)
   - Gives relief (0)
   - Don't know/doesn't apply (0)

   Score each answer according to the figure in brackets against it.

Warning

Patients and doctors do not agree on the meaning of 'heartburn'. Carlsson and colleagues, in their study of Swedish and UK patients,[21] found that, of those patients who said they suffered from 'a burning feeling rising from the stomach or lower chest up towards the neck', only 32% also said that they had heartburn. Conversely, 10% of those who denied that they had the 'burning feeling' described above, said they had heartburn.

Can GORD exist without heartburn and/or reflux?

Yes. The Montreal definition[1] stresses:
  (a) that epigastric pain can be the major symptom of GORD
  (b) that the chest pain of GORD can resemble cardiac pain without traditional heartburn and reflux
  (c) that the complications of GORD (stricture, Barrett's oesophagus) can be found in patients without heartburn or reflux.

How can heartburn be distinguished from ischaemic chest pain?

The problem tends to arise only in someone with no previous history of either. A patient in whom a pattern is already established will recognise whether this is the same as, or different from, their symptoms of angina or heartburn. In a patient in whom the chest pain is new, the distinction between the two can usually be made on the symptoms: heartburn tends to be related to meals, brought on by bending or lying down and be relieved by food or antacid. Ischaemic pain tends to be related to exertion or emotion, relieved by rest or glyceryl trinitrate (see *Angina*, p. 487). However, the existence of exercise-induced reflux complicates the situation.[1]

Does GORD cause symptoms outside the GI tract?

Yes. Chronic cough, chronic laryngitis and asthma are associated with GORD.[1] It is not clear whether the association is because of aspiration or via a neurogenic reflex. However, the diagnosis should not be hard, for two reasons:
- Extra-oesophageal syndromes are likely to be accompanied by overt symptoms of reflux and heartburn.
- GORD is unlikely to be the sole cause of the cough, laryngitis or asthma. Rather, it may trigger an exacerbation of symptoms in a patient who already has those conditions.

Does a prompt response to a proton pump inhibitor confirm a clinical diagnosis of GORD?

There is a strong clinical impression that GORD responds so promptly to a proton pump inhibitor (PPI) that this response can be used to confirm a clinical diagnosis of GORD. A study from Amsterdam in 1997[23] reported that a response to omeprazole 40 mg daily for 2 weeks was as sensitive and specific as pH monitoring in the diagnosis of GORD and a simple and inexpensive tool for the diagnosis of GORD. If the test was positive, the probability became 68% and if negative, it became 37%. However, the pre-test probability of GORD in the study was 55% so an improvement to 68% is unimpressive. The pre-test probability that this was not GORD was 45% so a decrease of this to 37% is equally unimpressive.

A recent meta-analysis of 15 studies[24] found that the test was capable of slightly refining the probabilities in the correct direction. The authors found a sensitivity of 78%, a specificity of 54%, hence an LR+ of 1.7, and LR− of 0.4. The implications of these figures are shown in Table 23.2. The results are statistically significant, but clinically are unlikely to be enough to alter management.

Table 23.2 The value of response to a PPI in the diagnosis of GORD, where the initial probability of GORD in a patient with dyspepsia is 25%[14–16]

Trial of PPI	Likelihood ratio	Probability of GORD after the trial of a PPI
Response	1.7	38%
No response	0.4	11%

Follow each row from left to right to see how the response to a PPI alters the probability of GORD.

Example

A 60-year-old man presents with an intermittent burning epigastric pain rising up into the chest that is relieved by food. It has been present on most days for the last 2 months and he has not previously suffered from it. There is no obvious precipitating cause.

Because of his age, and the persistence of new, unexplained symptoms, he is referred for urgent endoscopy, which is normal. The endoscopist recommends that he be managed for non-ulcer dyspepsia.

The GP remembers that the pre-test probability of GORD in someone with dyspepsia is about 20%. This is increased to 37% because of the good history of heartburn (Fig. 23.1) but is halved by the negative endoscopy. That still leaves a probability of GORD of 18.5%. The GP prescribes omeprazole 40 mg daily for 2 weeks. Symptoms resolve completely after 5 days but return 2 weeks after the end of the course. This positive test means that the probability of GORD is now about 28% (Fig. 23.2). Twenty-four-hour pH monitoring is not available locally.

The GP shares with the patient the diagnostic difficulty – he has an acid-related condition but whether it is functional dyspepsia or reflux is impossible to say. They decide not to test for *H. pylori* on the grounds that the small benefit from eradication in functional dyspepsia is outweighed by the risk of worsening GORD. The GP gives lifestyle advice appropriate for GORD and agrees to give omeprazole as needed at the lowest dose that contains symptoms.

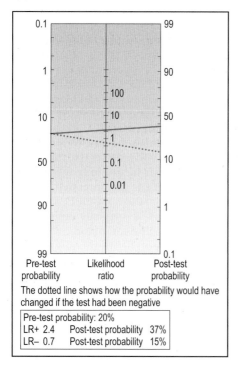

The dotted line shows how the probability would have changed if the test had been negative

Pre-test probability: 20%	
LR+ 2.4	Post-test probability 37%
LR– 0.7	Post-test probability 15%

Figure 23.1 The probability of oesophagitis before and after the detailed clinical assessment in the example above.

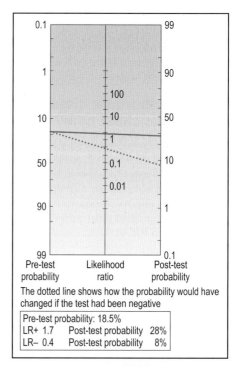

The dotted line shows how the probability would have changed if the test had been negative

Pre-test probability: 18.5%	
LR+ 1.7	Post-test probability 28%
LR– 0.4	Post-test probability 8%

Figure 23.2 The probability of oesophagitis before and after the omeprazole test in the example above.

Intermittent claudication

25

Use the history to distinguish the following:

(a) *Intermittent claudication*: pain in the calf, or occasionally buttock or thigh, which occurs on walking and is relieved by rest. It occurs at the same walking distance each time (see 'Peripheral vascular disease' below).[1]

(b) *Acute deep vein thrombosis*: pain usually in the calf which is worse on walking but still present at rest and associated with calf tenderness and swelling (see *The swollen leg*, p. 247).

(c) *Venous claudication*: usually due to past proximal deep vein thrombosis, it is described as a feeling that the whole leg will burst. It subsides only slowly with rest but faster if the leg is elevated.

(d) *Lumbar spinal stenosis*: poorly localised pain and weakness in one or both legs that is variable from day to day, which worsens if the spine is extended (as in walking or standing) and improves if the spine is flexed (as in sitting).

(e) *Joint or soft tissue problems* (muscle, tendons or ligaments): pain localised to the affected area and reproduced by moving the affected joint or tensing the affected muscle.

PERIPHERAL VASCULAR DISEASE (PVD)

KEY FACTS

- Classical intermittent claudication is a powerful predictor of the presence of PVD. Peripheral vascular disease may also present as atypical exertional leg pain or as rest pain or as ulceration of the foot.
- Absent foot pulses are a strong predictor of PVD. If the history is also suggestive, the diagnosis has been 'ruled in'. Other predictors (a femoral artery bruit, a cooler limb on the affected side and a prolonged venous filling time) may be useful if the foot pulses are present, although they are less sensitive tests than the foot pulses.
- The importance of the detection of PVD lies not only in the diagnosis of the cause of a patient's symptoms but in the opportunity it presents for the prevention of cardiovascular disease in all its manifestations.

A PRACTICAL APPROACH

- ⋆ Clarify the exact symptoms, in relation to timing, in relation to walking and what relieves the pain.
- ⋆ Ask about other risk factors, symptoms or conditions which are related to PVD (e.g. smoking, hypertension, diabetes, coronary heart disease).
- ⋆ Examine the leg and foot pulses and palpate the abdomen for an aortic aneurysm.
- ⋆ Measure the ankle brachial index (ABI) in all in whom you suspect PVD.
- ⋆ If PVD is confirmed by the above, assess the patient's risk of cardiovascular disease and manage accordingly.
- ⋆ Refer all who are sufficiently troubled by the claudication or whose leg is at risk.

Prevalence in the population

Peripheral vascular disease is present in 17% of people in Scotland aged 55–74.[2] Of these, 26% have intermittent claudication, i.e. 4.5% of the population aged 55–74. In this study, PVD was defined as an ABI <0.90. A study from the Netherlands found that PVD was present in 12.4% of people aged 40 to 78, of whom 69% were asymptomatic.[3]

Prevalence in primary care and barriers to diagnosis

A study from Minnesota found that 29% of older primary care attenders (age ≥70 or age ≥50 if they had diabetes or had smoked) had PVD as indicated by an ABI <0.90.[4] In 44% of these patients, PVD had not previously been diagnosed. In those in whom the diagnosis had already been made, 83% of the patients were aware of the diagnosis but only 49% of their current physicians were. The importance of this finding is that the detection of PVD, associated as it is with other manifestations of cardiovascular disease, allows preventative measures to be set in place before the development of symptoms. The Minnesota study reflects this. While 71% of the patients with known cardiovascular disease (CVD) were taking antiplatelet medication, only 54% of those with known PVD were and only 33% of those in whom PVD was a new discovery.

Ouriel, in an editorial, outlines the chain of events that leads to under-detection of PVD: doctors do not routinely ask about leg pains; even if they do, most patients with PVD do not have classic intermittent claudication; palpation of peripheral pulses is rarely performed; and even when it is, few GPs proceed to measurement of the ABI.[5]

Patients with asymptomatic PVD have a risk of CVD that is comparable to those with intermittent claudication.[6]

Does the history reliably indicate the diagnosis?

This question divides into three parts.

1. Is it possible to obtain a clear and reproducible history of intermittent claudication?

Yes. The essentials of the classical history have been encapsulated in the Edinburgh Claudication Questionnaire (Table 25.1), which has a sensitivity of 91% and a specificity of 99% *for intermittent claudication* (not for PVD) as determined by a physician on clinical assessment,[8] giving an LR+ of 130 and an LR– of 0.09.

In other words, the Edinburgh Claudication Questionnaire gives few false negatives and even fewer false positives, in deciding whether leg pain is intermittent claudication.

2. Does the history of intermittent claudication reliably indicate PVD?

No. There are too many other conditions which give similar symptoms. The history of intermittent claudication only moves the probability modestly in the direction of the diagnosis of PVD with an LR+ 3.3 (95% CI 2.3 to 4.8) (Table 25.2).[9]

3. Does the absence of intermittent claudication exclude the diagnosis of PVD?

No. The absence of claudication is virtually useless in excluding mild PVD. Using an ABI cut-

---

Table 25.1 Edinburgh Claudication Questionnaire[7]

Question	Positive answer
Do you get a pain or discomfort in your leg(s) when you walk?	Yes
Does this pain ever begin when you are standing still or sitting?	No
Do you get it if you walk uphill or hurry?	Yes
What happens to it if you stand still?	Usually disappears in 10 minutes or less
Where do you get this pain or discomfort?	Calf – definite claudication Thigh or buttock – atypical claudication Elsewhere – not claudication

A positive result is when all answers indicate claudication.

Table 25.2 Value of the symptom of intermittent claudication in the diagnosis of moderate to severe PVD, based on the risk in a Scotsman in late middle age who has *not* presented with leg pain[9]

Probability of PVD before taking the history	History	Likelihood ratio (95% CI)	Probability of PVD after the history (95% CI)
17%	Positive	3.3 (95% CI 2.3–4.8)	40%
	Negative	0.6 (95% CI 0.4–0.8)	11%

Follow each row from left to right to see how the presence or absence of intermittent claudication alters the probability of PVD.

off of <0.95 for the diagnosis of PVD, the LR– is 0.9 (95% CI 0.8 to 1.0). It is a little more useful in arguing against the presence of moderate to severe PVD (LR– 0.6 (95% CI 0.4 to 0.8)) (Table 25.2).[9]

If the patient has exertional leg pain which does not meet the criteria for intermittent claudication, could it be due to PVD?

Yes. Two studies from the USA compared patients with and without low ABIs.[10,11] A low ABI was significantly associated not only with classical symptoms of intermittent claudication but also with atypical exertional symptoms and with pain in the leg at rest. The atypical exertional symptoms included pain which did not show the typical timing or did not include the calf. Patients with critical leg ischaemia tend to feel rest pain in the foot rather than the leg. The pain is relieved if the legs are allowed to hang down, thereby improving the arterial flow.

Are risk factors for PVD important in the assessment?

Yes. They alter the probability of PVD in the patient under consideration, and so affect the post-test probability once the clinical assessment has been completed (Table 25.3). A history of ischaemic heart disease in a 60-year-old English patient, for instance, raises the probability of PVD from a baseline of 15% (midway between the Netherlands and Scotland) to 29%. This becomes the pre-test probability to which the likelihood ratios for the clinical assessment can be applied.

Combining symptoms and risk factors

A study from Dutch primary care has developed a decision rule which combines the result of the Edinburgh Claudication Questionnaire with a risk factor score:[13]

- *score 1* for each of: male sex; age 60–64; hypertension (adequately treated); hypercholesterolaemia
- *score 2* for each of: age 65–69; hypertension (not adequately treated)
- *score 3* for each of: age 70–74; ever smoked; a positive Edinburgh questionnaire
- *score 4* for: age 75–79
- *score 5* for age 80–84
- *score 6* for age ≥85
- *score 8* for current smoking.

The probability of PVD, as defined by an ABI <0.9, is shown in Table 25.4.

Does the examination reliably indicate the diagnosis?

Yes, but only if it is positive. Absence of foot pulses is a strong indicator of PVD (Table 25.5), although some patients without PVD have absent pulses. The dorsalis pedis (DP) pulse is impalpable in 8.1% of people without PVD, and the posterior tibial (PT) pulse in 2.9%, although the pulse can usually be identified by Doppler. See below for more discussion of the different predictive values of the foot pulses. In 0.7% of healthy people, both DP and PT pulses are absent. Conversely, some patients with PVD have palpable pulses, although they may disappear on exertion.

If the history suggests PVD, the finding of palpable pulses does not rule the diagnosis out; ABI measurement is needed.

The findings of different studies give the ranges of statistics in Table 25.5.[14]

Table 25.3 Risk factors for PVD and how they alter the probability that the patient has PVD, based on a baseline risk of 15%[12]

Risk factor	Present or absent	Likelihood ratio	Probability of PVD according to whether the risk factor is present or absent
Sex	Male	1.4	20%
	Female	0.7	11%
Age	Age ≥60	1.7	23%
	Age <60	0.4	7%
History of ischaemic heart disease	Yes	2.3	29%
	No	0.7	11%
History of cerebrovascular disease	Yes	3.5	38%
	No	0.9	14%
Diabetes	Yes	2.2	28%
	No	0.9	14%
Smoker	Yes	1.2	17%
	No	0.6	10%
Work involves little physical exertion	Yes	1.3	19%
	No	0.6	10%

Note. These risk factors are not independent of each other and their likelihood ratios cannot therefore be applied one after the other to reach a final figure for the probability of PVD. However, the more risk factors are present the more likely it is that the patient will have PVD.

Table 25.4 The probability of PVD according to the score using the Dutch decision rule[13]

Score	Probability of PVD
0–3	14.5%
13 or above	71%

Intermediate scores gave intermediate probabilities between those extremes.

Measuring the venous filling time

1. Lie the patient supine and identify a vein in the foot which stands out above the level of the skin on the affected leg.
2. Raise the leg to 45° for 1 minute.
3. Sit the patient up with the legs dangling over the side of the couch.
4. Measure the time before that vein starts to rise above the level of the skin. The test is positive if the time is >20 seconds.

Other points

- Note that other traditional signs have little value in the diagnosis. The capillary refill test, a foot that is blue or purple, the absence of hair on the lower leg or the finding of atrophic skin are weak predictors of PVD and add nothing to the much more powerful signs above.
- The finding of an absent pulse is highly reproducible, i.e. different examiners agree in their findings (kappa = 0.92). However, the finding of a *reduced* pulse leads to major disagreement between examiners (kappa = 0.01 for the popliteal and 0.15 for the femoral).[14] It is wiser to record a pulse as present or absent.
- In using the likelihood ratios in Table 25.5 in a patient who has more than one sign, it is essential to know whether the signs are independent of each other. Only if they are can the likelihood ratios be applied one after the other (see p. xxiii). Multivariate analysis shows that absent pulses, a prolonged venous filling time, a unilaterally cool limb and a femoral artery bruit are independent predictors of the presence of PVD.[14] However, the negative likelihood ratios of the femoral bruit, the prolonged venous filling time and the cool limb are so close to 1 that they can be omitted from the examination

Table 25.5 The probabilities of PVD according to the results of the physical examination, based on a probability, before the examination, of 15%

Finding	Whether positive or negative	Likelihood ratio	Probability of PVD after the examination
Foot pulses[14]	Abnormal	9.0–45	61–89%
	Normal	0.3–0.4	5–7%
Femoral pulse[12]	Absent	6.3	53%
	Present	0.9	14%
Femoral artery bruit[14]	Present	5.7	50%
	Absent	0.7	11%
Affected leg temperature compared to the other[14]	Cooler	5.8	51%
	The same	0.9	14%
Wounds or sores on the foot or toes[12]	Present	5.9	51%
	Absent	0.98	15%
Venous filling time[14]	Abnormal	3.6–4.6	39–45%
	Normal	0.8	12%

PVD was defined as an ABI <0.9, except in the study of the venous filling time in which PVD was diagnosed as ABI <0.5.

without loss, unless the diagnosis is in doubt. Then, *if they are found*, they shift the probability in favour of the diagnosis because of their high positive likelihood ratios.

● The pattern of the absent pulses indicates the site of obstruction. An absent femoral pulse indicates aorto-iliac obstruction and correlates with pain in the buttock and thigh as well as the calf. The absence of the popliteal and both foot pulses indicates femoro-popliteal obstruction, in which pain is confined to the calf. The absence of the foot pulses only indicates peroneo-tibial obstruction. Pain may be felt in the foot or not at all. It is a pattern almost confined to diabetes and the rare thromboangiitis obliterans.

Is an absent dorsalis pulse significant in the presence of a normal posterior tibial pulse?

Probably not, because of the frequent congenital absence of the dorsalis pedis pulse. A study from California[15] found that the LR+ and LR– for an absent or markedly reduced dorsalis pedis pulse were only 1.8 and 0.7 against likelihood ratios of 7.9 and 0.3 for an abnormal posterior tibial pulse.

Is the ABI diagnostic of PVD?

Yes, largely so, but the test must be performed properly (see box).

The accuracy of the test depends on the cut-off value used. With a cut-off of 0.97, the ABI is 96–97% sensitive and 94–100% specific for occlusion or at least 50% stenosis on angiography. If the more usual cut-off of 0.90 is used, the sensitivity will be lower (90%) but the specificity higher (98%) (LR+ 45; LR– 0.1).[4,14] Most patients with claudication have an ABI <0.8 and those with rest pain have an ABI <0.5. Gangrene tends to occur with an ABI <0.20.[8]

Measuring the ankle brachial index

1. Lie the patient supine.
2. Measure the systolic pressure in both arms in the usual way. If they differ, use the higher.
3. Put the cuff about 3 cm above the ankle on each side, inflate it and, using a handheld Doppler, measure the pressure at the point when the Doppler detects the return of the pulse. Measure the pressure in both posterior tibial and dorsalis pedis arteries. Use the higher.
4. The ABI is the ankle systolic pressure divided by the brachial systolic pressure.

Notes:

● A Doppler must be used to estimate the systolic pressure at the ankle but the method used to measure the brachial pressure does not seem to matter.[16]

● Two tests should be performed and the average used. There is an intra-observer variation of 12% when performed by doctors and nurses.[17]

● If the arteries at the ankle are non-compressible because of calcification, an abnormally high ABI will be obtained, usually >1.3. The test is invalid.

Example

A man aged 65 with a history of ischaemic heart disease presents with pain in the left leg on walking. His risk factors give him an initial probability of PVD of about 30% (see above). His history meets the criteria for intermittent claudication, raising the probability of PVD to 59% (Fig. 25.1).

However, after searching for his foot pulses carefully, his GP locates them. She considers them to be weak and is tempted to use this as evidence in favour of the diagnosis of PVD, but remembers in time that determination of weakness is too subjective to be useful. The presence of the pulses reduces the

probability of PVD to 30% (Fig. 25.2). He has no femoral bruit and the leg and foot looks and feels normal, but she knows that the negative likelihood ratios for these signs are too close to 1 to be useful.

She checks for other possible diagnoses and finds none; the calf is not tender, there is no arthritis or soft tissue tenderness. She arranges for her nurse to measure the ABI and is not surprised when the result proves to be 0.7 in the left leg, 0.8 in the right. His probability of PVD rises to 95% (Fig. 25.3) and she concludes that the diagnosis has been made.

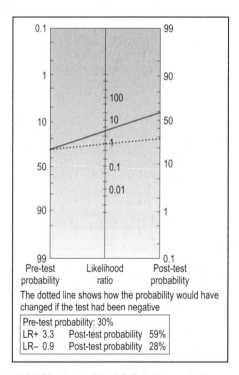

The dotted line shows how the probability would have changed if the test had been negative

Pre-test probability: 30%	
LR+ 3.3	Post-test probability 59%
LR– 0.9	Post-test probability 28%

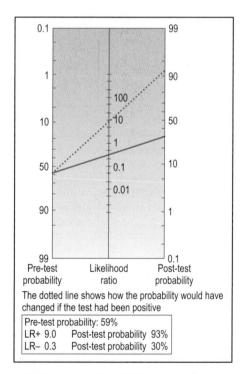

The dotted line shows how the probability would have changed if the test had been positive

Pre-test probability: 59%	
LR+ 9.0	Post-test probability 93%
LR– 0.3	Post-test probability 30%

Figure 25.1 The probability of PVD before and after obtaining the history of intermittent claudication in the example above.

Figure 25.2 The probability of PVD before and after the examination of the pulses in the example above.

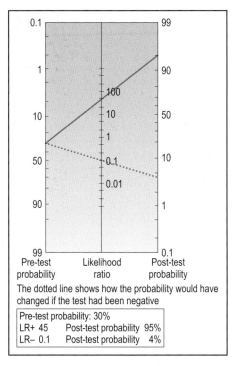

The dotted line shows how the probability would have changed if the test had been negative

Pre-test probability: 30%		
LR+ 45	Post-test probability	95%
LR− 0.1	Post-test probability	4%

Figure 25.3 The probability of PVD before and after the finding of a reduced ABI in the example on p. 168.

REFERENCES

1. Montgomery P, Gardner A. *The clinical utility of a six-minute walk test in peripheral arterial occlusive disease patients.* J Am Geriatr Soc 1998;46: 706–711.

2. Fowkes F, Housley E, Cawood E, et al. *Edinburgh Artery Study: prevalence of asymptomatic and symptomatic peripheral arterial disease in the general population.* Int J Epidemiol 1991;20:384–392.

3. Hooi J, Stoffers H, Kester A, et al. *Peripheral arterial disease: prognostic value of signs, symptoms, and the ankle-brachial index.* Med Decis Making 2002;22:99–107.

4. Hirsch A, Criqui M, Treat-Jacobson D, et al. *Peripheral arterial disease detection, awareness, and treatment in primary care.* JAMA 2001;286:1317–1324.

5. Ouriel K. *Detection of peripheral arterial disease in primary care.* JAMA 2001;286:1380–1381.

6. Hooi J, Stoffers H, Kester A, et al. *Risk factors and cardiovascular diseases associated with asymptomatic peripheral arterial occlusive disease. The Limburg PAOD Study.* Scand J Prim Health Care 1998;16:177–182.

7. Burns P, Gough S, Bradbury A. *Management of peripheral arterial disease in primary care.* BMJ 2003;326: 584–588.

8. Leng G, Fowkes F. *The Edinburgh Claudication Questionnaire: an improved version of the WHO/Rose Questionnaire for use in epidemiological surveys.* J Clin Epidemiol 1992;45:1101–1109.

9. Khan N, Rahim S, Anand S, et al. *Does the clinical examination predict lower extremity peripheral arterial disease?* JAMA 2006;295: 537–546.

10. McDermott M, Mehta S, Greenland P. *Exertional leg symptoms other than intermittent claudication are common in peripheral arterial disease.* Arch Intern Med 1999;159: 387–392.

11. McDermott M, Greenland P, Liu K, et al. *Leg symptoms in peripheral arterial disease.* JAMA 2001;286:1599–1606.

12. Stoffers H, Kester A, Kaiser V, et al. *Diagnostic value of signs and symptoms associated with peripheral arterial occlusive disease seen in general practice.* Med Decis Making 1997;17:61–70.

13. Bendermacher B, Teijink J, Willigendael E, et al. *Symptomatic peripheral arterial disease: the value of a validated questionnaire and a clinical decision rule.* Br J Gen Pract 2006;56: 932–944.

14. McGee S, Boyko E. *Physical examination and chronic lower-extremity ischemia.* Arch Intern Med 1998;158: 1357–1364.

15. Criqui M, Fronek A, Klauber M, et al. *The sensitivity, specificity, and predictive value of traditional clinical evaluation of peripheral arterial disease: results from noninvasive testing in a defined population.* Circulation 1985;3: 516–522.

16. Gardner A, Montgomery P. *Comparison of three blood pressure methods used for determining ankle/ brachial index in patients with intermittent claudication.* Angiology 1998;49:723–728.

17. Kaiser V, Kester A, Stoffers H, et al. *The influence of experience on the reproducibility of the ankle-brachial systolic pressure ratio in peripheral arterial occlusive disease.* Eur J Vasc Endovasc Surg 1999;18:25–29.

Lower urinary tract symptoms (LUTS) in men

26

KEY FACTS

- Lower urinary tract symptoms (LUTS) in men is a syndrome defined by symptoms. It is usually due to benign prostatic hyperplasia (BPH) but a small proportion of patients have chronic prostatitis, previous prostatic surgery, bladder abnormalities or a neurological cause for their symptoms.
- Symptoms correlate poorly with prostate size and with urinary flow rates. It is the symptoms that affect the patient's quality of life and which should guide management.
- Objective measures (e.g. prostate size and urine flow rate) are useful in predicting the likely need for surgery and in guiding the choice of drugs.

A PRACTICAL APPROACH

- ✱ Ask all eight questions of the International Prostate Symptom Score (IPSS). Men may not volunteer sensitive information (e.g. about urge incontinence) unless asked. Score the answers but, as well as the total score, note separately how bothered the patient is by his symptoms.
- ✱ Ask about pain, both during micturition and independent of it. Get the patient to be specific about where the pain is felt. If pain is significant, refer for an assessment of the possibility of prostatitis.
- ✱ Ascertain whether nocturia is the dominant symptom. If so, ask the patient to keep a 24-hour voiding diary to look for nocturnal polyuria.
- ✱ Examine the prostate digitally and the abdomen for retention.
- ✱ Examine the urine and send a midstream urine (MSU) for microscopy and culture, and blood for a serum creatinine.
- ✱ If the clinical picture is of uncomplicated BPH, no further attempts at diagnosis are needed, although the management of the patient may necessitate referral.

Prevalence

Approximately 25% of men aged 40 and over have lower urinary tract symptoms.[1] The prevalence increases with age so that 60% of men in their 60s report symptoms, compared to 14% in their 40s.[2]

LUTS is not to be confused with two other related entities:
- benign prostatic hypertrophy (BPH), a histological diagnosis found increasingly after the age of 30 so that it is present in 88% of men in their 80s[2]

■ the clinical finding of an enlarged prostate, found in 20% of men in their 60s and 43% of men in their 80s.[2]

While there is an association between symptoms and both the finding of an enlarged gland and the histological finding of hyperplasia, they are not necessarily associated. Symptoms occur in normal sized glands and enlarged hyperplastic glands are found in men without symptoms.

A further limitation of the traditional concept that symptoms are the result of bladder outflow obstruction due to an enlarged prostate is that symptoms correlate poorly with reduced urinary flow rates.[3]

Initial probabilities

It is tempting to assume that chronic LUTS, with no atypical features, is always due to BPH. However, a study of men aged 40–79 randomly selected from the community, the Olmsted County Study of Urinary Symptoms and Health Status among Men, found that 13.4% of men had conditions other than BPH that might give rise to LUTS:[4]

■ previous prostate cancer or surgery 7.8%
■ back surgery 4.8%
■ bladder surgery 1.3%
■ neurological conditions 1.4%.

These conditions were all evident from the history and their diagnosis will not be considered here.

Other possible diagnoses

■ *Bladder cancer or stone.* A Dutch study of 750 men with LUTS found 3 with bladder tumours and 49 with bladder stones (of whom only 1 needed treatment).[5] The study found no clinical predictors which might have enabled the GP to detect those men in whom BPH was not the cause of the symptoms.

■ *Chronic prostatitis* is suggested by urinary symptoms (dysuria, frequency, hesitancy, urgency, weak stream) accompanied by pain in the rectum, perineum, penis, testicles, lower abdomen or back, and pain on ejaculation (see below). The patient might feel unwell, with malaise and fatigue. The Olmsted County Study found that 2% of men aged 40 to 79 had prostatitis-like symptoms.[6] Among men aged 40 to 49, 14% had LUTS, which meant that roughly 1 in 7 of those had prostatitis-like symptoms, suggesting that prostatitis was the cause of their symptoms. In older men, the 2% with prostatitis are swamped by the greater numbers with BPH. By the age of 70 and over, fewer than 1 in 15 with LUTS has prostatitis-like symptoms.

The presence of LUTS is defined by the history

Symptoms are divided into voiding symptoms and filling symptoms.

Voiding symptoms:
■ hesitancy
■ weak stream
■ straining to void
■ terminal dribbling
■ a sensation of incomplete emptying
■ double voiding
■ overflow incontinence
■ acute retention.

Filling symptoms:
■ nocturia
■ frequency
■ urgency
■ urge incontinence.

Several *symptom scores* have been validated. Of these, the IPSS is the most commonly used and the simplest (see box opposite). This is a convenient way to record symptoms in a way that can be compared with future assessments. It allows the patient's symptoms to be graded according to severity as follows:[2]

■ 1–7: mild
■ 8–19: moderate
■ 20–35: severe.

In addition, the overriding question 8, about the effect of symptoms on the quality of life, should guide the clinician in management, since the syndrome is defined by its symptoms, not by the underlying pathology.

The International Prostate Symptom Score (IPSS)

1. Incomplete emptying
Over the past month, how often have you had a sensation of not emptying your bladder completely after you have finished urinating?

2. Frequency
Over the past month, how often have you had to urinate again less than 2 hours after you finished urinating?

3. Intermittency
Over the past month, how often have you found you stopped and started again several times when you urinated?

4. Urgency
Over the past month, how often have you found it difficult to postpone urination or felt sudden urges to urinate?

5. Weak stream
Over the past month, how often have you had a weak urinary stream?

6. Straining
Over the past month, how often have you had to push or strain to begin urination?

7. Nocturia
Over the past month, how many times did you typically get up to urinate from the time you went to bed at night to the time you got up in the morning?

8. Quality of life
If you were to spend the rest of your life with urinary conditions just the way they are now, how would you feel about it?

Score each question as follows: 'not at all' = 0; 'less than one time in 5' = 1; 'less than half the time' = 2; 'about half the time' = 3; 'more than half the time' = 4; 'almost always' = 5.

For question 7 the scores are: 'none' = 0; 'once' = 1; 'twice' = 2; 'three times' = 3; 'four times' = 4; 'five times or more' = 5.

For question 8 the scores are: 'delighted' = 0; 'pleased' = 1; 'mostly satisfied' = 2; 'no strong feelings either way' = 3; 'mostly dissatisfied' = 4; 'unhappy' = 5; 'terrible' = 6.

Three cautions in interpreting these symptoms

1. Nocturia. The symptom of nocturia may be misleading because of the phenomenon of nocturnal polyuria. A patient who fails to concentrate his urine at night may be troubled by nocturia without having any true lower urinary tract symptoms. It occurs in renal insufficiency, diabetes mellitus, diabetes insipidus, heart failure, leg oedema, sleep apnoea, and with certain drugs (digoxin, phenytoin, lithium, diuretics and excess vitamin D) as well as in those who drink too much fluid in the evening.

Suspect it in those who have nocturia out of proportion to other symptoms, or who report nocturia three or more times a night.

Confirm it with a 24-hour voiding diary, recording both the number of times urine is passed, and the volume each time. Nocturnal polyuria exists if >35% of the total 24-hour output is passed at night.[7]

2. Not all symptoms cause equal distress. A study of Swedish men found that a complaint of incontinence, not explicitly asked about in the IPSS, was associated with greater distress than any other symptom, while men could cope quite well with hesitancy and straining.[8]

3. Effect on the quality of life. The fact that there is only one 'quality of life' question in the IPSS means that the score tends to measure the physical facts of the patient's urinary symptoms rather than the emotional impact. As part of the Olmsted County Study, the impact of urinary symptoms on physical and mental aspects of health was measured.[9] Men were most affected by (in order of importance):

- role limitation due to physical problems
- fatigue
- role limitation due to emotional problems
- general perception of their health.

A clinician who focuses on the physical symptoms of LUTS may miss the impact they have on the patient's life and well-being.

Pain and discomfort in the distinction between prostatitis and BPH

* Ask whether the patient has pain, either when passing urine, or independently of micturition.

A study from the USA has defined the National Institutes of Health Chronic Prostatitis Symptom Index.[10] The authors caution against using it as a diagnostic tool; indeed the groups in which it was validated were not chosen randomly, and the problem of defining a gold standard for the diagnosis of prostatitis has not been solved.

Table 26.1 The value of symptoms in the diagnosis of prostatitis compared to BPH, based on a hypothetical pre-test probability of prostatitis of 10% in men with LUTS

Site, or timing, of pain or discomfort	Positive likelihood ratio (95% CI)	Probability of prostatitis
Tip of penis (other than when urinating)	22 (5.4–88)	78%
Perineum	8.9 (4.4–18)	52%
Testicles	4.5 (2.5–8.1)	35%
Lower abdomen	4.1 (2.7–6.5)	34%
On or after ejaculation	3.5 (2.4–5.2)	27%
Dysuria	1.9 (1.4–2.5)	20%

Likelihood ratios calculated from data from the work of Litwin and colleagues.[10]

However, examination of the performance of the index in men with a clinical diagnosis of prostatitis, compared to those with a diagnosis of BPH, gives some idea of the value of individual pain symptoms in the diagnosis of prostatitis. The absence of any of these symptoms does not argue hugely against the diagnosis of prostatitis and so negative likelihood ratios have not been given (Table 26.1).

Other lower urinary tract symptoms are common in both groups. Patients with prostatitis in the study were considerably more bothered by their symptoms than were those with BPH.

Diagnosis of prostatitis is difficult and important. If there are significant pain symptoms other than during micturition, and if the patient is sufficiently bothered by them, referral is needed. For more details of the diagnosis of chronic prostatitis, see *Dysuria and other acute urinary symptoms in men*, page 87.

The examination

Digital rectal examination allows the assessment of prostate size (as well as detecting changes suggestive of cancer (see *Prostate cancer*, p. 469). Prostate size correlates, though not completely, with the presence of BPH and the probability of progression towards the need for surgery. The finding of an enlarged prostate might also influence the choice of a 5α-reductase inhibitor.

A review from Texas has shown that the examiner tends to underestimate prostate size, especially when the prostate volume is >30 ml.[11]

The prostate may be tender in chronic prostatitis but an absence of tenderness does not argue against the diagnosis.

Abdominal examination is needed for the detection of the enlarged bladder of acute or chronic retention. The former will be acutely tender in a man in pain; the latter will be more flaccid and easily missed.

Investigations

Urine analysis. Testing for protein, microscopy for cells and culture are recommended to detect those men in whom LUTS indicate a urinary infection.[2] Testing for haematuria is unrewarding. It is common in BPH, and one large study found that it did not correlate with intravesical pathology.[5]

Serum creatinine. Eleven per cent of men presenting with LUTS have a raised serum creatinine, but in most cases it is due to nephropathy secondary to diabetes or hypertension.[12] In those with no underlying cause for renal impairment, an elevated serum creatinine does not correlate with severity of LUTS. Only in men referred for surgery are a clinically significant number found with renal insufficiency secondary to lower urinary tract obstruction.

Prostate specific antigen (see below).

Imaging of the urinary tract. There is no place for this in primary care in a patient with typical LUTS and a normal serum creatinine; indeed its value is doubtful in secondary care (other than transrectal ultrasound) in the absence of a residual urine.[2]

Uroflowmetry. This provides useful information and correlates well with symptoms.

The maximum urine flow rate gives useful information about which patients are likely to need surgery and who is likely to respond well to it.

Men with a flow rate <10 ml/s are likely to benefit from surgery and those with rates >15 ml/s are not; indeed they are unlikely to have bladder outflow obstruction.[2]

No studies have examined whether patients can perform this test reliably at home, but it does not seem beyond a man of reasonable intelligence, in possession of a measuring jug, marked in millilitres, and a watch. He should understand that he should start to collect the urine once he has reached his maximum flow and should stop before the stream starts to tail off. The same result from repeated measurements would suggest that his technique is reliable.

Other questions to which patients may want answers

What is the chance that the symptoms are due to cancer of the prostate?

Both LUTS and carcinoma of the prostate are common and any occurrence of the two together is likely to be coincidental. There is no evidence that carcinoma of the prostate is more common in men with LUTS than in those without, and in the UK, the prostate specific antigen (PSA) is not part of the work-up of a patient with LUTS, unless the rectal examination suggests a malignant gland.[13]

The UK position is that the PSA in this situation would be screening, not diagnosis, and the PSA does not meet criteria for adoption of a screening test (it has poor sensitivity and specificity, there is no evidence of benefit from the result and there is considerable opportunity for harm) (see *Prostate cancer*, p. 471). Poor specificity is especially likely in BPH where the enlarged gland itself causes a raised PSA.

European guidelines do recommend a PSA for men with LUTS if a diagnosis of prostate cancer

would alter management, but accept that not all urologists would include it in the work-up of LUTS.[2] In the USA, PSA is part of a screening programme for cancer of the prostate. As usual, when evidence is lacking, recommendations vary according to national temperament and the realities of the different health care systems.

What is the chance that the symptoms will progress so that I need surgery?

The tendency of age-related LUTS in men is for them to worsen over time. Progression is manifested by:

- falling maximum flow rate (Qmax)
- increasing residual volume
- increase in prostate size: over the age of 40 there is an annual increase in Caucasians of 1.6% but with considerable variation between individuals[14]
- deterioration in symptom score.

Different studies have proposed different prognostic features, according to what each study measured. The Baltimore Longitudinal Study of Aging,[15] using questionnaires and rectal examination, found that, of men aged 60 or older with a clinical diagnosis of BPH, 39% underwent surgery over 20 years of follow-up. The younger the man, the less likely surgery was over the next 20 years. The three factors (apart from age) that predicted the need for surgery were:

- weak urinary stream
- a feeling of incomplete voiding
- an enlarged prostate.

Men with one factor had a 9% risk of surgery over 20 years, those with two had a 16% risk and those with three had a 37% risk. However, even all three factors were less powerful as a predictor of surgery than being aged 60 or over (see above).

Am I going to go into acute retention?

The risk of acute retention increases with increasing age and with increasing severity of symptoms. The Olmsted County Study found an annual incidence of acute retention of 0.26% in men aged 40–49 with no, or only mild, symptoms. In men aged 70–79 with no, or mild, symptoms, it was 0.93%, and in men aged 70–79 with moderate or severe symptoms, it was 3.5%.[16] In men with an enlarged prostate (>30 ml), the risk was further increased 3-fold.

Example

A 72-year-old man presents, shortly after a hospital admission with heart failure, with worsening of his longstanding, but previously mild, lower urinary tract symptoms. He has mainly voiding symptoms of frequency and urgency and now he has nocturia three times a night. He is very bothered by this, giving him an IPSS of 14.

History, examination, and urine and blood tests are unremarkable. The prostate is not enlarged. The GP notes that the nocturia has worsened since the hospital admission and checks his medication. Sure enough, he has become muddled and is taking his diuretic at night. A change to taking it in the morning reduces his nocturia to once a night and increases his satisfaction hugely.

He asks whether he will ever need surgery and the GP reassures him. Although he is of an age when many men do, he has none of the bad prognostic features (poor stream, feeling of incomplete emptying, enlarged prostate), and now that the nocturia has been sorted out, there has been little change in his IPSS over the last 5 years.

REFERENCES

1. Crawford E. *Management of lower urinary tract symptoms suggestive of benign prostatic hyperplasia: the central role of the patient risk profile.* BJU Int 2005;95 (Suppl 4):1–5.

2. de la Rosette J, Madersbacher S, Alivizatos G, et al. *European Association of Urology guidelines on benign prostatic hypertrophy: European Association of Urology, 2006.* Online. Available: www.uroweb.org.

3. Madersbacher S, Klingler H, Djavan B, et al. *Is obstruction predictable by clinical evaluation in patients with lower urinary tract symptoms?* Br J Urol 1997;80:72–77.

4. Gades N, Jacobson D, Girman C, et al. *Prevalence of conditions potentially associated with lower urinary tract symptoms in men.* BJU Int 2005;95:549–553.

5. Ezz El Din K, Koch W, de Wildt M, et al. *The predictive value of microscopic haematuria in patients with lower urinary tract symptoms and benign prostatic hypertrophy.* Eur Urol 1996;30:409–413.

6. Roberts R, Jacobson D, Girman C, et al. *Prevalence of prostatitis-like symptoms in a community based cohort of older men.* J Urol 2002;168:2467–2471.

7. Marinkovic S, Gillen L, Stanton S. *Managing nocturia.* BMJ 2004;328:1063–1066.

8. Engstrom G, Walker-Engstrom M-L, Henningsohn L, et al. *Prevalence of distress and symptom severity from the lower urinary tract in men: a population-based study with the DAN-PSS questionnaire.* Fam Pract 2004;21:617–622.

9. Roberts R, Jacobsen S, Rhodes T, et al. *Natural history of prostatism: impaired health states in men with lower urinary tract symptoms.* J Urol 1997;157:1711–1717.

10. Litwin M, McNaughton-Collins M, Fowler FJ, et al. *The National Institutes of Health Chronic Prostatitis Symptom Index: development and validation of a new outcome measure.* J Urol 1999;162:369–375.

11. Roehrborn C. *Accurate determination of prostate size via digital rectal examination and transrectal ultrasound.* Urology 1998;51 (Suppl 4A):19–22.

12. Gerber G, Goldfischer E, Karrison T, et al. *Serum creatinine measurements in men with lower urinary tract symptoms secondary to benign prostatic hypertrophy.* Urology 1997;49:697–702.

13. PRODIGY. *Prostate – benign hyperplasia: Sowerby Centre for Health Informatics at Newcastle, 2006.* Online. Available: www.prodigy.nhs.uk/guidance

14. Rhodes T, Girman C, Jacobsen S, et al. *Longitudinal prostate growth rates during 5 years in randomly selected community men 40 to 79 years old.* J Urol 1999;161:1174–1179.

15. Arrighi H, Metter E, Guess H, et al. *Natural history of benign prostatic hypertrophy and risk of prostatectomy. The Baltimore Longitudinal Study of Aging.* Urology 1991;38 (Suppl 1):4–8.

16. Jacobsen S, Jacobson D, Girman C, et al. *Natural history of prostatism: risk factors for acute urinary retention.* J Urol 1997;158:481–487.

A lump in the neck

KEY FACTS

- In primary care, most swellings in the neck are cervical nodes; almost all swollen nodes are a reaction to infection; and most of those infections are self-limiting. The most common non-infectious swelling in the neck is the thyroid.
- The challenge is to detect the occasional lump that needs specific treatment, e.g. infection other than viral; the thyroid swelling that is associated with disturbed thyroid function or is malignant; or the node that is evidence of lymphoma, leukaemia or metastatic cancer.

A PRACTICAL APPROACH

This is suggested in the text below.

Common causes

(a) *Cervical lymph nodes.* Usually bilateral if due to generalised infection or infection in the pharynx; unilateral if due to a unilateral focus. Specific nodes have been described:

■ the Delphian node which lies in the midline just above the thyroid isthmus. It drains the thyroid and the larynx and so raises the possibility of carcinoma in those sites

■ Virchow's node: an enlarged left supraclavicular node, associated with thoracic, abdominal or pelvic malignancy.

(b) *The thyroid gland.* Two features distinguish it:

■ it lies in the front of the neck between the cricoid cartilage and the suprasternal notch, or in the side of the neck between the thyroid cartilage and the clavicle

■ it moves with the trachea on swallowing.

Observation with the neck in the normal position combined with palpation can detect goitre with a sensitivity of 43–82% and a specificity of 88–100%.[1] Using the mean of those figures gives a useful LR+ of 10 and a less useful LR– of 0.4. Imagine that the GP, faced with a swelling in the front of the neck of a 50-year-old man, considers that the probability that the swelling is a goitre is 50% (based on a prevalence of goitre in men of 5% and the fact that, at a quick glance, it looks like a goitre, which raises the probability to, say, 50%). More detailed observation and palpation will raise that probability to 91% if the examination is positive, although the probability of goitre remains as high as 29% even if examination suggests it is not a goitre.

(c) *Superficial lumps that are not specific to the neck,* e.g. sebaceous cyst, or carbuncle.

Uncommon causes

(a) *Thyroglossal cyst.* A tense or fluctuant non-tender swelling in the midline above the thyroid cartilage. The diagnosis is confirmed if the lump moves up when the patient protrudes the tongue. The absence of this sign does not exclude the diagnosis. However, if positive, the sign distinguishes the cyst from a midline thyroid nodule, which will move upwards on swallowing but not on protruding the tongue.

(b) *Branchial cleft cyst.* A tense, non-tender swelling anterior to the sternomastoid muscle at the level of the hyoid. It is less common than the thyroglossal cyst in the ratio of 1:3.

It often presents in early adult life. The diagnosis is made from its position – it emerges anterior to the upper third of the sternomastoid muscle, arising from beneath it – and from its feel: unless it has become infected it will feel cystic, 'like a half-filled hot water bottle'.[2]

(c) *Pharyngeal diverticulum.* It protrudes lateral to the trachea, enlarges after eating or drinking and can be emptied by pressure. The patient is usually elderly, and may report regurgitation of undigested food, bouts of coughing and gurgling in the neck. A barium swallow is needed to confirm the diagnosis.

(d) *Carotid body tumour.* This presents in middle age, grows very slowly, and is hard, oval and regular, hence the name 'the potato tumour'. It is positioned at the bifurcation of the carotid artery and transmitted pulsations from the artery can be felt.

Red flags

Refer urgently if the lump is:

(a) fixed to underlying tissue; or

(b) hard, rather than firm; or

(c) associated with hoarseness, dysphagia or other upper GI symptoms; or

(d) associated with neurological abnormalities; or

(e) fails to resolve in 3 weeks and the cause is not apparent;[3] or

(f) is present in a patient who is systemically unwell without obvious cause.

No other figures were found to enable the sensitivity or specificity of different signs to be calculated.

What is the cause of this patient's goitre?

The point prevalence of goitre in the UK: 23% in women and 5% in men.[4] In this study of nearly 3000 British adults, goitre was not associated with abnormal thyroid function.

Initial probabilities

Common:

(a) Simple diffuse goitre; develops at puberty, usually in girls.

(b) Multinodular goitre; present in 5% of women >50 years old.

Uncommon:

(a) Viral thyroiditis.

(b) Hashimoto's thyroiditis.

(c) Subacute (de Quervain's) thyroiditis. The thyroid is tender and the erythrocyte sedimentation rate (ESR) high.

(d) Postpartum thyroiditis.

(e) Graves' disease.

(f) Thyroid nodule (palpable in 1–5% of the population. The higher figure is found in older people and in women). The causes are:
  ■ 95% benign adenoma, a colloid cyst or part of a multinodular goitre
  ■ 5% carcinoma.

(g) Iodine deficiency – the commonest cause worldwide but rarely seen outside areas of iodine deficiency.

Diagnosing thyroid carcinoma clinically

Three physical signs strongly indicate carcinoma:[1]
■ vocal cord paralysis (LR+ 12)
■ cervical lymphadenopathy (LR+ 7.4)
■ fixation of the gland (LR+ 7.2).

The absence of these signs by no means excludes it (sensitivity <30%).

Three (or four) other factors increase the risk of carcinoma slightly:
■ a family history of medullary carcinoma
■ male sex: the risk that a nodule is malignant in a man is twice that in a woman
■ age: carcinoma is more common in younger patients
■ possibly irradiation: a history of irradiation to the thyroid may or may not increase the risk.[5]

The low sensitivity of the three signs of carcinoma means that a GP cannot reliably distinguish benign from malignant nodules and therefore must refer all new thyroid nodules.

No other figures were found to enable the sensitivity or specificity of different signs to be calculated.

What features assist the diagnosis of the cause of lymphadenopathy in the neck?

The problem with answering this question is that all studies are from specialist settings, to which only a small portion of patients with swollen nodes in primary care are referred.

Initial probabilities

■ Reactive lymphadenitis to bacterial or viral infection (either active, or past with residual enlargement)
■ Malignancy, whether lymphoma, leukaemia or a metastasis from a carcinoma or sarcoma
■ Inflammatory, e.g. sarcoidosis, rheumatoid arthritis.

The probabilities of these conditions in a patient in primary care can only be guessed very roughly from the findings of hospital clinics. In primary care, the proportion with reactive lymphadenitis is likely to be much higher than in secondary care, since most will have been diagnosed clinically by the GP and not referred.
● A US study of 105 children referred with lymphadenopathy found malignancy in 5% (lymphoma in three, one leukaemia and one rhabdomyosarcoma) with the rest benign, mainly reactive lymphadenitis.[6]
● A US study of 106 patients under 21 referred for lymphadenopathy (89% in the head or neck) also found that 5% were malignant (three lymphoma, two thyroid).[7]
● A study from Texas[8] of nodes at all sites (47% were cervical) and in all age groups, found that, in the 922 in whom a diagnosis could be made on fine needle biopsy, 64% were malignant. Of all enlarged nodes in the neck, supraclavicular nodes are most likely to be malignant.[8]

The probabilities can be adjusted according to three factors:
■ *Age.* These studies show that the probability of malignancy rises with age, from 5% in children to 64% when all age groups are combined. A study from Los Angeles found the frequency of malignancy in supraclavicular nodes to be 32% in those aged 40 and below, compared to 68% for those >40.[9]
■ *Ethnicity and location.* In a study of supraclavicular node biopsies in north India, 13.5% were tuberculous,[10] as were 14.5% in a series in South Korea.[11]
■ *HIV-positive* patients are more likely to have an infective cause. In the Los Angeles series, 14% of patients undergoing supraclavicular node aspiration were HIV positive: cultures for TB and atypical organisms are required.[9]

How can a diagnosis be made clinically?

No studies have examined this question. Traditional teaching is as follows:[2]

Define the site of the swollen nodes. Examine the patient from behind. Search specifically for nodes in each of the sites listed below.

If the swollen nodes are localised, search for a focus of infection (or, rarely, tumour). The search should show an understanding of which structures drain to which nodes.
■ *Supraclavicular nodes* drain the chest, breast, abdomen and pelvis. A US study of 152 supraclavicular node biopsies (57% of them on the left) found that 63% were malignant, and that almost all the malignancies from the abdomen and pelvis were left sided.[12] Malignancies from the thorax, head and neck lymphoma and leukaemia were equally distributed.
■ *Submandibular nodes* drain the eyelids, side of the nose and the lips, cheek and chin and the floor of the mouth.
■ *Submental nodes* drain the tongue, teeth and mouth.
■ *Occipital nodes* drain the scalp and are often enlarged bilaterally in rubella.
■ *The jugular chain of anterior cervical nodes* drains the mouth, tongue and throat. The 'tonsillar' node lies near the top of this chain.
■ *Nodes in the posterior triangle* drain the scalp.

If the lymphadenopathy is generalised, search for pointers to a cause, e.g. the tonsillar exudates of infectious mononucleosis, the rash of rubella.
Define the characteristics of the nodes.
■ Small, tender and mobile nodes suggest reactive lymphadenitis.
■ Hard, large nodes, especially if fixed to underlying tissue or to skin, suggest malignancy. The nodes of lymphoma are typically 'rubbery'.
Examine for hepatosplenomegaly unless a cause of the lymphadenopathy has already been found. If present, think of disseminated infection, inflammation or malignancy.
Ask about other symptoms. Dysphagia could indicate a primary carcinoma of the oesophagus; cough could indicate a carcinoma of the bronchus; malaise, night sweats and itching could indicate a lymphoma; bleeding and bruising could indicate leukaemia.

Investigations

Whether to investigate in primary care will depend on the findings so far.

If no local treatable cause has been found, the choice lies between immediate referral or initial investigations:

(a) full blood count, ESR, blood film

(b) chest X-ray

(c) serology for infectious mononucleosis, cytomegalovirus, toxoplasmosis, HIV infection.

Referral

The UK guidelines for the referral of a patient with lymphadenopathy and no evidence of previous local infection include the following:[13]

- persisting for 6 weeks or more
- increasing in size
- >2 cm in size
- widespread
- associated with splenomegaly, night sweats or weight loss.

REFERENCES

1. McGee S. *Evidence-based physical diagnosis.* Philadelphia: Saunders, 2001.

2. Clain A. *Hamilton Bailey's demonstration of physical signs in clinical surgery, 14th edn.* Bristol: John Wright and Sons, 1967.

3. NHS Executive. *Referral guidelines for suspected cancer.* London: Department of Health, 2000.

4. Vanderpump M, Tunbridge W, French J, et al. *The incidence of thyroid disorders in the community: a twenty-year follow-up of the Whickham Survey.* Clin Endocrinol 1995;43:55–68.

5. Dolan JG, Wittlin SD. *Thyroid nodules.* In: Black ER, Bordley DR, Tape TG, Panzer RJ, eds. Diagnostic strategies for common medical problems. Philadelphia: American College of Physicians, 1999:484–492.

6. Buchino J, Jones V. *Fine needle aspiration in the evaluation of children with lymphadenopathy.* Arch Pediatr Adolesc Med 1994;148:1327–1330.

7. Ponder T, Smith D, Ramzy I. *Lymphadenopathy in children and adolescents: role of fine-needle aspiration in management.* Cancer Detect Prev 2000;24:228–233.

8. Steel B, Schwartz M, Ramzy I. *Fine needle aspiration biopsy in the diagnosis of lymphadenopathy in 1103 patients. Role, limitations and analysis of diagnostic pitfalls.* Acta Cytol 1995;39:76–81.

9. Ellison E, LaPuerta P, Martin S. *Supraclavicular masses: results of a series of 309 cases biopsied by fine needle aspiration.* Head Neck 1999;21:239–246.

10. Gupta N, Rajwanshi A, Srinivasan R, et al. *Pathology of supraclavicular lymphadenopathy in Chandigarh, north India: an audit of 200 cases diagnosed by needle aspiration.* Cytopathology 2006;17: 94–96.

11. Na D, Lim H, Byun H, et al. *Differential diagnosis of cervical lymphadenopathy: usefulness of color Doppler sonography.* Am J Roentgenol 1997;168:1311–1316.

12. Cervin J, Silverman J, Loggie B, et al. *Virchow's node revisited. Analysis with clinicopathologic correlation of 152 fine-needle aspiration biopsies of supraclavicular lymph nodes.* Arch Pathol Lab Med 1995;119: 727–730.

13. The National Collaborating Centre for Primary Care. *Referral guidelines for suspected cancer in adults and children: 2004.*

Memory loss and dementia

Memory loss and mild cognitive impairment

- The complaint of memory loss is common. Studies in patients aged 65 and over give rates of complaints of memory loss of between 25% and 56%.[1] Rates tend to be higher in older people and in those with a lower level of education. Rates vary according to the tests used and whether depressed and cognitively impaired people are excluded.

- Memory loss is not a *necessary* feature of normal ageing, with the exception of some decline in rote learning.[2] When a patient, or especially the patient's family, complains of progressive memory loss, the main possibilities, if disease is present, are depression, anxiety,[3] age-associated memory impairment, mild cognitive impairment and dementia.

- About 40% of Americans >65 years old have age-associated memory impairment.[4] Only 1% progress to dementia annually. About 10% of Americans >65 years old have mild cognitive impairment and, of them, 15% develop Alzheimer's disease annually.[4]

- A complaint of memory loss is not a reliable guide to whether it is really present. Some studies have failed to show a relationship between a patient's complaint of memory loss and objective memory impairment, once those with dementia are excluded.[5] Conversely, of those shown by objective testing to have memory loss, only 6% have noticed it.[5]

- It is not clear whether a complaint of memory loss increases the likelihood that the patient has cognitive impairment. One study suggests that an older patient complaining of memory loss has a risk of being found to have cognitive impairment after 1 year follow-up that is almost five times that of those with no memory complaints.[1] Other studies have failed to find any predictive value in the complaint of memory loss[5] in non-demented patients.

- Patients who complain themselves are more likely to have depression than cognitive impairment.[1] Those in whom there is cognitive impairment are more likely to have mild cognitive impairment than dementia. When it is the family who brings the patient to the doctor's attention, the diagnosis is more likely to be dementia.

Testing for memory loss[6]

1. At the start, give the patient an address to remember (e.g. *42 West St*), plus the names of three objects (e.g. *cup, bell, door*).
2. Ask a number of questions: date, day, month, year, name of interviewer, the names of two prominent people.
3. Ask the patient to repeat the address and the three objects.

   Be aware that this is a crude test of memory. The patient's observations of memory impairment may still be correct, even if every one of these questions is answered correctly.

Assessment

* Make an objective assessment of the presence of poor short-term memory (see above).
* Ask about the patient's mental state:
  ■ 'Are you particularly worried at the moment? (see *Anxiety*, p. 328)
  ■ 'Have you been low, or have you lost interest in things recently?' (see *Depression*, p. 373). However, if depression is found, do not dismiss the possibility of co-morbid dementia; 12% of those with dementia are also depressed.[7]
* Check for cognitive impairment other than memory loss, and for dementia (see below).

Is this patient suffering from mild cognitive impairment?

Definitions vary and are arbitrary. It exists when there is either:

(a) objective evidence of at least moderate memory loss but cognition is otherwise normal and the patient's ability to function is unimpaired[2]; or

(b) mild memory loss plus mild cognitive impairment that falls short of dementia.

Assessment of the ability to function normally is subjective. A person in work with cognitive impairment might be judged to have dementia because of the interference of the condition with his or her job. Had that person retired, the diagnosis might have been mild cognitive impairment because of the lack of interference with daily life.

Prevalence

● Cognitive impairment is common in old age but not inevitable. In a study of 95 elderly Canadians, with a mean age of 84, who were cognitively intact at entry into the study, 51% developed cognitive impairment over follow-up of up to 13 years. Of those, 56% developed dementia at a mean of 2.8 years later.[8]

● Mild cognitive impairment will progress to dementia at a rate of 12% per year.[9]

● Patients with mild cognitive impairment should be screened for a reversible cause (see *Dementia*, p. 185). Treatment is more likely to reverse the impairment at this stage than if discovered later. Ironically, GPs tend to investigate patients with more advanced disease in whom the results are less likely to be useful.[10]

Does this patient have dementia?

KEY FACTS

- Up to 10% of people over 65 have dementia, as do up to half of those over 85.
- Informal assessment of cognitive function is unreliable. Formal tests are needed.
- The diagnosis of dementia requires deterioration in memory and at least one other area of cognition, such that the deterioration interferes with daily life. Formal testing should therefore cover memory, reasoning, visuospatial skills and the ability to function satisfactorily.
- The search for a cause should involve looking for:
  ■ disorders which mimic dementia, e.g. depression or delirium
  ■ disorders which cause dementia – the so-called 'reversible dementias'.

A simple battery of blood tests is probably adequate but a more energetic search for a cause might be made if the patient is younger than usual, if the history is shorter and if abnormal neurological signs are found.

- A special case is vascular dementia. If found, it is worth controlling blood pressure and other risk factors, both in the hope of limiting progression and of reducing the risk of coronary events.

Background

● A brief definition is that dementia exists when there has been a decline in memory and at least one other cognitive domain, e.g. language, visuospatial or executive function, sufficient to interfere with social or occupational function in an alert person, where the decline is not due to some other disorder. This is the essence of the DSM-IV definition.[11] The ICD-10 definition adds that the decline must have been present for 6 months, that there should be no clouding of consciousness and that there should be evidence of decline in emotional control, or motivation, or a change in social behaviour, e.g. emotional lability, irritability, apathy or coarsening of social behaviour.[12]

● The prevalence of dementia is 3–11% of those over 65, and 25–47% of those >85.[13] The wide ranges are due to different settings and definitions. Of those who are demented, the Rotterdam study[14] found that 72% had Alzheimer's disease, 16% had vascular dementia, 6% had the dementia of Parkinson's disease; 5% had other dementias. The older the patient, the more likely the diagnosis is to be Alzheimer's disease.

● Early diagnosis is important. It allows the family to plan for the future, allows early psychological and social interventions and allows drugs to be started at the phase of the illness when they are most effective.

● The possibility of dementia is usually raised by a report of memory loss. Such a report from the family is more reliable than a complaint by the patient.[15] A decline in function is a yet more reliable pointer.[16]

● Failure to recognise dementia is common. In different studies, dementia was not recognised by 21% of family members, by 22% of nurses[17] and by 25% of doctors.[18] Conversely, in a study of nuns in the USA,[17] the nurses overdiagnosed dementia in 16%. Doctors seem to be more specific. A study from Finland found that doctors in primary care missed half of the diagnoses of dementia (sensitivity 48%) but, if they did diagnose it, they were almost always right (specificity 99.6%).[10] Overall, >50% of patients with dementia have never been diagnosed.[13]

● There is no gold standard for the diagnosis. Even histology at autopsy correlates poorly with cognitive state.[18] A review of six different sets of criteria for the diagnosis in 1879 Canadians, aged 65 and older, found that they gave a diagnosis of dementia with a prevalence that ranged from 3.1% to 29.1%.[19] The DSM-IV definition comes midway in this range and is widely accepted.

The history

Ask about:
■ the rate of onset: a rapid onset suggests an acute confusional state
■ a past history, or present symptoms, of depression
■ a family history of dementia
■ current medical problems which could be contributing
■ current medication which could be contributing
■ a history of recent head trauma
■ delusions or hallucinations: auditory hallucinations point to a psychotic illness; visual hallucinations suggest an organic brain disorder including dementia with Lewy bodies; delusions, including paranoia, may occur late in any dementia
■ the degree of insight
■ memory loss
■ difficulty performing routine tasks
■ social function: does the patient take part in conversations and behave according to normal social conventions?

Brief examination

Note the following:
■ The state of alertness.
■ Is the patient well dressed and presented?
■ Are responses to questions appropriate?
■ Gait. Abnormal gait suggests hydrocephalus or cerebrovascular disease or dementia with Lewy bodies.
■ Blood pressure. Hypertension increases the probability of cerebrovascular disease.

■ Focal neurological signs. They are probably part of a cerebrovascular cause of the dementia but may be due to other CNS disorders.

Follow up any clues in the history by looking for relevant signs.

Assessment

Clinical judgement alone is unreliable. Formal testing is better but is insensitive to small changes.[20] A combination is needed. Different tests test for different aspects of impairment. It is best to combine at least two, and if possible four, complementary tests, e.g. the Abbreviated Mental Test Score (AMTS) and clock drawing[21] plus the report of an informant who knows the patient well.

Step 1. Cognitive testing

If sensitively introduced, almost all patients find testing acceptable – only 5% don't.[18] Introducing it as a memory test helps – loss of memory is (erroneously) accepted as part of growing old.

* Preliminary screen: two questions:
  1. tell the patient three words (e.g. *house, tree, car*) and ask them to recall them a few minutes later; and
  2. ask them where they are.

These are almost as specific as the full Mini Mental State Examination (MMSE) (sensitivity 98%, specificity 95%; LR+ 20; LR– 0.02).[15] Alternative preliminary screens are to ask the patient to spell WORLD backwards or to perform serial 7s.

* *Formal testing of cognition.* A number of instruments exist, of similar value. The AMTS (see below) has a sensitivity of 81% and a specificity of 84% (LR+ 5.1; LR– 0.2), judged against a diagnosis made using DSM criteria.[22] However, the clinician must be precise when scoring and resist the temptation to give the patient the benefit of the doubt. On a test, only 1 out of 104 doctors scored each item correctly and only 17 obtained the correct score, which in this study was 5.[23] Scores ranged from 3.5 to 9. Forty-one doctors incorrectly scored the patient as not impaired; 78 doctors gave half marks, which contributed to their inaccuracy.

The AMTS is less accurate than the MMSE but it is quicker, hence its widespread use in primary care.

The Abbreviated Mental Test Score

Ask the patient:

1. his or her age (*exact no. of years*)
2. the time (*to the nearest hour*)
3. to remember a simple address, e.g. 42 West St, and repeat it at the end of the test (*with no errors*)
4. the year (*current year*)
5. the place (*exact address or the name of the surgery or hospital*)
6. to identify two people present (*by name or role*)
7. their date of birth (*correct day and month*)
8. the dates of World War I (*1914 or 1918 is enough*)
9. the name of the monarch/head of state (*must be the current one*)
10. to count backwards from 20 to 1 (*with no mistakes, or with mistakes which the patient corrects spontaneously*).

Score the answers precisely, as indicated in the brackets, with 1 point for each correct answer. A score <7 suggests dementia.

Step 2. The clock drawing test

The clock drawing test (see below) tests for executive function deficit – which is missed by the AMTS. Its sensitivity is 87.5% and the specificity 82.3% (LR+ 4.9; LR– 0.1).[15]

The clock drawing test[21]

Give the patient a piece of paper on which is drawn an empty circle. Ask the patient to write in all the numbers on the face of a clock and draw in the hands to show the time at 10 to 2.

Complex scoring systems exist. The simplest is to say that the patient has passed the test if the numbers are correctly drawn and the time is correct. However, the specificity of this is likely to be low.

The simplest well-validated system is to ignore the hands and to divide the clock into four quadrants, based on wherever the patient has drawn the figure 12. Count the number of figures in each quadrant. If a figure is on a line, count it as being in the quadrant that is clockwise to the line. Score each quadrant separately. Score 1 if there are fewer or more than three figures in the quadrant but score 4 if there are too many or too few in the final quadrant. A score of 0–3 is normal; 4–7 suggests dementia.[24]

If formal scoring seems too complex, just make a judgement about whether the clock is normal or abnormal. This performs almost as well as the most complex formal scoring system.[25]

Step 3. Assessment of daily living

Deterioration in the following four domains of daily living are significantly associated with cognitive impairment.[26] Can the patient do the following without assistance?

(a) managing medication
(b) using the phone
(c) coping with a budget
(d) using transportation.

Inability to do at least one of these is 94% sensitive and 71% specific for dementia (LR+ 3.2; LR– 0.08).

Step 4. Informant's report

Ask the person closest to the patient. Using a formal questionnaire with which to question the informant in one study improved the sensitivity for the diagnosis of dementia from 76%, using the MMSE alone, to 93% when the informant's report was used as well.[27] The specificity, however, fell from 90% to 81%. Most of the required information will have been covered in the initial history and the assessment of daily living. The informant report alone had a sensitivity of 90% and a specificity of 65% (LR+ 2.6; LR– 0.2). Informal questioning may not produce such reliable results.

All patients should be assessed by a multidisciplinary team specialising in the assessment of dementia, if the GP's assessment suggests that dementia is present.[28]

Could the findings be due to some other disease that mimics dementia?

■ *Delirium* (see p. 55).
■ *Depression* may mimic dementia so closely that the condition is called 'pseudodementia'. Formal testing should help to distinguish the two. However, patients with 'pseudodementia' often have an underlying dementia which is exaggerated by the depression.[18]
■ *Substance-induced cognitive impairment.* Common substances to cause this are alcohol, psychotropic drugs, anticholinergics and anticonvulsants. As with depression and delirium, there is often a degree of underlying dementia which is unmasked by the drugs.
■ *Psychosis.*
■ *Conversion hysteria or factitious dementia,* in which the patient will perform poorly in some situations (e.g. formal testing) and well in others when not being 'tested'.

If dementia, is it secondary?

● With each new analysis the proportion of dementias described as reversible is revised downwards. Traditionally, 9% were referred to as 'reversible'.[29] However, only 5% are even potentially reversible: those due to drugs, metabolic or hepatic disease, hyponatraemia, calcium disorders, B_{12} deficiency, thyroid disease or hypoglycaemia.[30] Furthermore, only 0.6% of dementias actually improve and only half of those reverse completely.[29]

More recently, the 2006 SIGN guideline judges that reversible causes are present in <1% and doubts the value of any routine investigations in the absence of clinical pointers.[31]

- Patients with a reversible dementia have shorter histories, are less severe and show less cortical atrophy on CT scan.
- The usual recommendation is to check haemoglobin, erythrocyte sedimentation rate, urea and electrolytes, glucose, liver function tests, calcium, phosphate, thyroid function tests, B_{12} and urine analysis.[15] Testing for syphilis has been dropped in Western countries since there has not been a recorded case of syphilis-induced dementia in the last 20 years in the elderly.[18]
- The American Academy of Neurology now recommends CT or MRI for initial work-up of dementia.[7] The useful yield will be scant.[18]

If primary, what type is it?

The assessment of the type of dementia is the role of the specialist. A study from England and Wales[32] casts doubt on the traditional distinctions drawn between different aetiologies. In a series of 209 unselected autopsies of patients with a median age at death of 85 years, cerebrovascular changes were found in 78% and Alzheimer's disease (AD)-type changes in 70%. Only 100 of the patients were demented. Alzheimer's disease changes were found in 61% of demented and in 34% of non-demented patients. Vascular lesions were as common in demented and non-demented patients. Most patients who were demented had mixed disease. This challenges the idea of separate dementia types. However, an attempt to decide on the type of dementia is worthwhile as more treatments related to aetiology become available.

- *Alzheimer's disease* is characterised by a slow decline in all areas of cognitive function. The diagnosis becomes more likely the older the patient.
- *Vascular dementia* is suggested by a step-wise progression in a patient with known cardiovascular disease or risk factors for it. Focal neurological signs may be found. Treatment of hypertension can arrest or reverse decline.[18]
- *Lewy body dementia* is worth differentiating because of the poor prognosis and the importance of avoiding neuroleptics. The characteristic pointers are fluctuating cognition, visual hallucinations and features of Parkinson's disease.
- *Fronto-temporal dementias* often occur before the age of 65, with behavioural changes an early manifestation.

The SIGN guideline gives more detail about the different clinical manifestations.[31]

Example

An 80-year-old man presents for a medical examination to assess his fitness to drive. His probability of dementia, based on the population prevalence, is 20%. However, his daughter accompanies him and whispers that she has some concerns about his driving but is unable to say more in front of him. This raises the probability of dementia to, say, 30%. If he fails any one of the four tests (steps) described above, the probability of dementia is sufficiently high to need to be pursued further, with the following probabilities:

- failure on the two-question screening test: probability of dementia 90% (Fig. 28.1)
- failure on clock drawing: probability of dementia 68%
- failure on activities of daily living: probability of dementia 58%

- a more detailed formal account from the daughter in private suggesting dementia: probability of dementia 39%.

Failure of any one of these tests is therefore grounds for refusal of a driving licence and for referral for more detailed assessment.

Conversely, passing any one of these tests reduces the probability of dementia to between 1% for the screening questions and 11% for the clock drawing test. Passing more than one reduces the probability still further.

Note: These tests cannot be applied one after the other, using the post-test probability of the previous test as the new pre-test probability, because, with the possible exception of the clock drawing test, they are not independent of each other.

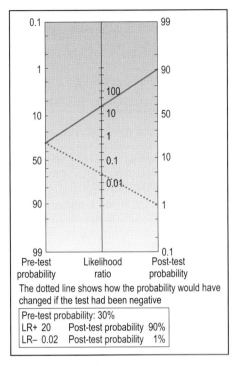

Figure 28.1 The probability of dementia before and after the two-question screening test in the example on p. 186.

REFERENCES

1. Jonker C, Geerlings M, Schmand B. *Are memory complaints predictive for dementia? A review of clinical and population-based studies.* Int J Geriatr Psychiatry 2000;15:983–991.

2. Knopman D, Boeve B, Petersen R. *Essentials of the proper diagnosis of mild cognitive impairment, dementia, and major subtypes of dementia.* Mayo Clin Proc 2003;78:1290–1308.

3. Dérouesne C, Lacomblez L, Thibault S, Leponcin M. *Memory complaints in young and elderly subjects.* Int J Geriatr Psychiatry 1999;14: 291–301.

4. Small G. *What we need to know about age related memory loss.* BMJ 2002;324:1502–1505.

5. Jungwirth S, Fischer P, Weissgram S, et al. *Subjective memory complaints and objective memory impairment in the Vienna-Transdanube aging community.* J Am Geriatr Soc 2004;52:263–268.

6. Geerlings M, Jonker C, Bouter L, et al. *Association between memory complaints and incident Alzheimer's disease in elderly people with normal baseline cognition.* Am J Psychiatry 1999;156:531–537.

7. Knopman D, DeKosky S, Cummings J, et al. *Practice parameter: diagnosis of dementia (an evidence-based review). Report of the Quality Standards Subcommittee of the American Academy of Neurology.* Neurology 2001;56:1143–1153.

8. Howieson D, Camicioli R, Quinn J, et al. *Natural history of cognitive decline in the old old.* Neurology 2003; 60:1489–1494.

9. Petersen R, Stevens J, Ganguli M, et al. *Practice parameter: early detection of dementia: mild cognitive impairment (an evidence-based review).* Neurology 2001;56:1133–1142.

10. Lopponen M, Raiha I, Isoaho R, et al. *Diagnosing cognitive impairment and dementia in primary health care – a more active approach is needed.* Age Ageing 2003;32:606–612.

11. American Psychiatric Association. *Diagnostic and statistical manual of mental disorders, 4th edn, text revision.* Washington DC: American Psychiatric Association, 2000.

12. WHO. *The ICD-10 Classification of mental and behavioural disorders: diagnostic criteria for research.* Geneva: World Health Organization, 1993.

13. Boustani M, Peterson B, Hanson L, et al. *Screening for dementia in primary care: a summary of the evidence for the US Preventative Services Task*

Force. Ann Intern Med 2003;138: 927–937.

14. Ott A, Breteler M, van Harskamp F, et al. *Prevalence of Alzheimer's disease and vascular dementia: association with education. The Rotterdam study.* BMJ 1995;310: 970–973.

15. Eccles M, Clarke J, Livingstone M, et al. *North of England evidence based guidelines development project: guideline for the primary care management of dementia.* BMJ 1998; 317:802–808.

16. Van Hout H, Vernooij-Dassen M, Hoefnagels W, et al. *Dementia: predictors of diagnostic accuracy and the contribution of diagnostic recommendations.* J Fam Pract 2002; 51:693–699.

17. Greiner L, Snowdon D. *Underrecognition of dementia by caregivers cuts across cultures.* JAMA 1997;277(22):1757.

18. Kaplan N, Palmer B, Vicioso B. *Dementia: when is it not Alzheimer disease?* Am J Med Sci 2002;324: 84–95.

19. Erkinjuntti T, Ostbye T, Steenhuis R, Hachinski V. *The effect of different diagnostic criteria on the prevalence of dementia.* N Engl J Med 1997;337:1667–1674.

20. Powlishta K, Von Dras D, Stanford A, et al. *The clock drawing test is a poor screen for very mild dementia.* Neurology 2002;59: 898–903.

21. Dysch L, Crome P. *Using the clock drawing task in primary care.* Geriatr Med 2003(Sept):75–80.

22. Antonelli I, Cesari M, Pedone C, et al. *Construct validity of the abbreviated mental test in older medical inpatients.* Dement Geriatr Cogn Disord 2003;15:199–206.

23. Holmes J, Gilbody S. *Differences in use of abbreviated mental test score by geriatricians and psychiatrists.* BMJ 1996;313:465.

24. Watson Y, Arfken C, Birge S. *Clock completion: an objective screening test for dementia.* J Am Geriatr Soc 1993;41:1235–1240.

25. Scanlan J, Brush M, Quijano C, et al. *Comparing clock tests for dementia screening: naive judgements vs formal systems – what is optimal?* Int J Geriatr Psychiatry 2002;17:14–21.

26. Barberger-Gateau P, Commenges D, Gagnon M, et al. *Instrumental activities of daily living as a screening tool for cognitive impairment and dementia in elderly community dwellers.* J Am Geriatr Soc 1992;40: 1129–1134.

27. MacKinnon A, Mulligan R. *Combining cognitive testing and informant report to increase accuracy in screening for dementia.* Am J Psychiatry 1998;155:1529–1535.

28. Royal College of Psychiatrists. *Consensus statement on the assessment and investigation of an elderly person with suspected cognitive impairment by a Specialist Old Age Psychiatry Service.* London: Royal College of Psychiatrists Council Report CR49, 1995.

29. Clarfield A. *The decreasing prevalence of reversible dementias: an updated meta-analysis.* Arch Intern Med 2003;163:2219–2229.

30. Katzman R, Rowe J. *Principles of geriatric neurology.* Philadelphia: FA Davis, 1992.

31. SIGN. *Management of patients with dementia.* Edinburgh: Scottish Intercollegiate Guidelines Network, 2006. Online. Available: www.sign.ac. uk.

32. Neuropathology Group of the MRC Cognitive Function and Ageing Study. *Pathological correlates of late-onset dementia in a multicentre, community based population in England and Wales.* Lancet 2001;357: 169–175.

Menorrhagia and other abnormal bleeding patterns

29

KEY FACTS

- The presentation of menorrhagia does not raise a suspicion of gynaecological cancer, nor of any other pathology where early detection is necessary.
- An enquiry should be made about other symptoms, which might raise such suspicion – other abnormal bleeding patterns, pelvic pain or dyspareunia. This search is mainly via the history but also by pelvic examination and a haemoglobin estimation.
- If menorrhagia is the only symptom, referral for investigation is only needed in those who fail to respond to medical treatment or who will not be satisfied without referral.

A PRACTICAL APPROACH

- * Attempt an objective assessment of the amount of blood lost by asking about clots, the frequency of pad changing, the need to change pads at night and the need for double pads.
- * At the same time, do not lose sight of the fact that the crucial factor is how troublesome the bleeding is to the patient.
- * Ask about other gynaecological symptoms: irregular bleeding, bloodstained discharge, post-coital bleeding, dyspareunia or pelvic pain.
- * Perform a pelvic examination and a speculum examination if a smear is due.
- * Check the haemoglobin.
- * Embark on medical management without further investigation unless the above approach has detected a pointer towards the need for further investigation.

Definition

- Menorrhagia has been arbitrarily defined as an average blood loss per period of at least 80 ml. This was chosen because it occurs in <5% of the Swedish menstruating population and is more than twice the mean loss.[1] However, it is of limited value clinically because:

    (a) patients have no idea how much blood they lose and doctors do not measure it except in a research setting[2]

    (b) it correlates poorly with whether women are bothered by their loss; in one study, 26% of women with a loss below 60 ml thought it was heavy while 40% of those with a loss >80 ml thought it was light or moderate[3]

    (c) it does not correlate with the likelihood of pathology being found nor of iron stores being low.

- A more meaningful concept is that menorrhagia represents regular menstrual bleeding which the patient finds too heavy, provided the doctor has checked that a complaint about heavy loss is not a surrogate for other problems.

- A further problem is that menorrhagia usually does not exist alone; there is considerable overlap between symptoms of heavy bleeding, pain and mood change. A study from Edinburgh of women referred to a gynaecological clinic because of menstrual problems found serious differences between the reason given by the GP for referral and that given by the patient.[4] In a quarter of cases, the patient and the GP disagreed about whether bleeding was the reason for referral (in the discordant cases, the GP was four times more likely than the patient to think that it was), while in a quarter of cases, they disagreed whether pain was the reason for referral (with the patient twice as likely to think that it was). The study was unable to show the reason for the discordance but suggests that a menstrual complaint is a complex of symptoms which tends to be reframed into a complaint of bleeding in the process of referral: a reframing which may lead to unnecessary surgery.

Prevalence

In the general population

A survey of 1513 British women aged 18 to 54 gave the figures in Table 29.1.[5]

In primary care

Five per cent of women aged 30 to 49 consult with menorrhagia.[6]

Initial probabilities

No studies have examined the initial diagnostic probabilities in women presenting with heavy periods in primary care. A study from secondary care[7] gave the following figures:

- dysfunctional uterine bleeding 61% (i.e. no pathology found on investigation)
- fibroids 11%
- others 28%:
  - (a) endometrial polyps
  - (b) endometriosis
  - (c) polycystic ovary syndrome
  - (d) anovulatory bleeding.

In addition, the following are possible causes:
- infection
- hypothyroidism
- a bleeding disorder
- post sterilisation
- endometrial cancer
- an intrauterine contraceptive device (IUD)
- endometrial hyperplasia.

Is a search for an underlying pathology worthwhile?

No, not in the absence of red flags.

One view of the possible pathologies is that, in menorrhagia without red flags (see below), fibroids, polyps, endometriosis and polycystic ovary syndrome, if found, are likely to be coincidental. These are common conditions, with fibroids being found in 10% of women over 40 and adenomyosis in up to half of postmortem specimens.[8] An IUD should be obvious and other conditions are so rare that they should not be pursued unless the history or examination suggests it. Furthermore, the finding of fibroids and polyps would not alter the management, which is, in the first instance, medical and may be conducted in primary care.

Table 29.1 Incidence and prevalence of menstrual complaints in the British population[5]

Complaint	Incidence in 1 year	Prevalence
Menorrhagia ('heavy periods')	25%	52%
Heavier than usual	21%	23%
Change in pattern of cycle	29%	32%
Short cycle	21%	24%
Long cycle	15%	22%
Intermenstrual bleeding	17%	14%
Post-coital bleeding	6%	6%
Prolonged periods	9%	9%

Another way of looking at the question is to note that the incidence of endometrial carcinoma from the age of 60 is 50 per 100 000 of the population. In younger women it is much more uncommon, being rare below age 35; <5 per 100 000 at age 45; and <10 per 100 000 at age 50. With 5% of women aged 30 to 49 consulting with menorrhagia, only 1 in 500 of them would expect to have a cancer and that woman would almost certainly have one or more red flags (see below), namely intermenstrual or irregular bleeding (or postmenopausal bleeding in the woman past the menopause).

The value of the history in assessment of menorrhagia

The following questions are useful in an assessment of the heaviness of the loss:[7]

■ *Do you pass clots?* If so, are they larger than a 50p piece (1.1 inches in diameter)? (odds ratio (OR) for a loss greater than 80 ml = 4.8. This means that the probability of true menorrhagia is increased nearly five times if the patient is passing large clots.)

■ *How often do you change your pad or tampon* at the height of the period? (If > hourly, OR for a loss greater than 80 ml = 3.1.)

■ *What is the total number of pads or tampons* you use in a period?

■ *Do you have to change the pad or tampon in the night?*

■ *Does the blood leak* onto underclothes or bedding?

■ *Do you need to wear two pads* or a pad and a tampon?

The patient should also be asked about the presence of red flags (see below).

Questions about her general health should reveal clues to hypothyroidism on the rare occasions in which it presents with menorrhagia. Questions to reveal a bleeding disorder should include whether periods have been heavy since puberty, and whether the patient bleeds readily in other situations.

Examination

The Royal College of Obstetricians and Gynaecologists (RCOG) guideline[6] recommends abdominal and pelvic examination but speculum examination only if a cervical smear is due. Where examination reveals a uterus that is >10 weeks in size or where there is a pelvic mass or tenderness, referral is indicated.

Investigations

✷ Check the haemoglobin. Anaemia is associated with a loss greater than 80 ml.

✷ If anaemic, check the serum ferritin.

No other investigations are indicated unless the history has revealed pointers to other diseases or to likely gynaecological pathology.

After the above steps have been taken

Women with clots greater than a 50p coin, who change pads or tampons more than hourly at the height of the period, and who have a low ferritin, have a 76% chance of having a loss greater than 80 ml. Does the size of the loss matter? It does not predict uterine pathology, iron status, or likely response to treatment. Its value to the GP is that it provides one piece of the jigsaw that is made up of events in the genital tract and the patient's reaction to those events. It is the interaction between those two features that determines whether a patient presents with menorrhagia.

The patient's perspective

The approach outlined above, that patients with menorrhagia should be treated symptomatically and only referred if the severity of their symptoms warrants it, may not be in accordance with the wishes of the patient. In a study of women referred with various bleeding disorders to an Edinburgh gynaecological clinic, 94% were glad they had been investigated. Indeed 34% of those in the lowest risk group (under age 40 with no risk factors) wished they had had more investigations.[9]

Referral

The referral guidance for menorrhagia from the National Institute for Health and Clinical Excellence is that women with menorrhagia should only be referred if:[10]

■ there is suspicion of underlying cancer, including persistent intermenstrual or post-coital bleeding; or

■ despite 3 months of drug treatment, heavy bleeding persists and is interfering with the quality of life. Failure of treatment is best based on the woman's own assessment; or

■ the patient wishes to explore the possibility of surgical intervention rather than persist with drug treatment; or

■ they have severe anaemia that has failed to respond to treatment.

Do risk factors for endometrial cancer alter this decision?

Risk factors are conditions which are associated with raised oestrogen levels: exogenous unopposed oestrogen administration, obesity, chronic anovulation, diabetes, oestrogen-secreting tumours and tamoxifen use. Risk of endometrial cancer is also raised in hereditary non-polyposis colorectal cancer. However, the increase in risk in these conditions is too small (e.g. tamoxifen increases the risk of endometrial cancer 2–3-fold) for investigation to be justified if it is not otherwise necessary.

Predictive value of red flags

Guidelines commonly recommend that referral should be considered in patients with abnormal bleeding,[6] namely:
■ intermenstrual bleeding
■ irregular bleeding
■ sudden change in the volume of blood lost
■ post-coital bleeding
■ dyspareunia
■ pelvic pain
■ premenstrual pain.

   However, the predictive value of these symptoms for cancer is low. A study from Finland examined the number of cancers detected over a mean follow-up of 7 years in 37596 women recorded as having abnormal bleeding when they presented for a routine cervical smear (Table 29.2). Women with an abnormal smear were excluded.[11]

   A note of caution should be sounded in relation to this study, on two counts:
1. Women did not present with these complaints, they were asked about problems when attending for a routine smear. Women with more alarming symptoms may have attended gynaecological clinics and so not attended the smear clinic.
2. They were only included in the study if their cervical smear was negative. Post-coital bleeding is a powerful predictor of cervical cancer if all women are included, with an odds ratio of 15. This risk did not show in this study because almost all those women would have had positive smears and been excluded.[11]

Studies from secondary care give higher predictive values for abnormal bleeding because patients have already been selected for referral by the GP. In these secondary care studies, postmenopausal bleeding carries the highest risk of cancer, but even then the probability is not high. One study from Switzerland found endometrial cancer in only 4.4%.[12] A study from secondary care in Taiwan found only 2.9% had endometrial cancer, although 7.6% suffered from either cervical intraepithelial neoplasia (CIN) III or cervical cancer[13] – diagnoses that can be made in primary care by inspecting the cervix and performing a smear.

Conclusion

It appears, and it comes as no surprise in view of the widespread nature of menstrual abnormalities, that only a small proportion of patients with menstrual complaints present in primary care and that GPs only refer a small proportion of them to specialist clinics. No study

Table 29.2 The increase in risk of gynaecological cancers in women with abnormal bleeding[11]

Bleeding abnormality	Prevalence of the symptom	The standardised incidence ratio (95% CI)*
Irregular bleeding	3.9%	1.2 (0.9–1.3)
Bloodstained discharge	1.1%	1.3 (1.0–1.8)
Postmenopausal bleeding	0.2%	1.8 (1.1–2.9)
All abnormal bleeding	5.9%	1.2 (1.1–1.4)

*This is the incidence of gynaecological cancers in patients with that abnormality over the expected incidence in the population. A standardised incidence ratio of 1.2, therefore, means that a woman with irregular bleeding has 1.2 times the risk of gynaecological cancer of the rest of the population of the same age and sex.

has explicitly studied this process nor analysed the factors which lead to such effective screening out of benign disorders.

The low positive predictive values of these symptoms confirm the UK recommendations for referral from the Department of Health:[14]

1. That, as far as bleeding abnormalities are concerned, women should be referred urgently for suspected cancer if there is:
   (a) postmenopausal bleeding in a woman not on HRT; or
   (b) persistent or unexplained bleeding that continues for >6 weeks after stopping HRT; or
   (c) postmenopausal bleeding in a patient on tamoxifen; or
   (d) vulval bleeding from a vulval ulcer; or possibly
   (e) persistent intermenstrual bleeding even with a negative pelvic examination.

2. That a pelvic examination including cervical smear should be performed when patients present with any of the following:
   (a) altered menstrual cycle
   (b) intermenstrual bleeding
   (c) post-coital bleeding
   (d) postmenopausal bleeding
   (e) vaginal discharge.

Example

A reclusive unmarried woman aged 40 presents with an infected finger and asks, in passing, whether heavy periods are a sign of cancer of the uterus. The GP is able to say that they are not. The patient then asks about heavy periods that are also irregular and the GP has to agree that that does raise the risk slightly. It does not require great acumen to guess that she is asking about her own symptoms and, having ascertained that this is the case, he suggests that he examine her to see if there are any grounds for concern. This she refuses utterly; she is terrified of being examined vaginally and wants no help with this fear. She does, however, want to know how great a risk she is running by not being investigated. The GP asks a few more questions: the blood loss does sound large; symptoms have developed gradually over months or even years; the cycle is irregular rather than regular with intermenstrual bleeding; and she is well in herself. She is neither obese nor diabetic and there is no family history of cancer. He is able to reassure her that the cancer risk is very small (the Finnish study above suggests <1 in 1000) but that examination might reveal a treatable cause such as a fibroid. She is unmoved in her refusal but agrees to a blood test for anaemia. The GP makes a note to continue to offer help with her fear of examination, and the other symptoms of anxiety that he suspects she has, as he gets to know her better.

REFERENCES

1. Warner P, Critchley H, Lumsden M, et al. *Menorrhagia II: is the 80 ml blood loss criterion useful in management of complaint of menorrhagia?* Am J Obstet Gynecol 2004;190:1224–1229.

2. O'Flynn N, Britten N. *Diagnosing menstrual disorders: a qualitative study of the approach of primary care professionals.* Br J Gen Pract 2004;54:353–358.

3. CRD. *The management of menorrhagia.* Centre for Reviews and Dissemination: Effective Health Care 1995;1(9).

4. Warner P, Critchley H, Lumsden M, et al. *Referral for menstrual problems: cross sectional survey of symptoms, reasons for referral, and management.* BMJ 2001;323: 24–28.

5. Shapley M, Jordan K, Croft P. *An epidemiological survey of symptoms of menstrual loss in the community.* Br J Gen Pract 2004;54:359–363.

6. RCOG Guideline Development Group. *The initial management of menorrhagia; a national evidence-based clinical guideline.* London: Royal College of Obstetricians and Gynaecologists, 1998. Online. Available: www.rcog.org.uk.

7. Warner P, Critchley H, Lumsden M, et al. *Menorrhagia I: measured blood loss, clinical features, and outcome in women with heavy periods: a survey with follow-up data.* Am J Obstet Gynecol 2004;190:1216–1223.

8. Pearce J. *Disturbances of the menstrual cycle.* In: Varma T, ed. Clinical gynaecology. London: Edward Arnold, 1991.

9. Critchley H, Warner P, Lee A, et al. *Evaluation of abnormal uterine*

bleeding: comparison of three outpatient procedures within cohorts defined by age and menopausal status. Health Technol Assess 2004;8(34).

10. National Institute for Clinical Excellence (NICE). *Referral advice 2001: Menorrhagia.* London: NICE. Online. Available: www.nice.org.uk. Reproduced with permission.

11. Viiki M, Pukkala E, Hakama M. *Bleeding symptoms and subsequent risk of gynecological and other cancers.* Acta Obstet Gynecol Scand 1998;77: 564–569.

12. Bachmann L, ter Riet G, Clark T, et al. *Probability analysis for diagnosis of endometrial hyperplasia and cancer in postmenopausal bleeding: an approach for a rational diagnostic workup.* Acta Obstet Gynecol Scand 2003;82: 564–569.

13. Lin H, Wu M, Shyu M, et al. *Clinical study of 381 postmenopausal bleeding patients.* J Formos Med Assoc 1993;92:241–244.

14. NICE. *Referral guidelines for suspected cancer.* London: National Institute for Health and Clinical Excellence, 2005. Online. Available: www.nice.org.uk.

30

Neck pain

Both acute and chronic neck pain are common. Their origin is usually presumed to be musculoskeletal and more detailed diagnosis is usually not possible. However, occasionally neck pain is due to more serious pathology:
■ infection
■ malignancy
■ trauma
■ disc or bony displacement with nerve root or cervical cord compression
■ haemorrhage, as in subarachnoid haemorrhage
■ generalised arthritis or another generalised condition.

Red flags are described to assist in the detection of these conditions, with decision rules for the detection of clinically important trauma following neck injury.

A PRACTICAL APPROACH

* Ask about trauma, other joint problems or muscle pains, general health and tingling or weakness in the arms or legs.
* Pursue any positive responses, including the use of a formal rule for the assessment of neck injury if there has been trauma.
* In the absence of any other pointers, explain that the nature of the musculoskeletal disorder will never be precisely defined and that investigation would be unlikely to make a diagnosis possible or alter treatment.

Population prevalence

● About two-thirds of people will experience neck pain at some time in their lives.[1,2] The point prevalence varies between studies. A recent Swedish study found that it was 43% (95% CI 41% to 44%) with the highest prevalence at age 55–64[3] and with 19% reporting chronic pain (continuous neck pain for >6 months).
● In the Netherlands, neck pain accounts for up to 2% of general practitioner consultations.[4]
● In the UK, about 15% of hospital-based physiotherapy, and, in Canada, 30% of chiropractic referrals, are for neck pain.[5,6]

Differentiating the possible causes

Attempts to diagnose the cause of neck pain are likely to be unsuccessful in the large majority of patients. Most will have pain for which no cause can be found; in others it will be due to cervical spondylosis or cervical disc disease. Differentiating these three is difficult, since X-ray changes of spondylosis are common after the age of 40 and correlate poorly with symptoms.[7] Magnetic resonance imaging (MRI) scan is needed for the visualisation of disc prolapse. In the absence of disc prolapse, a study of young adults found no correlation between MRI findings and the presence or absence of neck pain.[8] Furthermore, such differentiation would be unhelpful since, with the exceptions below, the treatment of neck pain (encouraging activity, avoidance of collars and early mobilisation or manipulation) is the same regardless of aetiology and duration.

Red flags

Check for the following red flags:
* *Is the patient unwell?* Fever raises the possibility of meningitis, a cervical abscess or cervical lymphadenopathy. Exhaustion, weight loss or a

past history of malignancy raise the possibility of a malignant cause. A history of drug misuse or of immunosuppression raises the possibility of atypical infections.

* *Has there been recent trauma?* Check the patient using the NEXUS criteria[9] and/or the Canadian C-spine rule[10] (see below). The latter has been shown to be more sensitive, though less specific, than physician judgement. In a Canadian study of 6265 patients, the physicians' judgement had a sensitivity of 92% and a specificity of 54% against a sensitivity of 100% and a specificity of 44% for the rule.[11] In a head-to-head study of the two rules, the Canadian C-spine rule was the more sensitive in the detection of clinically important injury (sensitivity 99.4% (95% CI 96 to 100) versus 90.7% (95% CI 85 to 94)).[10]

* *Does the patient have a more generalised disorder affecting the joints or soft tissues?* Specifically, rheumatoid arthritis predisposes to subluxation of the atlanto-axial joint, as does Down's syndrome. In ankylosing spondylitis, rigidity and kyphosis of the lumber and thoracic spine are likely to be obvious by the time the neck is involved. Jaw claudication would suggest that the neck pain might be due to giant cell arteritis.

* *Is there compression of the spinal cord?* Ask about difficulty balancing and walking; about difficulties using the hands; about bowel, bladder and sexual function. If any of these is positive, check for exaggerated reflexes in the lower limbs and depressed reflexes in the upper limbs. Look for up-going plantar reflexes. Check for Lhermitte's sign – an electric shock-like feeling down the spine on flexing the neck.

* *Is there nerve root compression?* Ask about pain, paraesthesiae or weakness in the upper limbs. If any of these is present, look for reduction in the following reflexes: biceps (C5 and 6); triceps (C7) and supinator (C6). In the absence of symptoms or of reflex abnormality, testing for weakness or sensory loss is unlikely to be rewarding. If you notice ptosis and miosis, check for Horner's syndrome which could be due to damage to the sympathetic innervation of the eye in the neck. It is likely to be associated with C8 and T1 nerve root signs,[12] i.e. weakness of finger flexion, abduction and adduction; and sensory loss on the medial border of the forearm and in the fourth and fifth fingers.

* *Was there a whiplash injury in the hours or days before the onset of pain?* Some studies find no correlation between a history of whiplash injury and the presence of neck pain; in others there appears to be a correlation.[3] The importance is medico-legal rather than that there are therapeutic implications.

* *Was the onset sudden and associated with headache, or loss of consciousness?* Subarachnoid haemorrhage is a possibility.

* *Is there evidence of a psychological component?* Depression may present in a somatic disguise. A patient who is 'catastrophising' the problem may benefit from a cognitive behavioural approach. Tests have been developed to act as pointers to the presence of abnormal illness behaviour[13] but a recent systematic review has cast doubt on their ability to distinguish organic from non-organic pain.[14]

Two other conditions may be distinguishable clinically:

■ *Torticollis*. The neck will be stiff and the head turned to one side, because of muscle spasm. It is not a diagnosis in itself since it is usually secondary to any of the (clinically undiagnosable) causes of neck pain.

■ *Fibromyalgia*, in which there will be trigger points in the neck and elsewhere (see *Fibromyalgia*, p. 388).

Investigations

Investigations are unlikely to be helpful in the absence of any red flag.

Referral

Grounds for referral in a patient with non-specific neck pain are:

1. early, for mobilisation or manipulation, to a physiotherapist, chiropractor or osteopath
2. after 6 weeks if symptoms are failing to settle and the patient is disabled by the pain and/or stiffness, to a rheumatologist for assessment.

The decision rules for neck trauma

The NEXUS criteria

NEXUS criteria for X-ray of the cervical spine after blunt trauma[9]

N – neurological examination: any focal deficit?

S – spine examination: any posterior midline tenderness of the cervical spine?

A – alertness: any alteration?

I – intoxication: any evidence?

D – distracting injury: any painful injury that might distract the patient from the pain of the cervical spine injury?

X-ray is needed if any of the criteria are present.

A positive answer to any of the five NEXUS questions means that the patient needs immediate referral for X-ray of the cervical spine, looking for fracture, dislocation or subluxation. The rule has a sensitivity for detecting clinically significant injury of 99.6% (95% CI 99.8% to 100%) and a specificity of 12.9%. In Hoffman's series of 34 069 patients of all ages who presented to 21 emergency departments across the USA with blunt neck trauma, the questions had the predictive values for cervical spine injury shown in Table 30.1. If only clinically significant injury was considered, the performance of the rule was even better, with a positive predictive value of 1.9% and a negative predictive value of 99.9% (95% CI 99.8% to 100%). The sensitivity of the rule would have been 100% had it not been for 2 patients who were missed; but one of them probably had an old fracture and in the other the rule seems to have been misapplied.[9] In Hoffman's series, use of the rule could have avoided X-ray in 12.6% of cases.

The Canadian C-spine rule (Fig. 30.1)

A Canadian study of 8283 patients with neck trauma found that the Canadian C-spine rule was 99.4% sensitive and 45.1% specific for clinically important injury (Table 30.2).[10] However, 10% of the patients could not be scored because the physician failed to evaluate the range of neck movement the full 45° to left and right. To be useful, the rule must be followed precisely.

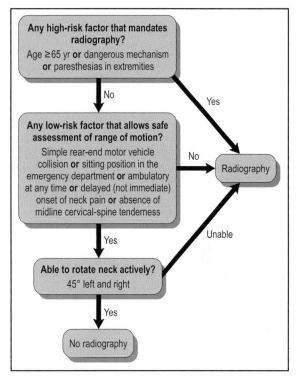

Figure 30.1 The Canadian C-spine rule. (Reproduced with permission from Stiell I, Clement C, McKnight R, et al. The Canadian C-spine Rule versus the NEXUS Low-Risk Criteria in Patients with Trauma. N Engl J Med 2003;349:2510–2518. Copyright © 2003 Massachusetts Medical Society. All rights reserved.)

Table 30.1 The performance of the NEXUS questions in the diagnosis of cervical spine injury[9]

Probability before the assessment	Score	Likelihood ratio	Probability of that condition after the assessment
2.4%	At least 1 positive	1.1	2.7%
	All negative	0.08	0.2%

Follow each row from left to right to see how the score alters the probability of cervical spine injury on X-ray.

Table 30.2 The performance of the Canadian C-spine rule in the diagnosis of clinically important injury to the cervical spine[10]

Probability before the assessment	Score	Likelihood ratio	Probability of that condition after the assessment
2.2%	Positive	1.8	4%
	Negative	0.01	0.01%

Follow each row from left to right to see how the score alters the probability of cervical spine injury on X-ray.

Example

A 45-year-old scaffolder comes with a 3-week history of neck pain and limitation of neck movements, especially on trying to look to the right. He is unable to work. He has not had it before and does not know what brought it on; it was there when he woke one morning. He has been to an osteopath with no benefit.

The GP confirms that neck movements are limited. She checks that he feels well in himself, that there was no trauma, that he has no other joint trouble, that he has no pain or weakness in the arms or legs. As he walked into the consulting room his gait had been normal. She feels she has excluded any serious condition.

She explains that it is impossible to say exactly what the musculoskeletal problem is, and that she cannot recommend anything better than the osteopath. He asks for an X-ray and she explains that, in the absence of a history of trauma and suspicion of a fracture, X-ray is unhelpful. However, she wants to see him in 3 weeks if he is not improving to reassess the situation.

REFERENCES

1. Cote P, Cassidy D, Carroll L. *The Saskatchewan health and back pain survey: the prevalence of neck pain and related disability in Saskatchewan adults.* Spine 1998;23:1689–1698.

2. Mäkelä M, Heliävaara M, Sievers K, et al. *Prevalence, determinants, and consequences of chronic neck pain in Finland.* Am J Epidemiol 1991;134: 1356–1367.

3. Guez M, Hildingsson C, Nilsson M, et al. *The prevalence of neck pain.* Acta Orthop Scand 2002;73:455–459.

4. Lamberts H, Brouwer H, Groen A, et al. *Het transitiemodel in de huisartspraktijk [Dutch].* Huisart Wet 1987;30:105–113.

5. Waalen D, White P, Waalen J. *Demographic and clinical characteristics of chiropractic patients: a 5-year study of patients treated at the Canadian Memorial Chiropractic College.* J Can Chiropract Assoc 1994;38:75–82.

6. Hackett G, Hudson M, Wylie J, et al. *Evaluation of the efficacy and acceptability to patients of a physiotherapist working in a health centre.* BMJ 1987;294:24–26.

7. Barry M, Jenner J. *ABC of rheumatology: pain in neck, shoulder and arm.* BMJ 1995;310:183–186.

8. Siivola S, Levoska S, Tervonen O, et al. *MRI changes of cervical spine in asymptomatic and symptomatic young adults.* Eur Spine J 2002;11:358–363.

9. Hoffman J, Mower W, Wolfson A, et al. *Validity of a set of clinical criteria to rule out injury to the cervical spine in patients with blunt trauma.* N Engl J Med 2000;343:94–99.

10. Stiell I, Clement C, McKnight R, et al. *The Canadian C-spine rule versus the NEXUS low-risk criteria in patients with trauma.* N Engl J Med 2003;349:2510–2518.

11. Bandiera G, Stiell I, Wells G, et al. *The Canadian C-spine rule performs better than unstructured physician judgement.* Ann Emerg Med 2003;42:395–404.

12. McGee S. *Evidence-based physical diagnosis.* Philadelphia: Saunders, 2001.

13. Sobel J, Sollenberger P, Robinson R, et al. *Cervical nonorganic signs: a new clinical tool to assess abnormal illness behavior in neck pain patients: a pilot study.* Arch Phys Med Rehabil 2000;81:170–175.

14. Fishbain D, Cole B, Cutler R, et al. *A structured evidence-based review on the meaning of nonorganic physical signs: Waddell signs.* Pain Med 2003;4:141–181.

Example–cont'd

To test for carpal tunnel syndrome he asks her to place her hand flat on the desk and then to raise her thumb against his resistance. It is definitely weaker on the right. He then tests for pain sensation with a sterile pin on the fingers. There is some diminution in sensation on the lateral three fingers.

The GP decides that his tentative diagnosis is carpal tunnel syndrome; she has the classic distribution, weakness of thumb abduction and diminution of pain sensation in the median nerve distribution.

When he gets home that night he works it out more thoroughly. Carpal tunnel syndrome was,

from the start, the most likely diagnosis, with a probability of, say, 15%, being commoner in a woman than a man. The classic distribution of symptoms increased the probability to 30%, the weakness of thumb abduction to 44% and the hypalgesia to 71% (Figs 31.1–31.3). He knows that it may not be correct to apply these likelihood ratios one after the other, since they have not been proved to be independent. But he is relieved to read that symptoms in all fingers and above the wrist are well described, even though there is no convincing explanation for them.

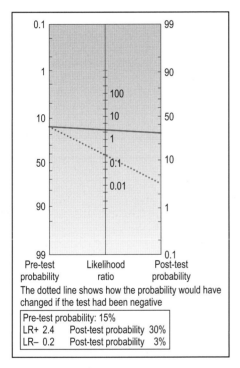

The dotted line shows how the probability would have changed if the test had been negative

Pre-test probability: 15%
LR+ 2.4   Post-test probability 30%
LR– 0.2   Post-test probability 3%

Figure 31.1 The probability of carpal tunnel syndrome before and after the question about the distribution of symptoms in the example above.

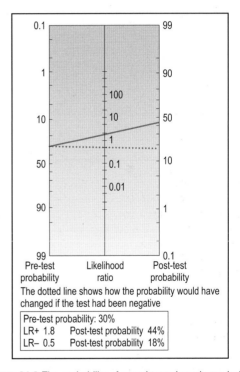

The dotted line shows how the probability would have changed if the test had been negative

Pre-test probability: 30%
LR+ 1.8   Post-test probability 44%
LR– 0.5   Post-test probability 18%

Figure 31.2 The probability of carpal tunnel syndrome before and after testing thumb abduction in the example above.

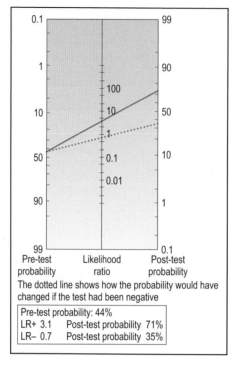

Figure 31.3 The probability of carpal tunnel syndrome before and after testing for hypalgesia in the median nerve distribution in the example on p. 203.

REFERENCES

1. McGee S. *Evidence-based physical diagnosis.* Philadelphia: Saunders, 2001.

2. Walker-Bone K, Palmer K, Reading I, Cooper C. *Soft-tissue rheumatic disorders of the neck and upper limb: prevalence and risk factors.* Semin Arthritis Rheum 2003;33: 185–203.

3. Ferry S, Pritchard T, Keenan J, et al. *Estimating the prevalence of delayed median nerve conduction in the general population.* Br J Rheumatol 1998;37:630–635.

4. D'Arcy C, McGee S. *Does this patient have carpal tunnel syndrome?* JAMA 2000;283:3110–3117.

5. Katz J, Stirrat C, Larson M, et al. *A self-administered hand symptom diagram for the diagnosis and epidemiological study of carpal tunnel syndrome.* J Rheumatol 1990;17: 1495–1498.

6. Ferry S, Silman A, Pritchard T, et al. *The association between different patterns of hand symptoms and objective evidence of median nerve compression.* Arthritis Rheum 1998;41:720–724.

7. Stevens I. *De Quervain's stenosing tenovaginitis.* In: Patient presentations in general practice. Roseville, NSW: McGraw-Hill Australia, 1999:529.

8. Elliott B. *Finkelstein's test: a descriptive error that can produce a false positive.* J Hand Surg 1992;17B: 481–482.

5. Zakrzewska J. *Diagnosis and differential diagnosis of trigeminal neuralgia.* Clin J Pain 2002;18: 14–21.

6. Nurmikko T, Eldridge P. *Trigeminal neuralgia – pathophysiology, diagnosis and current treatment.* Br J Anaesth 2001;87:117–132.

7. Pow E, Leung K, McMillan A. *Prevalence of symptoms associated with temporomandibular disorders in Hong Kong Chinese.* J Orofacial Pain 2001; 15:228–234.

8. Ciancaglini R, Radaelli G. *The relationship between headache and symptoms of temporomandibular disorder in the general population.* J Dent 2001;29:93–98.

9. Emshoff R, Rudisch A, Innerhofer K, et al. *Magnetic resonance imaging findings of internal derangement in temporomandibular joints without a clinical diagnosis of temporomandibular disorder.* J Oral Rehabil 2002;29: 516–522.

10. Madland G, Feinmann C. *Chronic facial pain: a multidisciplinary problem.* J Neurol Neurosurg Psychiatry 2001;71: 716–719.

Palpitations

- Most people who notice palpitations do not consult. Of those who do, about 20% are found to have a significant cardiac arrhythmia. Many others, with significant arrhythmias, do not notice them.
- The most common arrhythmias are extrasystoles and atrial fibrillation (AF). Also common is an undue awareness of the normal heartbeat.
- The history, examination and ECG make a diagnosis possible in the majority of cases although the likelihood ratios of the different findings have yet to be worked out. A minority of cases will need referral, either because of alarming aspects of the history (e.g. syncope, chest pain, breathlessness), or because a significant arrhythmia has been found, or suspected, which needs specialist assessment, or because a diagnosis has not been made.

A PRACTICAL APPROACH

- ★ Take a careful history, noting how the palpitations start and stop, whether rapid or slow, weak or powerful, what triggers them and how long they last.
- ★ Consider features of the patient that are relevant: age, the presence of heart disease or a tendency to somatisation.
- ★ Examine the pulse and the heart.
- ★ Order a 12-lead ECG. Look not only for an abnormal rhythm but for abnormalities specific for arrhythmia (e.g. a short PR interval and delta wave; or a long QT interval and abnormal T wave) as well as more general evidence of cardiac disease.
- ★ Make a preliminary diagnosis. Refer if unable to exclude cardiac disease and significant arrhythmias confidently.
- ★ Refer more readily if the patient is older, has cardiovascular disease, or if the palpitations happen at work, last for >5 minutes, or the abnormal rhythm is regular, starts and stops suddenly, and is very slow or very fast (>140/min).
- ★ Do not make a diagnosis of non-cardiac palpitations just because the patient has a psychiatric disorder; it may be coincidental.

Definition

Palpitations are a subjective phenomenon, being the unpleasant awareness of an abnormal heartbeat. The beat may be fast or slow, regular or irregular, momentary or sustained.

Prevalence

In the population

Each year, 2 to 3 people report a new onset of palpitations per 1000 of the population, with a point prevalence of diagnosed arrhythmias of 2%.[1]

Arrhythmias are hugely more common than this. A population study from Norway found that 74% of 54 patients who denied noticing palpitations in the last year had arrhythmias on a single 24-hour ECG monitor.[2]

In primary care

In a Dutch study, 625 patients, out of a population of nearly 50 000, consulted 27 GPs because of palpitations, over a period of almost 2 years, giving an annual incidence of 0.6%.[1]

Initial probabilities

Probabilities depend on the method used to make the diagnosis and the selectivity of the referring GPs in selecting patients for the study.

In a Dutch study in primary care, where the GP suspected an arrhythmia and where the diagnosis was made on *a single standard ECG*,[1] the following were found:
- significant cardiac arrhythmias: 6.6% (of which 70% were AF, and the rest were flutter, supraventricular tachycardia (SVT), chaotic atrial rhythm, sinus arrest and ventricular tachycardia (VT))
- insignificant cardiac arrhythmias: 19.5% (mainly extrasystoles, sinus bradycardia and sinus tachycardia)
- no arrhythmia found: 73.9%.

In a UK study in primary care, in which the diagnosis was made on *an event recorder during a bout of palpitations* over a 2-week period, the following were found:[3]
- significant cardiac arrhythmias: 19%
- insignificant cardiac arrhythmias: 11% (benign extrasystoles and sinus tachycardia)
- no arrhythmia found: 28%
- no palpitations occurred during the 2-week recording period: 42%.

The use of an event recorder as the gold standard makes the UK figures more likely to approximate to the true probabilities. Had a longer period of recording been used, the percentage of significant arrhythmias might well have been higher.

Studies from hospital settings yield higher percentages of patients with cardiac disease (43% in a study from Pittsburgh),[4] testifying to the fact that patients without cardiac disease are less likely to be referred to a specialist or to present in the emergency room.

How good are patients at detecting arrhythmias?

Patients are extraordinarily poor at detecting their arrhythmias.
- A study from New England of 137 patients who had arrhythmias while keeping a symptom diary and being continuously monitored found that 64% detected none of their arrhythmias, only 19% detected >1% and only 6% detected >10%.[5] None of the patients in whom atrial fibrillation was found detected it.
- A study from Norway found that 82 out of 97 patients monitored for 24 hours developed arrhythmias; none of them detected them.[2]

It may be that more serious arrhythmias are more likely to be detected, either as palpitations or as chest pain or syncope.
- In a series of 197 patients with sustained VT but without loss of consciousness, Brugada et al found that all 47 with VT but with otherwise normal hearts noticed palpitations. They also found that only 6 out of 97 with VT who had had a previous myocardial infarction noticed palpitations, and they postulate that left ventricular function must be good for the VT to be noticed by the patient.[6]

Can patients at least reliably report their heart rate? No. A study from Northampton[7] found that only 20% of patients complaining of palpitations could accurately report their heart rate over a short period when they were being monitored and asked to note their heart rate (heartbeat perception test).

Can a diagnosis of arrhythmia be made in primary care?

The history

Mayou et al[7] suggest the following features of the history are associated with a clinically significant arrhythmia:
- it starts and ends suddenly
- it is rapid
- if an ECG is taken during an attack it is abnormal.

Conversely, sinus tachycardia is likely to be the diagnosis if:
- the palpitation starts and ends gradually
- it occurs in situations of anxiety
- the beating is described as being forceful and regular
- the rate is <140 per minute.

Table 33.1 Correlation between the words used to describe palpitations and the arrhythmias found[5]

Symptom	Probability of an arrhythmia at the time	Type of arrhythmia (in those with that symptom and an arrhythmia)
'Stopping'	95%	VPC 100%
'Fluttering'	81%	VPC 58%; APC 39%; AT 2%
'Irregular'	78%	VPC 48%; APC 45%; AT 5%
'Jumping'	62%	VPC 86%; APC 14%; AT 0%
'Pounding' or 'vigorous'	39%	VPC 84%; APC 12%; AT 2%
'Racing'	21%	VPC 73%; APC 18%; AT 0%

VPC, ventricular premature contraction; APC, atrial premature contraction; AT, atrial tachycardia.

Certain features point to specific arrhythmias:
■ If the patient notices that a Valsalva manoeuvre will terminate the attack, this is probably an SVT.[8]
■ Extrasystoles are likely if the patient describes:
   (a) a flip-flopping in the chest
   (b) a sudden cessation of the heart for a second followed by a forceful beat.

However, the reliability of these features has not been tested.

The predictive values of the words patients use to describe their palpitations have been assessed in a study from New England[5] in which patients kept a symptom diary which was then compared with the results of continuous ECG monitoring. They found the positive predictive values shown in Table 33.1, i.e. each description had the probability shown in column 3 of being associated with an arrhythmia.

It is interesting to note that, in this study, in which 99 patients reported palpitations while being monitored, the report of 'stopping' was never associated with a prolonged pause or with bradycardia and 'racing' was never associated with tachycardia.

Other features that increase the probability that a report of palpitations indicates an arrhythmia

Apart from the patient's description of the palpitations, a number of features have, in different studies, been found to be significantly associated with arrhythmia:
■ older age[1]
■ male sex: odds ratio (OR) 2.6 (95% CI 1.2 to 5.4)[4]
■ the presence of cardiovascular disease: OR 3.5 (95% CI 1.6 to 7.8)[1,4]
■ palpitations that are regular[3] (although this is contradicted in the Pittsburgh study, which found that irregular palpitations were more likely to be due to cardiac disease[4]): OR 3.2
■ palpitations that are felt at work[3]
■ palpitations which last more than 5 minutes: OR 5.7 (95% CI 2.4 to 13.7)[4]
■ a lack of previous consultations for non-specific complaints[7]
■ no, or few, other complaints.[4]

The influence of psychiatric morbidity on the diagnosis

Patients with high scores on questionnaires for somatisation, hypochondria and psychiatric morbidity are more likely to complain of palpitations that are *not* confirmed by concurrent ECG monitoring than are patients with lower scores.

It is tempting to assume that a psychiatric diagnosis decreases the probability of an arrhythmia but such an assumption is dangerous. Various psychiatric diagnoses (panic attacks, panic disorder, anxiety disorder and depression) are more common in those who present with palpitations regardless of the final diagnosis. There is a trend for all of the above to be most common in those with sinus tachycardia and least common in those with significant arrhythmias, but in a study of 184 patients with palpitations in a cardiac clinic, the differences were not significant.[7]

A study of 107 consecutive patients with paroxysmal SVT found that 67% met the criteria for the diagnosis of panic disorder. That diagnosis may not be immediately obvious. Of the 59 patients in whom the diagnosis was not made at the first assessment, 54% subsequently received a diagnosis of panic, stress or anxiety disorder.[9]

13. Chen C, Bravata D, Weil E, et al. *A comparison of dermatologists' and primary care physicians' accuracy in diagnosing melanoma.* Arch Dermatol 2001;137:1627–1634.

14. English D, Burton R, Del Mar C, et al. *Evaluation of aid to diagnosis of pigmented skin lesions in general practice: controlled trial randomised by practice.* BMJ 2003;327:375–380.

15. Gachon J, Beaulieu P, Sei J, et al. *First prospective study of the recognition process of melanoma in dermatological practice.* Arch Dermatol 2005;141:434–438.

16. McGee R, Elwood M, Adam H, et al. *The recognition and management of melanoma and other skin lesions by general practitioners in New Zealand.* N Z Med J 1994;107:287–290.

17. Morris A, Gee B, Millard L. *Geometric cutaneous melanoma: a helpful clinical sign of malignancy?* Dermatol Surg 2003;29:827–828.

Pleuritic chest pain

- The commonest causes, musculoskeletal pain and chest infection, are usually obvious clinically.
- Pleuritic pain in the absence of pointers to these two common causes may pose a problem. Important diagnoses may not be accompanied by specific clinical signs and only referral to secondary care will clarify the situation. Disorders to consider, which may give rise to no clinical signs, are:
  - pneumothorax
  - pulmonary embolism
  - pleurisy due to viral infection or other systemic illness
  - Bornholm disease.

A PRACTICAL APPROACH

- ★ Look for an obvious clinical picture which would narrow down the possibilities, e.g. the fever and productive cough of a respiratory infection, or the pain on movement that was brought on by heavy lifting.

In the absence of an obvious cause, proceed methodically:

- ★ Look for risk factors for pulmonary embolism or pneumothorax.
- ★ Ask about other symptoms, especially cough and breathlessness.
- ★ Ask about the characteristics of the pain, especially what exacerbates it.

- ★ Examine the chest: skin, position of the tracheal, resonance, breath sounds, heart sounds, chest wall tenderness and axillary and supraclavicular nodes.

If the cause is still not clear, choose between the three options below, according to the situation:

- watchful waiting
- chest X-ray
- hospital referral (immediate or by outpatient appointment).

Definition

Pleuritic chest pain is pain in the chest which is worsened by breathing or coughing.

Note that not all pleuritic pain is felt in the chest. Pain originating from the pleura can also be felt outside the chest, because of the innervation of the parietal pleura.

Inflammation of the upper portion of the pleura will be felt in the chest. Inflammation of the lower portion, supplied by the lower six intercostal nerves, may also be felt in the upper abdomen. Inflammation of the central portion of the diaphragm, supplied by the phrenic nerve, will be felt in the neck and shoulder tip.[1]

Initial probabilities

The initial probabilities when a patient presents to the emergency department with pleuritic chest pain are as follows:
- *Musculoskeletal pain* 45% (see below).[2]
- *Chest infection* 22%.[2]
- *Pneumothorax* 7%.[2] This is commonest in males aged 10–30 with a second peak after age 55. Dyspnoea is usually present. Clinical signs may be obvious, or non-existent if the pneumothorax is small. Chest X-ray is diagnostic. See *Pneumothorax*, page 461.
- *Pleurisy without pneumonia* 6%.[2] A pleural rub may be present, distinguished by its unique quality (footsteps in snow, or a creaking door), and by being heard at the same point in each breath, often in expiration as well as inspiration.
- *Pulmonary embolism* (PE) 1%[2] to 21%.[3] The setting, and the investigations used, will determine the prevalence; in primary care, it is likely to be nearer 1% than 21%. See *Pulmonary embolus*, page 477.
- *Acute pericarditis* <1%.[2] The pain may worsen with inspiration and on lying flat. There may be dyspnoea. See *Pericarditis*, page 457.
- *Carcinoma*, primary or secondary.
- *Herpes zoster* (see below).
- *Bornholm disease* (epidemic pleurodynia) is uncommon. It may be associated with myocarditis or pericarditis which will complicate the clinical picture.

Is a chest X-ray likely to help?

It may, but it probably will not. It is likely to be normal in pulmonary embolism, chest wall pain, pericarditis, and possibly in pleurisy. It will probably be abnormal in acute respiratory infection but the diagnosis will usually have been made already on clinical grounds. It can be difficult to distinguish radiologically between infection and infarction; again the clinical picture will decide.

A small pneumothorax and malignant deposits in ribs are two conditions in which the diagnosis may be discovered unexpectedly on the chest X-ray.

Is this musculoskeletal pain?

It may arise from the chest wall or the thoracic spine (usually the costovertebral joints). It is worse on bending, twisting or lifting. There is usually a history of trauma or that the pain came on when exerting. Although it hurts to breathe or cough, the patient should not feel breathless when still.

The examination should include the following:
(a) Compression of the chest by pressing with both hands on the sternum; pain suggests that it originates from the chest wall.
(b) Palpation of the spine, chest wall and costosternal and sternoclavicular joints. This may localise the source of the pain. A specific syndrome is Tietze's syndrome, which is often associated with costosternal joint swelling as well as tenderness. It usually affects the second or third costosternal joints.

    However, chest wall tenderness is not specific for musculoskeletal pain; it may also be present in pulmonary embolism. In one series in the emergency department, it was found in 18% of patients with pleuritic pain, of whom 13% had a PE.[3]
(c) 'Springing' the ribs individually by pressing on them anteriorly one at a time, to detect rib fracture. Stress fractures of the ribs usually occur posterolaterally. The sixth is most commonly affected.[4]

Is this shingles (herpes zoster)?

The difficulty occasionally arises because the doctor fails to examine the chest for a rash in a good light; the early erythema which precedes the blisters can be missed. More usually, the pain is misdiagnosed in the days before the rash appears.

Clues are:
(a) the patient is unwell with a slight fever
(b) the axillary nodes are enlarged
(c) the pain is in the distribution of one or two dermatomes
(d) the pain is described in a way that suggests nerve pain: it is burning or shooting with paraesthesiae. Examination reveals sensory loss or distortion, with allodynia (a light touch is felt as painful).

The bottom line

Suspect a pulmonary embolus unless the history and examination make another cause much more likely.[1] Suspect an embolus even more readily in a patient at risk of venous thromboembolism and/ or one who is also breathless without chest signs.

REFERENCES

1. Jones K, Raghuram A. *Investigation and management of patients with pleuritic chest pain presenting to the accident and emergency department.* J Accid Emerg Med 1999;16:55–59.

2. Thomas L, Reichl M. *Pulmonary embolism in patients attending the accident and emergency department with pleuritic chest pain.* Arch Emerg Med 1990;8:48–51.

3. Hull R, Raskob G, Carter C, et al. *Pulmonary embolism in outpatients with pleuritic chest pain.* Arch Intern Med 1988;148:838–844.

4. Jensen S. *Musculoskeletal causes of chest pain.* Aust Fam Phys 2001;30: 835–839.

Rectal bleeding

KEY FACTS

- Rectal bleeding is common, although most people who experience it do not consult a doctor.
- Benign causes, e.g. haemorrhoids, fissure or diverticulitis, are more common than carcinoma. They may coexist with a carcinoma and mislead the GP as to the cause of the bleeding.

- A combination of symptoms, signs and investigations will have a major impact on an individual's risk that cancer is present.
- The role of the GP is to use that combination, taking into account both positive and negative findings, in order to decide whether to refer, to refer urgently or to recommend 'watchful waiting'.

A PRACTICAL APPROACH

- ★ Ask about the character of the bleeding, any change in bowel habit, abdominal pain, anal symptoms and weight loss.
- ★ Examine for an abdominal mass and perform a rectal examination, looking for anal abnormalities and for a rectal mass; 80% of rectal carcinomas can be detected on digital examination.[1]
- ★ Make a judgement about the need for referral based on the age of the patient, the presence of worrying symptoms or signs and the duration of symptoms. Assume the patient has a pre-test probability of serious disease of 2% and adjust it using the nomogram and likelihood ratios given below. Only refer if symptoms have been present for 6 weeks, unless the positive predictive value is very high.

- ★ Discuss the option of 'watchful waiting' in those in whom the probability of serious disease after examination is low (e.g. <2%). In one series of 8000 patients with rectal bleeding, the risk of cancer in patients without worrying symptoms or signs was 1:160.[2] Explain to the patient that, if referred, investigations are uncomfortable and carry their own risk.
- ★ Agree to refer a patient whose probability of serious disease is low but whose anxiety persists after explanation of the probabilities.
- ★ Reconsider the need for referral if the bleeding continues for more than 3 months.
- ★ Consider sending blood for haemoglobin, white blood cell count and erythrocyte sedimentation rate in patients in whom the decision about referral is not clear clinically.

Prevalence

In the general population

The prevalence of rectal bleeding in the general UK population is approximately 20% in any one year,[3–5] with 28% admitting to rectal bleeding at some time in their life.[5] A UK study asking about rectal bleeding in the last 6 months found a prevalence of 11.4%.[6] Most of these patients never consult a doctor about the bleeding.

As a complaint in primary care

This is the crucial statistic on which all subsequent estimates of disease probability are based, but it is hard to be sure of the true figure. For this chapter, an annual figure of 7 per 1000 patients[7] is used. A study recording only rectal bleeding in patients over age 34 found the comparable figure of 15 per 1000 per year.[8]

Initial probabilities in primary care

Colorectal adenoma or carcinoma

Eleven studies were identified in which an attempt was made to investigate all patients with rectal bleeding. Five UK studies found risks of colorectal carcinoma which varied from 2.4%[9] to 8%[10] in patients aged 40 and over. Studies from abroad ranged from a risk of 3.3% from the Netherlands[11] to 15% from Denmark.[12] All but one of these studies are vulnerable to selection bias; that is, they are dependent on general practitioners referring patients with rectal bleeding for investigation. It is inevitable that GPs would fail to refer some patients because they considered the bleeding too trivial to warrant investigation. The one study which avoided this bias was a case-control study from Exeter, in which the records of patients with colorectal cancer, and the records of controls, were searched for evidence of a complaint of rectal bleeding.[9] While this method has other problems, it seems likely that the true incidence of colorectal carcinoma in patients aged 40 and over with rectal bleeding is of the order of 2.4%.

Most studies which reported on adenomas found the same percentage with adenomas as with carcinoma.[8,10–16] That gives a risk of carcinoma or adenoma in a patient with rectal bleeding aged 40 or over of about 5%.

Non-malignant conditions

■ Haemorrhoids 16%[17]–28%[10]–29%[15]–79%[13]
■ Diverticular disease 1%[17]–5%[15]–16%[10]–26%[13]
■ Inflammatory bowel disease 2%[8]–3%[13]–4%[14]–9%[17]–11%[10,15]
■ Anal fissure 4%[15]–6%[13]–7%[17]
■ No cause found 11%[10]–61%.[17]

Other possible causes of rectal bleeding

■ Local causes: anal fistula, perianal inflammation, rectal prolapse, trauma
■ Gastroenteritis
■ Intestinal ischaemia
■ Recent bowel surgery
■ Arteriovenous malformation
■ Massive upper GI haemorrhage
■ Bleeding diathesis.

The clinical assessment for colorectal cancer

Tables 36.1 to 36.5 show how details of the history and a few investigations can alter the probability of colorectal cancer.

In Table 36.1, the predictive value of different symptoms in the diagnosis of cancer in patients with lower GI symptoms is shown. In this large study of 2268 patients referred to secondary care, among whom 95 had colorectal cancer (4.2%), no one symptom was strikingly useful, either in predicting or ruling out cancer.

A smaller UK study of patients presenting in primary care with rectal bleeding[8] found an overall rate of colorectal cancer, in the 83% who agreed to be studied, of 4.1%. The study examined the predictive value of *combinations* of symptoms and found them much more useful than single symptoms (see Table 36.2).

The symptom of a change in bowel habit can be analysed further (Table 36.3). A change towards more frequent and/or looser stools is most significant while a change towards harder and/or less frequent stools argues slightly against the diagnosis.

These figures become even more significant if all serious outcomes are considered (Table 36.4). **Combining the presence or absence of symptoms further**

These post-test probabilities (above) following a positive test are still low, while the post-test probabilities following a negative test are not

Table 36.1 The value of various clinical features in the diagnosis of colorectal cancer in patients referred from primary care with lower GI symptoms. The initial probability of colorectal carcinoma was 4.2%[18]

Symptom	Feature	LR (95% CI)	Probability of carcinoma after considering that feature
Age 60 or above	Present	1.8 (1.6–2.0)	7%
	Absent	0.3 (0.2–0.5)	1%
Blood mixed with stool	Present	2.7 (1.9–3.9)	13%
	Absent	0.8 (0.7–0.9)	4%
Dark blood	Present	2.3 (1.0–5.5)	11%
	Absent	0.96 (0.9–1.0)	4%
Loose motions	Present	1.9 (1.5–2.4)	9%
	Absent	0.7 (0.6–0.9)	4%
Constipation	Present	0.3 (0.1–0.8)	2%
	Absent	1.1 (1.1–1.2)	5%
Alternating loose and constipated stool	Present	0.96 (0.7–1.3)	5%
	Absent	1.0 (0.9–1.1)	5%
Increased frequency of stool	Present	1.8 (1.5–2.0)	9%
	Absent	0.5 (0.4–0.7)	3%
Bloodstained mucus	Present	3.6 (2.8–4.7)	16%
	Absent	0.7 (0.6–0.8)	3%
Abdominal pain	Present	0.6 (0.5–0.8)	3%
	Absent	1.4 (1.2–1.7)	7%
Weight loss	Present	2.2 (1.5–3.4)	11%
	Absent	0.9 (0.8–0.97)	4%
Fatigue	Present	0.8 (0.6–1.1)	4%
	Absent	1.1 (0.9–1.2)	5%

Follow each row from left to right to see how that feature alters the probability of cancer.
In Tables 36.1 to 36.5, the pre-test probabilities used will be those that were found in the studies being described.

Table 36.2 The effect of the addition of a further factor in a patient with rectal bleeding symptoms in the prediction of colorectal cancer where the prevalence of colorectal cancer is 4.1%[8]

Extra factor	Whether present or absent	LR (95% CI)	Probability of carcinoma (95% CI)
A change in bowel habit	Present	2.4 (1.9–2.7)	9% (7–10%)
	Absent	0.0 (0.0–1.1)	0% (0–4%)
No perianal symptoms	Present	2.9 (1.7–4.8)	11% (7–17%)
	Absent	0.5 (0.2–1.0)	2% (1–4%)
Age ≥60	Present	1.5 (1.0–2.2)	6% (4–8%)
	Absent	0.5 (0.2–1.4)	2% (1–5%)

Follow each row from left to right to see how the factor alters the probability of cancer.
NB. These statistics are derived from figures given in the article by Ellis and Thompson.[8] Note that none of the negative likelihood ratios reach statistical significance.

Table 36.3 Further analysis of the type of bowel change in the prediction of colorectal cancer where the prevalence of colorectal cancer is 4.1%[8]

Symptom	Whether present or absent	LR+ (95% CI)	Probability of carcinoma (95% CI)
Bleeding plus looser ± more frequent stools compared to constipation or no change	Present	3.2 (2.4–4.2)	12% (9–15%)
Bleeding plus harder ± less frequent stools compared to no change	Present	0.7 (0.1–4.4)	3% (1–16%)

Follow each row from left to right to see how the combination alters the probability of cancer. Thus constipation argues slightly against the diagnosis of carcinoma in patients with rectal bleeding but without reaching statistical significance.

Table 36.4 Combinations of symptoms in the prediction of colorectal cancer, polyp or proctocolitis in a patient presenting in primary care with rectal bleeding and whose initial probability of serious pathology is 12.8%[8]

Symptom	Whether present or absent	LR (95% CI)	Probability of serious pathology (95% CI)
Bleeding plus a change in bowel habit	Present	1.7	20% (16–25%)
	Absent	0.5	7% (4–11%)
Bleeding plus no perianal symptoms	Present	3.2	32% (24–41%)
	Absent	0.5	7% (5–10%)

Follow each row from left to right to see how the combination alters the probability of serious pathology.

negligible. A patient who presents in primary care with rectal bleeding and a change towards looser, more frequent stool still has a risk of colorectal cancer of only 12%. However, if the patient is at least 60 years old, the probability of cancer rises to 17% (see Fig. 36.1 of the example at the end of the chapter) and if no perianal symptoms are also present this rises to 37% (see Fig. 36.2 of the example). This explains the decision of the authors of the UK guidelines for urgent referral to propose a combination of symptoms and an age cut-off in their recommendations (see below).

Similarly, combining a series of negatives (rectal bleeding with no change of bowel habit, with perianal symptoms, in a patient aged <60), using the nomogram on page xxiv, produces a probability of cancer that moves from 4.1% to 2% to 1% to 0.5%.

It is interesting to note that the study found that other symptoms, usually thought to be sinister, were of no predictive value: dark blood, blood in the pan as well as on the paper, a large volume of blood, blood mixed with the stool.

Blood tests are usually ignored in the assessment of rectal bleeding. Table 36.5 shows that they are useful, indeed possibly more useful than symptoms.

Using the patient's age in assessing the probability of carcinoma

A cut-off of age 60. Wauters et al, in a study covering 83 890 patient years in primary care in Belgium,[19] found that the most useful age cut-off was 60. Out of 27 colorectal cancers in patients with rectal bleeding, only one occurred between ages 50 and 59 and only one below 50. In Wauters' study, the age of 60 or over has, for the diagnosis of cancer (compared to being aged <60), the following figures:

- LR+ 2.0 (95% CI 1.7 to 2.4)
- LR− 0.1 (95% CI 0.04 to 0.5).

Table 36.5 The value of investigations in the diagnosis of colorectal polyp or carcinoma[11] in a patient whose prior probability of carcinoma is 5%

Investigation	LR (95% CI)	Probability according to the test result (95% CI)
Anaemia	6.6 (1.7–26)	26% (12–50%)
No anaemia	0.7 (0.4–1.3)	4% (2–5%)
Raised ESR (>30)	10 (2.8–35)	34% (17–57%)
Normal ESR	0.6 (0.3–1.3)	3% (2–5%)
Raised WBC (>10^9/L)	7.5 (3.9–14)	28% (19–41%)
Normal WBC	0.3 (0.06–1.3)	2% (1–4%)

Follow each row from left to right to see how the investigation result alters the probability of polyp or cancer. ESR, erythrocyte sedimentation rate; WBC, white blood cell (count).

In other words, being aged 60 or over hardly increases a patient's risk of cancer, but being aged <60 hugely reduces it.

A cut-off of age 50. This is even less useful in increasing the probability of cancer but not significantly more useful in ruling it out:

- LR+ 1.6 (95% CI 1.4 to 1.8)
- LR– 0.09 (95% CI 0.01 to 0.6).

Implications in practice. In Wauters' study, a patient aged under 60 with rectal bleeding and no other symptoms and signs had a probability of cancer of 1% (95% CI 0% to 4%). This is much reduced but not negligible. A cost-effectiveness study of rectal bleeding in patients aged 25 to 45 found that the increase in life expectancy as a result of investigation was at a cost comparable to screening for colorectal cancer in an asymptomatic, but older, population.[20]

Value of a family history of colorectal carcinoma in assessing the probability of carcinoma

Not much, if any. It is clear that a family history increases the risk of a patient developing colorectal carcinoma. At the age of 40 to 59, the fact that one first-degree relative has colorectal cancer increases the risk by 1.7. If two or more have colorectal cancer, the risk increases by 2.75.[21] If one of those was aged <55 at the time of diagnosis or if only one first-degree relative had colorectal cancer diagnosed before age 45, the risk is increased 5-fold. Lifetime risks range from 10% for those with a single first-degree relative affected before the age of 45, to 50% in the first-degree relatives of those with familial adenomatous polyposis. However, in practice,

family history has not proved useful in the assessment of patients with symptoms,[11] possibly because the patient with a family history presents more readily with minor symptoms, so negating the increased risk, and if screening is being undertaken, those with early cancer have already been detected. Despite this, common sense dictates that a patient who has not been screened, whose symptoms do not appear trivial and who has a family history of colorectal carcinoma should be referred even more readily than one who has no such history.

Does the presence of anal pathology argue against there being concurrent colorectal malignancy?

Yes. If the patient has noticed an anal protrusion, the probability of an anal cause of the bleeding is increased 6-fold (OR = 6 (95% CI 2 to 15)).[22] However, this does not rule out the possibility that the bleeding is coming from a source higher in the bowel. One Australian study found that 16% of patients with haemorrhoids also had a colorectal source of bleeding and in 5% this was a malignancy.[22] Wrongly attributing bleeding to haemorrhoids is a common reason for a delayed diagnosis of cancer.[23]

Is faecal occult blood useful in the patient complaining of rectal bleeding?

It depends how it is done. The sending of six samples for occult blood testing is useful but rarely practised in primary care. The single test following rectal examination is more common[24] and is useless (see *Colorectal carcinoma*, p. 369).

Referral guidelines

The UK National Institute for Health and Clinical Excellence has highlighted the following categories as needing urgent referral (i.e. to be seen in under 2 weeks):[25]

Referral is urgent in patients with:
■ a right-sided abdominal mass clinically arising from the large bowel; or
■ a rectal (not pelvic) mass; or
■ rectal bleeding with a change in bowel habit to more frequent stools and/or increased frequency of defecation persisting for 6 weeks in a patient aged 40 or older; or
■ iron deficiency anaemia without obvious cause (haemoglobin <11 g/dl in men or <10 g/dl in non-menstruating women).

In patients over 60 years old, referral is urgent in any patient with:
■ rectal bleeding persisting for at least 6 weeks; or
■ change of bowel habit to looser stools and/or increased frequency of defecation persisting for 6 weeks (even without rectal bleeding).

The following, if there is no rectal or abdominal mass, are at very low risk of cancer:
■ those with rectal bleeding plus anal symptoms (e.g. pruritus, soreness, pain, lumps or prolapse)
■ those with a change in bowel habit in the direction of constipation
■ those with abdominal pain without clear evidence of obstruction.

Criticism has been made of two of these recommendations[7]: that a change of bowel habit in the direction of constipation should not necessarily influence the decision; and that it may be unnecessary to wait for a 6-week history before urgent referral when the patient has highly suggestive symptoms. However, in general the guidelines are supported by the likelihood ratios given in Tables 36.2 to 36.5.

General points

1. Individual characteristics in a patient with rectal bleeding only increase the risk of carcinoma modestly; a combination of symptoms is a more powerful predictor. A combination of a change to more frequent and looser stool in a patient aged over 60 with no perianal symptoms, for instance, is a powerful predictor of carcinoma.
   Conversely, the absence of these characteristics reduces the probability, such that, in a patient aged 50 with rectal bleeding but where the blood is not mixed with stool and there is no increased frequency of motions, the probability of carcinoma or polyp is reduced from 5% to 2% (calculated using the LR− figures from Table 36.1).

2. Symptoms need to be interpreted with care. An altered bowel habit in a patient with rectal bleeding is most significant if it is towards looser and/or more frequent stools. Abdominal pain argues (slightly) against the diagnosis of carcinoma but not if the pain is in the lower abdomen when its presence does not influence the diagnosis either way.

3. The probability of carcinoma can only be assessed if the history covers the relevant features, listed above, and an abdominal and rectal examination are performed. The situation in London in the 1980s, when fewer than half of patients referred with colorectal symptoms had had a rectal examination,[26] would not have permitted an accurate assessment of probabilities.

Example

A 65-year-old man presents with a history of 4 weeks of blood in the stool. On questioning, he does think his stool has been looser than usual. He is vague about the characteristics of the blood but he is clear that he is otherwise well. He has no anal symptoms.

The GP examines him and finds nothing wrong: specifically no pallor, and no mass in the abdomen or rectum. She explains that she wants a blood test for anaemia and that, whatever the result, she wants to refer him urgently for investigation. The GP plays down the risk of cancer, saying it will almost certainly turn out to be nothing serious. Afterwards she calculates the risk, making the assumption that his risk factors are independent of each other.

Rectal bleeding plus a change to looser stool has a risk of carcinoma of 12%. His age increases this to 17% (Fig. 36.1) and his lack of anal symptoms to 38% (Fig. 36.2). If she discovers that he is anaemic, the risk of carcinoma would rise to 70%.

- eye involvement
- runny nose
- whether the patient thinks this is an allergy.

For the GP, the likelihood ratios quoted in the review raise two questions: do they apply to patients presenting in primary care? and can they be applied sequentially? It may be that *either* a question about cats *or* one about trees may be used, but not both. Until these issues are resolved they are better taken as general indicators of usefulness rather than likelihood ratios to be used formally.

* *Examine* for
  (a) the typical swollen mucosa of allergic rhinitis
  (b) septal deformity, which suggests an alternative diagnosis
  (c) nasal polyps, which can cause rhinorrhoea and nasal obstruction mimicking rhinitis. They are no more common in patients with allergic rhinitis than in the general population, but they are more common in non-allergic rhinitis and non-allergic asthma.[18] An individual polyp could be an antrochoanal polyp, a benign massive polyp, or any of a number of very rare, benign or malignant tumours such as a juvenile nasopharyngeal angiofibroma,[19] or a nasopharyngeal carcinoma (which is commonest in the Chinese, who have an annual incidence of 20 per 100 000)[20] or an inverting papilloma, which is a benign, locally aggressive tumour of the nasal cavity and sinuses. The last named is very

uncommon but significant because of its tendency to recur and its association with squamous cell carcinoma.

* *Consider diagnostic tests for allergy.*
  (a) *Serological (radioallergosorbent testing (RAST)) tests* attempt to detect specific IgE that binds to common allergens, such as dust mites, pollens, animal proteins and mould spores.
  (b) *Skin prick tests* determine skin sensitivity to specific allergens (Table 37.5).

Because reported sensitivities and specificities of serological and skin tests vary widely, it is difficult to calculate the post-test probability of allergic rhinitis with any confidence.

Skin tests have specific problems:

- *False positive results* can occur from eczema, from placing the skin testing sites too close together, from using an excessively large test solution injection and from irritation caused by the skin test solution. In addition, the presence of specific IgE in the patient does not indicate disease because a patient could be sensitised but asymptomatic.

- *False negative results* can occur from poor skin testing technique and the recent use of antihistamines, tricyclic antidepressants or topical steroids. Each patient has his or her own characteristic skin reactivity, which can affect results as well.[17]

Combining history with allergy testing. A study from the Netherlands, in 365 patients in general practice aged 12 or over with chronic or recurrent nasal symptoms, found that the combination of

Table 37.5 Accuracy of selected skin tests and in-vitro tests for the diagnosis of allergic rhinitis, compared with clinical diagnosis.[17] Based on a pre-test probability of allergic rhinitis of 10% in a patient presenting with rhinorrhoea

Test	Allergen	Result	Likelihood ratio	Probability
Skin prick tests	Cat	Positive	3.6	29%
		Negative	0.5	5%
	Grass	Positive	6.8	43%
		Negative	0.3	3%
In-vitro tests (RAST)	Cat	Positive	3.4	27%
		Negative	0.5	5%
	Grass	Positive	4.6	34%
		Negative	0.4	4%
Phadiatop test	Multiallergen	Positive	3.9	30%
		Negative	0.3	3%

Follow each row from left to right to see how each test alters the probability of allergic rhinitis.

history and a single test (RAST or skin prick) permitted a diagnosis of nasal allergy with extraordinary accuracy.[21] The key question in the history was entirely about the timing of the symptoms:

- symptoms in spring or summer suggest tree, grass or weed allergy
- symptoms after certain household activities, e.g. bed making, suggest house dust mite allergy
- symptoms after contact with animals suggest allergy to animal dander.

Only in the case of mould allergy was there no characteristic timing.

A positive history, combined with a positive RAST or skin prick test, gave positive predictive values (PPV) of 100%. Confidence intervals were as wide as 59–100% (mould) or as close as 96–100% (housedust mite). The only exception was allergy to weed pollen, when the PPV was only 90% (95% CI 73 to 98%). The gold standard was the (inevitably imperfect) diagnosis of a panel of three experts. The RASTs were considered positive if class 1 or above; the skin prick tests if the mean weal diameter was at least 3 mm.

* *Once the diagnosis has been made*, classify the condition further according to duration and severity.

  Duration:
- *Intermittent*: occurring 4 days or less per week or for less than 4 weeks.
- *Persistent*: occurring more than 4 days per week and for more than 4 weeks.

  Severity:
- *'Mild'*, which has all of the following: normal sleep; normal daily activities, sport, leisure; normal work and school; and the symptoms are not troublesome.
- *'Moderate/severe'*, where one or more of the following occurs: abnormal sleep; impairment of daily activities, sport or leisure; problems caused at work or school; and troublesome symptoms.[22]

Is this non-allergic rhinitis?

The symptoms are similar to allergic rhinitis, but there is no pruritus and no evidence of allergic disease. It can be sporadic or perennial. It includes a highly diverse group of rhinitis syndromes united by their pervasive symptoms of clear rhinorrhoea or congestion with *less* prominent sneezing, nasal pruritus and conjunctival irritation.[23]

Types of non-allergic rhinitis:
- idiopathic or vasomotor rhinitis
- non-allergic rhinitis with eosinophilia
- rhinitis medicamentosa, caused by the persistent use of cocaine or over-the-counter nasal decongestants (e.g. Sinex or Otrivine)
- occupational rhinitis, due to exposure to airborne irritants or allergens in the workplace
- drug-induced rhinitis may be caused by a number of medications, including angiotensin-converting enzyme inhibitors, beta-blockers, chlorpromazine, aspirin, other NSAIDs and oral contraceptives
- structural problems, such as septal deviation or tumours
- granulomatous diseases (rarely) such as rhinoscleroma, sarcoidosis and tuberculosis.

In the absence of pointers to one of these specific subtypes, the diagnosis is made by the exclusion of infective and allergic causes of rhinorrhoea.

Ask about medication, occupational irritants, triggers that the patient has noticed and other illnesses. In separating allergic from vasomotor rhinitis the following symptoms have proved useful:[24]

(a) *Complaints*: among other symptoms there is no pain or fullness in the head in vasomotor rhinitis, while these, together with distress, occur in allergic rhinitis.

(b) *Timing*: unpredictable in vasomotor rhinitis, depends on exposure to stimuli. In allergic rhinitis it is seasonal depending on the causative allergens.

(c) *Age*: in vasomotor rhinitis, the onset is usually in middle age (>20 years) and symptoms do not abate with age, whereas the onset of the allergic rhinitis is at preschool age and symptoms tend to diminish after about the age of 60. In old age, senile rhinorrhoea may occur, probably due to a failure of vasomotor control of the mucosa.

(d) *Sense of smell*: usually not affected in vasomotor rhinitis but reduced or abolished in allergic rhinitis.

(e) *Nasal discharge*: very profuse, clear and watery in vasomotor rhinitis, but also mucopurulent with superinfection in allergic rhinitis.

(f) *Nasal examination (rhinoscopy)*: differences between the appearance of the mucosa are described but it is unlikely that a GP would be able to differentiate allergic from non-allergic rhinitis on rhinoscopy. The finding of one or more nasal polyps shifts the probabilities towards a non-allergic cause; see above.

Is this vasomotor rhinitis?

Ask whether the runny nose seems to be triggered by anything. It is believed to be a neurovascular response to stimuli acting on the nasal mucosa, and may be triggered by:

- emotion
- certain odours (e.g. perfumes, cigarette smoke, paint fumes, inks)
- alcohol
- spicy foods
- environmental factors such as temperature, barometric pressure changes and bright lights.

In one small study,[25] researchers concluded that autonomic system dysfunction is significant in patients with vasomotor rhinitis ($P < 0.005$). Possible compounding factors included previous nasal trauma and extra-oesophageal manifestations of gastro-oesophageal reflux disease.

Unilateral discharge

Two uncommon causes occur in infants and children.

1. Choanal atresia

Congenital blockage of the posterior choana prevents the normal nasal mucus stream from reaching the pharynx, resulting in anterior discharge. If infected, the discharge is mucopurulent. The condition occurs in 1 out of every 7000 to 8000 live births. Approximately 60% of reported cases are unilateral, with a right-sided predominance.

A simple test for unilateral choanal stenosis is to have the child attempt nose blowing with the opposite nostril occluded by external pressure. Failure to detect any air movement suggests complete obstruction. The differential diagnosis includes nasal septal deformity, nasal foreign body and choanal polyp. Failure to pass a catheter through the occluded nostril can be misleading in the older child because there is enough space in the nasal cavity for the catheter to curl without passing into the nasopharynx. The otolaryngologist can visualise the choanal closure with a small, flexible scope passed through the nostril. The CT scan is the preferred method to confirm a diagnosis of unilateral or bilateral choanal atresia.[26]

2. Foreign body in the nose

The patient, usually a child, has unilateral discharge which gradually becomes purulent. Recurrent unilateral epistaxis is also possible. The child may not volunteer the history of insertion but inspection with an auriscope will reveal the cause.

Cerebrospinal fluid leak

Aetiology[27]

(a) *Non-surgical trauma*: 80%. This is usually due to blunt trauma to the head, including fracture of the petrous temporal bone or other destructive processes in which CSF in the middle ear drains to the nose in the presence of an intact tympanic membrane.

(b) *Surgical trauma*: 16%. This is a sequel of skull-base surgery, commonly functional endoscopic sinus surgery (FESS), transphenoidal pituitary surgery, translabyrinthine acoustic schwannoma and mastoid surgery with an intact tympanic membrane

(c) *Non-traumatic causes*: 3–4%. These are usually destructive skull-base lesions, including neoplasms, or developmental defects of the ethmoid, sphenoid, frontal or petrous temporal bones with the formation of a meningocele or meningoencephalocele (with an intact tympanic membrane).

Diagnosis

Unless identified at the time of surgery, diagnosing a cerebrospinal fluid fistula can be difficult.

- *Beta-2 transferrin* in the fluid is the gold standard laboratory diagnosis for a CSF fistula. This protein is found in only three bodily fluids – CSF, perilymph and vitreous humour.[28]

- *A glucose oxidase test strip* is a traditional and rapid screening test. However, this has been found to be unreliable:

(a) False positive results may be caused by reducing substances present in lacrimal gland secretions and in nasal mucus; glucose at a concentration of as low as 5 mg/dl can lead to a positive result with this test.

(b) The presence of active meningitis can lower the glucose level in the CSF and may lead to false negative readings.

Despite these drawbacks, glucose testing can be used as a first-line diagnostic test in a patient with a history of craniofacial injury. However, all positive results should be confirmed with the more reliable beta-2 transferrin test.[29]

Whom to refer because of rhinorrhoea[30]

(a) Those who do not respond to maximal management by their general practitioner.

(b) Those with unilateral rhinitis; nasoendoscopy is needed.

(c) Allergic rhinitis with allergic conjunctivitis severe enough to be a candidate for topical steroids. Specialist supervision is necessary. Problems include steroid-induced glaucoma and inadvertent treatment of an eye infected with herpes simplex virus (dendritic ulcer).

(d) Severe allergic rhinitis in pregnancy. Pregnancy can cause or exacerbate rhinitis. However, not all drugs are suitable for use in pregnant women, so extra care should be taken when prescribing. Refer if the patient does not respond to maximal management.

(e) Ear, nose and throat referral is also recommended for:

- other unilateral nasal problems (e.g. obstruction), especially in children
- nasal perforations, ulceration or collapse
- bloodstained discharge
- crusting high in the nasal cavity
- recurrent infection
- periorbital cellulitis (admission is urgent).

Example

A 30-year-old factory worker attends with a complaint of a runny nose for about 3 months. When it started he thought it was a cold but he never had a sore throat, fever or other cold symptoms. The rhinorrhoea is clear and there has never been any facial or tooth pain.

The GP decides that there is nothing to suggest sinusitis but at this stage the probabilities of allergic and non-allergic rhinitis are about equal, i.e. each is 50%.

Further questions reveal that the eyes are never itchy, the discharge is constant and nothing seems to make it worse, certainly not pets or plants. He has never had an allergic condition in the past and there is no family history of asthma, eczema or hay fever.

Without formally calculating the new probabilities, the GP decides that this is very unlikely to be allergic rhinitis. She decides against any allergy tests on the grounds that even if they were positive she wouldn't believe them.

Had she made that calculation, she would have found that just four features in the history (being negative) reduced the probability of allergic rhinitis from 50% to 2%, assuming that they can be applied sequentially. These are, using the figures from the Seattle systematic review,[17] allergy to pollen or animals (LR− 0.1); previous history of asthma, eczema or allergic rhinitis (LR− 0.8); family history (LR− 0.7); and eye involvement (LR− 0.5).

She is right that a positive skin prick test, for instance, would probably be a false positive. With a positive likelihood ratio of about 6, the probability of allergic rhinitis in this patient, after a positive test, would still be only 12% (Fig. 37.1).

She is puzzled as to the type of non-allergic rhinitis. The lack of variation makes vasomotor rhinitis unlikely. He takes no medication. She asks about his work and learns that he started work in a plastics factory about a month before the symptoms started and, yes, the smell of the chemicals can be fairly strong.

The GP explains that nothing is certain at this stage but that nasal irritation from the chemicals at work is a possibility. She asks him to obtain details of the medical officer at work so that she can ascertain the type of chemicals used and the risk of an irritant rhinitis. Meanwhile, the patient is about to take his first holiday since starting work and she asks him to return afterwards to report whether the symptoms have abated.

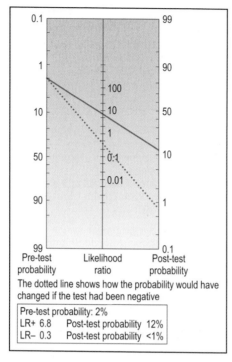

Figure 37.1 The probability of allergic rhinitis as a result of a skin pinprick test for grass in the example on p. 240.

REFERENCES

1. Johnston S, Holgate S. *Epidemiology of viral respiratory infections.* In: Myint S, Taylor-Robinson D, eds. Viral and other infections of the human respiratory tract. London: Chapman & Hall, 1996:1–38.

2. Day J, Briscoe M, Rafeiro E, et al. *Comparative clinical efficacy, onset and duration of action of levocetirizine and desloratadine for symptoms of seasonal allergic rhinitis in subjects evaluated in the Environmental Exposure Unit (EEU).* Int J Clin Pract 2004;58: 109–118.

3. Sibbald B, Rink E. *Epidemiology of seasonal and perennial rhinitis: clinical presentation and medical history.* Thorax 1991;46:895–901.

4. Agency for Healthcare Research and Quality. *Management of allergic and nonallergic rhinitis: Evidence Report/Technology Assessment Number*

54. AHRQ Publication No. 02-E024, Rockville, MD.

5. Dubreuil C, Gehanno P, Goldstein F, et al. *Treatment of acute maxillary sinusitis in adult outpatients: comparison of a five versus ten day-course of cefuroxime axetil.* Med Malad Infect 2001;31: 70–78.

6. Aitken M, Taylor J. *Prevalence of clinical sinusitis in young children followed up by primary care pediatricians.* Arch Pediatr Adolesc Med 1998;152:244–248.

7. National Institute of Allergy and Infectious Diseases. *The common cold, NIAID Fact Sheets.* NIAID, 2005. Online. Available: www.niaid.nih.gov/factsheets/cold.htm.

8. Mäkelä M, Puhakka T, Ruuskanen O, et al. *Viruses and bacteria in the etiology of the common*

cold. J Clin Microbiol 1998;36: 539–542.

9. Lindbaek M, Hjortdahl P. *The clinical diagnosis of acute purulent sinusitis in general practice – a review.* Br J Gen Pract 2002;52:491–495.

10. Lau J, Zucker D, Engels E, et al. *Diagnosis and treatment of acute bacterial rhinosinusitis.* Evidence Report/Technology Assessment No. 9. Rockville, MD: Agency for Health Care Policy and Research, 1999.

11. Williams JJ, Simel D. *Does this patient have sinusitis? Diagnosing acute sinusitis by history and physical examination.* JAMA 1993;270: 1242–1246.

12. Berg O, Carenfelt C. *Analysis of symptoms and clinical signs in the maxillary sinus empyema.* Acta Otolaryngol 1988;105:343–349.

13. Engels E, Terrin N, Barza M, Lau J. *Meta-analysis of diagnostic tests for acute sinusitis.* J Clin Epidemiol 2000;53:852–862.

14. Royal College of Radiologists. *Making the best use of a department of clinical radiology, 5th edn.* London: RCR, 2003.

15. Smolensky M, Reinberg A, Labrecque G. *Twenty-four hour pattern in symptom intensity of viral and allergic rhinitis: treatment implications.* J Allergy Clin Immunol 1995;95:1084–1096.

16. Van Cauwenburge P, Bachert C, Passalacqua G, et al. *Consensus statement on the treatment of allergic rhinitis.* European Academy of Allergology and Clinical Immunology. Allergy 2000;55: 116–134.

17. Gendo K, Larson E. *Evidence-based diagnostic strategies for evaluating suspected allergic rhinitis.* Ann Intern Med 2004;140:278–289.

18. Grigoreas C, Vourdas D, Petalas K, et al. *Nasal polyps in patients with rhinitis and asthma.* Allergy Asthma Proc 2002;23:169–174.

19. Duvall AJ, Moreano AE. *Juvenile nasopharyngeal angiofibroma: diagnosis and treatment.* Otolaryngol Head Neck Surg 1987;97:534–540.

20. World Health Organization. *Initiative for vaccine research (IVR).* Geneva: WHO, 2005. Online. Available: www.who.int/vaccine_ research/en/ (search on 'nasopharyngeal' and choose 'viral').

21. Crobach M, Hermans J, Kaptein A, et al. *The diagnosis of allergic rhinitis: how to combine the medical history with the results of radioallergosorbent tests and skin prick tests.* Scand J Prim Health Care 1998;16:30–39.

22. ARIA. *Allergic rhinitis and its impact on asthma.* Allergic Rhinitis and its Impact on Asthma Initiative, 2001. Online. Available: www.whiar. com.

23. Dykewicz M, Fineman S, Skoner D, et al. *Diagnosis and management of rhinitis: complete guidelines of the Joint Task Force on Practice Parameters in Allergy, Asthma and Immunology. American Academy of Allergy, Asthma and Immunology.* Ann Allergy Asthma Immunol 1998;81:478–518.

24. Nauman HE. *Differential diagnosis in otorhinolaryngology.* New York: Thieme, 1993:184–189.

25. Jaradeh S, Smith T, Torrico L, et al. *Autonomic nervous system evaluation of patients with vasomotor rhinitis.* Laryngoscope 2000;110: 1828–1831.

26. Dunham M. *Choanal atresia.* The Child's Doctor, 1998. Online. Available: www.childsdoc.org/fall98/ choanal/choanal.asp.

27. Beckhardt R, Setzen M, Carras R. *Primary spontaneous cerebrospinal fluid rhinorrhea.* Otolaryngol Head Neck Surg 1991; 104:425–432.

28. Constantino P, Janecka I. *Cranial-base surgery.* In: Bailey B, ed. Head and neck surgery – otolaryngology, 2 edn. Philadelphia: Lippincott-Raven, 1998:1848–1853.

29. Skedros D, Cass S, Hirsch BE, et al. *Beta-2 transferrin assay in clinical management of cerebral spinal fluid and perilymphatic fluid leaks.* J Otolaryngol 1993;22:341–344.

30. PRODIGY. *Allergic rhinitis.* PRODIGY, 2005. Online. Available: www.prodigy.nhs.uk/ guidance.asp.

38

Sleepiness

KEY FACTS

- Daytime sleepiness is very common, especially after a meal and in those with a sedentary lifestyle or who are bored. Most people with it do not suffer from a treatable disorder. In others, it is secondary to inadequate sleep, depression or sedative drugs.
- However, primary disorders occur and, of them, sleep apnoea is common.

A PRACTICAL APPROACH

- * *Assess whether the sleepiness suggests a disorder* or is within the normal range for that patient's age and level of activity. The Epworth Sleepiness Scale is a useful way of doing this.
- * *Identify, from the history, those with one of the 'primary' conditions*:
  - *obstructive sleep apnoea* (ask their partner about snoring, choking and stopping breathing during sleep)
  - *primary hypersomnia* (ask about difficulty waking up and sleepiness in the day severe enough to affect the person's life)
  - *narcolepsy* (ask whether the attacks are sudden, and whether there are other episodes that are linked with the condition: cataplexy, sleep paralysis, hallucinations on falling asleep, sleepwalking or automatic behaviour).
- * *Identify, from the history, those with one of the 'secondary' conditions*:
  - inadequate sleep
  - depression
  - drug use.

Prevalence

The prevalence of daytime sleepiness in the general population, based on a Dutch survey, is 15%.[1]

The prevalence as a presentation in primary care, and the frequency with which it is due to the different causes listed below, are unknown.

Diagnosis

Distinguish between:
- Sleepiness due to inadequate amounts of, or poor quality, sleep; see *Insomnia*, page 160.
- Sleepiness which is better described as fatigue. Ask whether the patient feels tired all the time, or feels tired after minimal exertion, whether mental or physical. If the answer is yes, proceed as for *Fatigue*, see page 110.
- Bouts of sleepiness in a person who seems to get enough sleep at night and who does not feel sleepy between bouts; see 'Is this narcolepsy?', below.
- Sleepiness in a person whose sleep is disturbed by episodes of apnoea or hypopnoea, see *Obstructive sleep apnoea*, page 439.
- Sleepiness associated with depression, see *Depression*, page 372.

■ Sleepiness due to drugs, e.g. sedatives, or to withdrawal from stimulant drugs such as cocaine or amfetamines.

■ Primary hypersomnia (see below).

Is this primary hypersomnia?

Prevalence

The prevalence in primary care is unknown. It is found in 10% of those who present to sleep clinics complaining of sleepiness.[2]

Definition

It is a condition of unknown aetiology characterised by persistent daytime sleepiness, and usually actual episodes of sleeping in the day, despite longer than average night-time sleep. It develops gradually in young adults and may continue indefinitely or resolve in middle age. It is often mistaken for laziness or for a lack of direction in life.

Diagnosis

■ Two features distinguish it from narcolepsy:
   (a) sufferers have difficulty waking
   (b) the daytime sleeps come upon the patient gradually, unlike the sudden onset of a bout of sleep in narcolepsy.

■ It is distinguished from 'normal' sleepiness by its severity. It leads to poor performance at work and an unsatisfactory personal life. In drivers, it is dangerous. An uncommon variant, the Kleine–Levin syndrome, is characterised by episodes of severe hypersomnia, lasting days or weeks, separated by months of normal functioning.

Refer those sufficiently troubled by symptoms that suggest primary hypersomnia. Specialist assessment and polysomnography usually allow a clear diagnosis to be made.

Is this narcolepsy?

Prevalence

Narcolepsy with cataplexy: 3–5 per 10 000 of the population.

Narcolepsy with or without cataplexy: 9–15 per 10 000.[3] Most UK GPs will therefore have at least one such patient but most will be undiagnosed. It is present in 1–2% of the first-degree relatives of those affected.

Definition

Narcolepsy is a chronic neurological disorder affecting sleep regulation. It is characterised by excessive daytime sleepiness and episodes of falling asleep in the day, sometimes in inappropriate circumstances. Certain bizarre features may be present:

■ *Cataplexy*, in which the patient suddenly loses motor function bilaterally at a moment of emotion – usually laughter, excitement or anger. Attacks usually last less than a minute. In a severe attack, the patient may fall and may twitch but will not lose consciousness.

■ *Sleep paralysis*, in which the patient cannot move for a few minutes on waking or on falling asleep.

■ *Hypnagogic hallucinations* (dream-like episodes when falling asleep).

■ *Disturbed sleep*, with behavioural abnormalities such as sleepwalking.

■ *Automatic behaviour*, in which a repetitive task is performed without full awareness while feeling sleepy.

Diagnosing narcolepsy from the history

∗ *Check that the patient suffers from daytime sleepiness, not just fatigue.* The Epworth Sleepiness Scale allows formal assessment of this (see box opposite). Using a cut-off of >10, the scale has a sensitivity of 93.5% and a specificity of 100% for narcolepsy, giving the very useful figures of an LR+ infinitely high (95% CI 8.4 to infinity) and an LR– 0.06 (95% CI 0.05 to 0.09) (although there is some doubt over these figures because cases and controls were from different studies). These are the likelihood ratios for the distinction between patients with narcolepsy and normal controls.[4] They cannot be used to distinguish narcolepsy from other sleep disorders.

∗ *Check for other causes of sleepiness* (see *Fatigue*, p. 111). This should include lack of sufficient sleep, depression, obstructive sleep apnoea, sedative drugs or a chronic medical condition.

∗ *Ask about the specific features* of the syndrome listed above. For instance, ask 'Do you ever develop sudden weakness in all limbs when you laugh or get emotional?'; 'Do you notice any odd things that happen when you are waking up or falling asleep?'; 'Do you sleepwalk?'

∗ *Ask about the age of onset.* The condition may start in childhood or in early middle age but a teenage or early adult onset is usual. Sleepiness in the theatre, in front of TV and after a meal, starting in late middle age or older, is unlikely to be narcolepsy.

* *Refer to a specialist* with an interest in sleep disorders any patient in whom narcolepsy is a possibility and another cause for the sleepiness does not seem more likely. No studies have been performed which allow a statistical approach to this decision. In practice, if the condition is interfering with the patient's life, referral is justified. The condition can interfere with school, work, driving and relationships and, once a diagnosis is made, treatment can alleviate the disability.

The Epworth Sleepiness Scale

* Ask: 'How likely are you to doze off or fall asleep in the following situations, in contrast to just feeling tired? This refers to your usual way of life in recent times. Even if you have not done some of these things, try to work out how they would have affected you.'
  - Sitting and reading
  - Watching TV
  - Sitting inactive in a public place (e.g. a theatre or a meeting)
  - As a passenger in a car for an hour without a break
  - Lying down to rest in the afternoon when circumstances permit
  - Sitting and talking to someone
  - Sitting quietly after a lunch without alcohol
  - In a car, while stopped for a few minutes in traffic.
* Score as follows:
  0 – would never doze
  1 – slight chance of dozing
  2 – moderate chance of dozing
  3 – high chance of dozing.
  A score >11 carries a high probability of a sleep problem, though not necessarily narcolepsy, provided simple causes, e.g. lack of sleep or depression, have been excluded.

Example

A 55-year-old man inexplicably drives his car into an oncoming vehicle and kills its driver. When he is discharged from hospital, on police bail, he consults his GP to ask whether the crash could have been due to narcolepsy. He has no memory of losing control of his vehicle, even though he received no head injury. He reports that he falls asleep easily when watching TV and has had previous experiences when driving when he has had to stop the car because he feels himself falling asleep. He says these episodes have been getting worse 'since he became middle-aged'.

His GP agrees that it is quite likely that the accident was caused by his falling asleep. She also works out that narcolepsy is not the most likely cause of his sleepiness. He's the wrong age, and further questioning fails to reveal any of the characteristic symptoms.

She tests him on the Epworth Sleepiness Scale, which confirms that he is excessively sleepy with a score of 13. He sleeps well at night and slept well the night before the accident. He is otherwise well.

She feels the diagnosis lies between 'normal' sleepiness and primary hypersomnia; a distinction which is especially important in view of the charge of dangerous driving that he faces. A further question reveals that he has difficulty waking in the morning, saying, 'Everyone knows I'm no good till I've had my second cup of coffee in the morning'. His wife confirms this and that she never suggests that they go to the theatre any more because he will fall asleep within minutes.

Although she cannot calculate the probabilities formally, the GP thinks that there is a good chance that this is primary hypersomnia and refers him for sleep studies.

REFERENCES

1. Rijsman R, Neven A, Graffelman W, et al. *Epidemiology of restless legs in the Netherlands.* Eur J Neurol 2004; 11:607–611.

2. American Psychiatric Association. *Diagnostic and statistical manual of mental disorders, 4th edn, text revision.* Washington DC: American Psychiatric Association, 2000.

3. Zeman A, Britton T, Douglas N, et al. *Narcolepsy and excessive daytime sleepiness.* BMJ 2004;329:724–728.

4. Johns M. *Sensitivity and specificity of the multiple sleep latency test (MSLT), the maintenance of wakefulness test and the Epworth sleepiness scale: failure of the MSLT as a gold standard.* J Sleep Res 2000;9:5–11.

The swollen leg (the unilaterally swollen leg of recent onset)

39

- Clinical examination is unreliable in the diagnosis of deep vein thrombosis (DVT); it can be improved by the use of a clinical score.
- In secondary care and in the emergency department, the combination of a low score and a negative D-dimer test reduces the probability of DVT to <1%. Further investigations may justifiably be omitted.

- However, in the one study performed in primary care, a low score plus negative D-dimer test gave a probability of DVT of 2.3%. This is a level at which the general practitioner would decide not to refer for further investigations only if there were some extra grounds or the patient was happy to accept a risk of missing a DVT of 1 in 43.

A PRACTICAL APPROACH

- ★ Check first that there is not some clear clinical picture other than a DVT: acute arthritis, cellulitis with fever, lymphoedema associated with lymph nodes in the groin or evidence of trauma.
- ★ Ask about issues that contribute to the Wells score: previous DVT, current cancer, immobilisation.
- ★ Look for swelling especially of the whole leg, tenderness at the site of the deep veins, pitting oedema, dilated superficial veins.

- ★ If there is swelling, measure the calf and compare it to the other side.
- ★ Calculate the patient's risk as low, moderate or high.
- ★ Perform a D-dimer test, if available, provided the risk, assessed clinically, is sufficiently low for a negative D-dimer to permit the patient to avoid referral.
- ★ Otherwise refer for imaging.

Initial probabilities

In the patient with a swollen leg, the initial probabilities are:
- deep vein thrombosis
- lymphoedema, usually due to tumour or post-irradiation
- cellulitis
- acute arthritis, e.g. gout
- superficial thrombophlebitis

- post-thrombotic syndrome
- chronic venous insufficiency
- venous obstruction without thrombosis
- ruptured Baker's cyst
- acute arterial ischaemia.

If there has been *trauma*, three other diagnoses are possible:
- haematoma
- torn gastrocnemius muscle
- fracture.

Note: These diagnoses are not mutually exclusive. For instance, DVT can coexist with trauma, venous insufficiency and obstructive lymphadenopathy.

It is not possible to give statistics for the prevalences of these conditions in the patient presenting in primary care with an acutely swollen leg, nor is there evidence about which features of the examination help to distinguish them. Sometimes the diagnosis is clear. The cold white pulseless leg of acute arterial ischaemia should be obvious, as should the fact that in acute arthritis the joint is the source of the pain and swelling. Other obvious diagnoses are cellulitis when there is high fever and a sharp-edged erythema, or lymphoedema when there are obviously pathological nodes in the groin. When there is doubt, it usually takes the form of the question: is this a deep vein thrombosis (DVT)? A ruptured Baker's cyst and low-grade cellulitis are notoriously difficult conditions to distinguish from DVT, and, because of the serious implications if the diagnosis of a DVT is missed, most research has focused on this question.

Is this a deep vein thrombosis?

Incidence: 1 in 1000 of the population per year. After the age of 70 the risk doubles.[1]
Prevalence of confirmed DVT: Among patients with a swollen and/or painful leg in whom the suspicion of DVT is sufficiently strong to be referred to secondary care: 25%.[2]
Risk factors for DVT: A study from French general practice found the following risk factors with their odds ratios (ORs) for DVT:[3]

(a)	plaster cast on leg	36
(b)	orthopaedic surgery	16
(c)	past history of venous thromboembolism (VTE)	16
(d)	pregnancy	11
(e)	general surgery	9
(f)	violent effort or muscular trauma	7.6
(g)	deterioration in general condition	5.8
(h)	immobilisation (confined to bed or armchair	5.6
(i)	venous insufficiency	4.5
(j)	chronic heart failure	2.9
(k)	obesity	2.4
(l)	travel by car, train or plane for at least 4 hours in the last 4 weeks	2.4
(m)	infectious disease	2.0
(n)	standing >6 hours a day	1.9
(o)	>3 pregnancies	1.7

Other risk factors with their ORs (95% confidence intervals)[4] not available from the above study are:

(a) family history of VTE (the OR is dependent on the precise details)
(b) male sex: 1.7 (1.4 to 2.0) although under the age of 50, DVT is more common in females (OR 1.8)[5]
(c) age: >60: 1.6 (1.3 to 1.9)
(d) cancer: 2.4 (1.9 to 2.8)
(e) systemic lupus erythematosus 4.4 (3.1 to 5.5)
(f) lower limb arteriopathy: 1.9 (1.3 to 2.5).

Making the diagnosis clinically

* *Refer certain patients* for imaging whose probability of DVT is so high that a low Wells score (see below) would not rule it out: patients who are pregnant; patients with previous VTE; and patients with symptoms or signs suggestive of a pulmonary embolus. Otherwise:
* Score the patient on the modified Wells score.[6] Score +1 for each of the following:
  (a) active cancer (treatment ongoing or within previous 6 months or palliative)
  (b) recently bedridden for >3 days or major surgery in the last 12 weeks requiring general or regional anaesthesia
  (c) localised tenderness in the deep vein system in calf and/or thigh
  (d) the entire leg is swollen
  (e) paralysis, paresis or recent plaster immobilisation of a lower limb
  (f) the calf circumference is >3 cm greater than the other side, measured 10 cm below the tibial tuberosity
  (g) unilateral pitting oedema
  (h) collateral superficial veins (other than varicose veins)
  (i) previous documented DVT.
  Score −2 if an alternative diagnosis is at least as likely.

The probability of DVT according to a patient's score is shown in Table 39.1. A recent meta-

Table 39.1 Interpretation of the Wells score in the original study,[7] where the pre-test probability of a DVT was 16%

Score	Probability of DVT	LR+ (95% CI) of the Wells score	% with DVT (95% CI) = post-test probability
≥3	High (vs. moderate or low)	15 (9.5–25)	75% (63–84%)
1–2	Moderate (vs. low)	2.3 (1.8–2.8)	17% (12–23%)
<1	Low (vs. high or moderate)	0.4 (0.2–0.6)	3% (1.7–5.9%)

Follow each row from left to right to see how the Wells score alters the probability of DVT from the baseline of 16%.
NB. Other symptoms and signs traditionally thought to be useful have been shown to be useless, e.g. pain, Homan's sign, erythema.[8]

Table 39.2 Probability of DVT using the Wells score in Dutch primary care,[9] where the overall probability of DVT was 29%

Wells score	Probability of DVT from Wells' study	% with DVT (95% CI) = post-test probability
≥3	High	37.5% (35.6–39.4%)
1–2	Moderate	16.5% (15.4–17.6%)
<1	Low	12.0% (10.9–13.1%)

analysis has revised these post-test probabilities to 53%, 17% and 5% for high, medium and low risk, respectively.[6] However, these patients were seen in secondary care. In primary care, the spectrum of patients may be different, as may the expertise of the clinicians; Wells' clinical assessments were made by a few trained research physicians. A study of 1295 patients in Dutch primary care with suspected DVT gives very different figures (Table 39.2).

This suggests that the Wells score cannot be used in primary care to exclude the diagnosis of DVT.

D-dimer test

If a D-dimer test is available
Patient with low probability of DVT

Perform it on all patients with a low clinical probability for DVT, using the likelihood ratios appropriate to the method used.

Refer for imaging (ultrasound or venography) if positive but reconsider if negative. In Wells' study, a low risk patient with a negative D-dimer test had a probability of DVT approaching zero.

Further investigations would only have shown a DVT in about 0.3%.[10] It would have been necessary to refer 333 such patients to find one positive.

However, as we have seen above, the situation in primary care is different. The authors of the Dutch study examined the probability of DVT in patients with various degrees of low Wells score and negative D-dimer test (Table 39.3).
Patient with moderate or high probability of DVT

Ask, would the results of the test alter the decision to refer?

■ A patient with very low probability (<0) and a negative D-dimer has a post-test probability of 1.4%. Whether to refer when the risk of DVT is this low (1 in 71) is something for clinician and patient to discuss.

■ A patient with moderate probability and a negative D-dimer has a post-test probability of 2.3%, or of 1.8% if a very sensitive cut-off is used (see below). Referral would be a matter of clinical judgement.

■ A patient with high probability and a negative test has a post-test probability of the order of 21%.[10] The patient would still need referral.

Table 39.3 Probability of DVT with a low Wells score plus a negative D-dimer test in Dutch primary care[9]

Wells score	D-dimer test	% with DVT (95% CI) = post-test probability
≤1	Negative	2.9% (2.5–3.3%)
≤0	Negative	2.3% (1.9–2.7%)
≤–1	Negative	1.4% (0.2–2.6%)

Table 39.4 Operating characteristics of the D-dimer test[6]

Pre-test probabilities	Sensitivity (95% CI%)	Specificity (95% CI%)	LR+ (95% CI%)	LR– (95% CI%)
Low	88 (81–92)	72 (65–78)	3.3 (2.6–4.1)	0.2 (0.1–0.3)
Moderate	90 (80–95)	58 (49–67)	2.1 (1.8–2.5)	0.2 (0.1–0.3)
High	92 (85–96)	45 (37–52)	1.6 (1.5–1.8)	0.2 (0.1–0.3)

If the patient would be referred whatever the result of the test, the test is clearly of no benefit in primary care.

If a D-dimer test is not available

Refer all those with a suspicion of DVT regardless of their Wells score unless the evidence is very strong that another condition is more likely than DVT; in which case, consider treating for that and keeping the patient under review. However, this is a dangerous area. Adding clinical judgement to the use of the Wells score does not appear to alter the overall accuracy.[11] It may be better at classifying as 'high probability' those subsequently shown to have a DVT but worse at classifying as 'low probability' those who do not.[12]

Operating characteristics of the D-dimer test

These depend on the type of assay, the cut-off level used and the prior probability of DVT. The most recent meta-analysis found the figures in Table 39.4.[6]

In other words, the negative likelihood ratio is more useful than the positive likelihood ratio. Put another way, the test can be used to exclude the diagnosis of DVT but not to confirm it.

Another meta-analysis found an even higher sensitivity and even lower specificity when the cut-off was set at 500 ng/ml: sensitivity 97%, specificity 35 to 45% (LR+ 1.5 to 1.8; LR– 0.09 to 0.07).[13]

Other points about the D-dimer test

- *False positives are common*, especially in cancer, infection, pregnancy and when there has been recent surgery, trauma, or haemorrhage (see box opposite). This may be why the specificity falls as the pre-test probability rises: these patients are more likely to have one of the conditions in which false positives occur.

- *False negatives are less common but may occur in old and small DVTs.* When a DVT is more than 15 days old, the value of the D-dimer test in ruling out the diagnosis starts to decline.[10] It may also be less sensitive in detecting DVT that is confined to the calf[10] and in patients already given heparin.

- *Agreement on the use of the D-dimer test has not yet been reached.* The US Agency for Healthcare Research and Quality reported in 2003 that the literature was too varied for them to come to conclusions about the accuracy of the test,[14] a view not shared by the later guideline from the British Society for Haematology.[10] Their guideline points out that sensitivity can approach 100% with almost all assays, provided a sufficiently low cut-off value is used, but with correspondingly low specificities (31% to 91%).[10]

False positives and false negatives in the D-dimer test

False positives occur in any situation where there is an increase in the formation and degradation of fibrin: infection, cancer, trauma, surgery, heart failure, renal failure, acute coronary syndrome, acute stroke, pregnancy, sickle cell crisis. It is unfortunate that these are the very situations in which DVTs are most likely to occur.

False negatives are uncommon. They occur in a few situations: when the thrombus is small, as in a small distal DVT; when the test is performed more than 11 days after the onset of thrombosis, and certainly after 15 to 20 days; in patients on heparin (although the test is usually still positive); and in patients with a poor fibrinolytic response.

Is there a better scoring system than the Wells score?

This question is raised by the poor performance of the score in primary care; but it seems that there is not. The authors of the Dutch study (above) found nine independent predictors of DVT in their sample, only some of which were the same as those of Wells, but their predictive power was no better than his score. Of those scored as low risk, 15% were found to have a DVT.[15]

Should the patient be screened for malignancy?

The fact that malignancy is a risk factor for DVT raises the question of whether a patient with a DVT and no apparent risk factor (an idiopathic DVT) should be screened for cancer. A study of 250 patients from Padua, Italy[16] found the following:

- At diagnosis, cancer was found in 3.3% of those with an idiopathic DVT, compared to none in those with a secondary DVT (i.e. where a risk factor was present).
- Over 2 years' follow-up, cancer developed in 7.6% of those with an idiopathic DVT compared to 1.9% of those with a secondary DVT (OR 2.3; 95% CI 1 to 5.2). These figures agree with those in a more recent primary care study.[17]
- Of the 35 patients with *recurrent* idiopathic DVT, 6 (17.1%) developed cancer.
- Overall, cancer was found in 10.5% of those with idiopathic cancer; almost all (9%) at presentation or within one year of the DVT.

The screening carried out in the Padua study was within the capacity of a primary care physician: history and examination (including pelvic, rectal and breast examinations), full blood count, erythrocyte sedimentation rate, urea and electrolytes, liver function tests, urinalysis and chest X-ray. More sophisticated tests were only used if the initial screen produced a positive. *Conclusion.* Relevant guidelines do not currently recommend screening for malignancy. It would detect cancer at an earlier stage but whether there is any benefit in terms of survival is unknown.[18] However, until that evidence becomes available, there seems to be a case for screening those with recurrent idiopathic DVT. Of the six cancers in those with recurrent idiopathic thrombosis in the Padua study, those in ovary, lung and prostate might have been detected by screening but not those in pancreas, stomach or brain.

Example

A stoical 55-year-old woman puts her foot down a rabbit hole when out walking. She is able to limp back to her car and drive home. Over the next few days the calf becomes increasingly swollen and bruised and she rests it, although she is able to put weight on the leg without pain.

After a week she visits the GP because the calf seems to be getting more painful rather than less. He finds extensive bruising over the calf which is tender (+1) and swollen (+1). There is moderate ankle oedema in that leg and foot (+1). He finds it difficult to decide whether all his findings are due to muscle trauma (−2) or whether she has now developed a DVT. A calculation of the Wells score shows that, despite the trauma, her risk of DVT is still moderate (17%). A negative D-dimer would only reduce this to 4% (Fig. 39.1), a level that the GP finds too high to ignore. He refers her for immediate imaging. His hunch is that the imaging will prove positive, because of the recent increase in her calf pain: a point in the history not allowed for in the Wells score.

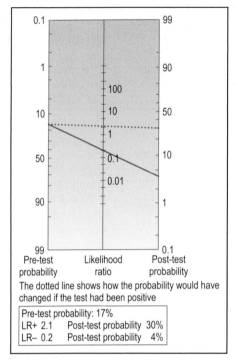

Figure 39.1 The probability of DVT before and after a D-dimer test in the example on p. 251.

REFERENCES

1. Bandolier. *DVTs and all that.* Bandolier 2003;April:110–112.

2. Wells P, Hirsh J, Anderson D, et al. *Accuracy of clinical assessment of deep-vein thrombosis.* Lancet 1997;345:1326–1330.

3. Samama M-M. *An epidemiological study of risk factors for deep vein thrombosis in medical outpatients. The Sirius Study.* Arch Intern Med 2000;160:3415–3420.

4. Anand S, Wells P, Hunt D, et al. *Does this patient have deep vein thrombosis?* JAMA 1998;279:1094–1099.

5. Silverstein M, Heit J, Mohr D, et al. *Trends in the incidence of deep vein thrombosis and pulmonary embolism.* Arch Intern Med 1998;158:585–593.

6. Wells P, Owen C, Doucette S, et al. *Does this patient have deep vein thrombosis?* JAMA 2006;295:199–207.

7. Wells P, Anderson D, Bormanis J, et al. *Value of assessment of pretest probability of deep-vein thrombosis in clinical management.* Lancet 1997;350:1795–1798.

8. Tovey C, Wyatt S. *Diagnosis, investigation and management of deep vein thrombosis.* BMJ 2003;326:1180–1184.

9. Oudega R, Hoes A, Moons K. *The Wells Rule does not adequately rule out deep venous thrombosis in primary care patients.* Ann Intern Med 2005;143:100–107.

10. British Society for Haematology. *The diagnosis of deep vein thrombosis in symptomatic outpatients and the potential for clinical assessment and D-dimer assays to reduce the need for diagnostic*

imaging. Br J Haematol 2004;124:15–25.

11. Kearon C, Ginsberg J, Douketis J, et al. *Management of suspected deep venous thrombosis in outpatients by using clinical assessment and D-dimer testing.* Ann Intern Med 2001;135:108–111.

12. Miron M, Perrier A, Bounameaux H. *Clinical assessment of suspected deep vein thrombosis: comparison between a score and empirical assessment.* J Intern Med 2000;247:249–254.

13. Kelly J, Rudd A, Lewis R, et al. *Plasma D-dimers in the diagnosis of venous thromboembolism.* Arch Intern Med 2002;162:747–756.

14. Segal J, Eng J, Jenckes M, et al. *Diagnosis and treatment of deep venous thrombosis and pulmonary embolism.* Evidence Report/Technology

Assessment No. 68. Rockville, MD: Agency for Healthcare Research and Quality, 2003.

15. Oudega R, Moons K, Hoes A. *Limited value of patient history and physical examination in diagnosing deep vein thrombosis in primary care.* Fam Pract 2005;22:86–91.

16. Prandoni P, Lensing A, Buller H, et al. *Deep-vein thrombosis and the incidence of subsequent symptomatic cancer.* N Engl J Med 1992;327: 1128–1133.

17. Oudega R, Moons K, Nieuwenhuis H, et al. *Deep vein thrombosis in primary care: possible malignancy?* Br J Gen Pract 2006;56: 693–696.

18. Robinson G. *Pulmonary embolism in hospital practice.* BMJ 2006;332: 156–160.

Syncope

- Vasovagal attacks are the commonest cause of syncope in the whole population. They are as common in the elderly as in the young, but the greatly increased risk of cardiac syncope in the older patient makes that the most likely diagnosis in those over 65.
- Decision rules have been formulated which show that the risk of a poor outcome in the weeks following an episode of syncope is almost entirely related to cardiac abnormalities which can be detected on history, examination or ECG.
- If the clinical assessment clearly points to a benign cause that can be managed in primary care, referral for further investigation is likely to produce results that, if positive, are false positives.

A PRACTICAL APPROACH

- *Check the history of the attack* for typical vasovagal symptoms, orthostatic hypotension, a seizure, palpitations, transient neurological symptoms or breathlessness. Ask about previous attacks and a history of cardiac disease.
- *Examine* the heart, the blood pressure (BP) lying, and see if the BP drops ≥20 mmHg on standing up.
- *Perform an ECG* unless the patient is <45 years old and the history strongly suggests a vasovagal attack.
- *Conclusion.* If there are clear pointers to a benign diagnosis and this is the first attack, referral is unnecessary. Referral is also likely to be unproductive if there are no pointers to any specific cause and the points below do not apply.

Refer if:
(a) there are pointers to a condition that needs specialist assessment (a history suggestive of a seizure, a transient ischaemic attack (TIA) or the finding of cardiac disease or an abnormal ECG); or
(b) the diagnosis is unclear and there have been recurrent attacks; or a single attack has occurred in a dangerous place or has caused injury.

Definition

Syncope is a sudden transient loss of consciousness and of postural tone, followed by spontaneous recovery, in the absence of head trauma.

Incidence and prevalence

The annual incidence of syncope in adults in the community (from the Framingham Heart Study) is 0.6%.[1] The incidence rises from the age of 70.

For patients aged 60–69 it is 0.5%; for those aged 70–79 it is 1.1%; for those aged 80 and above it is 1.8%.

Prevalence of different causes among patients in the community with syncope:[1]
 (a) Vasovagal attack (also called neurocardiogenic syncope): 21%.
 (b) Cardiac causes (arrhythmias, structural defects and ischaemia): 9%.
 (c) Orthostatic hypotension: 9%.
 (d) Medication (usually by causing orthostatic hypotension or arrhythmia): 7%.
 (e) Situational causes (e.g. cough syncope, micturition syncope, syncope associated with defecation or with swallowing): <1%.
 (f) Carotid sinus sensitivity. It is found in 39% of asymptomatic persons aged >65 and so its presence in a patient with syncope may be coincidental.[2] It is found in 20% to 40% of older patients referred with unexplained syncope.[3]
 (g) Psychiatric disorders (anxiety, panic, depression, conversion hysteria) are well known in tertiary centres but are rare as a cause of syncope in the community.
 (h) Cause unknown: 37%.

Other disorders which mimic syncope, with their prevalences among patients with transient loss of consciousness in the community, where known:
 (a) Seizure disorder: 5%.
 (b) Stroke or TIA: 4%.
 (c) Drop attacks, in which an older person, usually female, will suddenly drop to her knees and get up again without loss of consciousness.

Note. One patient may have several reasons for syncope. For instance, the fall of blood pressure in a patient with orthostatic hypotension may trigger a vasovagal attack.

Initial probabilities when a patient presents with syncope

No data exist for the incidence and prevalence of the different causes of syncope in primary care, but data from emergency departments[4,5] give figures similar to those for the population above, but with fewer of unknown cause (14%).

Emergency department studies also include diagnoses which would have been hard to make retrospectively in the community study, but which are made in patients who present acutely to emergency departments (e.g. pulmonary embolism 1%).[4]

Influence of age on the diagnostic probabilities

The patient's age will alter the above probabilities but not hugely. Younger patients with syncope will be even more likely to be suffering from vasovagal attacks while older patients will have a higher prevalence of cardiac disease, orthostatic hypotension and carotid sinus sensitivity.

A study of patients with unexplained syncope in secondary and tertiary care[6] found that the risk of a cardiac cause in those aged 65 and over was three times that of patients aged under 65 (34% vs. 12%), while the risk of vasovagal syncope was 16 times less (1% vs. 16%). However, neurally-mediated reflex syncope as a whole was common in both groups (55% in the older vs. 69% in the younger), with the older patients having more cases due to carotid sinus sensitivity (18% vs. 8%) and orthostatic hypotension (3% vs. 0.5%) and the younger patients having more situational syncope (10% vs. 4%).

Prognosis

An alternative approach to making an immediate specific diagnosis in primary care is to concentrate on the assessment of short-term prognosis. This is a way of ensuring that those at risk of serious outcomes from cardiac disease or stroke are referred promptly.

Those with syncope of cardiac origin have a 2-fold increase in their risk of death from any cause, mainly from coronary heart disease and stroke. However, the risk of death seems to be due to the underlying disease rather than the syncope.[7] Those with syncope of neurological origin have a 1.5-fold increase in the risk of death from any cause, mainly due to an increase in stroke risk. Other causes are not associated with a significant increase in the risk of death in the Framingham study, but those with syncope of unknown origin have a hazard ratio for death of 1.3 (95% CI 1.1 to 1.6), suggesting that in some the cause was cardiac or neurological.[1]

Table 40.1 The value of the San Francisco Syncope Rule in the prediction of a poor outcome in the 7 days following syncope[8]

Pre-test probability of a poor outcome	Score	LR	Probability of a poor outcome (95% CI)
12%	≥1	2.5	25% (20–30%)
	0	0.06	0.8% (0–2%)

Follow each row from left to right to see how the score alters the probability of a poor outcome.

The San Francisco Syncope Rule[8] states that a patient with *none* of the following will *not* have a serious outcome in the 7 days following syncope:

- abnormal ECG
- shortness of breath
- systolic BP <90 mmHg
- haematocrit <30%
- a history of congestive heart failure.

The rule is 96% sensitive and 62% specific, giving the figures in Table 40.1.

In other words, it is excellent at reassuring patients with none of the risk factors in the short-term but not so good at identifying those who will have a poor 7-day outcome.

The assessment in primary care

The clinical assessment in emergency departments and in secondary care yields the diagnosis in 32% to 75% of patients, according to different studies.[4] In a study of 788 patients presenting with syncope to the emergency department of the Hôpital Cantonal in Geneva,[4] 69% had a diagnosis that was strongly suspected after the initial examination. The two commonest causes made at the initial assessment were:

1. Vasovagal attack (38%). This is a diagnosis well worth making clinically in primary care. One study calculated that, in the USA, up to $16 000 (1993 prices) of unnecessary diagnostic tests may be performed on a patient who is ultimately diagnosed as having suffered a vasovagal attack.[9]

2. Orthostatic hypotension (24%). Of these, 38% were drug-related (80% of which were due to an ACE inhibitor); 22% were due to hypovolaemia; 12% had postprandial hypotension; 28% were idiopathic.

It is likely that the history and examination in primary care will be even more successful in making an initial diagnosis. Patients with the clearest clinical picture will never reach the emergency department or the syncope clinic, provided the diagnosis is benign, since the diagnosis will have been made by the patient, the family or the general practitioner.

Diagnosis from the history

In the history, the most important factors are the past history, the situation in which the attack occurred and an account from any witnesses. The patient's own history is least likely to be discriminatory, since most symptoms are non-specific. Dizziness before the attack and exhaustion afterwards are common to most episodes regardless of cause.

* *Diagnose a vasovagal attack* if there were premonitory symptoms (e.g. nausea, dizziness, yawning, blurred vision, everything seeming far away) and a precipitating event (e.g. fear, pain or standing in a hot room). There may be a history of other attacks in similar circumstances. Witnesses will comment on the patient's pallor, that consciousness was restored shortly after the patient fell or was laid down, and that there was no subsequent confusion or true drowsiness. The report of an abnormally slow weak pulse is confirmatory but not diagnostic: bradycardia occurs in some cardiac arrhythmias and in carotid sinus hypersensitivity. The patient will recall being soaked in sweat on regaining consciousness and often feeling nauseous or vomiting. The diagnosis is more likely if the first attack occurred at least 4 years before.[10]

* *Suspect orthostatic hypotension* if episodes of dizziness or loss of consciousness occur on standing up from the lying position, after food or during exercise (although this latter may also suggest a cardiac cause). It is more likely in the older person, in patients with diabetes, rheumatoid arthritis, Parkinson's disease or

Table 40.2 Predictors of cardiac syncope in patients aged ≥65 seen in secondary care with unexplained syncope, based on a pre-test probability of a cardiac cause of 34% in this study[6]

Predictor	Presence	LR (95% CI)	Probability of a cardiac cause
History of heart disease	Present	2.6 (2.1–3.2)	57%
	Absent	0.1 (0.04–0.2)	5%
Myoclonic movements during the event	Present	6.0 (2.3–16)	76%
	Absent	0.8 (0.8–0.9)	29%
Syncope during exertion	Present	15 (3.1–72)	89%
	Absent	0.9 (0.8–0.9)	32%
Syncope when supine	Present	7.0 (1.3–37)	76%
	Absent	0.9 (0.9–1.0)	32%

Follow each row from left to right to see how the factor alters the probability that the syncope has a cardiac cause.

stroke, and in those on drugs which cause hypotension (e.g. antihypertensives, tricyclic antidepressants, levodopa or phenothiazines). Because of the autonomic dysfunction there will be an absence of sweating, in contrast to the vasovagal attack.

✶ *Suspect a cardiac cause* if the patient is known to have cardiac disease.

■ *A history of cardiac disease* makes the diagnosis of a cardiac cause four times more likely, raising the probability in the general population from 4.8% in those without cardiovascular disease to 22% in those with cardiovascular disease.[1]

■ *The history of the attack* is less useful in establishing whether the cause is cardiac.

(a) Two Italian studies found that a cardiac cause is more likely if syncope occurred when supine or on exertion, if blurred vision preceded the loss of consciousness and if the patient is being seen within 4 years of the first episode.[6,10] (See Table 40.2 to see how some of these features affect the diagnostic probabilities in older patients.)

(b) However, a US study examined 19 symptoms in patients with syncope due to arrhythmia compared to controls and found that only an absence of nausea and/or vomiting before the loss of consciousness was significant, with an odds ratio of 7.1 (95% CI 1.6 to 33.3). Other symptoms, including chest pain, palpitations, a lack of prodrome or a duration of more than 2 minutes of unconsciousness, were unhelpful.[11]

■ *The report of an absent pulse* is not significant. Most lay observers cannot feel the pulse of a profoundly hypotensive person. A very slow pulse, if felt, could indicate a vasovagal attack, carotid sinus sensitivity or a bradyarrhythmia.

■ *Stokes–Adams attacks* are too rare to figure in these prospective studies but the pallor during the attack, followed by flushing as the patient recovers, is characteristic. It is unlikely to be specific, however, and may occur in any episode of unconsciousness where cardiac output falls suddenly and then rises equally suddenly.

In other words, in the older patient, a history of heart disease only doubles the probability that the syncope is cardiac; but the absence of such a history makes cardiac syncope very unlikely. Conversely, the absence of myoclonic jerks, syncope on exertion or when supine does not rule out a cardiac cause but their presence supports the diagnosis strongly. However, note that these factors lost their predictive power if the patient did not have heart disease.

✶ *Suspect a seizure* if there is a report of an aura, tonic-clonic movements, biting of the tongue, a blue face, prolonged disorientation or sleepiness after the attack, subsequent aching muscles or a duration of unconsciousness >5 minutes. Urinary incontinence is not a useful pointer.[7] Do not confuse myoclonal jerks, which can occur in syncope of any cause, with the tonic (forceful extension of the limbs) and clonic (more violent and repetitive) movements of a seizure. However, be aware that even clonic-tonic activity can occur in neurocardiogenic syncope. A Chicago study induced apparent tonic-clonic seizure-like activity in 5% of subjects who had a positive tilt table test.[12]

* *Suspect a stroke, TIA or subarachnoid haemorrhage* if there was unilateral numbness or weakness, visual loss, symptoms of vertebrobasilar ischaemia or severe headache, especially in a patient with no previous history of attacks.
* *Suspect carotid sinus syndrome* if attacks are precipitated by pressing on the neck, or turning the head wearing a tight collar. Most patients with the syndrome, however, give no such history[7] and most patients with proven carotid sinus sensitivity do not complain of syncope.[2]
* *Suspect a pulmonary embolus (PE)* if there was a sudden onset of dyspnoea with or without chest pain, and/or risk factors for PE were present.

The examination

* *Check the BP* sitting, then lie the patient down, examine the heart (see below), then repeat the BP lying then standing. Orthostatic hypotension is present if the systolic pressure falls ≥20 mmHg or the diastolic >10 mmHg. It is the cause of the syncope if the fall in BP is associated with symptoms. The patient should remain standing for 3 minutes with repeated BP readings (having been lying down for 5 minutes) before orthostatic hypotension can be ruled out. A fall of 10–19 mmHg is significant if it takes the systolic pressure below 90 mmHg (with or without symptoms). However, the lack of a fall in blood pressure does not rule the diagnosis out. It may vary with medication or with the time of day (being more common first thing in the morning) or it may occur up to 45 minutes after standing up.[13]
* *Examine the heart.* Cardiac disorders, apart from arrhythmias, particularly associated with syncope are aortic stenosis, pulmonary hypertension, heart failure or left ventricular systolic dysfunction, and any other condition associated with a fixed cardiac output.
* *Do not perform carotid sinus massage.* This is positive if massage for up to 5 seconds (on each side separately) leads to asystole for >3 seconds or drops the systolic pressure by >50 mmHg and is associated with syncope or presyncope. However, European guidelines require the use of continuous ECG and blood pressure monitoring as well as warning of the 0.45% risk of serious neurological complications.[7] Finally, the test, as described above, is neither sufficiently sensitive nor specific to be useful and should be performed using a tilt table. It is not therefore a test for primary care.

Investigations

ECG. In two studies, all the patients in whom extensive cardiovascular work-up found evidence of arrhythmia had an abnormal baseline ECG.[4,10] Particularly significant are:

(a) sinus pauses of at least 3 seconds (or at least 2 seconds if associated with symptoms)

(b) sinus bradycardia (<35 beats per minute or <40 if associated with symptoms)

(c) slow atrial fibrillation (AF) with R-R intervals of 3 seconds or more

(d) supraventricular tachycardia (SVT) of 180/min or more for at least 30 seconds or associated with hypotension

(e) second degree or complete atrioventricular (AV) block

(f) ventricular tachycardia (VT) with symptoms or lasting >5 seconds

(g) evidence of acute coronary syndrome.

Other tests would only rarely yield useful results. In an emergency department study:

(a) a blood sugar showed hypoglycaemia in 0.5%[4]

(b) the haemoglobin pointed to gastrointestinal haemorrhage in 0.3%.[4]

Syncope in the older patient

An older person has an annual risk of falling of 30% and up to 30% of these falls may be due to syncope.[14] They pose a special diagnostic problem because:

■ more than one factor often contributes to the episode (e.g. vasovagal attack due to postural hypotension, exacerbated by medication, plus poor balance)

■ the history is less often diagnostic than in the younger patient[6]

■ their risk of cardiac and of neurological disease is higher than the younger patient and so a precise diagnosis is more urgent.

A prediction rule that is older than the San Francisco Rule (see above) proposed only four risk factors for a poor prognosis of which age >45 was one.[15] The other three were an abnormal ECG, a history of congestive heart failure and a history of ventricular arrhythmia. The mortality over 1 year was 1% in those with a score of 0, 9% in those with a score of 1, rising to 27% in those with a score of 3 or 4.

Who needs specialist referral?

Refer if the initial assessment suggests a cause which requires investigation in secondary care. In the Geneva study,[4] 10% were referred because of clues in the initial examination. In 73% of these, the suspected diagnosis was confirmed. Seizures and stroke were the commonest diagnoses, followed by pulmonary embolism and aortic stenosis.

What if the initial assessment yields no strong clues as to the diagnosis?

This is likely to be the case in 24%.

Who needs cardiological referral?

Anyone with a pointer towards cardiac disease in the clinical assessment or the ECG.

Evidence from studies examining the benefit of cardiological assessment:

- Extensive work-up in the Geneva study[4] revealed a probable cause in 25% of patients. None of the patients who were free from cardiac disease clinically and who had a normal ECG was found to have a cardiac cause for their syncope. The LR+ (for clinical assessment plus ECG) was not impressive at 1.9 (95% CI 1.6 to 2.3) but the LR– seems extraordinarily useful at 0.0 (95% CI 0.0 to 0.7), although the confidence interval is disappointingly wide because the study was not large.

- Similar results come from a study of emergency department and secondary care patients from Italy, in whom the clinical absence of heart disease allowed exclusion of a cardiac cause for syncope in 97% of patients (see Figure 40.1).[10] The presence of heart disease was 95% sensitive and 55% specific for a cardiac cause; LR+ 2.1 (95% CI 1.82 to 2.42); LR– 0.09 (95% CI 0.04 to 0.24). In their series, the post-test probability of a cardiac cause if the clinical assessment suspected heart disease was 39%. In other words, the patient still probably did not have a cardiac cause for syncope but further investigation would be needed to separate those patients from those who did. If the clinical assessment found no suspicion of heart disease, the probability of a cardiac cause was 3% (4 cases); 3 of these 4 cases had a history of palpitations before the loss of consciousness. Therefore, if the patient has no evidence of heart disease clinically, including ECG, and no history

of palpitations before losing consciousness, referral to a cardiologist can be omitted (but with the knowledge that 1% of cases of cardiac syncope will be missed).

Considering all relevant studies, the finding of no clinically evident cardiac disease and a normal ECG virtually rules out a cardiac cause for the syncope. Only patients with cardiac disease or an abnormal ECG need cardiological referral.

Who needs referral for a tilt table test?

The test is less valuable than cardiological assessment. The principle behind the test is that tilting the patient head up at 70° for 40 minutes will reveal whether a person has a propensity towards the abnormal autonomic reaction of a vasovagal attack. A positive tilt test is one where the blood pressure falls or the heart slows or both. It does not completely rule in, or out, a vasovagal attack (sensitivity 30% to 85%; specificity 80% to 90%) as the cause of the syncope.[16] Therefore only refer if the diagnosis of vasovagal attack is possible but not definite *and* it is important to establish the diagnosis as firmly as possible; for instance, because of recurrent attacks, or one attack associated with injury or a motor vehicle accident or occurring in a high-risk setting.[16] Testing for carotid sinus sensitivity can be performed at the same time.

Three rarities not to be missed

Hypertrophic cardiomyopathy, which may be familial, with a prevalence of 1:500 to 1:5000.[17] Refer if there is a family history or non-specific ECG abnormalities, e.g. atrial fibrillation or some degree of heart block.

Brugada syndrome: a familial condition of ventricular tachyarrhythmias in patients with normal hearts and associated with sudden death.[17] Refer if there is a family history of cardiac arrest or sudden death, or because of the characteristic ECG finding of right bundle branch block and ST elevation in V1–V3.

Drug-induced arrhythmias in patients on drugs that prolong the QT interval, e.g. terfenadine. Refer if the QT interval is greater than 0.45 seconds.

Example

A 42-year-old woman presents with three episodes of loss of consciousness in the last 10 years. All have occurred in a theatre or cinema when relaxing after a particularly fraught day. Each time there have been the same warning signs (an indescribable feeling that something is wrong and an urge to get out of her seat) and on returning to consciousness she has been sweating profusely and then vomits. The patient had considered them to be 'faints' until the third attack when a doctor sitting nearby commented that she was pulseless during the attack. She now fears that she suffers from recurrent cardiac arrests.

The GP finds her well, with nothing to find on examination and with a normal ECG. He is confident that these are vasovagal attacks, because of the long timescale, the fact that they always occur in the same situation, the characteristic history and the normal examination and ECG. Figure 40.1 shows the power of the clinical assessment in ruling out a cardiac cause.

The patient and her family are not reassured. The GP guesses that a cardiological opinion will agree with his but that it will prove no more reassuring than his opinion. He refers her for a tilt table test. After 10 minutes in the tilt position her symptoms are reproduced exactly and she is convinced that the diagnosis of a vasovagal attack is correct. The GP subsequently looks up the sensitivity of the tilt table test (mean value 57%) and realises that using it to reassure the patient was a gamble (Fig. 40.2). A negative test was quite possible and while it would not have deflected him from the diagnosis of vasovagal attacks it would have further convinced her that he was wrong.

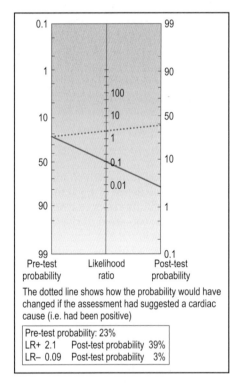

The dotted line shows how the probability would have changed if the assessment had suggested a cardiac cause (i.e. had been positive)

Pre-test probability: 23%	
LR+ 2.1	Post-test probability 39%
LR– 0.09	Post-test probability 3%

Figure 40.1 The probability of a cardiac cause of syncope before and after the clinical assessment (history, examination and ECG) in the example above.[10]

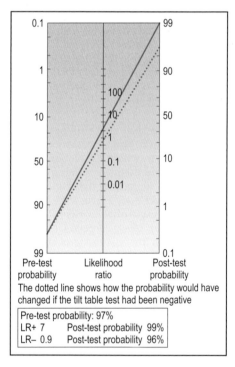

The dotted line shows how the probability would have changed if the tilt table test had been negative

Pre-test probability: 97%	
LR+ 7	Post-test probability 99%
LR– 0.9	Post-test probability 96%

Figure 40.2 The probability that the syncope was vasovagal before and after the tilt table test in the example above.[10]

REFERENCES

1. Soteriades E, Evans J, Larson M, et al. *Incidence and prognosis of syncope.* N Engl J Med 2002;347: 878–885.

2. Kerr S, Pearce M, Brayne C, et al. *Carotid sinus hypersensitivity in asymptomatic older persons: implications for diagnosis of syncope and falls.* Arch Intern Med 2006;166: 491–492.

3. Kumar N, Thomas A, Mudd P, et al. *The usefulness of carotid sinus massage in different patient groups.* Age Ageing 2003;32:666–669.

4. Sarasin F, Louis-Simonet M, Carballo D, et al. *Prospective evaluation of patients with syncope: a population-based study.* Am J Med 2001;111:177–184.

5. Ammirati F, Colivicchi F, Santini M. *Diagnosing syncope in clinical practice. Implementation of a simplified diagnostic algorithm in a multicentre prospective trial – the OESIL 2 Study.* Eur Heart J 2000;21:935–940.

6. Del Rosso A, Alboni P, Brignole M, et al. *Relation of clinical presentation of syncope to the age of patients.* Am J Cardiol 2005;96: 1431–1435.

7. Brignole M, Alboni P, Benditt L, et al. *Guidelines on management (diagnosis and treatment) of syncope.* Eur Heart J 2001;22:1256–1306.

8. Quinn J, Stiell I, McDermott D, et al. *Derivation of the San Francisco Syncope Rule to predict patients with short-term serious outcomes.* Ann Emerg Med 2004;43:224–232.

9. Calkins H, Byrne M, el-Atassi R, et al. *The economic burden of unrecognised vasodepressor syncope.* Am J Med 1993;95:473–479.

10. Alboni P, Brignole M, Menozzi C, et al. *Diagnostic value of history in patients with syncope with or without heart disease.* J Am Coll Cardiol 2001;37:1921–1928.

11. Oh J, Hanusa B, Kapoor W. *Do symptoms predict cardiac arrhythmias and mortality in patients with syncope?* Arch Intern Med 1999;159: 375–380.

12. Passmore R, Horvath G, Thomas J, et al. *Clinical spectrum and prevalence of neurologic events provoked by tilt table testing.* Arch Intern Med 2003;163:1945–1948.

13. Cheshire W. *Delayed orthostatic hypotension: is it worth the wait?* Neurology 2006;67:8–9.

14. Strickberger S, Benson D, Biaggioni I, et al. *AHA/ACCF scientific statement on the evaluation of syncope.* Circulation 2006;113: 316–327.

15. Martin T, Hanusa B, Kapoor W. *Risk stratification of patients with syncope.* Ann Emerg Med 1997;29: 459–466.

16. Fenton A, Hammill C, Rea R, et al. *Vasovagal syncope.* Ann Intern Med 2000;133:714–725.

17. Plunkett A, Hulse J, Mishra B, et al. *Variable presentation of Brugada syndrome: lessons from three generations with syncope.* BMJ 2003;326: 1078–1079.

Tinnitus

KEY FACTS

- Tinnitus is common. Most patients can be assessed and managed in primary care with referral to an audiologist for provision of a hearing aid if necessary.
- Almost all patients will be aged >55 and complaining of bilateral tinnitus of gradual onset. The likely cause is presbyacusis, or, in a patient with a history of prolonged exposure to noise, noise-induced hearing loss (NIHL).[1]
- If no atypical features are detected in the history and examination, and clinical tests confirm a bilateral sensorineural hearing loss, referral is only needed if the hearing loss warrants a hearing aid, or if the tinnitus is interfering with the quality of life, or if the patient would be entitled to compensation if the diagnosis of occupational NIHL were confirmed.

A PRACTICAL APPROACH

- ★ Ask about the character and duration of the tinnitus and whether unilateral or bilateral.
- ★ Ask about deafness and vertigo and about a family history of tinnitus.
- ★ Examine the ear, test for deafness even if the patient denies it and, if present, check whether it is conductive or perceptive with the Rinne test.
- ★ Decide which diagnosis best fits the pattern of symptoms and signs:
  - ■ Continuous tinnitus, associated with bilateral perceptive deafness, suggests presbyacusis or NIHL.
  - ■ Continuous tinnitus, associated with unilateral perceptive deafness, raises the possibility of acoustic neuroma.
  - ■ Continuous tinnitus, associated with conductive deafness, raises the possibility of otosclerosis or other middle ear disease.
- ■ Intermittent tinnitus, associated with perceptive deafness, in a younger person, raises the possibility of Ménière's disease.
- ■ Pulsatile blowing or clicking noises suggest objective tinnitus.
- ★ In all cases of chronic tinnitus, assess what effect it is having on the patient's mental state.
- ★ Refer for further investigation those with:[2]
  - (a) persistent unilateral tinnitus, or tinnitus in association with unilateral sensorineural hearing loss
  - (b) onset at a young age (for instance <50 years old)
  - (c) vertigo
  - (d) middle ear disease
  - (e) a family history of otosclerosis
  - (f) objective tinnitus.

Prevalence

Twenty-five per cent of the UK population (15 million people) have experienced tinnitus at some stage in their lives, and 6% of the UK population (3.6 million) suffer moderate to severe tinnitus. Eight per cent of the population consult their GP about tinnitus at some point in their life and 2–4% are referred to a specialist.[3] In 0.5% of the population, it is severe enough to interfere with their ability to lead a normal life.[4] It is most prevalent between 40 and 70 years of age, it is more common in men than in women, and occasionally can occur in children. The severity of tinnitus varies from an occasional awareness of a noise in one or both ears, to an unbearable sound that drives some people to contemplate suicide.[5]

Initial probabilities

No studies have assessed the prevalence of causative conditions in patients presenting with tinnitus in primary care. A French study of patients seen in a tinnitus clinic[6] found the following:

- noise-induced hearing loss (NIHL) 32%
- presbyacusis 23%
- Ménière's disease 32%.

In primary care, the prevalence of Ménière's disease will be much lower (see below) and that of presbyacusis higher. The older the patient, the more unlikely any condition other than NIHL and presbyacusis becomes.

Of the rarer conditions, an idea of the likely incidence in primary care of two of them can be roughly estimated, based on the fact that 8% of the population consult a doctor about tinnitus at least once in a lifetime. Over a 40-year adult lifespan, this equates to an adult consultation rate for tinnitus of 0.2% annually. Ménière's disease occurs in 1 in 10 000 of the population and acoustic neuroma in 1 in 100 000, and so their prevalence among consulters with tinnitus will be of the order of 1 in 200 and 1 in 2000 respectively:

- Ménière's 0.5%
- acoustic neuroma 0.05%.

Other uncommon causes are:

- otosclerosis: in an Australian study, 65% with confirmed clinical otosclerosis had tinnitus[7]
- ototoxic medication
- psychological disorders
- head injury

- temporomandibular joint (TMJ) dysfunction (possibly not causative, see below)
- infections affecting the eighth nerve or the central nervous system
- other systemic disease
- vascular disorders of the head and neck
- soft tissue disorders of the middle ear, eustachian tube or palate.

Step 1. The initial assessment

The history

1. *What is the character of the tinnitus?* A high-pitched continuous sound suggests NIHL or presbyacusis. A continuous low-pitched noise, with roaring exacerbations during attacks of vertigo, is characteristic of Ménière's disease. Clicking and banging suggests middle ear or palatal disease. An intermittent scratching, worsened by pressing on the ear, suggests a problem in the external auditory canal. A pulsating sound raises the possibility of objective tinnitus from a vascular disorder of the head or neck.

2. *Was the onset acute or gradual?* Sudden onset suggests acoustic trauma, infection or ototoxicity from a chemical agent. A gradual onset, presenting many years later with no other symptoms except deafness, suggests NIHL or presbyacusis.

3. *Is it bilateral?* In NIHL and presbyacusis, tinnitus is usually bilateral. Acoustic neuroma is unilateral in 95% of cases. Ménière's disease is likely to be unilateral in the early years.

4. *Is the patient deaf? If so, is the deafness unilateral or bilateral?* Conductive deafness suggests a problem in the external or middle ear; sensorineural deafness suggests a lesion of the cochlea or eighth nerve. For the differentiation between these, see page 52.

5. *Are there other symptoms?* Intermittent vertigo suggests Ménière's disease. Persistent vertigo suggests a progressive neurological lesion.

The examination

1. *Look in the ear.* Wax, if found, will probably not be the cause of the tinnitus but it will be necessary to remove it in order to examine the drum.

2. *Test for deafness* on both sides. The whisper test has been validated for use in primary care[8] (see p. 52).

3. *If deafness is found,* determine whether it is conductive or perceptive[9] (see p. 52).

Step 2. Refining the possibilities suggested by the initial assessment

Is it due to noise-induced hearing loss (NIHL)?

- Noise-induced hearing loss is suggested by bilateral deafness of gradual onset with a history of long-term exposure to noise, usually at work. Occasionally it is sudden in onset following more dramatic acoustic trauma and then may be unilateral.
- In those with noise-induced hearing loss (NIHL) and tinnitus, the tinnitus is not necessarily due to NIHL. A Polish study has estimated that noise is the cause of tinnitus in only 60% of cases of those with NIHL who had tinnitus.[10] In a study of Ministry of Defence staff with NIHL in whom the hearing loss was asymmetrical, 2.5% were found to have an acoustic neuroma.[11]
- In those in whom the tinnitus is due to NIHL, the longer the exposure to noise, the more likely it is that the tinnitus will be continuous. Of those exposed for 11–15 years, 20–42% have occasional tinnitus, and 8–15% of those exposed to noise for 20–30 years have continuous tinnitus.[12]

Audiometry: For practices with an audiometer or open access to audiometry, NIHL initially shows a notch at 4000 Hz, typically in both ears in chronic cases. Later, low frequencies are affected.

Is it due to presbyacusis?

Presbyacusis is suggested by bilateral deafness of gradual onset without a history of long-term exposure to noise. Rinne's and Weber's tests confirm that the hearing loss is sensorineural. The patient is likely to be over 50 years old. As with NIHL, the presence of tinnitus does not necessarily mean that it is due to the presbyacusis, but in the absence of other pointers, it is likely.

Audiometry: Bilateral symmetrical sensorineural hearing loss (SNHL), showing a high tone loss, or a flat pan-cochlear hearing loss, and a characteristic sloping curve, with a linear increase of hearing loss above 1000 Hz.

Is it due to Ménière's disease?

The diagnosis depends on the presence of all three of the following:[13]

1. at least two spontaneous episodes of vertigo lasting at least 20 minutes each
2. sensorineural hearing loss
3. tinnitus and/or a feeling of fullness in one or both ears.

However, the difficulty for the GP is that the patient may present with tinnitus and deafness years before the first episode of vertigo; and in these early years the deafness and tinnitus may be unilateral. In such cases, it is more accurate to refer the patient who meets the referral criteria below on the grounds of 'unilateral sensorineural deafness and tinnitus for investigation' rather than '? Ménière's disease'. Other pointers to the diagnosis are that the patient is likely to be aged 20 to 50, and that the tinnitus is fluctuating.

Audiometry: In the early phases and in disease-free intervals, the hearing is normal. In the later stages, there is fluctuating deafness in the low tones. In the end stage, the deafness is severe, pan-cochlear but usually unilateral.

Is it due to otosclerosis?

The following are the key questions:

1. Is there a chronic progressive subjective tinnitus?
2. How old is the patient? The maximum incidence is between 20 and 40 years old.
3. Is there a family history of otosclerosis? A positive family history is found in a quarter of cases.[14]
4. Is the patient male or female? Females are affected twice as often as males. Furthermore, once otosclerosis is present, a woman is more likely than a man to experience tinnitus.[7]
5. Is there an obstetric history? Pregnancy coincides with a period of progression of clinically manifest otosclerosis in half of all female patients.
6. Is there a conductive hearing loss? Conductive hearing loss is found in 80% of patients. In some cases, the disease causes cochlear degeneration, giving a sensorineural hearing loss as well. Mixed deafness is found in 15%, and pure SNHL in 5%.[15]

Audiometry: 80% of cases show conductive deafness. There is often a characteristic notch of the bone conductive curve at 2000 Hz (the Carhart notch).

Is it due to an acoustic neuroma (AN)?

- The first symptom is usually tinnitus. Tinnitus may be present for months or years before hearing loss or vertigo is noticed. The tinnitus is unilateral in 95% of cases. It is continuous and less disturbing than the tinnitus of Ménière's disease.[16]
- It is rare: annual incidence 1:50 000 to 1:100 000 of the population.[17] In patients with neurofibromatosis type 2, it may be bilateral. Do not dismiss the possibility of AN because the patient is elderly. A series from Denmark found a median age of 55.[18]
- Acoustic neuroma can be suspected, but not diagnosed, in primary care. What is needed is an understanding of the need to refer all patients with unilateral sensorineural hearing loss, even though 90% will be found not to have serious pathology (see below).
- Using MRI in patients with asymmetrical sensorineural hearing loss, a study from San Diego, California found an acoustic neuroma in 7.7%, with other significant lesions in 2.2%. Asymmetrical sensorineural hearing loss was defined as at least 15 dB asymmetry in two or more frequencies or at least 15% asymmetry in speech discrimination scores.[19] A study of unilateral sensorineural hearing loss from Ohio found 5.2% with AN and 6.5% with other significant lesions of the cerebellar-pontine angle, inner ear or brain.[20] The finding of serious pathology in 10% of those with unilateral sensorineural hearing loss appears to be consistent.

Is it due to ototoxicity?

Currently, almost every major group of medication includes one or more compounds with ototoxic properties.[21] Ototoxicity may affect hair cells, the eighth cranial nerve or their central nervous connections. The damage manifests itself as hearing loss, vertigo or tinnitus. Deafness is always bilateral.

Some culprits are:
- *antibiotics*: aminoglycosides, erythromycin, tetracyclines, vancomycin
- *anti-inflammatories*: NSAIDs, aspirin
- *chemotherapeutic agents*: bleomycin, cisplatin (the incidence of tinnitus in patients given cisplatin in clinical studies varies between 7%[22] and 38%[23]), methotrexate
- *cardiac drugs*: beta-blockers, loop diuretics
- *antimalarials*: chloroquine, quinine
- *heavy metals*: mercury, lead
- *tricyclic antidepressants*.

Is it due to a psychological disorder?

- *Somatisation*. Tinnitus may be a somatic manifestation of a psychological disorder. The tinnitus is likely to be genuine but the emphasis that the patient places on it is increased by the underlying psychological problem.
- *Hallucinatory tinnitus* may be a part of psychotic illness. Patients who report hearing voices are not usually thought to be suffering from tinnitus but a patient who reports hearing a drill boring into the brain might give rise to diagnostic confusion.

Is it objective tinnitus?

Objective tinnitus is a rare but significant subsection. It may be apparent to the observer as well as to the patient. Patients with objective tinnitus typically have a vascular abnormality, neurological disease or eustachian tube dysfunction.[24] If the patient's description suggests it, listen with the stethoscope to the neck, and over the ear and eye.[25] The tinnitus may be:
- *Pulsatile*: carotid stenosis, arteriovenous malformations, vascular tumours (e.g. glomus jugulare), valvular heart disease (usually aortic stenosis), states of high cardiac output (anaemia and drug-induced high output).[26,27]
- *Muscular/anatomical*: palatal myoclonus, spasm of stapedius or tensor tympani muscle, patulous eustachian tube.

Patients with a patulous eustachian tube may hear blowing sounds within the ear synchronised with breathing. It may develop after significant weight loss. Patients may have awareness of their own voice (autophony). The tinnitus may disappear with Valsalva's manoeuvre or when the patient lies down with the head in a dependent position.

Other causes

Other causes of tinnitus which the GP should only consider if the history already points in that direction are:
- *Head injury*. Neurological disorders or head trauma have been implicated in 5% to 10% of patients reporting tinnitus.[5]
- *Multiple sclerosis*.
- *Thyroid disease and other systemic illnesses*. Various metabolic abnormalities may be found in patients with tinnitus. In a Polish study, 34% of patients

with tinnitus were found to suffer from systemic diseases: hypertension (47%), hypercholesterolaemia (41%), rheumatic diseases (22%) and diabetes (16%).[28] With the possible exception of myxoedema, it is unlikely that there is a causative link with the tinnitus.

- *Temporomandibular joint dysfunction.* There is often said to be a correlation between tinnitus and disorders of the TMJ; 7% of patients with TMJ dysfunction complain of tinnitus, which is no higher than in the general population. The association is therefore not causative.[29]
- *Post-dural puncture.*[30]

The patient's perspective

Tinnitus may cause disruption of sleep patterns, an inability to concentrate and depression.[31] Conversely, depressed patients, particularly those with sleep disturbances, may focus on their tinnitus more than patients who are without an underlying psychological disorder.

Every assessment of a patient with tinnitus should include an assessment of the patient's mental state. The patient may have severe tinnitus and be suffering badly – even be suicidal – because of it; or the tinnitus may be mild but the patient's reaction to it is more disabling than it need be because of poor coping mechanisms.

Reasons for specialist referral[32]

Suspicion of underlying disease:
- persistent (>3 months) unilateral tinnitus
- unilateral or asymmetrical sensorineural deafness (acute and chronic)
- associated conductive deafness or another disease of the ear
- objective tinnitus.

Specialist management needed because of the severity of the condition:
- tinnitus intrusive enough to interfere with daily activities
- tinnitus with hearing loss that would benefit from a hearing aid
- tinnitus associated with severe anxiety.

Example

A 55-year-old orchestral musician presents with a gradual onset of left-sided deafness and tinnitus. He is not seeking treatment and he is clear that it is noise induced – he is an oboist and has sat with the trumpets playing into his left ear for 30 years – but he wants it documented because of the possibility of compensation.

The GP confirms that the drum is normal. The whisper test shows bilateral deafness, but considerably more on the left. The Rinne test is positive (air conduction better than bone conduction) on both sides, and in Weber's test the sound is heard on the right.

The GP explains that the findings fit with a diagnosis of noise-induced hearing loss but that they are more asymmetrical than she would expect – the noise from the trumpets would only have been slightly greater on the left than the right. She wants to refer him for investigation in case there is another cause as well. He is alarmed at this suggestion and wants to know what else it could be. She says there is a small possibility, no more than 5%, of either a benign tumour of the nerve, or early Ménière's disease.

The specialist agrees that investigations are justified and they confirm the diagnosis of NIHL.

REFERENCES

1. Roy D, Chopra J. *Tinnitus: an update.* R Soc Health 2002;122: 21–23.

2. Kaufman JA. *Tinnitus, otalgia, and facial paralysis.* In: Kaufman JA, ed. Core otolaryngology. Philadelphia: Lippincott, 1990:125–129.

3. The British Tinnitus Association website: www.tinnitus.org.uk.

4. MRC Institute of Hearing Research. *Epidemiology of tinnitus.* Ciba Found Symp 1981;85:16–34.

5. Schleuning AJ 2nd. *Management of the patient with tinnitus.* Med Clin North Am 1991;75:1225–1237.

6. Nicolas-Puel C, Faulconbridge RL, Guitton M, et al. *Characteristics of tinnitus and etiology of associated hearing loss: a study of 123 patients.* Int Tinnitus J 2002;8:37–44.

7. Gristwood RE, Venables WN. *Otosclerosis and chronic tinnitus.* Ann Otol Rhinol Laryngol 2003;112: 398–403.

8. Pirozzo S, Papinczak T, Glasziou P. *Whispered voice test for screening for hearing impairment in adults and*

Table 42.2 Symptoms useful in the diagnosis of Parkinson's disease[12] where the initial probability is 13%

Symptoms	Presence	Likelihood ratio	Probability of PD according to whether the feature is present or absent
Tremor	Present	1.3–17	16–72%
	Absent	0.2–0.6	3–8%
Face less expressive	Present	2.1	24%
	Absent	0.5	7%
Loss of balance	Present	1.6–6.6	19–50%
	Absent	0.3–0.4	4–6%
Change in speech (softer)	Present	3.4	34%
	Absent	0.5	7%
History of falls	Present	0.7	9%
	Absent	3.2	32%

Follow each row from left to right to see how each symptom alters the probability of PD.
Note that a history of falls seems to argue against the diagnosis of PD.

Special tests in suspected Parkinson's disease

The glabellar tap
Tap lightly with the finger on the patient's forehead (glabella) at about two taps per second. A normal response is to blink for the first few taps and then stop blinking. In Parkinson's disease the patient will continue to blink for longer than that, sometimes for as long as the tapping continues. Note: a false negative result may occur in a patient on levodopa; a false positive can occur if the examiner's hand is not kept above the patient's line of vision.

The heel–toe test
Ask the patient to walk, placing the heel of one foot immediately in front of the toes of the other. Failure to perform this is not specific to Parkinson's disease but it can be useful to demonstrate an abnormality of gait when, unstressed, gait appears normal.

Testing for rigidity
Rigidity is present when there is increased muscle tone with the following characteristics:

- resistance to passive movement is the same regardless of whether the limb is moved slowly or quickly
- flexor and extensor tone are the same
- there is no weakness.

Cogwheel rigidity may be present but its absence is not significant. Conversely, the presence of the clasp-knife phenomenon, in which resistance suddenly ceases as extension of a limb nears completion, argues strongly for the presence of spasticity, not rigidity.

Testing for bradykinesia
Ask the patient to tap on the table with each finger in turn, then to tap repeatedly with each heel in turn. The asymmetrical nature of PD means that each limb must be tested.

Refer all patients with a provisional diagnosis of PD to a neurologist. The distinction between PD and, especially, secondary parkinsonism can be difficult.

Is this essential tremor?

Defining diagnostic criteria for ET has proved difficult and two published definitions differ considerably.[8] Both rely on the importance of excluding other causes of tremor. A further difficulty is that Parkinson's disease and dystonia are found in patients with ET more often than would be expected by chance (in 6.1% and 6.9% respectively).[8]

The diagnosis is made on a few positive features. The tremor:

- is present at rest and worsens with voluntary movement.

- may be as slow as the tremor of PD or faster, but never as fast as the fine tremor of hyperthyroidism.

Table 42.3 The value of asking about difficulty with certain tasks in the diagnosis of Parkinson's disease,[12] when the initial probability is 13%

Symptoms	Presence	Likelihood ratio	Probability of PD according to whether the feature is present or absent
Turning in bed	Present	13	66%
	Absent	0.6	8%
Opening jars	Present	6.1	48%
	Absent	0.3	4%
Rising from a chair	Present	1.9–5.2	22–44%
	Absent	0.4–0.6	6–8%

Follow each row from left to right to see how each symptom alters the probability of PD.

Table 42.4 Signs useful in the diagnosis of Parkinson's disease[12] when the initial probability is 13%

Signs	Presence	Likelihood ratio	Probability of PD according to whether the sign is present or absent
Rigidity + bradykinesia	Present	4.5	40%
	Absent	0.1	1%
Tremor, rigidity + bradykinesia	Present	2.2	25%
	Absent	0.5	7%
Micrographia	Present	2.8–5.9	29–47%
	Absent	0.3–0.4	4–6%
Shuffling gait	Present	3.3–15	33–69%
	Absent	0.3–0.5	4–7%
Glabellar tap	Present	4.5	40%
	Absent	0.1	1%
Difficulty in walking heel to toe	Present	2.9	30%
	Absent	0.3	4%
Dementia	Present	3.2	32%
	Absent	0.5	7%

Follow each row from left to right to see how each sign alters the probability of PD.

■ often begins in one limb but becomes bilateral. The Sicilian study found that 87% involved one or more limbs, with involvement of the head alone (3%) or the head and limbs (10%) being less common.[2] When the head is involved, the tremor may be horizontal (no–no) or vertical (yes–yes).

■ is worsened by anxiety, anger, fatigue and, in 2 out of 3 patients, is improved within 1 hour of taking alcohol or a beta-blocker.

■ may start at any time in adult life with peaks of onset between ages 15–20 and 50–70. An early onset therefore argues in favour of ET against PD.

■ is found in other family members. However, the lack of a family history does not disprove the diagnosis. Studies have found a family history in 17 to 100% according to the intensity of the search.[8]

There should be no other neurological symptoms or signs. As a minimum, test for postural instability and gait.

Is this cerebellar disease?

✱ Test for ataxia.[13] Tests usually performed are:
■ the finger–nose–finger test, in which the patient touches the examiner's finger, then his

own nose, then the examiner's finger. In ataxia, the patient misjudges the distance and may overshoot, undershoot and show intention tremor, where increasing tremor is seen as the finger approaches its target.

■ the heel–knee–shin test, in which the patient, lying down, places one heel on the opposite knee then slides it down the shin. The same problems occur as described above, and also 'decomposition of movement' in which the patient performs one part of a complex movement, then another, rather than all together.

■ rapid alternating movements. Clapping is the easiest movement to test for dysdiadochokinesis.

✱ Test for nystagmus.

✱ Test for postural stability.

The sensitivity and specificity of these tests have not been established. The clinical impression is that if the above tests are performed by a clinician with experience of both positives and negatives, they are unlikely to miss a case.

Example

A 73-year-old woman who lives alone presents to a GP in a remote rural practice with a slow tremor of both hands. More striking to the GP is the fact that her voice has changed and that there is marked rigidity of all four limbs and spine. She agrees she is having difficulty walking but blames it on her recent falls. The GP feels confident that this is Parkinson's disease and is tempted to agree to her request to be treated without referral, because of the length of the journey to see a neurologist. However, caution prevails and he arranges an early appointment. He is surprised to learn that the diagnosis is progressive supranuclear palsy. He had failed to notice the extensor plantar responses and the loss of vertical eye movements. He makes arrangements for her care rather than expecting a dramatic response to levodopa.

REFERENCES

1. Rajput A, Offord K, Beard C, et al. *Essential tremor in Rochester, Minnesota: a 45-year study.* J Neurol Neurosurg Psychiatry 1984;47: 466–470.

2. Salemi G, Savettieri G, Rocca W, et al. *Prevalence of essential tremor: a door-to-door survey in Terrasina, Sicily.* Neurology 1994;44:61–64.

3. Louis E, Ottman R, Hauser W. *How common is the most common adult movement disorder? Estimates of the prevalence of essential tremor throughout the world.* Mov Disord 1998;13:5–10.

4. Smaga S. *Tremor.* Am Fam Physician 2003;68:1545–1552.

5. de Rijk M, Tzourio C, Breteler M, et al. *Prevalence of parkinsonism and Parkinson's disease in Europe: the* EUROPARKINSON *Collaborative Study. European Community Concerted Action on the Epidemiology of Parkinson's disease.* J Neurol Neurosurg Psychiatry 1997;62: 10–15.

6. MacDonald B, Cockerell O, Sander J, et al. *The incidence and lifetime prevalence of neurological disorders in a prospective community-based study in the UK.* Brain 2000;123:665–676.

7. Meara RJ, Bisarya S, Hobson JP. *Screening in primary health care for undiagnosed tremor in an elderly population in Wales.* J Epidemiol Community Health 1997;51:574–575.

8. Jankovic J. *Essential tremor: clinical characteristics.* Neurology 2000; 54(11 Suppl 4):S24.

9. Hughes A, Daniel S, Lees AJ. *Improved accuracy of clinical diagnosis of Lewy body Parkinson's disease.* Neurology 2001;57:1497–1499.

10. Schrag A, Ben-Shlomo Y, Quinn N. *How valid is the clinical diagnosis of Parkinson's disease in the community?* J Neurol Neurosurg Psychiatry 2002;73:529–534.

11. Ben-Schlomo B, Sieradzan K. *Idiopathic Parkinson's disease: epidemiology, diagnosis and management.* Br J Gen Pract 1995;45: 261–268.

12. Rao G, Fisch L, Srinivasan S, et al. *Does this patient have Parkinson disease?* JAMA 2003;289:347–353.

13. McGee S. *Evidence-based physical diagnosis.* Philadelphia: Saunders, 2001.

43

Vaginal discharge

KEY FACTS

- The extent to which women seek medical advice for vaginal discharge is highly variable, and many have normal discharge on examination.
- Sexually transmitted infections (STIs) may coexist with, but are not the commonest causes of, vaginal discharge. The risk of an STI should be assessed and screening offered in this context if risk factors for STIs are present.
- *Candida albicans* colonisation is a normal finding in the absence of symptoms.
- *Symptoms and signs are useful in the clinical diagnosis of discharge:*
  - Candidal infection is more likely in the presence of itching, erythema or a 'cheesy' discharge, and when the patient and doctor cannot detect an odour.

- Bacterial vaginosis is more likely in the presence of vaginal pH ≥4.7, a watery discharge and when the patient and doctor can detect an odour.
- *A high vaginal swab (HVS) is useful in the detection of Candida, streptococcal infection, and Trichomonas vaginalis if the high vaginal swab is fresh. It is generally not helpful in confirming the presence or absence of other STIs.*
- Pelvic infection should be considered postpartum, post-abortion and post-instrumentation when abnormal vaginal discharge is associated with additional symptoms and signs.
- Neoplasia is an uncommon cause of vaginal discharge.

A PRACTICAL APPROACH

- ★ Ask what concerns the patient; e.g. is it the discharge or concern about sexually transmitted infection (STI)?
- ★ Assess the risk factors for STI.
- ★ Ask specifically about itch, odour, type of discharge and previous infections.
- ★ Examine and note the type of discharge, odour, and signs of vulval inflammation. Perform a pelvic examination, looking for a foreign body or cervical erosion.

- ★ Send a high vaginal swab (HVS) in transport medium for culture for *Candida* and *Streptococcus*.
- ★ If the clinical picture suggests bacterial vaginosis, send an air-dried HVS (or a smear, according to the laboratory's preference).
- ★ Send endocervical and urethral swabs if at risk of STIs.

Background

- The complaint of abnormal vaginal discharge is common in primary care. However, the degree to which women consider their vaginal secretions to be abnormal, or seek medical advice about it, is highly variable, and influenced by their concerns about potential causes such as sexually transmitted infection (STI).[1] The characteristics of vaginal discharge vary across the menstrual cycle, both in women with and in women without vaginal infections.
- Vaginal discharge can occur in the presence or absence of STI, and with or without associated genital symptoms. Presentation with a chief complaint of vaginal discharge is not itself strongly suggestive of STI,[2] and consideration of other aspects of the history, and risk assessment for STI, are necessary.
- Colonisation with *Candida albicans* is a normal finding in the absence of symptoms, and does not require treatment.

Prevalence

- A study of 229 women of reproductive age attending primary care in Sweden who had not reported vaginal discharge found the following vaginal isolates:[3]
  - *Candida albicans* 19.2%
  - *Trichomonas vaginalis* 0.4%
  - bacterial vaginosis was identified in 8.3%.
- 15% of attendees at routine family planning clinics report the symptom of vaginal discharge on questioning.[4]

Initial probabilities

The initial probabilities when a woman presents in primary care complaining of increased or abnormal vaginal discharge have been considered in two studies.

- In a Scandinavian study of 101 primary care attendees complaining of vaginal discharge *or* offensive odour, the following were found:[5]
  - bacterial vaginosis 34%
  - candidal infection 23%
  - *Chlamydia trachomatis* 15%
  - *Trichomonas vaginalis* 9%
  - herpes simplex virus 7%
  - gonococcal infection 1%.
- In another Scandinavian study, among 361 primary care attenders complaining of vaginal discharge, the following were found:[3]

  - bacterial vaginosis 35.7%
  - *Candida* 31.3%
  - *Trichomonas vaginalis* 2.8%.
- The prevalence of beta-haemolytic streptococci in women complaining of vaginal discharge is less clear.

Do risk factors alter these probabilities?

The prevalence of the major causes of actual, or perceived, abnormal vaginal discharge vary markedly worldwide: these include the presence of *Trichomonas vaginalis*, pregnancy, bacterial vaginosis and the use of vaginal products (such as douches or herbs). In a UK setting, consideration of other symptoms and of demographic and behavioural risk factors help to assess the likelihood of sexually transmitted infection and less common causes of discharge. There is a lack of data on how such factors affect the probability of various diagnoses in the UK primary care setting.

The probability of the presence of a sexually transmitted infection is increased by:
  - younger age (<25 years)[6]
  - a new sexual partner in the past 3 months[6]
  - a history of contact with an STI[7]
  - Afro-Caribbean ethnicity.[6,8]

  Note: STIs can coexist with other causes of vaginal discharge, without themselves causing discharge or other symptoms. In a primary care setting, 16% of women microbiologically diagnosed with bacterial vaginosis or candidal infection (which are not sexually transmitted) will also have a sexually transmitted infection.[5]

  The probability of candidal infection is increased by:
  - pregnancy (prevalence 23% in the third trimester)[9]
  - diabetes mellitus.

Do the specific symptoms assist the diagnosis?

Symptoms in the diagnosis of candidal infection and bacterial vaginosis

A review of the literature on the relation between vaginal symptoms and candidal infection and bacterial vaginosis suggests that the presence or absence of itching, malodorous discharge or a watery discharge may be helpful in distinguishing these diagnoses[2,10] (Tables 43.1 and 43.2).

Table 43.1 The value of symptoms in the diagnosis of candidal infection,[10] based on a prevalence of candidal infection of 20% in women complaining of discharge

Symptom or absence of symptom	Presence of symptom	LR (95% CI). A range may be given	Probability of candidal infection according to presence or absence of the symptom
Itching	Yes	1.4 (1.2–1.7) to 3.3 (2.4–4.8)	26–45%
	No	0.2 (0.05–0.7) to 0.8 (0.7–0.9)	5–17%
NO odour perceived by patient	Yes	1.6 (1.1–2.4) to 2.1 (1.5–3.0)	29–34%
	No	0.3 (0.2–0.8) to 0.5 (0.2–1.0)	7–11%
Redness/erythema	Yes	2.0 (1.5–2.8)	33%
	No	0.8 (0.8–0.9)	17%
'Cheesy' discharge	Yes	2.4 (1.4–4.2)	37%
	No	0.5 (0.3–0.9)	11%
Discharge NOT watery	Yes	1.5 (1.2–1.9)	27%
	No	0.1 (0.02–0.8)	2%
Complaint of 'another candidal infection'	Yes	3.3 (1.2–9.1)	45%
	No	0.7 (0.5–1.0)	15%

Follow each row from left to right to see how each symptom alters the probability of candidal infection.
Adapted from Anderson MR et al. Evaluation of vaginal complaints. JAMA 2004; 291: 1368–1379. Copyright © 2004, American Medical Association. All rights reserved.

The probability of vaginal discharge being caused by other infections

- The symptoms of bacterial vaginosis are similar to those of the STI *Trichomonas vaginalis*, which is uncommon in the UK but common worldwide.[11,12]
- The specific complaint of 'abnormal yellow discharge'[2] is associated with the presence of chlamydial or gonococcal infection, while a complaint of painful genital skin lesions suggests genital herpes.[2]
- *Pelvic infection* includes pelvic inflammatory disease, post-abortal sepsis, puerperal sepsis and postoperative sepsis. The probability of pelvic inflammatory disease as a cause of vaginal discharge is linked to the probability of STI (see above) and the presence of additional symptoms and clinical signs including: lower abdominal pain, intermenstrual bleeding, recent onset of deep dyspareunia, adnexal tenderness and cervical excitation pain.[13]
- *Endometritis* may result in abnormal vaginal discharge, lower abdominal pain and associated features of pelvic infection.
- Gram-positive cocci may be seen on microscopy and beta-haemolytic streptococci may be identified by culture. These organisms may be a commensal in asymptomatic women but can also be pathogenic after surgical abortion, miscarriage, vaginal delivery or caesarean section.
- *Streptococcal infection* can cause symptomatic discharge in peri- or postmenopausal women. It is underdiagnosed in postmenopausal diabetic women, accounting for 52% of vaginal discharge by contrast with only 22% due to candidal infection.[14]
- *Uncommon causes of discharge* are: primary syphilis, *Escherichia coli*, non-specific vaginal infections and desquamative inflammatory vaginitis.

Consider the possibility of non-infective causes of vaginal discharge

The diagnosis will be based on the patient's history, and may be further supported by examination findings (see below).

- *Normal discharge*: many women report concerns about their vaginal discharge at a time of concern about STIs, and may have normal discharge.[1]
- *Cervical secretions* due to ectropion, endocervical polyp or primary herpes simplex affecting the cervix.
- *Allergic responses* (history of douching or other topical preparations) or *chemical irritation*.
- *Foreign body* (condom, tampon, intrauterine device or other).
- *Uncommon causes include*: physical trauma, vault granulation tissue, vesicovaginal fistula, rectovaginal fistula, neoplasia.

Table 43.2 The value of symptoms in the diagnosis of bacterial vaginosis,[10] based on a prevalence of bacterial vaginosis of 35% in women complaining of discharge

Symptom or absence of symptom[10]	Presence of the symptom	LR (95% CI)	Probability of bacterial vaginosis according to presence or absence of the symptom
Increased discharge	Yes	1.8 (1.2–2.8)	49%
	No	0.6 (0.4–0.9)	24%
Odour perceived by patient	Yes	1.6 (1.3–2.0)	46%
	No	0.07 (0.01–0.5)	4%
NO itching	Yes	1.6 (1.0–2.4)	46%
	No	0.6 (0.4–1.0)	24%

Follow each row from left to right to see how each symptom alters the probability of bacterial vaginitis.
Adapted from Anderson MR et al. Evaluation of vaginal complaints. JAMA 2004; 291: 1368–1379. Copyright © 2004, American Medical Association. All rights reserved.

Table 43.3 The value of signs in the diagnosis of candidal infection,[10] based on a prevalence of candidal infection of 20% in women complaining of discharge

Sign	Presence or absence	LR (95% CI). A range may be given	Probability of candidal infection according to presence or absence of the sign
Thick, curdy or flocculent discharge	Yes	2.7 (1.3–5.5) to 130 (19–960)	40–97%
	No	0.3 (0.2–0.4) to 0.9 (0.8–0.9)	7–18%
'Vulvar inflammation' and/or specific signs of inflammation including oedema, erythema, fissures and excoriations*	Yes	2.1 (1.5–2.8) to 8.4 (2.3–31)	34–68%
	No	0.7 (0.6–0.8)	15%
Curdy discharge plus itch	Yes	150 (20–1000)	97%
	No	0.2 (0.1–0.4)	5%
Odour as perceived by clinician as NOT 'fishy'	Yes	2.9 (2.4–5.0)	42%
	No	0.03 (0–0.5)	1%

*These can also occur in trichomoniasis, which is uncommon in the UK.
Follow each row from left to right to see how each sign alters the probability of candidal infection.
Adapted from Anderson MR et al. Evaluation of vaginal complaints. JAMA 2004; 291: 1368–1379. Copyright © 2004, American Medical Association. All rights reserved.

Is the examination helpful?

Characteristics of the discharge

The finding of a discharge on examination does not itself distinguish between candidal infection and bacterial vaginosis (BV).[10] However, certain types of discharge favour one or the other. Vulval inflammation favours candidal infection while a 'high cheese' smell favours BV and a fishy smell argues against candidal infection (Tables 43.3 and 43.4).[10] The combination of curdy discharge and itch almost always indicates *Candida*.

Table 43.4 The value of signs in the diagnosis of bacterial vaginosis,[10] based on a prevalence of bacterial vaginosis of 35% in women complaining of discharge

Sign	Presence or absence of the sign	LR (95% CI)	Probability of bacterial vaginosis according to presence or absence of the sign
Discharge that is other than normal	Yes	1.1 (1.0–1.2)	37%
	No	0.1 (0.01–0.9)	5%
Profuse discharge	Yes	3.0 (0.3–28)	62%
	No	0.98 (0.9–1.0)	35%
Discharge that is NOT white	Yes	2.0 (1.4–2.8)	52%
	No	0.5 (0.4–0.7)	21%
A 'high cheese' smell	Yes	3.2 (2.1–4.7)	63%
	No	0.3 (0.2–0.4)	14%

Follow each row from left to right to see how each sign alters the probability of bacterial vaginosis.
Adapted from Anderson MR et al. Evaluation of vaginal complaints. JAMA 2004; 291: 1368–1379. Copyright © 2004, American Medical Association. All rights reserved.

- Data on the relation between vaginal discharge and pathology of the *upper* reproductive tract (such as pelvic inflammatory disease, gonorrhoea and chlamydial infection) derives from populations at higher risk of sexually transmitted infections than most UK primary care populations.[2] Patients can, and frequently do, have more than one cause of vaginal discharge, while vaginal discharge is often *not* a symptom of a coexisting STI. Studies relating to developing countries have evaluated the sensitivity, specificity and positive predictive value (PPV) of testing and treatment algorithms (such as those of WHO) against actual microbiological diagnoses, for their capacity to exclude treatable STI. This approach does not yield data on sensitivity, specificity or PPV of approaches to diagnosis and treatment applicable to the UK primary care setting. However, it is interesting to note that the presence of 'yellow vaginal discharge' was associated with the identification of cervical chlamydial or gonorrhoea infection (odds ratio (OR) 2.9) and negatively associated with candidal infection (OR 0.64).

- Examination may reveal other physical causes of discharge, such as cervical ectopy, granulation tissues or fistulae. The appearance of the vagina may suggest douching or the use of foreign substances.

What tests are useful?

A high vaginal swab sent for culture and sensitivity, specifically to include beta-haemolytic streptococci and *Candida* species can confirm the diagnosis of these treatable microbial infections. However, note that:

- This swab is *not* useful in making or excluding the diagnosis of STI, and its processing varies between laboratories.[15]

- The rate of isolation of *Gardnerella vaginalis* is similar in women with and without bacterial vaginosis.[3]

- *Trichomonas vaginalis* may be identified on a high vaginal swab, but requires a fresh sample both for microscopy and for culture.

- As noted previously, *Candida* species may be a frequent finding in asymptomatic women. A positive culture for *Candida* species does not confirm that candidiasis is the cause of vaginal discharge, particularly when additional symptoms and signs suggestive of candidiasis are absent (see Tables 43.1 and 43.3).

Bacterial vaginosis can be formally diagnosed using:

1. *Hay–Ison criteria* based upon grading the appearance of a Gram-stained slide of vaginal secretions sampled from the posterior fornix. The appearance is scored from 0 to 4, with grade 2 suggestive of BV and grade 3 diagnostic. A dry slide of vaginal discharge can also be Gram stained at the laboratory, to make a microbiological diagnosis of BV.

2. *Amsel criteria.* Three of the four Amsel criteria must be present to make the diagnosis. The criteria are:

Table 43.5 Value of vaginal pH in the diagnosis of bacterial vaginitis,[16] based on a prevalence of bacterial vaginosis of 35% in women complaining of discharge

Vaginal pH	Likelihood ratio	Probability after the test
≥4.7	2.0	52%
<4.7	0.07	4%

- thin white homogeneous discharge
- vaginal pH > 4.5
- clue cells present on microscopy
- fishy odour on adding 10% potassium hydroxide (KOH).

The KOH test is now less frequently performed in clinical practice for health and safety reasons and, as this means one criterion is not taken into consideration, there is a move towards using Hay–Ison grading.

3. *Measurement of pH of vaginal fluid* (taking care not to raise the pH through lubricants, and avoiding use of samples taken at the time of menses when vaginal pH is raised) may be a useful test in *excluding* bacterial vaginosis. Using the presence of clue cells on Gram staining as a diagnostic gold standard, Eschenbach et al[16] measured vaginal pH in non-menstruating women who were not infected with *Trichomonas vaginalis*. The results (see Table 43.5) demonstrate that vaginal pH may be useful in excluding, but not in confirming, a diagnosis of bacterial vaginosis. Whatman pH indicator paper (narrow range pH 4.0–7.0) is available in the UK from Whatman International Ltd (www.whatman.com).

The problem of making the diagnosis of BV in primary care in the UK

Most of the literature relating to the specificity and sensitivity of tests for bacterial vaginosis assumes the availability of near patient microscopy, which, though commonly used in US office gynaecology and in UK genitourinary medicine clinics, is not generally available in UK primary care.[17,18] Some laboratories routinely Gram stain an air-dried HVS, allowing diagnosis of BV according to the Hay–Ison criteria. If yours does not, consider sending an air-dried smear of discharge on a slide for microscopy (after checking with the laboratory that they are willing to perform this).[18]

Further tests in those at high risk of STI

Risk factors are:

Age. All women under 25 are at increased risk for *Chlamydia* and gonorrhoea. Prevalence rates for chlamydial infection of approximately 10% have been noted among women under 25 years old screened in primary care,[6] and *Chlamydia* testing (endocervical and urethral swabs) in addition to appropriate testing to diagnose the cause of their vaginal discharge should be offered.

Following delivery and instrumentation. The risk of pelvic inflammatory disease is increased postpartum, following termination of pregnancy and in the 20 days following fitting of an intrauterine contraceptive device (IUD). These women should also be offered *Chlamydia* testing if not previously screened for this infection prior to abortion or IUD insertion. A high vaginal swab should also be sent for culture and sensitivity, looking for beta-haemolytic *Streptococcus* infection.

Example

A woman aged 23 attends for the first time for the fitting of an IUD. Her GP examines her prior to the fitting and notices a foul smelling, profuse creamy vaginal discharge. He asks her about this and she agrees that she has been a bit 'whiffy' recently. She has not noticed any irritation or other symptoms. Examination does not reveal any inflammation and bimanual pelvic examination is normal.

The GP explains that he suspects that there is infection in the vagina and that he is unhappy fitting an IUD until it is sorted out. He adds that he doesn't suspect *Chlamydia* but offers it as a screening test anyway, to which she agrees. He takes a high vaginal swab (marking the form '?BV ?TV') and separate

endocervical swabs for gonococcal culture and for *Chlamydia* nucleic acid amplification testing (NAAT). They agree on alternative contraception meanwhile.

The GP strongly suspects BV. The prevalence in women not complaining of discharge is 8% (see above), which is raised to 22% by the smell (Fig. 43.1) and to 46% by the profuse discharge (Fig. 43.2). The absence of other typical candidal features raises the probability of BV even further. Candidal infection is virtually ruled out by the clinical picture; any *Candida* found on the swab would be incidental. If *Chlamydia* is also found, it, too, would be coincidental but would need treating in view of the planned IUD insertion.

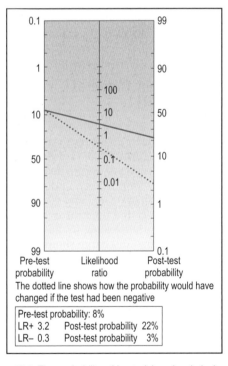

The dotted line shows how the probability would have changed if the test had been negative

Pre-test probability: 8%	
LR+ 3.2	Post-test probability 22%
LR– 0.3	Post-test probability 3%

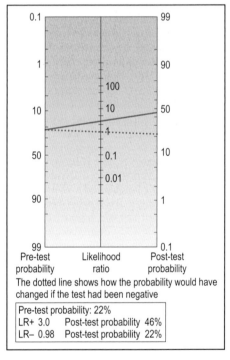

The dotted line shows how the probability would have changed if the test had been negative

Pre-test probability: 22%	
LR+ 3.0	Post-test probability 46%
LR– 0.98	Post-test probability 22%

Figure 43.1 The probability of bacterial vaginosis before and after the discovery of the smell in the example above.

Figure 43.2 The probability of bacterial vaginosis before and after the finding of profuse discharge in the example above.

REFERENCES

1. Bro F. *Vaginal discharge in general practice – women's perceptions, beliefs and behaviour.* Scand J Prim Health Care 1993;11(4):281–287.

2. Ryan CA, Courtois BN, Hawes SE, et al. *Risk assessment,* *symptoms, and signs as predictors of vulvovaginal and cervical infections in an urban US STD clinic: implications for use of STD algorithms.* Sex Transm Infec 1998;74 (Suppl 1): S59–76.

3. Bro F. *Vaginal microbial flora in women with and without vaginal discharge registered in general practice.* Dan Med Bull 1989;36:483–485.

4. Barrett H, Browne A. *Health, hygiene and maternal education:*

evidence from *The Gambia*. Soc Sci Med 1996;43(11):1579–1590.

5. Wathne B, Holst E, Hovelius B, et al. *Vaginal discharge – comparison of clinical, laboratory and microbiological findings*. Acta Obstet Gynecol Scand 1994;73:802–808.

6. LaMontagne DS, Fenton KA, Randall S, et al, on behalf of the National Chlamydia Screening Steering Group. *Establishing the National Chlamydia Screening Programme in England: results from the first full year of screening*. Sex Transm Infect 2004;80:335–341.

7. Pimenta JM, Catchpole M, Rogers PA, et al. *Opportunistic screening for genital chlamydial infection. II: Prevalence among healthcare attenders, outcome, and evaluation of positive cases*. Sex Transm Infect 2003;79:22–27.

8. Low N, Sterne JA, Barlow D. *Inequalities in rates of gonorrhoea and chlamydia between black ethnic groups in south east London: cross sectional study*. Sex Transm Infect 2001;77:15–20.

9. Paavonen J, Heinonen PK, Aine R, et al. *Prevalence of nonspecific vaginitis and other cervicovaginal infections during the third trimester of pregnancy*. Sex Transm Dis 1986;13: 5–8.

10. Anderson MR, Klink K, Cohrssen A. *Evaluation of vaginal complaints*. JAMA 2004;291(11): 1368–1379.

11. Health Protection Agency Centre for Infections. *Mapping the issues*. HIV and other sexually transmitted infections in the United Kingdom: 2005.

12. Cassell JA, Mercer CH, Sutcliffe L, et al. *Trends in sexually transmitted infections in general practice 1990–2000: population based study using data from the UK general practice research database*. BMJ 2006;332: 332–334.

13. Simms I, Warburton F, Westrom L. *Diagnosis of pelvic inflammatory disease: time for a rethink*. Sex Transm Infect 2003;79(6):491–494.

14. Rowe BR, Logan MN, Farrell I, et al. *Is candidiasis the true cause of vulvovaginal irritation in women with diabetes mellitus?* J Clin Pathol 1990; 43:644–645.

15. Jungmann E, Johnson AM, Ridgway G, et al. *How useful are high vaginal swabs in general practice? Results of a multicentre study*. Int J STD AIDS 2004;15: 238–239.

16. Eschenbach DA, Hillier S, Critchlow C, et al. *Diagnosis and clinical manifestations of bacterial vaginosis*. Am J Obstet Gynecol 1988; 158(4):819–828.

17. Royal College of Obstetricians & Gynaecologists, British Association for Sexual Health and HIV. *The management of women of reproductive age attending non-genitourinary medicine settings complaining of vaginal discharge*. J Fam Plann Reprod Health Care 2006;32:33–42; quiz 42.

18. Royal College of General Practitioners Sex Drugs and HIV Task Group and British Society for Sexual Health and HIV. *Sexually transmitted infections in primary care*. 2006.

44

Weight loss

KEY FACTS

- Unintentional weight loss is common, especially in the older person.
- In most, the cause will be obvious: either coexistent physical or mental illness or a psychosocial problem.
- Those without an obvious cause can be adequately assessed in primary care with a simple protocol (outlined below) which will diagnose most of those who have a detectable cause.

A PRACTICAL APPROACH

- ★ Ask about diet, eating habits, the enjoyment of food.
- ★ Ask about other symptoms, other illnesses and about drugs, including those bought over the counter.
- ★ Check formally for depression and, in older patients, for dementia.
- ★ Examine in a focused way, bearing in mind the commonest organic causes of weight loss, cancer and gastrointestinal (GI) disorders, as well as hyperthyroidism and neurological problems.
- ★ Perform the tests listed in the text below.
- ★ Act on any abnormality even if it does not seem, in itself, to point to a diagnosis. To give two examples:
  (a) the vague symptom of fatigue, with weight loss, is a powerful predictor of cancer

  (b) a person with weight loss and a lactate dehydrogenase >500 IU/L has a probability of cancer of >90% even when all other tests are normal.
- ★ If the above approach yields no clues, discuss with the patient and/or the family whether to pursue further investigations. In a quarter of patients with weight loss seen in primary care, no cause can be found over a 2-year follow-up. The next step would be invasive (upper and lower GI endoscopy) and unlikely to reveal serious disease in a person who has no other symptoms, signs or abnormal investigations. On the other hand, a policy of watchful waiting carries a risk of missing a cancer. No prospective studies have examined this risk in a patient in primary care and no figure for this risk can be given.

This chapter deals solely with *unintentional* weight loss.

Definition

A commonly accepted definition is the loss of at least 5% of body weight in 6 months, although some studies have used 7.5% and 1 year as criteria. A study from Seattle of men aged 65 and over found that a loss of 4% over 1 year was the best cut-off point in the identification of those with an increased risk of mortality.[1]

Prevalence

In the general population

The prevalence in the whole population is unknown. In the Seattle study of men aged 65 and over, 7.8% lost at least 5% in one year and 13.1% lost at least 4% in one year. Studies of patients in residential care find that 50% to 65% have lost at least 5% of body weight in 6 months.[2]

As a presentation in primary care

A US study from family practices in Georgia, of patients aged 63 and over, reviewed those in whom a weight loss of 7.5% over 6 months was recorded and in whom there was no obvious known cause.[3] Only 0.45% met the criteria.

Initial probabilities in a patient with involuntary weight loss

The Georgia study from family practice found the following conditions in 45 older patients with weight loss:[3]
- depression 18%
- cancer (lung 3, colon 1, pancreas 1, breast 1, prostate 1) 16%
- gastrointestinal causes other than cancer 11%
- hyperthyroidism 9%
- medication (thyroxine, nitrofurantoin, theophylline, procainamide) 9%
- neurological (Alzheimer's disease 2, cerebrovascular disease 1) 7%
- tuberculosis 2%
- poor nutritional intake 2%
- cholesterol phobia 2%.

After 2 years of investigation and observation, the cause remained unknown in 24%.

These figures are similar to those reported from secondary care[4] except that the proportion with thyrotoxicosis tends to be lower in secondary care, possibly because it had already been detected in primary care.

Other causes mentioned in secondary care studies that do not appear in the Georgia study are:[2]
- heart failure
- chronic lung disease
- diabetes
- Parkinson's disease
- uraemia
- anxiety
- alcoholism and drug misuse
- AIDS.

Note that occult malignancy, i.e. malignancy that is not obvious at the initial evaluation, is uncommon but not rare. The primary care study from Georgia detected 1 patient with cancer that had been missed at the initial assessment of 45 patients (although, given the small numbers, that 1 case does represent 14% of all those whose weight loss was due to cancer).The study from secondary care in California found four cancers that had been missed at the first assessment, out of 59 patients with a physical cause of their weight loss.[4] All four had lung cancer, of which two had been seen on chest X-ray (CXR) but attributed to old infection, one had a hilar mass that was missed on CXR and a fourth whose initial CXR was normal.

Frail elderly patients are a special case and may have more than one cause for their weight loss. Robbins has coined the concept of 'The 9 Ds' to make this point:[5]

dentition	dysgeusia	dysphagia
diarrhoea	disease (chronic)	depression
dementia	dysfunction	drugs

Dysgeusia is the loss of a normal sense of taste. Dysfunction refers to social causes of weight loss, e.g. loss of a spouse who used to prepare the meals, or mobility problems that make shopping difficult.

The clinical assessment

The history

The Georgia study found that the history detected the majority with psychiatric disorders. The secondary care study from California found that nearly half of patients had symptoms which pointed to the cause.
* Check that weight loss has indeed taken place. Some studies find that in about a quarter of patients who claim to have lost weight, the claim does not stand up to examination. Because of this, it has been suggested that two of the following should be present:[4]
  (a) clothes are looser
  (b) the weight loss is confirmed by a family member
  (c) the patient can specify how many kilos (or pounds) have been lost.

  Older patients can look cachexic because of the age-related loss of facial fat. Anecdotal evidence suggests that, in men who wear belts, those who

have not had to tighten their belt have not lost a significant amount of weight.[6]
* Ask about other symptoms, especially fatigue, appetite, bowel disturbance and cough.
* Ask about other coexisting conditions.
* Ask about diet, smoking and alcohol use.
* Check the medication as drugs can affect appetite or eating. Tricyclic antidepressants and anticholinergics can make chewing difficult because of a dry mouth; digoxin and ACE inhibitors can cause alterations in taste; NSAIDs and theophylline can cause dyspepsia and nausea.
* Assess the patient's mental state, both mood and cognition. Assess these formally (see pp. 373 and 182).
* Assess the patient's social situation. Ask who prepares the food.

The examination

The Georgia study found three out of seven cancers on examination. However, none of the four patients with thyrotoxicosis were detected.[3]
* In addition to examining the heart, lungs and abdomen, check the neck, axillae and groins for lymph nodes, and the breast or prostate for masses.

* Look for clues as to alcohol or drug misuse and assess thyroid status.

Combining the history and examination

The California study found that six clinical features were significant independent predictors of a physical cause of weight loss (Table 44.1).

Note that the most powerful predictor of physical disease is the presence of fatigue, and that the examination contributes relatively little to the total score.

Using the score

A score of 9 or above argues against a physical cause for the weight loss with a sensitivity of 97% and a specificity of 72%, giving these figures for the likelihood ratios: LR+ 3.4; LR– 0.05. In other words, the score only misses 3% with a physical cause of weight loss, but 17% of positives are false positives.

Using the figure from primary care that 58% of those older patients presenting with weight loss have a physical cause for it,[3] Table 44.2 shows the probability of physical disease if this decision rule is applied.

While a score below 9 is a powerful predictor of physical disease, a score of 9 or above does not

Table 44.1 Independent predictors of a physical cause of weight loss[4]

Clinical feature	Score
Less than 20 pack years of smoking	+3
No decrease in activities due to fatigue	+5
Patient complains of nausea/vomiting	–3
Recent improvement in appetite	–2
Cough that has recently changed	–1
Physical examination suggests a physical cause	–1
Correction factor	+8
Possible total	16

Table 44.2 Probability of physical disease as the cause of weight loss after the use of the Californian score

Score	Pre-test probability	Likelihood ratio (95% CI)	Post-test probability (95% CI)
<9	58%	3.4 (2.0–6.00)	86% (78–92%)
9 or over	58%	0.05 (0.01–0.2)	8% (2–26%)
Follow each row from left to right to see how the score alters the probability of physical disease being present.			

sufficiently rule it out to omit investigations in these patients.

Note also that it does not distinguish psychiatric disease from other non-physical causes.

Investigations

A consensus exists that the following is a reasonable basic screen:[2-5,7]
- full blood count and erythrocyte sedimentation rate
- urea and electrolytes, liver fuction tests, thyroid function tests, random glucose
- urine analysis
- stool occult blood
- chest X-ray.

The value of investigations

A Spanish study of 328 patients with weight loss, in whom the initial assessment had failed to find a cause, found the following:[8]
- malignancy in 35%
- psychiatric disorders in 24%.

Five independent predictors of malignancy were used to make a decision rule (Table 44.3).

A score of 0 or 1 was found to affect the probability of malignancy very little but more extreme scores were more powerful (Table 44.4).

Table 44.3 Independent predictors of cancer in patients in whom clinical assessment has not revealed a cause for weight loss[8]

Clinical feature	Score
Age >80	+1
Serum albumin >3.5 mg/dl	−2
White blood cell count >12 000 × 10^9/L	+1
Alkaline phosphatase >300 IU/L	+2
Lactate dehydrogenase >500 IU/L	+3

Referral for specialist assessment

Patients with abnormal findings, and possibly those in whom no cause has been found, are likely to need referral to secondary care. Secondary care studies have shown how useful referral is, but that may be because the initial assessment in primary care was inadequate. A French study of 77 very old patients in secondary care being investigated for weight loss found that gastroscopy led to a diagnosis in 46 compared to CXR in 17 and abdominal ultrasound in 15.[9]

Upper and lower GI endoscopy is likely to be the most useful investigations but no studies have reported on its value in the patient whose clinical assessment and investigations give no suggestion of a GI problem.

General points

Several general points about the assessment of weight loss can be made:
(a) The amount of weight loss is unhelpful in deciding on the probability of physical illness, once the cut-off point has been reached.[3]
(b) A failure to regain weight on prolonged follow-up is not evidence of a physical cause.[1]
(c) If there is coexistent illness, it can be difficult to decide if the weight loss is due to the condition. It is easier if the weight loss occurred at a time when the condition was unstable.[4] However, some patients are stable, but still sufficiently ill to lose weight. A review of a large trial of patients with heart failure found weight loss of at least 5% of body weight in 42% of patients, who were not necessarily poorly controlled. The weight loss was not due to diuresis since the patients were free from oedema on entry to the trial.[10]

Table 44.4 The value of the Spanish decision rule in the diagnosis of cancer in patients with weight loss in whom the diagnosis is not clear on initial clinical assessment

Score	Probability of cancer before applying the rule	Likelihood ratio	Probability of cancer after applying the rule
>1	35%	28	94%
<0	35%	0.07	4%

Follow each row from left to right to see how the score alters the probability of cancer being present.

REFERENCES

1. Wallace J, Schwartz R, LaCroix A, et al. *Involuntary weight loss in older outpatients: incidence and clinical significance.* J Am Geriatr Soc 1995; 44:465–466.

2. Bouras E, Lange S, Scolapio J. *Rational approach to patients with unintentional weight loss.* Mayo Clin Proc 2001;76:923–929.

3. Thompson M, Morris L. *Unexplained weight loss in the ambulatory elderly.* J Am Geriatr Soc 1991;39:497–500.

4. Marton K, Sox H, Krupp J. *Involuntary weight loss: diagnostic and prognostic significance.* Ann Intern Med 1981;95:568–574.

5. Robbins L. *Evaluation of weight loss in the elderly.* Geriatrics 1989;44:31–34, 37.

6. Winfield R. *Weight loss and the belt.* Ann Intern Med 1973;79: 910.

7. Huffman G. *Evaluating and treating unintentional weight loss in the elderly.* Am Fam Physician 2002;65: 640–650.

8. Hernandez J, Matorras P, Riancho J, et al. *Involuntary weight loss without specific symptoms: a clinical prediction score for malignant neoplasm.* Q J Med 2003;96:649–655.

9. Fauchais A, Puisieux F, Bulckaen H, et al. *Unexplained weight loss in the elderly: role of gastric fibroscopy, study of a cohort of 77 patients with a 13 month follow-up.* Rev Med Interne 2001;22:11–19.

10. Anker S. *Prognostic importance of weight loss in chronic heart failure and the effect of treatment with angiotensin-converting-enzyme inhibitors: an observational study.* Lancet 2003;361:1077–1083.

PART TWO

Disorders

Acute coronary syndrome

45

Once the possibility of acute coronary syndrome (ACS) has been raised, usually by a complaint of chest pain:
- The details of the history only alter the probabilities slightly.
- The physical examination is usually negative. If present, three signs argue in favour of ACS: hypotension, crackles and a third heart sound.

A normal examination does not alter the probabilities either way.
- The classic ECG changes of infarction are very useful in establishing the diagnosis, while a normal ECG argues usefully against it, though not enough to ignore a suggestive clinical picture.

A PRACTICAL APPROACH

- ∗ Make a decision about the need for immediate admission on the history. In general, all patients with a new episode of acute chest pain lasting >15 minutes need hospital assessment unless a number of features (the character of the pain, the lack of risk factors, another more likely diagnosis and a normal ECG) argue strongly against the diagnosis of acute coronary syndrome.
- ∗ Examine the patient mainly to look for complications of infarction (heart failure,

shock) or for pointers to an alternative diagnosis. Only make this examination if it does not substantially delay the arrival of the patient at a facility where acute intervention is possible.
- ∗ Perform an ECG, for diagnostic purposes, in those whose history raises the possibility of ACS but where that possibility is so small that admission would not be justified if the ECG were normal.

Definitions

- 'Acute coronary syndrome' (ACS) covers the spectrum of conditions from myocardial infarction (MI) with ST elevation at one end to unstable angina at the other. In primary care, the distinction between different entities within the syndrome is not hugely important since the management (immediate admission) is the same.
- 'Unstable angina' exists where there has been an abrupt change in symptoms such that angina is occurring at rest or at significantly lower levels of

activity, or that the frequency, duration or severity of attacks has substantially worsened. The recent onset (in the last 2 months) of severe angina should also be considered to be unstable.

Prevalence

- The prevalence of treated coronary heart disease in primary care in England and Wales is 3.7% (males) and 2.2% (females).[1] Of the US population, 0.4% present to an emergency department annually with a myocardial infarction and double that number present with unstable angina.[2]

- The prevalence of ACS among patients presenting with chest pain in primary care is 1.5%[3] to 5%,[4] although if the presentation takes the form of an emergency call, the prevalence is likely to be nearer 33%, of whom one-third are suffering from a myocardial infarction (see *Chest pain*, p. 33).

General principles of the diagnosis from the history

- *A history of chest pain* is usually the symptom that raises the possibility of ACS.
- The issue for the general practitioner in the emergency situation is not necessarily to diagnose acute myocardial infarction (AMI) but to judge whether the clinical picture, plus ECG changes if performed, allow the diagnosis to be ruled out. The GP is therefore interested in aspects of the clinical picture with high sensitivity, i.e. low negative likelihood ratios. No single aspect of the clinical picture meets this requirement, although a combination plus a normal ECG may.
- *Can ACS be diagnosed from the history?* The *presence* of acute chest pain is more important than its characteristics. Traditional teaching stresses the characteristic nature of the pain, e.g. that it is usually crushing and central, and studies have indeed shown that certain features are significantly more common in patients with ACS than in those subsequently shown not to be suffering from ischaemic pain. *However, if present, these characteristic features only alter the probability slightly.*
- *Example:* a study of patients presenting to an Austrian emergency department with chest pain[5] found that the characteristic history of crushing, squeezing or burning central chest pain, with or without radiation to the neck, jaw, back, shoulders, arms, wrists or epigastrium, and lasting >20 minutes, had a sensitivity of 85% and a specificity of 52% for AMI. This gives an almost useless LR+ of 1.8 (95% CI 1.1 to 2.8) and a more useful LR– of 0.3 (0.1 to 0.5). This means that, if present, the probability of AMI rises from, say, 10% (assuming it was an emergency call) to 16% and, if absent, it falls to 3%. Alone, these changes are insufficient to alter the course of action. Of them, radiation of pain to the *right* arm seems, contrary to traditional teaching, to be the single most useful characteristic (see below).
- *If symptoms of excessive autonomic activity* were present (nausea, vomiting or sweating), the specificity of the history in the Austrian study above rose to 63%; but requiring these extra symptoms dropped the sensitivity to 65%.[5]

- *The pain is usually symmetrical.* A patient may use the gesture of a clenched fist to describe the pain; a finger pointed at one site argues against the diagnosis.
- *Certain features militate against the diagnosis* of ischaemic pain. Lee and colleagues in Boston found that, of 596 patients with chest pain, if the pain was sharp or stabbing, there was no prior history of angina or MI, and chest pain could be reproduced by chest wall palpation or was pleuritic or had a positional component, none had ACS.[6] However, *individual* atypical features do not rule out the diagnosis. Lee found that 22% of patients presenting to the emergency department with sharp or stabbing pain had ACS, 16% had pain that was affected by position and 11% were tender to palpation (see below).[6]
- Other features of the history that militate against a diagnosis of ACS are those that point to other systems: a feeling of a lump in the throat, an acid taste, acid reflux, over-fullness after eating, pain that wakes the patient at night, cough.
- *The presence of risk factors* increases the probability of ACS but probably less than the physician, used to their value in predicting long-term coronary heart disease (CHD) risk, would expect. A study of 10 689 patients with chest pain found that age, gender, diabetes and a past history of CHD were significantly associated with current ACS in patients with chest pain[7] but with LR+s of between 1.1 (for male sex) and 2.2 (past history of MI), and LR–s between 0.9 (female sex) and 0.5 (no past history of angina). Individual risk factors would not greatly alter the probabilities but the presence of several would substantially increase the probability of ACS.
- Finally, it must be recognised that a small number of patients with ACS suffer no pain. The event is either undiagnosed or comes to the attention of the physician because of a complaint of malaise, fever or, in the elderly, confusion, stroke or syncope. In patients over the age of 85, these atypical presentations are the rule.[8] Even younger patients may not be particularly troubled by the pain. Short cites the example of a nurse who worked for a day despite the pain of a myocardial infarction and a man of 41 who played a game of badminton despite it.[9]

Statistics relating to aspects of the history

A meta-analysis of the predictive value of different features of the history shows how they contribute to the diagnosis of ACS.[10]

Unfortunately for the GP they are mainly derived from emergency departments and specialist units; equivalent data for primary care do not exist. The data in Tables 45.1 to 45.3 are derived from this meta-analysis and are (mainly) arranged in decreasing order of sensitivity. Post-test probabilities are based on a prevalence of ACS of 1.5% of those presenting with chest pain in primary care.[3]

A further useful pointer was detected in a study from Aberdeen, Scotland.[9] If the patient who has had a previous infarct or angina indicates that the present pain is in the same site, or below it, the probability that the present pain is ischaemic is increased (Table 45.4).

Atypical presentations pose difficulties in diagnosis. While more often due to causes other than myocardial ischaemia, they may be the sole manifestation of it.

■ *Dyspnoea* is the only complaint of 4% to 14% of patients with acute MI and of 5% with unstable angina.[2]

Table 45.1 Six features of chest pain that increase the probability of ACS based on a pre-test probability of 1.5%

Symptom	Presence	Likelihood ratio	Probability of ACS
Central pain	Present	1.1	2%
	Absent	0.3	0.5%
Crushing pain	Present	1.6	2%
	Absent	0.6	1%
Any radiation	Present	1.3	2%
	Absent	0.3	0.4%
Radiates to left	Present	1.2	2%
	Absent	0.6	1%
Radiates to right	Present	6.7*	9%
	Absent	0.7	1%
Lasts >1 hour	Present	1.1	2%
	Absent	0.8	1%

*Based on small numbers. 95% CI for LR+ = 3.0 to 15.
Follow each row from left to right to see how the symptom alters the probability of ACS.

Table 45.2 Four features of chest pain that reduce the probability of ACS based on a pre-test probability of 1.5%

Symptom	Presence	Likelihood ratio	Probability of ACS
Sharp pain	Present	0.4	0.7%
	Absent	1.3	2%
Pain that alters with change of position	Present	0.3	0.5%
	Absent	1.3	2%
Tenderness to palpation	Present	0.2	0.3%
	Absent	1.6	2%
Pleuritic pain*	Present	0.2	0.3%
	Absent	1.2	2%

*Figures relate to MI only.
Follow each row from left to right to see how the symptom alters the probability of ACS.

Table 45.3 Three other features of the history that increase the probability of ACS based on a pre-test probability of 1.5%

Symptom	Presence	Likelihood ratio	Probability of ACS
Past history of CHD	Present	1.2	2%
	Absent	0.8	1%
Sweating*	Present	2.1	3%
	Absent	0.6	1%
Nausea or vomiting	Present	1.8	3%
	Absent	0.8	1%

*Figures relate to MI only.
Follow each row from left to right to see how the symptom alters the probability of ACS.

Table 45.4 Relationship of pain to previous ischaemic pain

Symptom	Presence	Likelihood ratio	Probability of ACS
Pain in same site or below it	Present	3.7	10%
	Absent	0.02	<0.1%

Follow each row from left to right to see how the symptom alters the probability of ACS.
Based on a pre-test probability of ACS of 3% (raised because of the previous history, see above).

- *Nausea or vomiting* may be the main complaint. In a study of patients presenting with nausea or vomiting to US emergency departments, 15% had acute ischaemia (11% AMI, 4% unstable angina).[2]
- *Other symptoms* (fatigue, weakness, dizziness, confusion) occur in 11% to 40% of patients with AMI.[2]

The physical examination

Examination is generally unrewarding in acute ischaemia, unless there is associated arrhythmia. Blood pressure may be higher or lower than normal for that patient. A normal respiratory rate decreases the probability of infarction.[2] Short found that, in 456 patients examined up to 14 days after the infarction, the examination was usually normal but, if present, tachycardia, bradycardia, breathlessness, hypotension and arrhythmia were all significantly associated with the presence of an infarct.[9] A later US study[7] found that the presence of crackles (wherever they were heard in the lungs) slightly increased

the probability that the patient had ACS (LR+ 1.4 (95% CI 1.3 to 1.5); LR– 0.9 (95% CI 0.9 to 0.9)).

An earlier meta-analysis[11] found three features of the examination that were associated with positive likelihood ratios greater than 2 in the diagnosis of MI (Table 45.5).

No study has shown whether these three findings are independent. Assuming they are and all three are present, they increase the probability of MI usefully. If the history leads the clinician to an assessment that the probability of MI is 50%, these findings will increase it to 72% then to 90% then to 96%. If absent, they are less useful, reducing the probability to 41% then to 39% and then to 39% only.

The ECG

The 12-lead ECG is traditionally important in the diagnosis of acute MI.[2] The Heart Technology Assessment (HTA) meta-analysis found that three features of the ECG had an LR+ greater than 3 (Table 45.6).[10]

Table 45.5 Signs associated with acute MI[11] based on a pre-test probability of 1.5%

Sign	Presence	LR+	Probability of ACS
Crackles in the lungs	Present	2.1	3%
	Absent	0.8	1%
Third heart sound	Present	3.2	5%
	Absent	0.9	1%
Hypotension (systolic ≤80)	Present	3.1	4%
	Absent	0.97	1%

Follow each row from left to right to see how the finding alters the probability of ACS.

Table 45.6 Useful ECG indicators of AMI, based on a pre-test probability of 1.5%

ECG feature	Presence	Likelihood ratio	Probability if present
ST elevation	Present	13	17%
	Absent	0.5	1%
Q waves	Present	5.0	7%
	Absent	0.5	1%
ST depression	Present	3.1	5%
	Absent	0.6	1%

NB. All changes should occur in at least 2 leads from the same vascular territory. A significant Q wave is at least 1 mm deep and at least 0.03 seconds in duration. ST elevation or depression should be at least 1 mm in limb leads and at least 2 mm in chest leads.

Note that, while these ECG changes are useful if present, they hardly reduce the probability of AMI if absent.

In practice, the ECG of a patient with acute chest pain falls into one of three categories: normal, equivocal and classic.

1. *The normal ECG* is useful in excluding an AMI (Table 45.7).[10]
2. *The equivocal ECG* is of no use in the diagnosis either way. A study from Boston of patients with acute chest pain in the emergency department divided the normal ECG into two categories: the completely normal ECG, and the ECG with abnormalities that did not meet the above criteria for Q waves or ST elevation or depression.[6] These abnormalities included Q waves less than 1 mm deep, ST elevation or depression of less than 1 mm and changes that are known to be old. Table 45.8 shows that a

Table 45.7 Role of the normal ECG in the exclusion of AMI[10] based on a pre-test probability of 1.5%

ECG feature	LR	Probability of AMI
Normal	0.14	0.2%
Abnormal	1.6	2%

totally normal ECG is useful in ruling out ACS but an ECG with non-specific changes is no help in ruling ACS in or out.

3. *Clear ECG changes of infarction* are extraordinarily helpful in making the diagnosis, if present, but not so useful if absent (Table 45.9).[10]

Table 45.8 The normal and the non-specifically abnormal ECG in the diagnosis of ACS[6] based on a pre-test probability of 1.5%

ECG	LR	Probability of AMI
Completely normal	0.08	0.02%
Not completely normal	1.4	2%
Normal or equivocal	0.7	1%
Abnormal	8.7	13%

Table 45.9 The value of the classical ECG picture of AMI[10] based on a pre-test probability of 1.5%

ECG	LR	Probability of AMI
Judged to show infarction	145	69%
No clear changes of infarction	0.6	1%

However, *two factors* limit the value of the ECG studies above for primary care:

1. *Spectrum bias*. The patients seen in primary care with chest pain have a probability of ACS that is 25 times less than that in the emergency department. Those extra patients in primary care may have characteristics that alter the predictive value of the ECG.
2. *Lower expertise*. GPs may be even less expert than the physicians in cardiac trials. A study of US emergency physicians showed that they misread as normal 41% of abnormal ST segments and 36% of abnormal T waves and misread as abnormal 14% of normal ST segments and 17% of normal T waves.[12] Yet they are likely to see abnormal ECGs more often than are GPs.

Alternatively, it may be that GPs do significantly better. A more recent study from the Netherlands found good agreement on ECG interpretation between GPs and a cardiologist.[13] GPs who are not confident in their interpretation of sophisticated changes can use the fact that a *completely* normal ECG when the patient first presents with chest pain is a powerful predictor of the absence of ACS.

In conclusion, the ECG is only likely to alter management in cases where the diagnosis is in doubt. A classic history, giving, say, a 90%

probability of ACS, requires admission. A normal ECG would only reduce this probability to 56% and admission would still be needed. An abnormal ECG would increase the probability of ACS to 94%, which would not be a useful gain.

However, if, from the history, the diagnosis is in doubt with a probability of, say, 5%, a normal ECG would reduce that to virtually zero (<1%). Conversely, an ECG with an abnormal T wave would increase it to 7% and an ECG with ST elevation ≥1 mm would increase it to 13% and suggest that immediate admission was justified. An ECG with non-specific changes would leave the diagnosis in the same doubt as before.

The role of the ECG in determining which patients are suitable for thrombolysis is a different matter.

Another exercise in combining the history and a normal ECG. The Multicenter Chest Pain Study of patients presenting to US emergency departments with chest pain assessed the post-test probabilities for four features of the history and a normal ECG. For a female under 60 years old with chest pain that did not radiate to the arm, shoulder, neck or jaw and who did not describe the pain as a pressure, and whose ECG was normal, the probability of acute MI was zero. For a man aged >60 with pain that he described as a pressure and which radiated, the probability of acute MI was 26% despite a normal ECG. Non-specific ST or T wave changes produced a similar result.[14]

What ECG changes suggest infarction?[15]

■ *A pathological Q wave* has a duration of ≥0.04 s (1 small square) or has a depth that is more than a quarter of the height of the R wave in that lead. Ignore Q waves in AVR and III.

■ *A pathological R wave* is less tall than it should be, i.e. there are taller R waves either side of it in adjacent precordial leads.

■ *An ST segment* is elevated if it is >1 mm (1 small square) above the isoelectric line. In infarction, the ST segment is convex upwards. Depression of the ST segment occurs:

    (a) in subendocardial infarction, and

    (b) in leads that are opposite to those that show elevation.

■ *An abnormal T wave* is one where it is flat or biphasic or inverted (i.e. it goes in the opposite direction to the QRS in that lead). It is less specific for infarction than the other changes, although a deep symmetrical inverted T wave is suggestive.

How can different features of the clinical assessment and the ECG be combined? Answer: with difficulty.

- *Using the likelihood ratios.* The clinician cannot assume that different features are independent of each other and apply one likelihood ratio after another. While one aspect of the history (e.g. radiating chest pain) may well be independent of an aspect of the examination (e.g. hypotension) or of the ECG (e.g. pathological Q waves), two aspects of the history (e.g. radiating chest pain and crushing pain) may not predict an MI better than one or other of them.
- *Clinical decision rules* have been developed and validated to give the clinician an idea of the predictive value of combinations of features.[11,16] Their scoring systems can be complex, or, if only a few predictive features are chosen, they seem arbitrary. Even used properly, their benefit is marginal. A study from the Boston group using the majority of the clinical pointers above, plus ECG findings, as a computer-based protocol compared the protocol to the clinical judgement of emergency department physicians. The protocol had only a slightly higher specificity for the diagnosis of MI (74% for the protocol versus 71% for the physicians) with an equivalent sensitivity (88% for the protocol versus 87.8% for the physicians).[17]

Other issues

The impact of serum troponin estimation on the diagnosis of AMI

In 2000, the European Society of Cardiology and the American College of Cardiology proposed new criteria for the diagnosis of AMI: a typical rise and fall of biochemical markers, including troponin, plus at least one of the following: ischaemic symptoms, development of pathological Q waves, ischaemic ST segment changes (elevation or depression), or a coronary intervention.[18] The previous WHO definition required at least two of the following: typical symptoms, evolving ECG changes that included Q waves, and a creatinine kinase more than twice the upper limit of normal.[18]

This new European definition would have led, in part of Scotland, to a 58% increase in the diagnosis of AMI,[19] and in Warwickshire, England, to a 27% increase.[20] The patients diagnosed in Scotland as a result of the new criteria tended to be older (median age 74 vs. 68) and were more likely to be female (47% vs. 38%) than under the old criteria.

How to understand a specialist decision that a patient with a raised troponin level does not have ACS

The serum troponin is so sensitive and specific for myocardial damage that, in practice, a patient with a normal troponin level, taken at least 8 hours after the onset of pain, has not sustained an AMI (see the new definition of AMI above). However, the troponin level is so sensitive for myocardial damage that it is raised in situations in which the myocardium is damaged other than AMI: heart failure, left ventricular hypertrophy, myocarditis, shock, pulmonary embolism, cytotoxic drugs, renal failure, defibrillation or cardioversion. Check that another cause of myocardial damage does not better explain the raised troponin before questioning the diagnosis that an AMI has not occurred.

Does a response to glyceryl trinitrate (GTN) indicate acute coronary syndrome?

No. A study of 459 patients presenting with chest pain to an emergency department of Johns Hopkins Hospital, Baltimore found that a response to GTN was useless in the prediction of ACS.[21] It relieved chest pain in 35% of those subsequently found to have active coronary artery disease and in 41% of those without it. Glyceryl trinitrate is known to relieve oesophageal and smooth muscle spasm; this may explain the benefit in those without coronary artery disease. Conversely, GTN would not be expected to help those in whom a fixed coronary occlusion has occurred. It is likely, therefore, that this result does not undermine the strong clinical impression that response to GTN is useful in the diagnosis of *stable* angina.

How does the patient's age affect the predictive power of the clinical presentation of ACS?

Older patients with ACS are less likely to present with typical symptoms than younger patients. Furthermore, older patients are more likely than younger patients to have symptoms suggestive of ACS, and even to have typical ECG changes, when they are *not* suffering from ACS. The Chest Pain Study Group analysed 7734 patients presenting with acute chest pain.[22] Table 45.10 shows the likelihood ratios and frequencies for certain features in those with and without ACS according to age.

Table 45.10 shows that most predictors of ACS lose some of their power as the patient ages. A history of CHD even begins to argue *against* the

Clinical feature	LR+ age <65	LR+ age ≥65	Frequency of the feature in those aged <65	Frequency of the feature in those aged ≥65
Male gender	1.5	1.3	ACS 74% Non ACS 51%	ACS 52% Non ACS 39%
History of CHD	1.3	0.9	ACS 39% Non ACS 29%	ACS 55% Non ACS 61%
Pain felt as pressure	1.6	1.2	ACS 68% Non ACS 42%	ACS 63% Non ACS 50%
New ECG changes of infarction or ischaemia	5.8	3.2	ACS 80% Non ACS 13%	ACS 78% Non ACS 24%

Table 45.10 The significance of different clinical features in younger and older patients[22]

diagnosis of ACS in the older patient because most patients with non-ACS chest pain have such a history.

How do all these findings relate to primary care?

Patients with chest pain in primary care are a different group from those in emergency departments and secondary care; and GPs are different from hospital physicians. The GP is usually best served by understanding the relative predictive power of the different features above and coming to an informal decision about the probability of ACS, as shown in the example below.

The HTA meta-analysis of the overall ability of the emergency department physician to diagnose ACS, as judged by the decision to admit, shows an LR+ of 2.5 and an LR– of 0.08.[10] Since studies show that the pre-test probability of ACS in patients presenting to emergency departments is of the order of 40%,[6] these likelihood ratios are appropriate; 63% of admitted patients will have ACS and only 5% of those sent home will have ACS. However, in primary care, with a pre-test probability of 1.5%, these figures would be disastrous, with only 4% of admitted patients having ACS, although, of course, even fewer (0.1%) would be missed.

GPs must be using other criteria and thresholds for the diagnosis on which hospital-based studies are not able to throw light.

Example

A 45-year-old woman consults her GP urgently because of 4 hours of increasingly severe central chest pain radiating to both arms. She describes it as 'squeezing'. There is nothing else of relevance in the history, specifically no family history of coronary heart disease. The GP is aware that, before he heard the history, her chance of developing acute coronary syndrome that year was low: 1% of the population, but, he estimates, 0.1% of women aged 45. However, once a patient presents with chest pain, the probability of MI is nearer 5%, even if her age and sex make 1% a more likely figure.

Initially the history is highly suggestive of ischaemic cardiac pain. From memory, he recalls that the character of the pain isn't very useful (the LR+ for constricting pain is 1.6 and for central pain 1.1) but that radiation that includes the right arm (LR+ 6.7) is more useful. Applied successively, these likelihood ratios raise the probability of ACS from 1.0% to 1.9%, then to 2.0% then to 12%. However, this GP is a sceptic when it comes to the application of likelihood ratios based on patients seen in secondary care. GPs refer patients because they have constricting central chest pain; the usefulness of the symptoms may well have been 'used up' in the selection of patients for referral (see p. x). He decides that his clinical estimate of her probability of ACS from the history is more like 50%.

On examination, she has a tachycardia, which has no predictive power, and is sweating, which brings the probability of MI to 70%. She is, however, very anxious and the GP feels that the anxiety could well account for the tachycardia and the sweating.

Example–cont'd

The ECG shows none of the characteristic changes of infarction but the ST segments are depressed by 1 mm over the left ventricle (LR+ 3.1, see Table 45.6) raising the probability from 50% to 76% (Fig. 45.1) (or from 70% to 87% if he had decided to include the sweating).

The GP recalls that a totally normal ECG is very useful in ruling out ACS (LR– 0.08) and would have reduced the probability in this case from 50% to 8%. Even then her risk of ACS would have been high enough to admit her, so he does not have to worry whether he has been overgenerous when measuring the depth of her ST depression.

He admits her immediately to the local coronary care unit but is a little surprised to hear that she has been discharged after serial ECGs showed no change and troponin levels were normal. At the same time he receives a call to visit her at home because the pain is continuing. He considers what other serious causes of chest pain are possible; dissecting aneurysm comes to mind. He also recalls the severity of the disability that can come from a diagnosis of non-cardiac pain, as well as the breakdown in trust that can easily follow when the patient remains convinced that the cause is cardiac. He puts aside more time than usual for the visit.

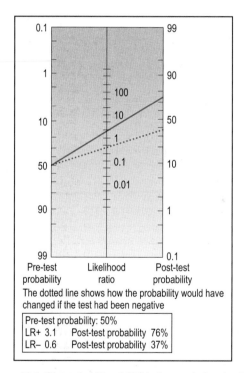

The dotted line shows how the probability would have changed if the test had been negative

Pre-test probability: 50%	
LR+ 3.1	Post-test probability 76%
LR– 0.6	Post-test probability 37%

Figure 45.1 The probability of AMI before and after the ECG in the example above.

REFERENCES

1. Key Health Statistics from General Practice. *Prevalence of treated coronary heart disease per 1000 patients.* London: Office for National Statistics, 1998.

2. Pope J, Selker H. *Diagnosis of acute cardiac ischaemia.* Emerg Med Clin North Am 2003;21:27–59.

3. Klinkman M, Stevens D, Gorenflo D. *Episodes of care for chest pain: a preliminary report from MIRNET.* J Fam Pract 1994;38:345–352.

4. Buntinx F, Knockaert D, Bruyninckx R, et al. *Chest pain in general practice or in the hospital*

emergency department: is it the same? Fam Pract 2001;18:586–589.

5. Mair J, Smidt J, Lechleitner P, et al. *A decision tree for the early diagnosis of acute myocardial infarction in nontraumatic chest pain patients at hospital admission.* Chest 1995;108:1502–1509.

6. Lee T, Cook E, Weisberg M, et al. *Acute chest pain in the emergency room. Identification and management of low-risk patients.* Arch Intern Med 1985;145:65–69.

7. Pope J, Ruthazer R, Beshansky J, et al. *Clinical features of emergency department patients presenting with symptoms suggestive of acute cardiac ischemia: a multicenter study.* J Thrombos Thrombol 1998;6:63–74.

8. Bayer A, Chadha J, Farag R, Pathy M. *Changing presentation of myocardial infarction with increasing old age.* J Am Geriatr Soc 1986;34:263–266.

9. Short D. *Diagnosis of slight and subacute coronary attacks in the community.* Br Heart J 1981;45:299–310.

10. Mant J, McManus R, Oakes R, et al. *Systematic review and modelling of the investigation of acute and chronic chest pain presenting in primary care.*

Health Technology Assessment: NHS R&D HTA Programme, 2004. Online. Available: www.ncchta.org.

11. Panju A, Hemmelgarn B, Guyatt G, et al. *Is this patient having a myocardial infarction?* JAMA 1998;280:1256–1263.

12. Jayes RJ, Larsen G, Beshansky J, et al. *Physician electrocardiogram reading in the emergency department – accuracy and effect on triage decisions: findings from a multicenter study.* J Gen Intern Med 1992;7:387–392.

13. Rutten F, Kessels A, Willems F, et al. *Electrocardiography in primary care: is it useful?* Int J Cardiol 2000;74:199–205.

14. Rouan G, Lee T, Cook E, et al. *Clinical characteristics and outcome of acute myocardial infarction in patients with initially normal or non-specific electrocardiograms.* Am J Cardiol 1989;64:1087–1092.

15. Rowlands D. *The electrocardiogram.* In: Ledingham J, Warrell D, eds. Concise Oxford textbook of medicine. Oxford: OUP, 2000.

16. Ebell M. *Evidence-based diagnosis.* New York: Springer, 2001.

17. Goldman L, Cook E, Brand D, et al. *A computer protocol to predict myocardial infarction in emergency department patients with chest pain.* N Engl J Med 1998;318:797–803.

18. McKenna C, Forfar J. *Was it a heart attack?* BMJ 2002;324:377–378.

19. Pell J, Simpson E, Rodger J, et al. *Impact of changing diagnostic criteria on incidence, management, and outcome of acute myocardial infarction: retrospective cohort study.* BMJ 2003;326:134–135.

20. Trevelyan J, Needham E, Smith S, et al. *Sources of diagnostic inaccuracy of conventional versus new diagnostic criteria for myocardial infarction in an unselected UK population with suspected cardiac chest pain, and investigation of independent prognostic variables.* Heart 2003;89:1406–1410.

21. Henrikson C, Howell E, Bush D, et al. *Chest pain relief by nitroglycerin does not predict active coronary artery disease.* Ann Intern Med 2003;139:979–986.

22. Solomon C, Lee T, Cook E, et al. *Comparison of clinical presentation of acute myocardial infarction in patients older than 65 years of age to younger patients: the multicenter chest pain study experience.* Am J Cardiol 1989;63:772–776.

46

Acute respiratory infections

Introduction

Acute respiratory infections may be classified in several different ways: by their symptoms (fever, sore throat, cough, ear pain, runny nose); by their clinical manifestations (coryza, pharyngitis, tonsillitis, epiglottitis, otitis media, influenza, bronchitis, pneumonia); or by causative organism. Furthermore, their symptoms and sometimes the whole clinical picture may be shared by conditions that are not infections (asthma, allergic rhinitis). Some of this complexity is shown in Figure 46.1.

Elucidating the exact location or responsible organism is usually clinically unhelpful. In this chapter, we focus on diagnostic questions that have the greatest impact on the patient with an acute respiratory infection. Sometimes the question is important because it affects the management of the illness (for example *Does this patient have pneumonia? Is this asthma or acute bronchitis?*); sometimes it is because the infection can have important sequelae (*streptococcal infection*); and finally there is the potentially extremely important question of *identifying possible cases of avian influenza*.

Does this patient have pneumonia?

KEY FACTS

- The reason for identifying patients with pneumonia is to identify those patients who may benefit from an antibiotic.
- None of the clinical symptoms and signs is able to rule in or rule out the diagnosis. Traditional signs, e.g. dullness to percussion and crackles, increase the probability of pneumonia only slightly and reduce it even less if absent.
- Even the global assessment after the history and examination is at best only moderately good at ruling pneumonia in or out.

- Laboratory values, such as erythrocyte sedimentation rate, C-reactive protein and full blood count, contribute only modestly to the diagnosis.
- Investigating, with a chest X-ray (CXR), only those patients who have a reasonable probability of pneumonia is a question of finding a balance between the risk of missing some pneumonias against that of over-investigation.
- Diagnosing community acquired pneumonia may not be necessary anyway.

A PRACTICAL APPROACH

* In a patient with an acute respiratory infection, use the history and examination to assess the probability that pneumonia is present. However, bear in mind that even a positive assessment carries a probability of pneumonia of only 13%.
* Decide on the need for a CXR. The minimum is to X-ray only those in whom there is reason to

think that, if pneumonia is present, the prognosis is poor: those with tachypnoea, hypotension, hypothermia or co-morbid disease. A more investigative stance would be to X-ray all those in whom the clinical assessment suggests pneumonia, in the knowledge that the number needed to test will be 8 (i.e. 7 out of 8 X-rays will be normal).

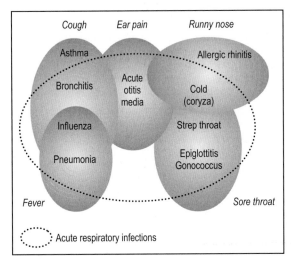

Figure 46.1 The way we classify acute respiratory infections is overlapping and confusing.

Pre-test probability of pneumonia

The prevalence of pneumonia in a patient population can vary enormously. A review of data from the US National Ambulatory Medical Care Survey from 1980 to 1994 showed that 5% of patients who presented to a primary care provider with an acute cough were diagnosed with pneumonia.[1] Similarly, in a study of previously well patients presenting to a general practitioner in the UK with acute cough, 6% met CXR criteria for pneumonia.[2] These two studies suggest that over a longer time period and wide patient population, the prevalence of pneumonia in patients with acute cough stays fairly constant at about 5%, but the time of year, the mix of patients and many other factors can cause large variations around this level.

The diagnostic accuracy of symptoms and signs

The problem of the lack of a 'gold standard'
Establishing the clinical features that identify patients with pneumonia is difficult because of the lack of a reference test (a 'gold standard') that clearly differentiates patients with pneumonia from patients that do not have pneumonia. Pathological organisms cannot be identified in up to 50% of those with pneumonia, even with extensive diagnostic testing.[3] Because of this, CXR changes are the most common reference standard in diagnostic accuracy studies, although the way these changes are defined varies between studies and there are also questions about the accuracy of even this test.[4] Nevertheless the CXR reference standard is the best we have, so we use it to study published estimates for the positive and negative likelihood ratios of clinical symptoms and signs for the presence of pneumonia in adults and children (Tables 46.1 and 46.2).

● The clinical studies suggest that no single sign or symptom can be used to rule in or rule out the diagnosis of pneumonia in adults. A recent study using a reference standard of biological evidence of bacterial lower respiratory tract infection also showed that no single sign or symptom was able to predict the presence of a bacterial infection.[18]

● Combinations of clinical features may be more clinically useful. However, even the doctor's global judgement after the full history and examination was, at best, only moderately useful at ruling out the diagnosis in one study (LR– 0.3, 95% CI 0.1 to 0.7),[10] and was poor in another (LR– 0.9, 95% CI 0.8 to 1.1).[8] If, after the history and clinical examination, the overall impression is that the patient does *not* have pneumonia, assuming a pre-test probability of 5%, the probability of pneumonia falls to <2%.[10] No

Example

A boy of 18 presents with a sore throat 2 days before an important examination. His GP doesn't use any of the clinical prediction rules formally, partly because she can't remember how to score them and partly because she is sceptical about their apparent accuracy. She has, however, a shrewd idea of which symptoms and signs predict streptococcal infection and which do not.

She notes that his youth is in favour of streptococcal infection, although not as much as if he were under 15. Everything else, however, is against it: there are no exudates, no fever, no recent known exposure to streptococcal infection, no tender glands, no tonsillar swelling. He even has a cough and runny nose and a relatively long course: the symptoms have been developing over 5 days.

The GP does not have access to a rapid antigen test. She reckons that the probability of streptococcal infection is in the region of 1% and that if she took a throat swab and it was positive it would probably be a false positive. She tells her patient that his chance of responding to penicillin is less than his chance of being brought out in a rash by it. He agrees to continue to suck (sugar-free) lozenges.

How can we diagnose acute otitis media (AOM)?

KEY FACTS

- Diagnosis is important in the ill child (with high fever or vomiting), the child under 2 years old and the child with bilateral infection. Diagnosis also allows for a subsequent check for residual deafness.
- The presence, or absence, of earache helps to rule in, or rule out, the diagnosis, but is less helpful in younger children.
- A red, cloudy, bulging or immobile ear drum helps to confirm the diagnosis.
- Crying is not the *cause* of a red ear drum.[40]

A PRACTICAL APPROACH

- * Assess the child's symptoms and general condition.
- * Examine both ear drums.
- * Treat a pink, rather than red, drum as normal unless the drum is abnormal in some other way (e.g. cloudy, retracted or bulging).

Definition and causative organisms

Acute otitis media is the presence of a middle ear effusion in conjunction with the rapid onset of one or more signs or symptoms of inflammation of the middle ear.[41]

The most common bacterial pathogens are *Streptococcus pneumoniae*, non-typeable *Haemophilus influenzae* and *Moraxella catarrhalis*,[42] but childhood vaccination against pneumococcal disease and *Haemophilus influenzae* b may have changed the frequency of causative pathogens in recent years.[43] Infection with these organisms is not specific for the ear, and will frequently cause overlapping or sequential infection in other areas of the respiratory tract.

Why does diagnosis matter?

- Overall, trials of antibiotics to treat AOM suggest only a modest benefit, with the number of patients who have pain at 2 to 7 days being reduced from 22% to 16%.[44] The possible benefits of antibiotics are also offset by an almost equivalent risk of side effects, such as nausea, vomiting and diarrhoea. In some parts of the world (especially Scandinavia and the Netherlands), antibiotics are rarely used for acute otitis media. In others (especially the USA), they are still the norm.
- In some groups of patients, the benefit of antibiotics is more marked: e.g. children under 2 years of age, children with high fever, those who are vomiting or who have bilateral disease.[45–47]
- Accurate diagnosis of an ill child helps to reduce parental concern.
- Diagnosis allows the primary care team to check that the transient deafness associated with AOM does settle. If it does not, the child's language acquisition or education may suffer unless measures are taken to compensate for this (such as ensuring talking is louder, hearing aids provided temporarily, or even referral for grommet tympanotomy).

The initial probability of AOM

By the age of 2 years, over 90% of children have had at least one episode of AOM and more than half have had two or more episodes. In a survey of children presenting to ambulatory care offices in the USA, AOM was present in about 20% of children 0–5 years of age, 10% of children 6–10 years of age and 5% of children 11–15 years of age.[48]

The diagnostic accuracy of the history and examination for AOM

Although the gold standard for the diagnosis of AOM is based on findings from tympanocentesis, most studies of diagnostic accuracy have compared the clinical features of AOM against findings on pneumatic otoscopy.[49] Almost all of these studies have been conducted in paediatric or otolaryngology settings, and therefore they may be less accurate in primary care settings where the incidence is lower. It is well recognised that misdiagnosis of AOM is common in the community.[50]

See Table 46.7 for the contribution made by symptoms and signs to the diagnosis of AOM.

Comments

● Earache is one of the most helpful clinical features in diagnosing AOM, but is unlikely to be identified in young children, and is therefore less helpful and less accurate in younger children.
● Symptoms and signs that do not help to diagnose AOM are vomiting, cough and rhinitis.

Table 46.7 Diagnostic accuracy of the history and examination for AOM (the most useful features are in bold)

	LR+ (range)	LR− (range)
Symptoms		
Ear pain[51–53]	**3.0–7.3**	**0.4–0.6**
Fever[51–53]	0.8–2.6	0.3–1.4
Signs		
Cloudy[54]	**6.7**	**0.4**
Distinctly red[54]	**3.0**	**0.8**
Bulging[54]	**13.7**	**0.6**
Retracted[54]	1.6	0.9
Impaired mobility[54]	**3.4**	**0.1**

These LRs for signs differ from those calculated in a recent systematic review in which rather different results from a paediatrician and an ear, nose and throat surgeon were combined.[55] We have used the figures for the paediatrician as being nearer to those likely in general practice.

Example

A child aged 3 is brought by her mother because she has been febrile and has cried all the previous night. She is rubbing both ears and her mother is convinced that this is an ear infection.

Examination reveals two normal drums and a slightly runny nose.

The GP reckons that, with an initial probability of 20%, the normal drums reduce this to <2%. His experience tells him that rubbing the ears is not specific for ear infection and he has never found any research evidence to alter that view.

He explains to the mother that this is likely to be an upper respiratory viral infection and that paracetamol is the best treatment.

Can avian influenza be differentiated from human forms?

KEY FACTS

● Avian flu cannot be reliably distinguished clinically from other forms of influenza.

A PRACTICAL APPROACH

★ Suspect it in a patient who has close contact with birds, especially ill birds, who presents with fever, especially if there are respiratory or gastrointestinal symptoms.

Avian influenza A (H5N1) virus is a highly pathogenic virus that spreads quickly through bird flocks with a mortality rate approaching 100%. Cases in humans have been reported since 1997, with an upsurge of human cases reported by the WHO since January 2004. Currently the spread of H5N1 virus from person to person has been limited (if at all) and all cases have involved close contact with an infected bird, mostly in previously healthy children and young adults. In recent outbreaks among humans in Asia and Europe, the mortality rate among patients hospitalised with the disease has been >50%[56] and the majority of patients have developed severe bilateral pneumonia requiring ventilatory support. However, it is possible that the cases described so far are only the most severely ill; those with more trivial infections are less likely to have been examined by health authorities.

From the current limited series of hospital cases, there were no clinical features that distinguished avian flu from other severe cases of influenza. Among 12 patients with influenza A H5N1 virus infection identified by virus isolation, the common presenting complaint for all patients was fever. Eight had symptoms or signs of upper respiratory tract infections and five had clinical and radiological evidence of pneumonia at presentation.[57] In addition to respiratory symptoms, a large proportion of patients also reported gastrointestinal symptoms such as diarrhoea, vomiting and abdominal pain, which are common in children with human influenza, but not in adults. In some cases, diarrhoea and fever were the dominant symptoms. Unlike human infections with H7 or H9 viruses, conjunctivitis was not prominent in H5N1-infected patients.

The diagnosis is confirmed by polymerase chain reaction detection of viral nucleic acids in throat swabs, sputum or tracheal aspirates.

REFERENCES

1. Metlay J, Fine M. *Testing strategies in the initial management of patients with community-acquired pneumonia.* Ann Intern Med 2003;138:109–118.

2. Macfarlane J, Holmes W, Gard P, et al. *Prospective study of the incidence, aetiology and outcome of adult lower respiratory tract illness in the community.* Thorax 2001;56:109–114.

3. British Thoracic Society Standards of Care Committee. *BTS guidelines for the management of community acquired pneumonia in adults.* Thorax 2001;56(Suppl 4):IV 1–164.

4. Hopstaken R, Witbradd T, van Engelshoven J, et al. *Inter-observer variation in the interpretation of chest radiographs for pneumonia in community-acquired lower respiratory tract infections.* Clin Radiol 2004;59(8):743–752.

5. Gennis P, Gallagher J, Falvo C, et al. *Clinical criteria for the detection of pneumonia in adults: Guidelines for ordering chest roentgenograms in the emergency department.* J Emerg Med 1989;7:263–268.

6. Diehr P, Wood R, Bushyhead J, et al. *Prediction of pneumonia in outpatients with acute cough: a statistical approach.* J Chronic Dis 1984;37:215–225.

7. Heckerling P, Tape T, Wigton R, et al. *Clinical prediction rule for pulmonary infiltrates.* Ann Intern Med 1990;113:664–670.

8. Hopstaken R, Muris J, Knottnerus J, et al. *Contributions of symptoms, signs, erythrocyte sedimentation rate, and C-reactive protein to a diagnosis of pneumonia in acute lower respiratory tract infection.* Br J Gen Pract 2003;53:358–364.

9. Singal B, Hedges J, Radack K. *Decision rules and clinical prediction of pneumonia: evaluation of low-yield criteria.* Ann Emerg Med 1989;18:13–20.

10. Lieberman D, Shvartzman P, Korsonsky I, et al. *Diagnosis of ambulatory community-acquired pneumonia. Comparison of clinical assessment versus chest X-ray.* Scand J Prim Health Care 2003;21:57–60.

11. Lynch T, Platt R, Gouin S, et al. *Can we predict which children with clinically suspected pneumonia will have the presence of focal infiltrates on chest radiographs?* Pediatrics 2004;113:186–189.

12. Mahabee-Gittens M, Grupp-Phelan J, Brody A, et al. *Identifying children with pneumonia in the emergency department.* Clin Pediatr 2005;44:427–435.

13. Redd S, Patrick E, Vreuls R. *Comparison of the clinical and radiographic diagnosis of paediatric pneumonia.* Trans R Soc Trop Med Hyg 1994;88:307–310.

14. Harari M, Shann F, Spooner V. *Clinical signs of pneumonia in children.* Lancet 1991;338:928–930.

15. Lozano J, Steinhoff M, Ruiz J, et al. *Clinical predictors of acute radiological pneumonia and hypoxaemia*

at high altitudes. Arch Dis Child 1994;71(4):323–327.

16. Leventhal J. *Clinical predictors of pneumonia as a guide to ordering chest roentgenograms.* Clin Pediatr 1992;21:730–734.

17. Taylor J, Del Beccaro M, Done S, et al. *Establishing clinically relevant standards for tachypnea in febrile children younger than 2 years.* Arch Pediatr Adolesc Med 1995;149:283–287.

18. Hopstaken R, Stobberingh E, Knottnerus J, et al. *Clinical items not helpful in differentiating viral from bacterial lower respiratory tract infections in general practice.* J Clin Epidemiol 2005;58:175–183.

19. Margolis P, Gadomski A. *Does this infant have pneumonia?* JAMA 1998;279:308–313.

20. van der Meer V, Neven A, van den Broek P, et al. *Diagnostic value of C reactive protein in infections of the lower respiratory tract: systematic review.* BMJ 2005;331:26.

21. Flanders S, Halm E. *Guidelines for community-acquired pneumonia. Are they reflected in practice?* Treat Respir Med 2004;3:67–77.

22. Hopstaken R, Coenen S, Butler C. *Treating patients not diagnoses: challenging assumptions underlying the investigation and management of LRTI in general practice.* J Antimicrob Chemother 2005;56: 941–943.

23. Classification Committee of the World Organisation of Family Doctors. *ICPC-2 international classification of primary care,* 2nd edn. Oxford: Oxford University Press, 1998.

24. Jones BF, Stewart MA. *Duration of cough in acute upper respiratory tract infections.* Aust Fam Physician 2002;31:971–973.

25. Glasziou P. *Twenty year cough in a non-smoker.* BMJ 1998;316:1660–1661.

26. Thiadens H, Postma D, de Bock G, et al. *Asthma in adult patients presenting with symptoms of acute*

bronchitis in general practice. Scand J Prim Health Care 2000;18:188–192.

27. Edwards C, Osman L, Godden D, et al. *Wheezy bronchitis in childhood. A distinct clinical entity with lifelong significance?* Chest 2003;124:18–24.

28. Jonsson J, Gislason T, Gislason D, et al. *Acute bronchitis and clinical outcome three years later: prospective cohort study.* BMJ 1998;317:1433–1440.

29. Smucny J, Flynn C, Becker I, Glazier R. *Beta-2-agonists for acute bronchitis.* The Cochrane Database of Systematic Reviews 2004 (Issue 1. Art No.: CD001726.pub2. DOI: 10.1002/14651858.CD001726.pub2.).

30. Del Mar C, Glasziou P, Spinks A. *Antibiotics for sore throat.* The Cochrane Database of Systematic Reviews 2004 (Issue 2. Art. No.: CD000023. DOI: 10.1002/14651858. CD000023.pub2.).

31. Randolph M, Gerber M, DeMeo K, et al. *Effect of antibiotic therapy on the clinical course of streptococcal pharyngitis.* J Pediatr 1985;106:870–875.

32. Ebell M, Smith M, Barry H, et al. *Does this patient have strep throat?* JAMA 2000;284:2912–2918.

33. Lindbaek M, Hoiby E, Lermark G, et al. *Clinical symptoms and signs in sore throat patients with large colony variant beta-haemolytic streptococci groups C or G versus group A.* Br J Gen Pract 2005;55:615–619.

34. Centor R, Witherspoon J, Dalton H, et al. *The diagnosis of strep throat in adults in the emergency room.* Med Decis Making 1981;1:239–246.

35. McIsaac W, Goel V, To T, et al. *The validity of a sore throat score in family practice.* Can Med Assoc J 2000;163:811–815.

36. Hoffmann S. *The throat carrier rate of group A and other beta hemolytic streptococci among patients in general practice.* Acta Pathol Microbiol Immunol Scand 1985;93:347–351.

37. Gunnarsson R, Holm S, Soderstrom M. *The prevalence of beta-*

haemolytic streptococci in throat specimens from healthy children and adults. Implications for the clinical value of throat cultures. Scand J Prim Health Care 1997;15:149–155.

38. Stewart M, Siff J, Cydulka R. *Evaluation of the patient with sore throat, earache and sinusitis: an evidence-based approach.* Emerg Med Clin North Am 1999;17: 153–187.

39. Dagnelie C, Barteline M, van der Graff Y, et al. *Towards a better diagnosis of throat infections (with group A beta-haemolytic streptococcus) in general practice.* Br J Gen Pract 1998;48:959–962.

40. Yamamoto L, Sumida R, Yano S, et al. *Does crying turn tympanic membranes red?* Clin Pediatr (Phila) 2005;44:693–697.

41. Clinical Evidence. *Acute otitis media.* BMJ Publishing Group, 2005. Issue 14.

42. Klein J. *Otitis media.* Clin Infect Dis 1994;19:823–833.

43. Cripps A, Otczyk D, Kyd J. *Bacterial otitis media: a vaccine preventable disease?* Vaccine 2005;23:2304–2310.

44. Glasziou P, Del Mar C, Sanders S, Hayem M. *Antibiotics for acute otitis media in children.* The Cochrane Database of Systematic Reviews 2004 (Issue 1. Art.No.:CD000219. DOI:10.1002/14651858. CD000219. pub2.).

45. Appelman C, Claessen J, Touw Otten F, et al. *Co-amoxiclav in recurrent acute otitis media: placebo controlled study.* BMJ 1991;303:1450–1452.

46. Burke P, Bain J, Robinson D. *Acute red ear in children: controlled trial of non-antibiotic treatment in general practice.* BMJ 1991;303:558–562.

47. Little P, Gould C, Moore M, et al. *Predictors of poor outcome and benefits from antibiotics in children with acute otitis media: pragmatic randomised trial.* BMJ 2002;325:22.

48. Marcy M. *Management of acute otitis media.* Rockville, MD: Agency

for Healthcare Research and Quality, 2001:1–159.

49. Pirozzo S, Del Mar C. *Otitis media.* In: Moyer V, ed. Evidence based pediatrics and child health. London: BMJ Books, 2004.

50. Asher E, Leibovitz E, Press J, et al. *Accuracy of acute otitis media diagnosis in community and hospital settings.* Acta Paediatr 2005;94:423–428.

51. Invargsson L. *Acute otalgia in children – findings and diagnosis.* Acta Paediatr Scand 1982;71:705–710.

52. Heikkinen T, Ruuskanen O. *Signs and symptoms predicting acute otitis media.* Arch Pediatr Adolesc Med 1995;149:26–29.

53. Niemela M, Uhari M, Jounio-Ervasti K, et al. *Lack of specific symptomatology in children with acute otitis media.* Pediatr Infect Dis J 1994;13:765–768.

54. Karma P, Penttila M, Sipila M, et al. *Otoscopic diagnosis of middle ear effusion in acute and non-acute otitis media. I. The value of different otoscopic findings.* Int J Pediatr Otorhinolaryngol 1989;17:37–49.

55. Rothman R, Owens T, Simel D. *Does this child have acute otitis media?* JAMA 2003;290:1633–1640.

56. World Health Organization. *Avian influenza ('bird flu') – Fact sheet, 2006.

57. Yuen K, Chan P, Peiris M. *Clinical features and rapid viral diagnosis of human disease associated with avian influenza A H5N1 virus.* Lancet 1998;351:467–471.

47

Alcohol misuse

- Up to 9% of primary care attenders are dependent or problem drinkers, a problem that is frequently denied by the patient and undetected by the GP.
- While asking whether a person is drinking over the recommended limits usually elicits a negative answer, three simple questions have useful sensitivity and specificity for problem drinking.
- Case-finding is recommended in most countries; that is, asking about alcohol when the possibility is raised by some aspect of the clinical situation. In New Zealand, routine 3-yearly questioning is recommended.
- In those who screen positive, more detailed questioning can establish whether misuse is present and, if so, the degree.
- Blood tests may play a small part in confirming the diagnosis, but not in rejecting it. They can be useful in demonstrating to the patient that alcohol is having a harmful effect on the body.

A PRACTICAL APPROACH

- * Be alert to the possibility of problem drinking in various situations:
  - when the patient has behaviour that may be associated with problem drinking (e.g. frequent job losses, inability to keep appointments, domestic violence)
  - when the patient belongs to a high-risk group (e.g. bar staff, males living alone, the bereaved)
  - when the patient has a condition associated with hazardous drinking (e.g. hypertension, impotence or depression)
  - when blood tests reveal an unexpected macrocytosis, elevated liver enzymes or a raised uric acid.
- * Ask about alcohol with the Audit-C questionnaire or a similar tool.
- * Discuss the result with the patient to elicit more information.
- * If high alcohol use is confirmed, ask questions designed to ascertain whether the patient is dependent, or whether the intake affects the ability to function in life.
- * Palpate for an enlarged liver.
- * Check the full blood count and liver enzymes including gamma-glutamyl transferase.

Background

- The level of at-risk drinking in Western societies is so high that the regular screening of all teenagers and adults might prove worthwhile. The New Zealand guidelines[1] recommend a 3-yearly screening for everyone over age 14.
- GPs in the Netherlands are aware of only one-third of their patients who are abusing or dependent on alcohol.[2]
- However, while GPs accept the importance of counselling patients with problem drinking, a study from Denmark shows how difficult some GPs find it to discuss the issue with problem drinkers who have been detected as a result of a screening questionnaire.[3]

Prevalence

Alcohol dependence or harmful use of alcohol is present in about 6% of attenders in primary care in the Western world.[4] Many more will be drinking excessive amounts of alcohol that put them at risk of harm. Individual studies give different rates. A study from Holland found that 8.9% of 1992 randomly selected GP attenders suffered from alcohol abuse or dependence in the previous year (male to female ratio = 2.8:1).[2] Of the men, roughly equal numbers were dependent on alcohol (6.1%) and abusing alcohol without dependence (7.6%). Binge drinking occurred at least weekly in 12.1% of men and 1.2% of women. Older people have a similar prevalence, and in them, the effect on their physical health is likely to be greater than in the young.[5]

Definitions

- *Dependence* means physiological dependence, manifested by compulsive use, tolerance and withdrawal symptoms.
- *Abuse*, or *problem drinking* means use of alcohol which causes social or interpersonal problems (e.g. poor work performance, violence in the family, driving while drunk) without dependence.
- *High alcohol intake* or *hazardous drinking*, without abuse or dependence, means drinking above the *Health of the Nation* targets[6,7]: for men, no more than 4 units a day or 21 units a week; for women, no more than 3 units a day or 14 units a week. In the

UK, 28% of men and 11% of women exceed these levels.[8]

Calculating alcohol intake

1 unit = 10 g ethanol = half a pint of beer, a single measure of spirits or a 125 ml glass of 8% wine. A bottle of 13.5% wine = 10 units, a bottle of sherry = 15 units, a bottle of spirits (75 cl) = 30 units. The number of units in a drink may be calculated by the formula:

$$\text{Units} = \frac{\text{volume (in ml) times \% alcohol}}{1000}$$

Thus, a 440 ml can of extra strong beer is 4 units, a 125 ml glass of 12% wine is 1.5 units.

Targeted screening (also called 'case-finding')

When a patient presents with symptoms that raise the possibility of dependence or problem drinking, ask about alcohol intake without simply asking how many drinks a week the person takes.

The Audit-C questionnaire[9] is a validated tool (see box on p. 314). A score of 5 or more for a man is 78% sensitive and 75% specific for an alcohol problem.[2] This gives the likelihood ratios and post-test probabilities shown in Table 47.1. Note that these figures still mean that a man who scores 5 or over, and whose pre-test probability of an alcohol problem is only average, has a post-test probability that is still only 33%. In other words, two-thirds of men who score 5 or over will be neither abusing alcohol nor dependent on it. Higher scores increase the probability of an alcohol problem. Four per cent of male problem drinkers will be missed by the test, using a cut-off of 5.

Table 47.1 Value of the Audit-C questionnaire in the diagnosis of an alcohol problem in men, based on a pre-test probability in primary care of 14%[2]

Score	Likelihood ratio (95% CI)	Probability of an alcohol problem
8 or over	8.5 (6.1–12)	58%
5 or over	3.1 (2.7–3.6)	33%
4 or below	0.3 (0.2–0.4)	4%

The Audit-C questionnaire for alcohol abuse or dependence

1. How often do you have a drink containing alcohol?

Score: 0 for never

1 for once a month or less

2 for 2–4 times a month

3 for 2 or 3 times a week

4 for 4 or more times a week.

2. How many drinks containing alcohol do you have on a typical day when you are drinking?

Score: 0 for 1–2

1 for 3–4

2 for 5–6

3 for 7–9

4 for 10 or more.

3. How often do you have 6 or more drinks on one occasion?

Score: 0 for never

1 for less than monthly

2 for monthly

3 for weekly

4 for daily or almost daily.

For women, it is only 50% sensitive (although 93% specific) and a score of 4 or more should prompt further questioning.[2] In a woman with a score of 5 or more, the probability of an alcohol problem is only 23% (Table 47.2).

Table 47.2 Value of the Audit-C questionnaire in the diagnosis of an alcohol problem in women, based on a pre-test probability in primary care of 4%[2]

Score	Likelihood ratio (95% CI)	Probability of an alcohol problem
8 or over	54 (17–171)	69%
5 or over	7.4 (5.1–10.7)	23%
4 or below	0.5 (0.4–0.7)	2%

Other points

- The oft-quoted CAGE questionnaire appears to be the least useful of all the screening instruments in current use.[2]

- A briefer test is to ask a single question:[10] 'When was the last time you had more than 5 drinks in a day (4 drinks for women)?' When the test is considered positive if the answer is 'within the last 3 months', the sensitivity and specificity for dependence, abuse or hazardous drinking (i.e. a wider group than those assessed against the Audit-C above) were 85% and 70% for men (LR+ 2.8; LR– 0.2) and 82% and 77% for women (LR+ 3.6; LR– 0.2).

If the screening test is positive:

* Take a full history of the patient's alcohol use and its consequences, including questions related to the ICD-10 criteria for alcohol dependence (see box opposite).

* Consider alcohol as a cause of 'black-outs', accidents, obesity, pancreatitis, dyspepsia, impotence, anxiety, depression, insomnia, a poor employment record, or a criminal record.

* Be aware of risk factors, such as employment in the licensing trade, a family history of alcohol problems, a lack of social support.

* Examine for hepatosplenomegaly and signs of cirrhosis.

* Take blood for:

   (a) *a full blood count* (for macrocytosis)

   (b) *liver function tests*, including gamma-glutamyl transferase (γGT). Note that the γGT is raised in only one-third of those with an alcohol problem, and that a raised level is not specific for alcohol abuse.[11] However, a raised mean cell volume (MCV) and a raised γGT together detect 75% of problem drinkers.[8]

* A more detailed biochemical screen, using 10 tests,[12] has achieved a sensitivity of 98% and a specificity of 95% for heavy drinkers. By far the most significant predictors of heavy drinking were a raised chloride and low sodium. Other components of the index were high levels of the following: the ratio of direct to total bilirubin, high density lipoproteins, monocytes, phosphate, platelets, aspartate transaminase, mean corpuscular haemoglobin and a low blood urea.

* Ask the patient to keep a drink diary for the next week to confirm the amount drunk.

ICD-10 criteria for the diagnosis of alcohol dependence (modified):[13]
At least 3 of the following must have been present for at least one month or for shorter periods repeatedly over at least 12 months:

1. strong desire or sense of compulsion to take alcohol
2. impaired capacity to control alcohol-taking behaviour in terms of onset, termination or levels of use
3. physiological withdrawal state when alcohol use is reduced or stopped; or use of alcohol to relieve or avoid withdrawal symptoms
4. evidence of tolerance to the effects of alcohol
5. other pleasures or interests being given up or reduced because of alcohol use
6. persistent alcohol use despite clear evidence of harmful consequences.

ICD-10 criteria for the diagnosis of harmful alcohol use:[13]

(a) clear evidence that alcohol is responsible for (or is substantially contributing to) physical or psychological harm
(b) the nature of the harm is clearly identifiable and specified
(c) the pattern of use has persisted for at least one month or has occurred repeatedly within the 12-month period
(d) the subject does not fulfil criteria for dependence.

Reproduced with the permission of WHO.[14]

Example

A 35-year-old manager of a firm of solicitors comes twice to ask for a certificate for a few days off work because he can't cope. On the second occasion the GP remembers that she had been asked to provide a medical report the year before in connection with a drink/driving offence. She asks if alcohol is a problem and he says it is not, though he admits to enjoying a drink. She hopes to disarm him by admitting that she too has something to drink every night after work and finds it hard to envisage a meal without wine. Within a minute she has the history that he and his wife drink a bottle of wine each evening and that he drinks most of it, which equates to an Audit-C score of at least 5. The GP reckons that his probability of having an alcohol problem, either dependence or problem drinking, has risen from a baseline of 14%

for a man in primary care to, say, 30% because of the driving conviction and the difficulties at work, to 57% as a result of the positive Audit-C test (Fig. 47.1). However, he remains resistant to the idea that alcohol could be contributing to his difficulties.

He does, however, mention the GP's line of questioning at home, because his wife telephones in confidence to report that he is drinking considerably more than he has admitted. Sometimes he falls asleep in front of the television after a heavy night's drinking, comes to bed at 3 in the morning and then feels too rough to go to work the next day. The GP is now clear that alcohol is the problem and plans to renew the discussion when he attends in a week's time.

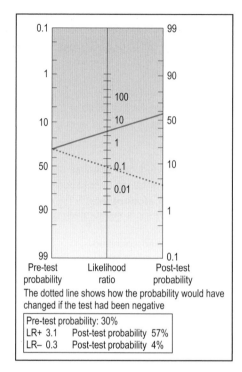

Figure 47.1 Nomogram to show the performance of the Audit-C questionnaire for the detection of an alcohol problem in the example on p. 315.

REFERENCES

1. National Health Committee (New Zealand). *Guidelines for recognising, assessing and treating alcohol and cannabis abuse in primary care*, 1999. Online. Available: www.nzgg.org.nz.

2. Aertgeerts B, Buntinx F, Ansoms S, et al. *Screening properties of questionnaires and laboratory tests in the detection of excessive drinking*. Br J Gen Pract 2001;51:206–217.

3. Beich A, Gannik D, Malterud K. *Screening and brief intervention for excessive alcohol use: qualitative interview study of the experiences of general practitioners*. BMJ 2002;325:870–872.

4. Goldberg D, Lecrubier Y. *Forms and frequency of mental disorders across centres*. In: Ustun T, Sartorius N, eds. Mental illness in general health care. An international study. New York: John Wiley, 1995:324–334.

5. O'Connell H, Chin A-V, Cunningham C, et al. *Alcohol use disorders in elderly people – redefining an age old problem in old age*. BMJ 2003;327: 664–667.

6. Department of Health. *The Health of the Nation: a strategy for health in England and Wales*. London: HMSO, 1992.

7. Inter-Departmental Working Group. *Sensible drinking*. London: HMSO, 1995.

8. Ashworth M, Gerada C. *Addiction and dependence – II: Alcohol*. BMJ 1997;315:358–360.

9. Editor. *Editor's note*. Br J Gen Pract 2001;51:409.

10. Canagasaby A, Vinson D. *Screening for hazardous or harmful drinking using one or two quantity-frequency questions*. Alcohol Alcohol 2005;40:208–213.

11. Bernadt MW, Mumford J, Taylor C, et al. *Comparison of questionnaire and laboratory tests in the detection of excessive drinking and alcoholism*. Lancet 1982;1:325–328.

12. Hartz AJ, Guse C, Kajdacsy-Balla A. *Identification*

of heavy drinkers using a combination of laboratory tests. *J Clin Epidemiol* 1997;50(12):1357–1368.

13. Piccinelli M, Tessari E, Bortolomasi M, et al. *Efficacy of the alcohol use disorders identification test as a screening tool for hazardous alcohol intake and related disorders in primary care: a validity study.* BMJ 1997;314:420–424.

14. WHO. *The ICD-10 classification of mental and behavioural disorders: diagnostic criteria for research.* Geneva: World Health Organization, 1993.

48

Anaemia

- Symptoms of anaemia are non-specific (e.g. tiredness or breathlessness).
- The sign of pallor is unreliable. Conjunctival pallor may be useful if present but it does not argue against the diagnosis of anaemia if absent.
- Most patients with anaemia are discovered as a result of a blood test; a haemoglobin (Hb) should be ordered in those with symptoms (as above) or with conditions which have worsened where that worsening could be a result of anaemia (e.g. worsening of heart failure or angina).
- Once discovered, the challenge is to find the cause. GPs in the UK omit further investigations in one-third of patients without an apparent reason.[1]

A PRACTICAL APPROACH

* Categorise into microcytic, macrocytic or normocytic anaemia according to the red cell indices.

In microcytic anaemia
* Check the serum ferritin. If low, confirm the diagnosis of iron deficiency with a trial of iron.
* If iron deficiency is confirmed, refer for GI investigations. Half will have GI disease and, of those, a fifth will have cancer. However, omit referral of menstruating women unless there are pointers to GI disease. Check the endomysial antibodies instead.
* If ferritin is normal, or if it is low but the haemoglobin does not rise with oral iron, check for chronic disease.
* In patients whose ethnic origin puts them at risk, and whose ferritin is normal, test for thalassaemia and haemoglobinopathy.

In macrocytic anaemia
* Check the serum B_{12} and the red cell folate. Also ask about alcohol intake, and check liver function (LFTs) and thyroid function tests (TFTs).
* Confirm a suspicion of pernicious anaemia with parietal cell and intrinsic factor antibodies.
* If a low red cell folate is found, look for evidence of poor nutrition. If nutrition is adequate, look for another cause.
* If B_{12} and folate are normal, look for other causes, e.g. drugs that cause macrocytosis, or malignancy.

In normocytic anaemia
* Look for evidence of chronic disease. However, iron, B_{12} and folate deficiency will all show normocytosis in the early stages: perform the investigations listed under those sections above as well.

If it is neither of these, is it secondary to chronic disease?

The history and examination are very likely to reveal this but, if not, check renal, liver and thyroid function, and the erythrocyte sedimentation rate (ESR) and chest X-ray (CXR) for tuberculosis in those at high risk.

If the diagnosis is still not clear

Refer to a haematologist. Bone marrow examination may be needed to establish the diagnosis of sideroblastic anaemia.

Macrocytosis

(MCV >95 fl and/or MCH >34 pg)[12]

> **Work-up of macrocytosis:** serum B_{12}, red cell folate, reticulocyte count, LFTs, TFTs. If B_{12} is low, check parietal cell and intrinsic factor antibodies.

- A normal MCV does not rule out folate or B_{12} deficiency. It may be normal in pernicious anaemia (PA)[29] and it may be artificially depressed if there is coincidental iron deficiency or thalassaemia. In such cases, the presence of hypersegmented neutrophils is more sensitive for the detection of megaloblastic anaemia.
- Conversely, a raised MCV is not at all specific for megaloblastic anaemia.

Pre-test probabilities

1. Major elevation of MCV (>130 fl):
   (a) vitamin B_{12} deficiency
   (b) folate deficiency.
2. Moderate elevation of MCV (>115 fl):
   (a) vitamin B_{12} deficiency
   (b) folate deficiency
   (c) liver disease
   (d) alcohol misuse
   (e) malignancy.

   A study of mixed inpatients and outpatients from New Haven, Connecticut[30] found that half their patients with an MCV >115 fl had deficiency of folate (31%) or B_{12} (13%) or both (6%); 15% had liver disease, 11% had alcohol misuse without liver disease, and 24% had another condition, of which nearly one-third were malignant. However, in developed countries in which foods are now fortified with folic acid (from 1998 in North America), folic acid deficiency is much less common.

3. Modest elevation of MCV (95–115 fl):
   (a) alcohol misuse; this is the cause in Finland in 80% of men and 46% of women with macrocytosis[31]
   (b) pernicious anaemia and other causes of B_{12} deficiency (6%)[31]
   (c) folate deficiency (4%)[31]
   (d) liver disease
   (e) myelodysplasia
   (f) blood loss or haemolysis with release into the bloodstream of immature red cells
   (g) hypothyroidism
   (h) chronic respiratory failure
   (i) HIV infection
   (j) drugs:[32]
   - antifolates, e.g. methotrexate
   - purine analogues, e.g. azathioprine
   - pyrimidine analogues, e.g. zidovudine
   - ribonucleotide reductase inhibitors, e.g. hydroxyurea
   - anticonvulsants: phenytoin, phenobarbital
   - others: metformin, colchicine
   (k) no cause found: 21%.[31]

These prevalences vary with age. A study of US outpatients aged >65 found biochemical B_{12} deficiency in 15%.[33] Decrease in gastric acid, as well as the increasing incidence of PA, appear to be responsible.

Clues to the diagnosis

(a) *From the history*: alcohol intake, malnutrition, a vegan diet, chronic haemolytic anaemia, inflammatory bowel disease, previous gastric or small bowel surgery, long-term use of acid suppressant therapy.
(b) *From the examination*: peripheral neuropathy, spinal cord disease, cognitive impairment; depression.
(c) *From the blood film*: hypersegmented neutrophils, cytopenia.

Tests

(a) *Serum B_{12}*.[32] False positives (i.e. low levels) occur in:
   - pregnancy
   - oral contraceptive use
   - partial gastrectomy
   - folate deficiency
   - strict vegetarians
   - normal people.

These false positives are likely to occur in those with mildly low B_{12} levels (100 to 250 ng/L). Using a cut-off of 100 improves specificity but reduces sensitivity from near 100% to 65% (and see box below).

(b) *Parietal cell antibodies*: sensitivity 84% but not at all specific; they are present in 5% to 22% of the general population.

(c) *Intrinsic factor antibodies*: sensitivity 50% but highly specific. A positive therefore establishes the diagnosis.

(d) Only refer for a *Schilling test* for pernicious anaemia if the diagnosis is still unclear.

(e) *Serum folate* is not useful; it is too dependent on dietary intake.

(f) *Red cell folate*. If red cell folate is low, look for malnutrition, increased requirements, e.g. pregnancy or haemolytic anaemia, or malabsorption. However, a low B_{12} will depress red cell folate (by impeding entry of folate into the cells).

A *therapeutic trial* is rarely necessary but, if conducted, give small doses of B_{12} then folate. Look for an increase in the reticulocyte count one week after the administration of each.

Interpreting the serum B_{12} result[34]

The following difficulties complicate the interpretation of a serum B_{12} level:

(a) It measures total, not active, B_{12}. Falsely low levels occur when the cobalamin-carrier protein level is low, as in women using oral contraception.

(b) Levels correlate poorly with symptoms and signs. Clinically significant deficiency may occur with a normal B_{12} level.

(c) There is no clear cut-off between normal and abnormal levels.

(d) The reference range varies between laboratories. In a laboratory with a normal range of 150–600 pmol/L (roughly = ng/L), the probabilities are as follows:

Serum B_{12} (pmol/L)	Probability of symptomatic deficiency
<75	high
75–150	moderate
150–220	low (3–5% of cases)
>220	rare (0.2% of cases)

Normal sized cells

(MCV 77–95 fl)

Work-up of normochromic anaemia: blood film, ESR, urea and electrolytes, LFTs, serum ferritin, B_{12}, red cell folate and endomysial antibodies.

The main probabilities

■ Acute blood loss, suggested by the history and examination

■ Chronic disease, suggested by the history and examination and the screening tests listed under microcytic anaemia

■ Renal failure

■ Liver failure

■ Early iron deficiency

■ Mixed iron and folate or B_{12} deficiency

■ Unsuspected coeliac disease, although macrocytosis is more common (see above)

■ Myelodysplasia suggested by neutropenia and thrombocytopenia

■ Hypoplastic or aplastic anaemia

■ Haemolytic anaemia suggested by a blood film showing reticulocytes, spherocytes or other abnormal red cells; increased urinary urobilinogen; raised serum bilirubin; raised lactate dehydrogenase; and a low haptoglobin level.[3]

Example

A 55-year-old ex-smoker is referred to his GP by the Blood Transfusion Service (BTS). They had found an Hb of 10.8 g/dl when he volunteered to give blood. He admits to feeling more tired than usual for a few months but denies other symptoms. There is no relevant past history and he takes no drugs. Examination reveals no enlarged nodes, and no abnormal abdominal masses. The report from the BTS showed indices within the normal range, although they were towards the lower end of the normal range for MCV and MCHC.

The GP orders the screening investigations for normochromic normocytic anaemia (see above). She is aware that the diagnosis is probably either iron deficiency or anaemia secondary to chronic disease and that these two possibilities are equally likely. The only abnormalities in the screening tests were a serum ferritin of 45 and an ESR of 50.

The GP feels she is not much further forward. The ferritin is within the laboratory's normal range but she is aware that it is borderline low and so is moderately predictive of iron deficiency. However, the raised ESR suggests an inflammatory condition. This could be the cause of the anaemia; or the patient could be iron deficient with a ferritin that is misleadingly elevated in the presence of coincidental inflammation.

She decides to investigate both possibilities at the same time, starting with a CXR and a prostate specific antigen (PSA), to cover the two commonest cancers for his age, sex and smoking history, and referring him at the same time to a gastroenterologist. Colonoscopy revealed a carcinoma of the ascending colon.

The anaemia responds completely to excision of the carcinoma and administration of oral iron. To what extent the anaemia was due to iron deficiency and to what extent due to malignancy was never resolved.

REFERENCES

1. Yates J, Logan E, Stewart R. *Iron deficiency anaemia in general practice: clinical outcomes over three years and factors influencing diagnostic investigations.* Postgrad Med J 2004;80:405–410.

2. WHO. *Nutritional anaemias: Report of a WHO Scientific Group.* Geneva: World Health Organization, 1968.

3. Tefferi A. *Anemia in adults: a contemporary approach to diagnosis.* Mayo Clin Proc 2003;78:1274–1280.

4. Chaves P, Xue Q-L, Guralnik J, et al. *What constitutes normal hemoglobin concentration in community-dwelling disabled older women?* J Am Geriatr Soc 2004;52:1811–1816.

5. Goddard A, McIntyre A, Scott B. *Guidelines for the management of iron deficiency.* Gut 2000;46 (Suppl 3–4):1–5.

6. Challand G, Michaeloudis A, Watfa R, et al. *Distribution of haemoglobin in patients presenting to their general practitioner, and its correlation with serum ferritin.* Ann Clin Biochem 1990;27:15–20.

7. De Maeyer E, Adiels-Tegman M. *The prevalence of anaemia in the world.* World Health Stat Q 1985;38:302–316.

8. Nardone D. *Usefulness of physical examination in detecting the presence or absence of anemia.* Arch Intern Med 1990;150(1):201–204.

9. Sheth T, Choudhry N, Bowes M, et al. *The relation of conjunctival pallor to the presence of anemia.* J Gen Intern Med 1997;12:102–106.

10. Kahn R, Romslo I, Lamvik J. *Anemia in general practice.* Scand J Clin Lab Invest Suppl 1990;200:41–45.

11. Hin H, Bird G, Fisher P, et al. *Coeliac disease in primary care: case finding study.* BMJ 1999;318:164–167.

12. Griner PF. *Microcytosis.* In: Black ER, Bordley DR, Tape TG, Panzer RJ, eds. Diagnostic strategies for common medical problems, 2nd edn. Philadelphia: American College of Physicians, 1999.

13. Kirkeby OJ, Fossum S, Risoe C. *Anaemia in elderly patients. Incidence and causes of low haemoglobin concentration in a city general practice.*

Scand J Prim Health Care 1991;9(3):167–171.

14. Booth IW, Aukett MA. *Iron deficiency anaemia in infancy and early childhood.* Arch Dis Child 1997;76:549–554.

15. James JA, Laing GJ, Logan S. *Changing patterns of iron deficiency anaemia in the second year of life.* BMJ 1995;311:230.

16. Griner PF, Oranburg PR. *Predictive values of erythrocyte indices for tests of iron, folic acid, and vitamin B12 deficiency.* Am J Clin Pathol 1978;70(5):748–752.

17. Provan D, Krentz A. *Oxford handbook of clinical and laboratory investigation.* Oxford: Oxford University Press, 2002.

18. Guyatt GH, Patterson C, Ali M, et al. *Diagnosis of iron deficiency anemia in the elderly.* Am J Med 1990;88:205–209.

19. Duncan J. *Positive diagnosis of anaemia of chronic disease (letter).* BMJ 2006;333:972.

20. Jamison JR. *Differential diagnosis for primary practice.*

Edinburgh: Churchill Livingstone, 1999.

21. Galloway M, Smellie W. *Investigating iron status in microcytic anaemia.* BMJ 2006;333:791–793.

22. Ioannou GN, Rockey DC, Bryson CL, Weiss NS. *Iron deficiency and gastrointestinal malignancy: a population-based cohort study.* Am J Med 2002;113:276–280.

23. Stellon AJ, Kenwright SE. *Iron deficiency anaemia in general practice: presentations and investigations.* Br J Clin Pract 1997;51(2):78–80.

24. Bampton PA, Holloway RH. *A prospective study of the gastroenterological causes of iron deficiency anaemia in a general hospital.* Aust N Z J Med 1996;26(6):793–799.

25. Black DA, Fraser CM. *Iron deficiency anaemia and aspirin use in old age.* Br J Gen Pract 1999;49(446):729–730.

26. Sayer J, Donnelly M, McIntyre A, et al. *Barium enema or colonoscopy for the investigation of iron deficiency anaemia?* J R Coll Physicians Lond 1999;33:543–548.

27. Marx J. *Iron deficiency in developed countries: prevalence, influence of lifestyle factors and hazards of prevention.* Eur J Clin Nutr 1997;51:491–494.

28. Reilly J, Cawley J. *Haematological disease.* In: Axford J, ed. Medicine. Oxford: Blackwell Science, 1996:11.29–30.

29. Carmel R. *Pernicious anemia: the expected findings of very low serum cobalamin levels, anemia and macrocytosis are often lacking.* Arch Intern Med 1988;148:1712–1714.

30. McPhedran P, Barnes MG, Weinstein JS, Robertson JS. *Interpretation of electronically determined macrocytosis.* Ann Intern Med 1973;1973:677–683.

31. Seppa K, Heinila K, Sillanaukee P, Saarni M. *Evaluation of macrocytosis by general practitioners.* J Stud Alcohol 1996;57(1):97–100.

32. Lancet J, Rapoport A. *Macrocytosis.* In: Black ER, Bordley DR, Tape TG, Panzer RJ, eds. Diagnostic strategies for common medical problems. Philadelphia: American College of Physicians, 1999.

33. Pennypacker L, Allen R, Kelly J, et al. *High prevalence of cobalamin deficiency in elderly outpatients.* J Am Geriatr Soc 1992;40:1197–1204.

34. Guidelines and Protocols Advisory Committee. *Investigation and management of vitamin B12 and folate deficiency: British Columbia Medical Association*, 2003. Online. Available: www.hlth.gov.bc.ca/msp/protoguides/gps/index.html.

Step 2. More detailed questioning for specific anxiety syndromes

The gold standard for the diagnosis of mental disorders is the in-depth clinical interview conducted by an experienced clinician. What follows is based on the ICD-10 classification of mental disorders[23] (reproduced with the permission of WHO). Its weakness is that, designed as it is for research purposes, it puts disorders into categories when, by their nature, those disorders have infinite variety. These classifications should not, therefore, be applied in cookbook fashion, but used as a support to the physician's clinical judgement. The problem for this book is that that judgement cannot be neatly described nor validated.

Is this an acute stress reaction?

The ICD-10 criteria are as follows:[23]
A. The patient must have been exposed to an exceptional mental or physical stressor.
B. Exposure to the stressor is followed by an immediate onset of symptoms (within 1 hour).
C. At least four of the symptoms listed in the box opposite must be present, at least one of which must be from items (1) to (4).
D. If the stressor is transient or can be relieved, the symptoms must begin to diminish after not more than 8 hours. If exposure to the stressor continues, the symptoms must begin to diminish after not more than 48 hours.
E. The reaction must occur in the absence of any other concurrent mental or behavioural disorder in ICD-10 (except generalised anxiety disorder and personality disorders), and not within 3 months of the end of an episode of any other mental or behavioural disorder.

Is this an adjustment disorder?

The ICD-10 criteria for this are:[23]
A. The onset of symptoms must occur within 1 month of exposure to an identifiable psychosocial stressor, not of an unusual or catastrophic type (which rather suggests the possibility of PTSD).
B. The individual manifests symptoms or behaviour disturbance of the types found in any of the affective disorders but the criteria for an individual disorder are not fulfilled.

The definition goes on to point out that symptoms of anxiety may be mixed with other emotions, e.g. depression and anger.

It may be hard to decide whether the reaction is within the normal range of human emotions or whether it amounts to a disorder. In making this decision, two questions are useful:
1. Is there more distress than would be expected?
2. Is there significant impairment in the person's ability to function, either socially or at work?

In addition, the patient should not have another disorder which explains the symptoms; they should not be due to bereavement; and, once the stress has terminated, symptoms should subside within 6 months.

When is anxiety bad enough to warrant the diagnosis of an anxiety disorder?

The ICD-10 definition lists the following symptoms of anxiety:[23] (Some anxiety disorders require the presence of at least two, some at least four.)

Autonomic arousal symptoms
(1) Palpitations or pounding heart, or accelerated heart rate
(2) Sweating
(3) Trembling or shaking
(4) Dry mouth (not due to medication or dehydration)

Symptoms involving chest and abdomen
(5) Difficulty in breathing
(6) Feeling of choking
(7) Chest pain or discomfort
(8) Nausea or abdominal distress (e.g. churning in stomach)

Symptoms involving mental state
(9) Feeling dizzy, unsteady, faint, or light-headed
(10) Feelings that objects are unreal (derealisation), or that the self is distant or 'not really here' (depersonalisation)
(11) Fear of losing control, 'going crazy' or passing out
(12) Fear of dying
(13) Hot flushes or cold chills
(14) Numbness or tingling sensations

For the diagnosis of generalised anxiety disorder, eight other symptoms are described:
(15) Muscle tension or aches and pains
(16) Restlessness and inability to relax
(17) Feeling keyed up, on edge or mentally tense
(18) A sensation of a lump in the throat, or difficulty in swallowing
(19) Exaggerated response to minor surprises or being startled
(20) Difficulty in concentrating, or mind 'going blank', because of worrying or anxiety
(21) Persistent irritability
(22) Difficulty in getting to sleep because of worrying

Reproduced with permission of the WHO

Is this post-traumatic stress disorder (PTSD)?

The most threatening types of trauma (rape, attempted homicide, suffering a terrorist attack, being a refugee) have associated rates of PTSD approaching 50% and above.[7]

The ICD-10 classification describes five criteria for the diagnosis of PTSD:

A. The patient must have been exposed to a stressful event or situation (either short- or long-lasting) of exceptionally threatening or catastrophic nature, which would be likely to cause pervasive distress in almost anyone.

B. There must be persistent remembering or 'reliving' of the stressor in intrusive 'flashbacks', vivid memories or recurring dreams, or in experiencing distress when exposed to circumstances resembling or associated with the stressor.

C. The patient must exhibit an actual or preferred avoidance of circumstances resembling or associated with the stressor, which was not present before exposure to the stressor.

D. Either of the following must be present:

   1. inability to recall, either partially or completely, some important aspects of the period of exposure to the stressor

   2. persistent symptoms of increased psychological sensitivity and arousal (not present before exposure to the stressor); shown by any two of the following:

      (a) difficulty in falling or staying asleep

      (b) irritability or outbursts of anger

      (c) difficulty in concentrating

      (d) hypervigilance

      (e) exaggerated startle response.

E. Criteria B, C and D must all be met within 6 months of the stressful event or of the end of the period of stress (although a later onset is not impossible).

Other points about PTSD

● A self-assessment questionnaire has been developed, using similar criteria.[24] When symptoms from B, C and D are present, it has a sensitivity of 86% and specificity of 80% for diagnosing PTSD, with a structured interview as the 'gold standard' (LR+ 4.3; LR− 0.18).

● Patients with the above symptoms who are seen within 1 month of the trauma are better described, at that stage, as having an acute stress disorder.

● PTSD is often missed in primary care because patients present, not with the classical symptoms, but with complaints of fatigue, insomnia, myalgia, headache or poor concentration. In addition, other disorders are often present (e.g. depression, anxiety or substance misuse) which mask the diagnosis of PTSD. The California study (above) found that 61% of those with PTSD had a major depressive illness and 39% had a generalised anxiety disorder.[3]

Is this generalised anxiety disorder (GAD)?

Generalised anxiety disorder is defined as follows:[23]

A. There must have been a period of at least 6 months with prominent tension, worry and feelings of apprehension about everyday events and problems.

B. At least four of the symptoms listed in the box on p. 331 must be present, at least one of which must be from items (1) to (4).

C. The disorder does not meet the criteria for panic disorder, phobic anxiety disorders, obsessive-compulsive disorder or hypochondriacal disorder.

D. The anxiety disorder is not due to a physical disorder, such as hyperthyroidism, an organic mental disorder or a psychoactive substance-related disorder, such as excess consumption of amfetamine-like substances or withdrawal from benzodiazepines.

Differentiating worry from generalised anxiety

Severe worry is common; but most severe worriers do not suffer from a psychiatric disorder. There seems to be a continuum on which severe worriers lie, with GAD at one end. There are two ways in which those with pathological worry (GAD) can be distinguished from severe worriers who are not ill:[25]

   (a) severe worriers without GAD may answer positively to any or most of the questions above; but are not likely to answer positively to all of them

   (b) when questioned in more depth, severe worriers without GAD tend to have symptoms that are less intense that those with GAD.

✱ When asking the questions above, ask them in an open-ended way, e.g. on how many days have you worried excessively in the last 6 months? Rather than 'Have you worried on most days in the last 6 months?' Those with high levels of worry are more likely to answer 'yes' to the second question than they are to answer '4 or more days a week' to the first.[25] Using a closed question, i.e. expecting the answer 'yes' or 'no', can therefore lead to the overdiagnosis of GAD.

Is this a phobia?

The ICD-10 criteria for the diagnosis of *specific phobia* are as follows:[23]

A. Either of the following must be present:
   (1) marked fear of a specific object or situation not included in agoraphobia or social phobia
   (2) marked avoidance of a specific object or situation not included in agoraphobia or social phobia.

   Among the most common objects and situations are animals, birds, insects, heights, thunder, flying, small enclosed spaces, the sight of blood or injury, injections, dentists and hospitals.

B. Symptoms of anxiety (see above) in the feared situation must have been manifest at some time since the onset of the disorder. They must include at least two of the symptoms listed in the box on p. 331, of which one must be from items (1) to (4).

C. Significant emotional distress is caused by the symptoms or by the avoidance, and the individual recognises that these are excessive or unreasonable.

D. Symptoms are restricted to the feared situation or contemplation of the feared situation.

When describing their fears, patients may recall that the original fear was of a specific threat (e.g. that the aircraft will crash) but that this has been overtaken by fears about the panic attack itself – that they will faint, vomit or lose control in some other way.

Social phobia is present if the fear is due to certain social or performance situations and the patient is focusing on the humiliation or embarrassment that he or she will feel on being the centre of attention. The phobia worsens as the person becomes more fearful because others will detect that fear.

Agoraphobia is present if the fear is that the patient will develop symptoms of anxiety or panic in a place where escape is difficult or embarrassing; or where help may not be available if they develop symptoms (e.g. fainting or diarrhoea) due to anxiety. In agoraphobia, the fear will relate to all situations which share the same features (e.g. all situations where the person can be seen by strangers). If the fear is restricted to one situation only, then this is a specific phobia rather than agoraphobia. To meet criteria for agoraphobia, the ICD-10 definition requires that the phobia relate to at least two of the following:
- crowds
- public places
- travelling alone
- travelling away from home.

Is this panic disorder?

Most people who have panic attacks do not have panic disorder. This term means that recurrent unexpected panic attacks occur and that they have disturbed the person's life for at least 1 month.

The ICD-10 criteria for the diagnosis of panic disorder are as follows:[23]

A. The individual experiences recurrent panic attacks that are not consistently associated with a specific situation or object and that often occur spontaneously (i.e. the episodes are unpredictable). The panic attacks are not associated with marked exertion or with exposure to dangerous or life-threatening situations.

B. A panic attack is characterised by all of the following:
   (1) it is a discrete episode of intense fear or discomfort
   (2) it starts abruptly
   (3) it reaches a maximum within a few minutes and lasts at least some minutes
   (4) at least four of the symptoms listed in the box on page 331 must be present, one of which must be from items (1) to (4).

Other points about panic disorder

- The attacks should not be due to a medical condition or a drug, nor better accounted for by another mental disorder, e.g. a phobia, obsessive-compulsive disorder, PTSD or separation anxiety disorder. Some patients also have panic attacks that are not unexpected (i.e. the patient can identify the trigger) but if unexpected attacks are also present, then panic disorder is present.
- *Co-morbidity.* Patients with panic disorder often become demoralised. Major depressive disorder has been found in 10–65%[14]; in some, it precedes the first panic attack. Other anxiety disorders may be present (generalised anxiety disorder in up to 30%, specific phobias in up to 20% and obsessive-compulsive

disorder in up to 10%).[14] The precise diagnosis is important: each mental disorder has a different prognosis and management.

■ *A family history.* A first-degree relative with panic disorder increases the probability that an individual will develop the condition 8-fold. However, most patients with the disorder do not have an affected relative, so family history is not useful in the diagnosis.

Is this obsessive-compulsive disorder (OCD)?

The ICD-10 criteria are as follows:[23]

A. Either obsessions or compulsions (or both) are present on most days for a period of at least 2 weeks.

B. Obsessions (thoughts, ideas or images) and compulsions (acts) share the following features, all of which must be present:

(1) They are acknowledged as originating in the mind of the patient, and are not imposed by outside persons or influences.

(2) They are repetitive and unpleasant, and at least one obsession or compulsion that is acknowledged as excessive or unreasonable must be present.

(3) The patient tries to resist them (but resistance to very longstanding obsessions or compulsions may be minimal). At least one obsession or compulsion that is unsuccessfully resisted must be present.

(4) Experiencing the obsessive thought or carrying out the compulsive act is not in itself pleasurable. (This should be distinguished from the temporary relief of tension or anxiety.)

C. The obsessions or compulsions cause distress or interfere with the patient's social or individual functioning, usually by wasting time.

D. The obsessions or compulsions are not the result of other mental disorders, such as schizophrenia and related disorders or mood (affective) disorders.

Patients with OCD go to some lengths to conceal their symptoms. The UK NICE guideline recommends that patients at risk of OCD be asked six case-finding questions:[19]

■ Do you wash or clean a lot?

■ Do you check things a lot?

■ Is there any thought that keeps bothering you that you would like to get rid of but cannot?

■ Do your daily activities take a long time to finish?

■ Are you concerned about putting things in a special order or are you very upset by mess?

■ Do these problems trouble you?

Patients at risk of OCD are those with another anxiety disorder, with depression, with alcohol or another substance misuse, with body dysmorphic disorder or with an eating disorder.

Is this body dysmorphic disorder (BDD)?

This is a condition in which the person is preoccupied with an imagined defect in his or her appearance, or, if the defect is real, the person's reaction to it is excessive. Patients with BDD spend excessive amounts of time examining themselves, picking at lesions, using various camouflaging techniques and consulting beauty and health professionals. The UK NICE guideline recommends that patients in whom the possibility of BDD is raised be asked five case-finding questions:[19]

■ Do you worry a lot about the way you look and wish you could think about it less?

■ What specific concerns do you have about your appearance?

■ On a typical day, how many hours a day is your appearance on your mind? (more than 1 hour a day is considered excessive).

■ What effect does it have on your life?

■ Does it make it hard to do your work or be with friends?

Patients at risk of BDD are those with social phobia, with depression, with alcohol or another substance misuse, with obsessive-compulsive disorder or with an eating disorder. The diagnosis should also be considered in those seeking help because of apparently minor physical blemishes.

Is this substance-induced anxiety?

Some substances cause anxiety by a direct physiological effect, either by intoxication or during withdrawal. Common examples are alcohol, amfetamines, cocaine and cannabis. Anxiety can be the result of too much thyroxine and can occur in the withdrawal from anxiolytics or hypnotics, when it may be difficult to distinguish from the original anxiety for which they were prescribed.

- A normal peak flow or spirometry at a consultation does not exclude the diagnosis of asthma.
- Children under 6, and some elderly or disabled patients, cannot reliably use a peak flow meter or spirometer. Assessment has to be based on symptoms.
- In patients with asthma over the age of 50, even if they can use the tests reliably, variability is less than that seen in younger patients.[18]

Techniques

Peak flow
* Instruct the patient to:
  1. Set the indicator to zero; assume a comfortable posture; hold the meter with the fingers away from the gauge; take a deep breath; and blow as fast and hard as possible.
  2. Take three readings each time and record the highest. If the readings vary by more than 20 L/min do three more readings. Take the highest of all six readings.
  3. If the patient needs to use an inhaler, take the readings first.

Reversibility test using a beta$_2$-agonist
* Record the baseline PEFR or FEV$_1$. Give a dose of a beta$_2$-agonist. Repeat the PEFR or FEV$_1$ 15 minutes later.

Reversibility test using oral steroids
* The procedure and measurements are the same except that prednisolone 30 mg per day is given for 2 weeks.

Response to exercise
* Record the baseline PEFR or FEV$_1$. Ask the patient to run for 6 minutes then repeat the recording every 10 minutes for 30 minutes.

Further testing

This can be useful in cases of doubt.
- In a UK study,[11] methacholine airway responsiveness diagnosed asthma with a sensitivity of 91% and a specificity of 90% (LR+ 9.1, LR– 0.1). Sputum eosinophilia was 72% sensitive and 80% specific (LR+ 3.6, LR– 0.3). The combination of the two was 100% sensitive for the diagnosis of asthma (all asthmatics had a positive response to one or other test) while none of those without asthma were positive for both.
- *Tests of allergy* give variable results according to the test and the subjects. Blood eosinophilia, in the

UK study above, was 21% sensitive but 100% specific (LR+ infinitely high, LR– 0.8) for the diagnosis of asthma. In an Israeli study of young adults with suspected asthma, skin prick tests were 91% sensitive but only 52% specific (LR+ 1.9, LR– 0.2).[19] In a Swiss population study, they were only 65% sensitive and 78% specific (LR+ 3.0, LR– 0.5) for current allergic asthma.[20] If a patient with asthma demonstrates a skin response to an allergen, the patient's asthma is not necessarily caused or exacerbated by that allergen: it is better considered as a more general indicator of atopy.[21] In the Swiss population study,[20] a positive skin prick test to at least one of eight aero-allergens only carried a positive predictive value for current allergic asthma of 5%. A negative test is, however, more useful in ruling asthma out; it has a negative predictive value of 99%. In other words, if it is negative, the probability of asthma is only 1%.
- Allergy tests can be added to other tests with benefit. A study of Dutch children aged 6 found that a positive test for specific IgE to three common allergens carried an odds ratio of 18.7 (95% CI 5.4 to 64.3) for the diagnosis of asthma, and that the test was an independent predictor of asthma, adding useful information to the history and to reversibility testing.[22]
- In conclusion, allergy tests are not necessarily positive in patients with asthma, but SIGN recommends that a negative test in a child should prompt consideration of alternative diagnoses.[1]
- *Chest X-ray* is only useful in the diagnosis of other conditions that might be confused with asthma.

Referral for diagnosis

* Do not make the diagnosis of asthma in patients with complicated histories or unexpected signs on examination. The following merit referral:

In children:
  (a) a history of symptoms that have been present from birth, especially if there has been a persistent wet cough, suggesting cystic fibrosis.
  (b) an abnormal cry which suggests a laryngeal problem.

In children and adults:
  (a) inspiratory stridor or a change in voice which suggests a laryngeal problem.
  (b) focal chest signs which suggest infection; when symptoms are longstanding, this may be bronchiectasis or TB.

Occupational asthma

- Only 2–6% of asthma in the UK is occupational; but asthma is so common that this amounts to 50 new cases per million adults per year. In Finland, the incidence has been estimated at 140 per million working people per year.[23]
- The common allergens vary from country to country. In Finland, animal allergens contribute 70% of cases against 17% in the UK and <3% in New Jersey, USA.[23] In the UK, the four most at-risk professions, in descending order, are: spray painting, plastics manufacture, chemical processing and baking.

To diagnose it:

- * Ask all working asthmatics whether their symptoms are worse on workdays than at weekends or holidays. If they are:
- * Ask the patient to record four peak flow readings a day, spread through the day, for 3 days at work. Each recording should be the best of three attempts. Repeat the recordings in 2 subsequent weeks. The patient should also record the peak flow on four occasions (at the same times of day) for a total of 9 days when at home (at weekends or during holidays). A study from Canada found that serial peak flow recordings by the patient were 73% sensitive for occupational asthma and 100% specific.[24] Peak flow recording forms can be downloaded from www.occupationalasthma.com.
- * If the peak flow readings at work are worse, refer for further confirmation of the diagnosis and assessment of the responsible allergen. If peak flow readings are the same at work and at home, still consider referring if the history is suggestive. A bronchial provocation test may be justified because of the poor sensitivity of serial peak flow readings. No one test is both sensitive and specific for occupational asthma.[25] Referral to a specialist with an interest in asthma and/or allergy is necessary in view of the importance of the diagnosis.
- * Do not dismiss the possibility of occupational asthma because no allergen can be implicated. The patient may have asthma which is exacerbated by dust or fumes at work without a specific immune response being present.
- * Some sophistication is required in the interpretation of the history and of the readings. Occupational asthma may not develop for years after exposure begins.[26] Airways obstruction due to occupational asthma may continue for some hours or even days after the patient leaves work. Only readings taken on days of no work should be considered to be representative of 'non-

exposure'. Even then, some patients will show no improvement on 1–2 days off work, but improve on holiday. However, many patients' airways obstruction improves on holiday for reasons unconnected to occupational asthma. Finally, do not dismiss the possibility of occupational asthma because the patient has left the job that seemed to be associated with it, without improving. Symptoms can continue for years after the allergen has been removed.[23]

- * One study of patients with suspected occupational asthma showed a tendency for the patient to falsify readings.[27] Only 49% of recorded figures were accurate and 28% were totally invented by patients.

A cautionary tale in interpreting the literature

In a study from Quebec,[28] patients referred with suspected occupational asthma were asked whether their symptoms worsened, or were only present, at work; and whether their symptoms improved over a weekend away from work. These two questions had LR+s of 1.1 and 1.4 respectively and LR−s of 0.7 and 0.5 respectively. Only a positive answer to the question about improvement at weekends reached statistical significance (and none of the values are clinically significant). However, these two questions should not be discarded in the *screening* for occupational asthma. All the patients tested in this study were already suspected of having occupational asthma. It is very likely that the diagnosis was suspected because these two questions had already been asked by the referrer and so their value had been 'used up' in primary care.

Alternative diagnoses

Older children and adults	Pre-school children
Respiratory infection	Bronchiolitis and other
COPD	respiratory infections
Heart failure	Foreign body
Foreign body	Cystic fibrosis
Cancer	Laryngeal disorders
Bronchiectasis	Allergic bronchopulmonary
Pulmonary embolus	aspergillosis
Interstitial lung disease	Gastro-oesophageal reflux
Gastro-oesophageal reflux	Tumours
Panic disorder	Heart failure

Pre-school children with wheeze

Pre-school children with wheeze present greater diagnostic problems than adults. Several syndromes have been identified:[29]

■ *Transient early wheezing.* It has no association with later asthma and usually resolves by the age of 3.

■ *Non-atopic wheezing (wheezy bronchitis).* It is not associated with a personal or family history of atopy, except by chance, but is more common in children who were premature, and who are exposed to tobacco smoke. It becomes more pronounced with viral respiratory infections and may be only manifest then. It responds less well to treatment than asthma.

■ *Asthma.* More than half of all those who develop asthma start to wheeze before the age of 3. Asthma that starts this early is almost always associated with atopy.

Confirmatory tests are not possible, because such young children cannot cooperate with lung function tests.

Example 1

A 45-year-old man presents with 'asthma' which has begun a year before. The diagnosis was made by a previous general practitioner on the basis of a history of wheeze and breathlessness on exertion. The symptoms always come on at the same level of exertion. He thinks his inhaler helps. There is no other relevant history. The GP's immediate thought is that the breathlessness is probably due to overweight and lack of fitness rather than asthma, and that the inhaler appears to help because he stops exerting to use it, as well as because of a placebo effect.

Using the likelihood ratios from the Swiss study in Table 50.1, the GP calculates that the symptoms of wheeze and dyspnoea only raise his probability of asthma from 2.3% to 24% (Fig. 50.1).

Spirometry is normal, but he was not wheezing at the time so this is not very helpful. Using the figures from the UK study of patients with mild asthma between attacks, the probability drops slightly to 20% (Fig. 50.2).

Reversibility testing is not appropriate in a patient with normal baseline spirometry, so the GP decides on two further tests. The patient is wearing trainers, so she sends him to run round the block and to come back when he's really breathless. His spirometry is unchanged. The probability of asthma drops to 15% (Fig. 50.3).

She also asks him to chart his peak flow readings over 2 weeks. They vary from day to day but the characteristic saw tooth pattern of diurnal variation is missing. This result drops the probability of asthma to 11% (Fig. 50.4).

The GP explains that the tests for asthma are negative, which makes asthma unlikely but does not rule it out. They agree a compromise: she agrees to renew the prescription for the inhaler and he agrees to a weight loss and fitness programme. Neither is optimistic about the outcome.

Example 2

A 16-year-old girl presents with a 3-month history of night-time cough. There is a parental history of asthma. Examination is normal. Spirometry is normal and there is no response to inhaled salbutamol. Peak flow readings at home show 15% diurnal variation.

Her initial probability of asthma is 10% (the population prevalence for her age), which is increased to, say, 50% by the suggestive, but not diagnostic, personal and family history. The normal spirometry and lack of response to inhaled salbutamol has no effect on the probability since they are very likely to be normal in someone with mild symptoms that only occur at night. The diurnal variation is suggestive of asthma but does not reach the 20% level. However, these cut-offs are arbitrary. The fact that there is some diurnal variation is important, even though the specificity of a 15% variation will be, say, 70% rather than 90%. This reduces the LR+ to 2 and the probability of asthma rises to about 70%.

The diagnosis is therefore likely but not proven and a therapeutic trial of salbutamol inhaler at night or even a 2-week course of steroids is justified.

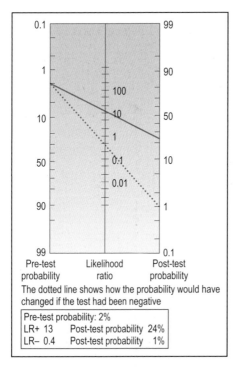

Figure 50.1 The probability of asthma before and after the history of wheeze and dyspnoea is obtained in example 1 on p. 343.

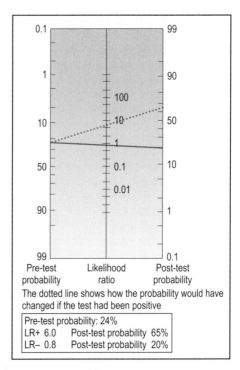

Figure 50.2 The probability of asthma before and after the negative spirometry in example 1 on p. 343.

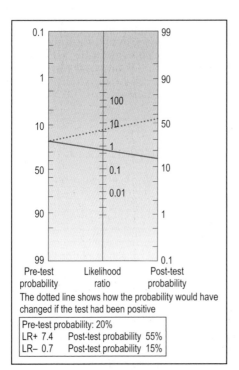

Figure 50.3 The probability of asthma before and after the lack of reversibility on exercise in example 1 on p. 343.

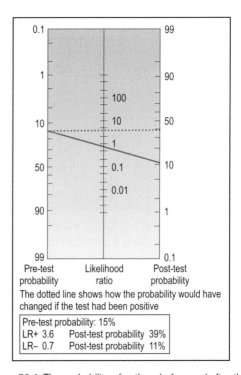

Figure 50.4 The probability of asthma before and after the lack of diurnal variation in example 1 on p. 343.

REFERENCES

1. Scottish Intercollegiate Guidelines Network, The British Thoracic Society. *British guideline on the management of asthma.* Thorax 2003;58(Suppl 1).

2. Rees J. *ABC of asthma: prevalence.* BMJ 2005;331:443–445.

3. Department of Health. *Health survey for England 1996.* London: HMSO, 1996.

4. Montnemery P, Hansson L, Lanke J, et al. *Accuracy of a first diagnosis of asthma in primary health care.* Fam Pract 2002;19:365–368.

5. Ward D, Halpin D, Seamark D. *How accurate is a diagnosis of asthma in a general practice database? A review of patients' notes and questionnaire-reported symptoms.* Br J Gen Pract 2004;54:753–758.

6. Baumann U, Haerdi E, Keller R. *Relations between clinical signs and lung function in bronchial asthma: How is acute bronchial obstruction reflected in dyspnea and wheezing?* Respiration 1986;50:294–300.

7. Sistek D, Tschopp J-M, Schindler C, et al. *Clinical diagnosis of current asthma: predictive value of respiratory symptoms in the SAPALDIA study.* Eur Respir J 2001;17:214–219.

8. Holleman D, Simel D. *Does the clinical examination predict airflow limitation?* JAMA 1995;273:313–319.

9. King D, Thompson B, Johnson D. *Wheezing on maximal forced exhalation in the diagnosis of atypical asthma.* Ann Intern Med 1989;110:451–455.

10. Siersted H, Mostgaard G, Hyldebrandt N, et al. *Interrelationships between diagnosed asthma, asthma-like symptoms, and abnormal airway behaviour in adolescence: the Odense Schoolchild Study.* Thorax 1996;51:503–509.

11. Hunter C, Brightling C, Woltmann G, et al. *A comparison of the validity of different diagnostic tests in adults with asthma.* Chest 2002;121:1051–1057.

12. Kunzli N, Stutz E, Perruchoud A, et al. *Peak flow variability in the SAPALDIA study and its validity in screening for asthma-related conditions.* Am J Respir Crit Care Med 1999;160:427–434.

13. Aggarwal A, Gupta D, Kumar V, Jindal S. *Assessment of diurnal variability of peak expiratory flow in stable asthmatics.* J Asthma 2002;39:487–491.

14. Gannon P, Newton D, Pantin C, Burge P. *Effect of the number of peak expiratory flow readings per day on the estimation of diurnal variation.* Thorax 1998;53:790–792.

15. King D. *Asthma diagnosis by spirometry: sensitive or specific?* Aust Fam Physician 1998;27:183–185.

16. Goldstein M, Veza B, Dunsky E, et al. *Comparisons of peak diurnal expiratory flow variation, postbronchodilator FEV1 responses, and methacholine inhalation challenges in the evaluation of suspected asthma.* Chest 2001;119:1001–1010.

17. Kesten S, Rebuck A. *Is the short-term response to inhaled beta-adrenergic agonist sensitive or specific for distinguishing between asthma and COPD?* Chest 1994;105:1042–1045.

18. Lewis S, Weiss S, Britton J. *Airway responsiveness and peak flow variability in the diagnosis of asthma for epidemiological studies.* Eur Respir J 2001;18:921–927.

19. Graif Y, Yigla M, Tov N, Kramer M. *Value of a negative aeroallergen skin-prick test result in the diagnosis of asthma in young adults.* Chest 2002;122:821–825.

20. Tschopp J, Sistek D, Schindler C, et al. *Current allergic asthma and rhinitis: diagnostic efficiency of three commonly used atopic markers (IgE, skin prick tests, and Phadiatop). Results from 8329 randomised adults from the SAPALDIA Study.* Allergy 1998;53:608–613.

21. Bowton D, Fasano M, Bass D. *Skin sensitivity to allergen does not accurately predict airway response to allergen.* Ann Allergy Asthma Immunol 1998;80:207–211.

22. Eysink P, ter Riet G, Aalberse R, et al. *Accuracy of specific IgE in the prediction of asthma: development of a scoring formula for general practice.* Br J Gen Pract 2005;55:125–131.

23. Meredith S, Nordman H. *Occupational asthma: measures of frequency from four countries.* Thorax 1996;51:435–440.

24. Leroyer C, Perfetti L, Trudeau C, et al. *Comparison of serial monitoring of peak expiratory flow and FEV1 in the diagnosis of occupational asthma.* Am J Respir Crit Care Med 1998;158:827–832.

25. Beach J, Rowe B, Blitz S, et al. *Diagnosis and management of work-related asthma*: Evidence Report/Technology Assessment: Number 129, 2005. Online. Available: www.ahcpr.gov.

26. Malo J, Ghezzo H, D'Aquino C, et al. *Natural history of occupational asthma: relevance of type of agent and other factors in the rate of development of symptoms in affected subjects.* J Allergy Clin Immunol 1992;90:937–944.

27. Malo J, Trudeau C, Ghezzo H, et al. *Do subjects investigated for occupational asthma through serial peak expiratory flow measurements falsify their results?* J Allergy Clin Immunol 1995;96:601–607.

28. Malo J, Ghezzo H, L'Archeveque J, et al. *Is the clinical history a satisfactory means of diagnosing occupational asthma?* Am Rev Respir Dis 1991;143:528–532.

29. Martinez F. *Development of wheezing disorders and asthma in preschool children.* Pediatrics 2002;109:362–367.

Benzodiazepine dependence

Prevalence

Studies of patients in primary care show that, of those who take benzodiazepines, the proportion who develop dependence is 47% in the Canary Islands,[1] 40% to 52% in Dutch general practice[2] and over 50% in rural Australia.[3] A US population study of people aged 15 to 54 found that 9.2% were using benzodiazepines and that 1.2% of those studied were dependent.[4] This lower figure for the proportion that is dependent in the population is not surprising; attenders in primary care are more likely to have problems than the general population.

Definition

The ICD-10 classification[5] defines benzodiazepine dependence as a syndrome which typically includes:

1. a strong desire to take the drug
2. difficulties in controlling its use
3. persisting in its use despite harmful consequences
4. higher priority given to drug use than to other activities and obligations
5. increased tolerance
6. sometimes, a physical withdrawal state.

The *ICD-10 Diagnostic Criteria for Research* tries to quantify the diagnosis by requiring that at least three of the above should have been present together for at least a month, or, if persisting for periods of less than a month, should have recurred together repeatedly within a 12-month period.[6] Inevitably arbitrary, this cut-off is useful for research but less useful in clinical practice.

Who is at risk of dependence?

- Suspect it in those who have taken a benzodiazepine for >1 month, especially those from high-risk groups.

A study from the Canary Islands of patients who had taken a benzodiazepine for >1 month found that dependence was more likely in those:
- of low educational background
- middle aged
- separated
- unemployed.

However, multivariate logistic regression analysis showed that only three variables were closely related to dependence:

- dose
- duration
- concomitant use of antidepressants.[1]

Above all, suspect it in those who obtain or have obtained their own supplies; or who are alcohol or multi-drug users.[7]

It is almost certain to be present in those who are members of a tranquilliser self-help group.[2]

Patient awareness of dependence

The patient may not be aware that dependence has developed. A study of long-term users in the Canary Islands found that 40% of those with a diagnosis of dependence, using the gold standard of the Composite International Diagnostic Interview administered by a psychiatrist, thought they were not dependent. Conversely, 11.5% of those who were judged not to be dependent thought they were.[8]

Screening for dependence

The Severity of Dependence Scale (SDS) has been validated as a screening test for benzodiazepine dependence in regular benzodiazepine users. It should be administered when the patient is symptom free. Using the gold standard of the Composite International Diagnostic Interview administered by a psychiatrist, in a study of 100 long-term users attending an outpatient mental health clinic in the Canary Islands,[8] the SDS was found to be 97.9% sensitive and 94.5% specific for dependence, using a threshold where a score of 7 or over was positive. These figures give the probabilities shown in Table 51.1.

The Severity of Dependence Scale (SDS)[9] (reproduced with permission of Blackwell Publishing)

In the last month:

1. did you think your use of tranquillisers was out of control?

2. did the prospect of missing a dose make you anxious or worried?

3. did you worry about your use of tranquillisers?

4. did you wish to stop?

5. how difficult would you find it to stop or go without your tranquillisers?

Scoring:

Score up to 3 for each question as follows:

- 'never'/'almost never' = 0
- 'sometimes' = 1
- 'often' = 2
- 'always'/'almost always' = 3.

For question 5, the corresponding answers are 'not difficult' = 0, 'quite difficult' = 1, 'very difficult' = 2, impossible' = 3.

A score of 7 or over is a positive result.

Even if a GP decides not to use the SDS formally, it is a useful guide to the sort of questions that are likely to reveal unsuspected dependence.

Confirming the diagnosis

Ask the patient about their relationship to the benzodiazepine along the lines of the definitions of dependence (above). Questions that ask about specific details rather than about general concepts are more likely to yield meaningful answers. For instance, ask 'Do you think about the medication at times in the day other than when you take it?' rather than 'Do you think you are psychologically dependent on the drug?'

The Benzodiazepine Dependence Self-Report Questionnaire has divided these questions into four categories:

- problematic use (e.g. 'Do you think the medication is destroying your life?')
- preoccupation (e.g. 'Do you feel safer when you have your medication with you?')
- lack of compliance (e.g. 'Do you ever take more medication than is written on the label?')
- withdrawal (e.g. 'Do you feel irritable or restless when you use less medication or stop?').

The full questionnaire asks 20 questions and has been validated.[10] It can be found on http://baserv.uci.kun.nl/~kan/Bendep-SRQ.html.

Confirmation of the diagnosis of dependence allows the GP to tailor the withdrawal programme to the patient.

Table 51.1 Value of the SDS in the diagnosis of dependence in a benzodiazepine user

Probability before the assessment	SDS score	Likelihood ratio (95% CI)	Probability of dependence after the assessment
50%	≥7	18 (5.6–56)	95%
	<7	0.02 (0.0–0.15)	2%

Follow each row from left to right to see how the SDS alters the probability of dependence in a benzodiazepine user.

Example

A 45-year-old woman has been taking nitrazepam 10 mg at night for 7 years, starting after a bereavement. She resists any suggestion that she try to sleep without it. On questioning, according to the SDS, she scores 7. She admits that the prospect of missing a dose would always worry her (3) and that she would find it very difficult to stop (3). She knows this because she has tried to do without it because she thought that being on a sedative for so long was bad for her (1).

The positive SDS raises her probability of dependence from a baseline of 50% to 95%.

(Fig. 51.1). Armed with this understanding, the GP says it would be unusual if she were able to stop without any adverse effects; that it is not her fault; and that very slow reduction will make coming off the nitrazepam possible, and indeed easier now than later. Reassured by this supportive approach, the patient admits that, when especially tense, she has taken extra doses of nitrazepam and then suffered insomnia and agitation the next day when she has had to go without.

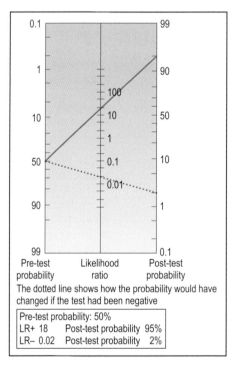

The dotted line shows how the probability would have changed if the test had been negative

Pre-test probability: 50%	
LR+ 18	Post-test probability 95%
LR– 0.02	Post-test probability 2%

Figure 51.1 The probability of benzodiazepine dependence according to the response to the SDS where the initial probability of dependence is 50%.[8]

REFERENCES

1. de las Cuevas C, Sanz E, de la Fuente L. *Benzodiazepines: more 'behavioural' addiction than dependence.* Psychopharmacology 2003;167: 297–303.

2. Kan C, Breteler M, Zitman F. *High prevalence of benzodiazepine dependence in out-patient users, based on the DSM-III-R and ICD-10 criteria.* Acta Psychiatr Scand 1997;96:85–93.

3. Lyndon R, Russell J. *Benzodiazepine use in a rural general practice population.* Aust N Z J Psychiatry 1988;22:293–298.

4. Anthony J, Warner L, Kessler R. *Comparative epidemiology of dependence on tobacco, alcohol, controlled substances, and inhalants: basic findings from the National Comorbidity Survey.*

Exp Clin Psychopharmacol 1994;2: 1–24.

5. WHO. *International statistical classification of diseases and related health problems,10th revision.* Geneva: World Health Organization, 2003. Online. Available: www.who.int.en (search on 'ICD 10').

6. WHO. *The ICD-10 classification of mental and behavioural disorders: diagnostic criteria for research.* Geneva: World Health Organization, 1993.

7. Kan C, Hilberink S, Breteler M. *Determination of the main risk factors for benzodiazepine dependence using a multivariate and multidimensional approach.* Compr Psychiatry 2004; 45:88–94.

8. de las Cuevas C, Sanz E, de la Fuente J, et al. *The Severity of Dependence Scale (SDS) as screening test for benzodiazepine dependence: SDS validation study.* Addiction 2000;95: 245–250.

9. Gossop M, Darke S, Griffiths P, et al. *The Severity of Dependence Scale (SDS): psychometric properties of the SDS in English and Australian samples of heroin, cocaine and amphetamine users.* Addiction 1995;90:607–614.

10. Kan C, Breteler M, van der Ven A, et al. *Cross-validation of the benzodiazepine dependence self-report questionnaire in outpatient benzodiazepine users.* Compr Psychiatry 2001;42:433–439.

52

Chronic fatigue syndrome

- The diagnosis of chronic fatigue syndrome (CFS) should be a positive one based on the characteristic symptoms, with the exclusion of other disorders as a necessary, but not defining, condition.
- Of those symptoms, the most characteristic is fatigability: that is, not just tiredness but a prolonged increase in exhaustion which occurs *after* mental or physical exertion, usually with a delay between the exertion and the onset of exhaustion.

- The fatigue affects the whole body, with both physical and mental manifestations. A less global picture is unlikely to be CFS.
- Although a final diagnosis cannot, by definition, be made until symptoms have been present for 6 months, a working diagnosis of CFS should be made much earlier, say at 6 to 12 weeks.[1] Other disorders should have been excluded by the 6-week stage.

A PRACTICAL APPROACH

- ★ Consider the diagnosis in a patient complaining of fatigue, including those with intermittent problems with cognitive function, apparent recurrent upper respiratory infections or numerous new autonomic complaints such as irritable bowel and irritable bladder syndromes.
- ★ Ask systematically about all features of the syndrome, along the lines of the Canadian Working Case Definition.
- ★ Check for evidence of another mental or physical disorder that would better explain the symptoms or which might coexist.

- ★ In the absence of clues to an alternative diagnosis, perform a small battery of tests. Avoid further investigations unless there is clear justification for them.
- ★ Refer to a physician with a special interest in CFS those in whom the diagnosis is in doubt or who are unable to accept the diagnosis without a specialist opinion.

Prevalence

The point prevalence in a primary care population in the UK using the Oxford criteria below is 0.6% (95% CI 0.2 to 1.5).[2]

Defining CFS

There are five main operational definitions of CFS.[3] Two are described here:

1. *The Oxford criteria*[4] are that CFS is present if the patient has severe disabling fatigue affecting both mental and physical functioning which has not always been present but which has been present for at least 6 months. There should be no known physical cause, and psychosis, bipolar affective disorder, eating disorder and organic brain disease must have been excluded.

2. *The Canadian Working Case Definition.*[5] This is the only definition intended for clinical, rather than research, use:

Essential criteria:

- *Fatigue*, which may be physical and/or mental; must be new; and must be bad enough to reduce the patient's activity by at least 50%.

- *Post-exertional malaise and/or fatigue.* The crucial point is the patient's muscular and/or mental fatigability with delayed recovery, often over more than 24 hours. The deterioration may occur some hours after the exertion.

- *Two or more neurological/cognitive manifestations*: confusion; impaired concentration and short-term memory; disorientation; difficulty with processing information, categorising and word retrieval; perceptual and sensory disturbances, e.g. spatial instability and disorientation and inability to focus vision. Other manifestations are ataxia, muscle weakness and fasciculation, and overload phenomena, e.g. photophobia, hypersensitivity to noise, emotional overload.

- *At least one symptom from two of the following three categories*:

1. *Autonomic manifestations*: orthostatic hypotension and/or tachycardia; light-headedness; extreme pallor; nausea and irritable bowel syndrome; irritable bladder syndrome; palpitations; exertional dyspnoea.

2. *Neuroendocrine manifestations*: loss of thermostatic stability; intolerance of extremes of heat and cold; loss or increase of appetite and/or weight; worsening of symptoms with stress.

3. *Immune manifestations*: tender lymph nodes; recurrent sore throat; recurrent flu-like symptoms; general malaise; new sensitivities to food, medication and/or chemicals.

- It should have been present for at least 6 months, usually has a discrete onset and is not due to another disease.

Almost always present:

- *Sleep dysfunction*; it may be unrefreshing with altered diurnal rhythm and be reduced or increased in amount.

- *Pain* in joints or muscles or headaches.

Note: This summary omits some details of the definition, for which it is necessary to consult the original article.

Note that these are operational criteria; that is, they enable patients, clinicians and researchers to talk about a group of patients who meet these criteria, without any assumption that CFS exists as a single disease rather than as a group of symptoms. It is not possible to assess their reliability since no gold standard exists for the diagnosis.

History, examination and investigations

* Check the history to see if the patient meets the above criteria. The key feature in the history is not just that the patient feels tired but that the tiredness worsens excessively after minimal physical or mental exertion.[6] The delay between the exertion and the worsening of symptoms is characteristic[1] and may be as long as 24 hours.

* Check clinically for a physical disorder which would exclude the diagnosis of CFS. A routine physical examination is unlikely to be helpful if the history has not provided any clues. The yield in one study of fatigue was 2%.[7,8] Examination for thyroid disease and neurological disorders might occasionally prove useful.

* Check the history, looking for a definite psychiatric diagnosis which would exclude the diagnosis of CFS. Note, however, that a psychiatric disorder may exist alongside CFS.

* Check the following investigations, if they have not already been done:[9]
   - full blood count, erythrocyte sedimentation rate
   - liver function tests, urea and electrolytes
   - thyroid stimulating hormone, creatine kinase
   - urine protein and sugar.

* The UK Royal Colleges warn against further investigation which is likely to be fruitless and which will delay the negotiation of a management plan. However, it would not be excessive to check, in addition, calcium, phosphate, magnesium, anti-nuclear antibodies

(ANA), rheumatoid factor (RF) and ferritin.[5] The yield from laboratory investigations is unlikely to be high: 5%,[7] 8%,[10] 9%.[11]

* Refer for specialist investigation if the examination suggests the possibility of an alternative diagnosis, e.g. if there are neurological symptoms or signs that are fixed, or there is a history of a tick bite or of exposure to TB. A sleep study may be needed if there is a history of waking in the morning with the bed clothes in a mess, or a partner reports episodes of apnoea (see *Obstructive sleep apnoea*, p. 439).

Conditions to bear in mind when conducting the above clinical examination and investigations

■ *Endocrine disorders*: Addison's disease, Cushing's syndrome, thyroid disorders, diabetes

■ *Haematological disorders*: anaemia, iron deficiency or iron overload

■ *Neurological disorders*: multiple sclerosis, Parkinson's disease, myasthenia gravis, B_{12} deficiency

■ *Rheumatological disorders*: rheumatoid arthritis, polymyalgia rheumatica, fibromyalgia

■ *Infectious diseases*: AIDS, TB, chronic hepatitis, Lyme disease

■ *Others*: cancer; obstructive sleep apnoea.

Characteristic symptoms which permit a positive early working diagnosis of CFS[1,5]

1. *Fatigue.* Patients may feel tired all the time or have recurrent bouts of fatigue. Compare the patient's activity level to what was normal for them before the illness.

2. *Post-exertional fatigue or malaise.* The most characteristic feature of the condition is the worsening of mental and/or physical fatigue after exertion, including mental exertion. As well as fatigue, flu-like symptoms may follow exertion. The exacerbation may not start until the next day and usually lasts at least 24 hours.

3. *Cognitive impairment.* This may take the form of poor concentration, reduced attention span, impaired short-term memory, difficulty remembering words, inability to organise thoughts and spatial disorientation. It will tend to worsen when concentrating for more than a short while, for instance during the clinical interview. Patients report visual disturbances, especially loss of depth perception, difficulty focusing and even inability to make sense of more than one portion of the visual field at a time.

4. *Overload phenomena* occur. Patients may be hypersensitive to light or sound or other sensory input. They may not be able to hear conversation because they cannot blank out background noise. They can only cope with one thought at a time and easily become emotionally overloaded. Overload can lead to a 'crash' in which they may be unable to think or move or speak.

5. *Motor impairment.* Patients may become clumsy, or ataxic, with specific muscle weaknesses. Balance may be poor and true vertigo may occur. They may lose their ability to perform skilled tasks, for instance brushing their teeth.

6. *Pain* may be felt in the muscles, joints or head. It may have a neuropathic quality. It often follows no anatomical pattern, giving rise to the erroneous diagnosis that it is psychogenic; 75% have muscular tender points characteristic of fibromyalgia.

7. *Sleep* is disturbed in 95% of patients. Sleep is unrefreshing, the normal sleep rhythm is disturbed and patients may sleep more or less than before they became ill.

8. *Orthostatic intolerance.* Hypotension (a fall of >20 mmHg systolic pressure) and tachycardia (>120 beats per minute) may occur on standing. Often they only occur after the patient has been standing for at least 10 minutes (i.e. the autonomic nervous system fatigues).

9. *Temperature control* may be impaired. The body temperature may fluctuate during the day and, after exertion, may go down rather than up. The patient may feel inappropriately hot, or cold; one part of the body may feel hot while another part feels cold, in a way that cannot be explained anatomically.

10. *Recurrent sore throat* is common with lymphadenopathy and flu-like symptoms. The throat may feel sore but the throat looks normal.

11. *Gastrointestinal disturbances*: the patient suffers from nausea, anorexia, abdominal distension or cramps, excessive wind and constipation.

12. *Intolerance* to alcohol, certain foods and some medications including immunisations.

The Canadian Expert Medical Consensus Panel makes the further point that the diagnosis is best arrived at, not by seeing whether the patient fits a template, but by understanding the complex whole of the patient's symptoms as they vary from day to day and month to month. If there is an overall coherent pattern that is characteristic of CFS, the diagnosis is very likely. In the absence of such coherence, the diagnosis is in doubt.

Patients with CFS are more likely to suffer from certain other conditions than the general population. Their presence should not be allowed to hide the fact that the patient also has CFS. They are:

■ fibromyalgia: approximately 75% of patients with CFS meet the criteria for fibromyalgia as well[5]

■ psychiatric disorders: depression, anxiety, and somatisation disorder.

Does a history of severe infection at the onset of the illness increase the probability that the patient has chronic fatigue syndrome?

Yes. A study from Australia has shown that a cohort of patients infected with Epstein–Barr virus, *Coxiella burnetii* or Ross River virus had a prevalence of chronic fatigue syndrome 6 months later of 11%.[12] The risk of developing the syndrome was related to the severity of the original illness and not to one or other organism. The authors suggest that the same will be found to apply to infection with other organisms as further research is reported.

REFERENCES

1. Working Group on CFS/ME. *A report to the Chief Medical Officer of an independent working group.* London: Department of Health, 2002:1–82.

2. Lawrie SM, Pelosi AJ. *Chronic fatigue syndrome in the community: prevalence and associations.* Br J Psychiatry 1995;166:793–797.

3. Mulrow CD, Ramirez G, Cornell JE, Allsup K. *Defining and managing chronic fatigue syndrome: Agency for Healthcare Research and Quality,* 2001. Online. Available: www.ahrq.gov.

4. Sharpe M, Archand L, Banatvala J. *Chronic fatigue syndrome: guidelines for research.* J R Soc Med 1991;84:118–121.

5. Carruthers B, Jain A, De Meirleir K, et al. *Myalgic encephalomyelitis/ chronic fatigue syndrome: clinical*

working case definition, diagnostic and treatment protocols. J Chronic Fatigue Syndr 2003;11:7–115.

6. Wessely S. *Chronic fatigue: symptom and syndrome.* Ann Intern Med 2001;134(9 part 2 Suppl): 838–843.

7. Ebell M. *What is a reasonable initial approach to the patient with fatigue?* J Fam Pract 2001;50:16; discussion 16–17.

8. Lane TJ, Matthews DA, Manu P. *The low yield of physical examinations and laboratory investigations of patients with chronic fatigue.* Am J Med Sci 1990;299(5):313–318.

9. UK Royal Colleges. *Chronic fatigue syndrome: report of a joint working group of the Royal Colleges of Physicians, Psychiatrists and General*

Practitioners. London: Royal College of Physicians, Royal College of Psychiatrists, Royal College of General Practitioners, 1996.

10. Sugarman JR, Berg AO. *Evaluation of fatigue in a family practice.* J Fam Pract 1984;19(5):643–647.

11. Ridsdale L, Evans A, Jerrett W, et al. *Patients with fatigue in general practice: a prospective study.* BMJ 1993;307:103–106.

12. Hickie I, Davenport TA, Wakefield D, et al. *Post-infective and chronic fatigue syndromes precipitated by viral and non-viral pathogens: prospective cohort study.* BMJ 2006;333:575–578.

Chronic obstructive pulmonary disease (COPD)

53

KEY FACTS

- Symptoms are neither sensitive nor specific for the diagnosis of COPD.
- Examination is likely to be normal in all but advanced cases.
- Peak flow testing will miss 1 in 10 cases and overdiagnose COPD even more often.

- Spirometry, including measurement of the FEV_1/FVC, is needed in those in whom the suspicion of COPD is raised, either by early symptoms or by a history of smoking.

A PRACTICAL APPROACH

- Suspect the diagnosis in anyone with dyspnoea and/or productive cough whose symptoms began after the age of 45, do not show much variability, and who has a history of smoking.
- Check for signs that support the diagnosis: wheeze, an over-inflated chest, a maximum laryngeal height ≤4 cm.

- Confirm it with spirometry: a FEV_1/FVC <70% with less than 15% reversibility.
- If the diagnosis is confirmed, check haemoglobin and body mass index and check the chest X-ray to exclude other pathologies.

Definition

Chronic obstructive pulmonary disease is a chronic, slowly progressive disorder characterised by airways obstruction (FEV_1 <80% predicted and FEV_1/FVC <70%) which does not change markedly over several months. The obstruction is largely fixed although there may be a reversible component.[1]

Prevalence

Prevalence is 4% (3% chronic bronchitis, 1% emphysema).[2] For smokers, the risk of developing COPD over 25 years is 35%, with 25% having clinically significant disease.[3] Heavier smokers carry the greater risk; in those who quit, it is reduced. For non-smokers, aged 30 to 60, the risk of any COPD over 25 years of follow-up is 4%.

The diagnostic problems

- Clinical diagnosis is unreliable. In a study from Spain, 172 patients with suspected COPD were examined in a pulmonary clinic. The clinical impression of the specialist missed 17% of cases (as defined by lung function tests) and overdiagnosed 19% (sensitivity 83%, specificity 81%; LR+ 4.3, LR– 0.2). Junior doctors tended to perform even worse although the difference was not statistically significant.[4]

• Symptoms suggest the possibility of COPD but are not sufficiently specific to confirm it, nor sensitive enough not to miss it. The symptom-based definition of COPD ('cough and sputum for at least 3 months of 2 consecutive years in the absence of other diseases'[5]) includes too many patients with no evidence of airways obstruction; and it is airways obstruction, not sputum production, that is associated with mortality.[1]

• Different physicians vary in their interpretation of signs (i.e. precision is poor). In a study from Colorado,[6] only moderate agreement was found between four physicians in judging whether patients had an increased percussion note (kappa (κ) = 0.31), cardiac dullness (κ = 0.49) and reduced breath sounds (κ = 0.47), although agreement was better on whether wheezes were present (κ = 0.69).

• Symptoms, signs and abnormal lung function tests are most likely to be present in patients with moderate to severe disease – the very group in whom the diagnosis is most obvious. In mild cases, the sensitivity of the signs and symptoms and lung function tests will be less than stated.

• At the severe end of the spectrum, while it will be obvious that the patient has airways obstruction, the distinction based on symptoms and signs between chronic asthma and COPD may be hard.

History and examination

Accuracy of the diagnosis of COPD from the history

Factors in the history which raise the possibility of COPD are:

■ regular sputum production
■ cough
■ dyspnoea
■ wheeze
■ recurrent respiratory infections
■ a smoking history
■ older age.

However, questioning along these lines is neither sensitive nor specific for COPD. A study in Belgian primary care found that a questionnaire designed to detect COPD administered to patients aged 35–70 was only 58% sensitive and 78% specific.[7] The questionnaire asked about cough, dyspnoea, wheeze and nasal allergy, currently or in the last year.

These results gave an LR+ of 2.7 (95% CI 2.4 to 3.1), which only raised the probability of COPD if

positive from 7% to 18%. The LR– was 0.5 (95% CI 0.5 to 0.6), which only reduced the probability to 4%. More sophisticated questioning is needed.

More detailed studies have derived likelihood ratios for individual factors in the history (Tables 53.1 and 53.2). Table 53.1 shows that a history of prolonged heavy smoking is paramount and that daily production of a substantial amount of sputum is also useful (as is the fact that the patient thinks he or she has COPD). However, the absence of any one of these factors is not very useful in arguing against the diagnosis.

The accuracy of the diagnosis of COPD from the examination

The examination in mild COPD is usually normal. The most specific signs (wheeze, decreased cardiac dullness, hyper-resonance) are usually absent. More advanced cases are more likely to have signs. The most advanced cases present a spectrum of signs with *blue bloaters* (cyanosed, not particularly breathless, with cor pulmonale) at one end and *pink puffers* (thin, breathless but with normal arterial oxygen tension) at the other. The clinical picture of a breathless patient with a hyperinflated chest who breathes through pursed lips, using the accessory muscles of respiration, with wheeze or with an ominously silent chest, is striking but is found in a minority of those with COPD (Table 53.3).

How to combine predictive factors from the history and examination

An international study of 309 patients with and without COPD gave the following statistics which were not dependent on setting (primary, secondary or tertiary care).[8] The gold standard for the diagnosis was FEV_1 and FEV_1/FVC ratio both less than the 5th centile. Using other lung function definitions made little difference to the results. Likelihood ratios (LRs) were adjusted for confounding from related diagnostic elements.

The presence of four factors:

■ age ≥45
■ patient thinks COPD is present
■ smoker of >40 pack years, and
■ maximum laryngeal height ≤4 cm

Table 53.1 The value of factors in the history that have been found to be predictive of the diagnosis of COPD (in order of the value of the LR+) based on a pre-test probability of 4%

Factor in the history	Presence	Likelihood ratio (95% CI)	Probability of COPD
Smokers of >70 pack years*[6]	Present	8.0 (2.5–25)	25%
	Absent	0.6 (0.4–0.9)	2%
Self-reported history of COPD[8]	Present	7.3	23%
	Absent	0.5	2%
Sputum production of ≥1/4 cupful a day[6]	Present	4.0 (1.9–8.3)	14%
	Absent	0.8 (0.7–0.96)	3%
Male sex[8]	Present	1.3 (1.1–1.6)	5%
	Absent	0.7 (0.6–0.9)	3%
Age ≥45[8]	Present	1.3	5%
	Absent	0.4	2%
Smokers who have smoked for at least a year[8]	Present	1.2 (1.0–1.5)	5%
	Absent	0.7 (0.5 to 0.9)	3%

Follow each row from left to right to see how the presence or absence of the factor alters the probability of COPD. Those likelihood ratios without confidence intervals are the result of multivariate analysis.
*A pack year is 20 cigarettes smoked each day for 1 year.

Table 53.2 Symptoms associated with airways obstruction (although not necessarily distinguishing COPD from asthma) based on a pre-test probability of 4%

Symptom	Presence	Likelihood ratio (95% CI)	Probability of COPD
Exertional dyspnoea[9]	Present	2.2	8%
	Absent	0.8	3%
Any dyspnoea[9]	Present	1.2	5%
	Absent	0.5	2%
Cough[9]	Present	1.8	7%
	Absent	0.7	3%

Follow each row from left to right to see how the presence or absence of the factor alters the probability of COPD.

gave an LR+ of 220 and an LR– of 0.1. This would change the probability of COPD from the population baseline of 4% to 90% if all four factors were present and reduce it to 0.4% if all were absent.

In that study, other features of the history and examination (gender, wheezing) were statistically significant in distinguishing COPD from other patients but not clinically useful, having unadjusted LRs of 1.3 and 0.7 (male and female) and 2.7 and 0.7 (wheezing present and absent).

A later study from the same group has refined the factors that contribute independently to the diagnosis of COPD down to three (Table 53.4).[10]

Table 53.3 Signs which suggest airways obstruction based on a hypothetical probability of 50% arrived at from the history

Sign	Presence	Likelihood ratio	Probability of COPD
Wheeze[8,9]	Present	36	97%
	Absent	0.8	44%
Decreased cardiac dullness[9]	Present	10	91%
	Absent	0.9	47%
Hyper-resonance[9]	Present	4.8	83%
	Absent	0.7	41%
Paradoxical movement of the lateral rib margin[4]	Present	4.1	80%
	Absent	0.5	33%
Decreased breath sounds[9]	Present	3.7	79%
	Absent	0.7	41%
Maximum laryngeal height ≤4 cm*[8]	Present	2.8	74%
	Absent	0.8	44%

Follow each row from left to right to see how the presence or absence of the sign alters the probability of COPD.
*Maximum laryngeal height is measured from the suprasternal notch to the top of the thyroid cartilage at the end of expiration.

Table 53.4 Factors contributing to the diagnosis of COPD on multivariate analysis

Factor	Adjusted LR+	Adjusted LR–
FET* ≥9 seconds	4.6	0.8
Self-reported history of COPD	4.4	0.5
Wheezing	2.9	0.8
All three present	59	0.3†

*Forced expiratory time.
†All three factors absent.

Lung function tests

- Spirometric values are part of the definition of COPD; yet they are abnormal in asthma and normal in some patients with early COPD. Their positive and negative likelihood ratios have been estimated at no higher than 5 and no lower than 0.6 respectively.[2] Distinguishing COPD from asthma also requires a consideration of the clinical features (Table 53.5).
- Spirometry by GPs can detect early COPD. A study in Belgium of 3158 patients aged 35 to 70 found that 7.4% of them, not known to have respiratory disease, had COPD defined by a FEV_1/FVC <88.5% of predicted value in men or <89.3% in women.[7]
- Reversibility testing and tests of bronchial hyper-responsiveness are needed to distinguish COPD from asthma. A study of patients aged 50 and over in London with a diagnosis of asthma in general practice found that a third of them had COPD;[12] that is, they had airways obstruction which did not achieve 15% improvement following nebulised salbutamol (see *Asthma*, p. 337).

Table 53.5 Clinical features that help to distinguish COPD from asthma[11]

Feature	COPD	Asthma
Age at onset	Almost always >45	Any age from childhood onwards
Time course	Slowly progressive	Sudden onset, episodic
History of atopy	Not necessarily	Often
Smoking history	Almost always	Not necessarily
Regular productive cough	Almost always	Usually not
Level of breathlessness	Constant	Variable
Woken at night by symptoms	Uncommon	Common

- Spirometry must include the FEV_1/FVC. The distinction between restrictive and obstructive defects can be missed by the FEV_1 alone.[13]
- The peak expiratory flow rate (PEFR) is not sufficient for the diagnosis of COPD. Spirometry detects the collapse of small airways while the PEFR measures the calibre of large airways. Data from the NHANES III study show that PEFR is only 89% sensitive and 76% specific for the diagnosis of COPD made by spirometry.[14] That the PEFR is inadequate in the diagnosis of COPD appears to be borne out by the Colorado study which found that adding a peak flow reading, with a cut-off of 200 L/min, did not improve the accuracy of the diagnosis of COPD (defined by spirometry) over history and examination.[6]

Further investigations are recommended at the time of initial diagnosis,[11] although their value has not been formally assessed:

- Chest X-ray to exclude other pathologies
- Haemoglobin for anaemia or polycythaemia
- Body mass index
- α_1-Antitrypsin level in those with COPD under age 45, especially if they are non-smokers or have a strong family history. A level <15–20% of the normal limits is highly suggestive of homozygous α_1-antitrypsin deficiency.[15]

Example

A 60-year-old male smoker of a pack a day with a history of productive cough for >5 years has noticed that he is breathless on exertion. As an older man with a smoking history, his initial probability of COPD is, say, 20%, based on the lifetime prevalence of smokers. A similar result would be reached by applying sequentially the small likelihood ratios for age, sex and smoking to the population prevalence of 4%. The probability rises to 35% because of the exertional dyspnoea (Fig. 53.1) and then to 49% because of the cough (Fig. 53.2). Examination is normal. At a relatively early stage of the disease, this does not reduce the probability. His FEV_1/FVC is 55–60% on three attempts, confirming airways obstruction. This raises the probability of COPD to 83% (Fig. 53.3). The GP considers that this establishes the diagnosis of COPD. With no hint of variability from the history, it would be justified not to perform reversibility testing in order to establish the diagnosis, although it might be useful in deciding on management.

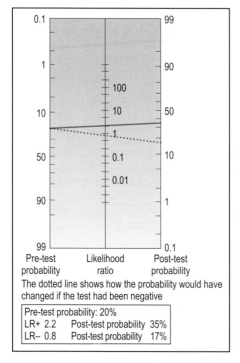

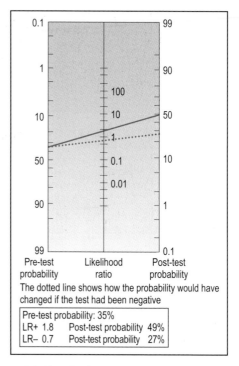

Figure 53.1 Alteration in the probability of COPD because of exertional dyspnoea in the example on p. 358.

Figure 53.2 Alteration in the probability of COPD because of the presence of cough (without copious sputum) in the example on p. 358.

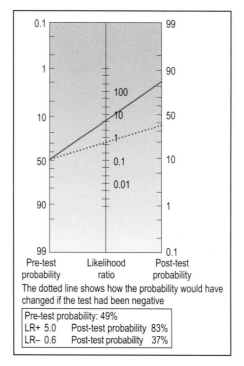

Figure 53.3 Alteration in the probability of COPD as a result of the FEV$_1$/FVC in the example on p. 358.

REFERENCES

1. The COPD Guidelines Group. *BTS guidelines for the management of chronic obstructive pulmonary disease.* Thorax 1997;52:Suppl 5.

2. Tan C, Mayewski R. *Chronic obstructive lung disease.* In: Black E, Bordley D, Tape TG, Panzer RJ, eds. Diagnostic strategies for common medical problems. Philadelphia: American College of Physicians, 1999:360–368.

3. Lokke A, Lange P, Scharling H, et al. *Developing COPD: a 25 year follow up study of the general population.* Thorax 2006;61:935–939.

4. Garcia-Pachon E. *Paradoxical movement of the lateral rib margin (Hoover sign) for detecting obstructive airways disease.* Chest 2002;122:651–655.

5. Medical Research Council. *Definition and classification of chronic bronchitis for clinical and epidemiological purposes.* Lancet 1965;1:775–779.

6. Badgett R, Tanaka D, Hunt D, et al. *Can moderate chronic obstructive pulmonary disease be diagnosed by historical and physical findings alone?* Am J Med 1993;94:188–196.

7. Buffels J, Degryse J, Heyrman J, Decramer M. *Office spirometry significantly improves early detection of COPD in general practice.* Chest 2004;125:1394–1399.

8. Straus S, McAlister F, Sackett D, et al. *The accuracy of patient history, wheezing, and laryngeal measurements in diagnosing obstructive airways disease.* JAMA 2000;283:1853–1857.

9. Holleman D, Simel D. *Does the clinical examination predict airflow limitation?* JAMA 1995;273:313–319.

10. Straus S, McAlister F, Sackett D, et al. *Accuracy of history, wheezing, and forced expiratory time in the diagnosis of chronic obstructive pulmonary disease.* J Gen Intern Med 2002;17:684–688.

11. National Institute for Clinical Excellence. *Chronic obstructive pulmonary disease.* Thorax 2004;59 (Suppl 1):1–232.

12. Griffiths C, Feder G, Wedzicha J, et al. *Feasibility of spirometry and reversibility testing for the identification of patients with chronic obstructive pulmonary disease on asthma registers in general practice.* Respir Med 1999;93:903–908.

13. Chavannes N. *The necessity for spirometry in the primary care management of COPD.* Prim Care Respir J 2004;13:11–14.

14. Jackson H, Hubbard R. *Detecting chronic obstructive pulmonary disease using peak flow rate: cross sectional survey.* BMJ 2003;327:653–654.

15. American Thoracic Society. *Standards for the diagnosis and management of patients with COPD.* American Thoracic Society, 2004.

Coeliac disease in adults (gluten intolerance) | 54

- Coeliac disease is largely undiagnosed because of the non-specific nature of the symptoms.
- Serological tests are extraordinarily accurate; but, in a person whose risk of coeliac disease is no higher than the population average, a positive test still means that the person probably does not have coeliac disease.

A PRACTICAL APPROACH

- Perform serological tests in patients:
  - (a) with suggestive symptoms: fatigue, weight loss, diarrhoea; or
  - (b) with otherwise unexplained findings of anaemia, malabsorption, osteoporosis or osteomalacia; or
  - (c) with a family history of coeliac disease.
- Be alert to the possibility of coeliac disease in patients with insulin-dependent diabetes and thyroid disease – conditions in which the incidence of coeliac disease is thought to be raised.
- Refer all those with positive serology to a gastroenterologist.
- If there is any delay in the patient being seen, check full blood count, B_{12}, ferritin, serum albumin, calcium, alkaline phosphatase, and a dual energy X-ray absorptiometry (DEXA) bone scan.

Prevalence

The prevalence in the UK is 1 in 300 (0.3%).[1] However, screening populations with highly sensitive serological tests has produced higher figures for Finland (2.5%; although only 0.5% of the population are diagnosed) and the USA (1%; where only 0.05% of the population are diagnosed).[2] Even within Europe, the prevalence varies using modern serological tests, being as low as 0.5% in Germany, where <0.1% of the population are diagnosed.[2]

The problem with diagnosis prompted by symptoms

Fatigue is reported in 80–90% and diarrhoea in 75–80% of adults with untreated coeliac disease.[1] Weight loss is common. Less common symptoms are reduced fertility, ataxia or symptoms related to osteoporosis.

The problems are 2-fold:
- in many patients, symptoms are too mild for them to present
- if they do present, no symptom is specific (see *Fatigue*, p. 110 and *Diarrhoea*, p. 58).

In a UK primary care study from Oxfordshire,[3] only 30 out of 1000 patients with reason to suspect coeliac disease were found to have the condition (Table 54.1). Furthermore, it is likely that most of those 30 would not have been diagnosed had they not been part of the study. Only 1 in 6 with the condition presented with gastrointestinal symptoms.

The problem with diagnosis prompted by presence of related diseases

Coeliac disease has been reported to have a prevalence of 6–8% in insulin-dependent diabetes and a lesser, but raised, prevalence in thyroid disease.[4] However, the Oxfordshire study found only one case out of 157 with diabetes or thyroid disease, which is not significantly above the prevalence in the general population.

Signs

There are none.

Investigations

■ *Endomysial antibodies (EMA).* Modern refinements have improved hugely on older versions of the tests and a meta-analysis has now found that it has a sensitivity of 97% and a specificity of 99%.[5] These give the extraordinarily useful likelihood ratios of LR+ 97 and LR– 0.03. The implications of these figures are shown in Table 54.2.

One reason for a false negative test is that it measures IgA and will be falsely negative in the 2% of the UK population who are IgA deficient. These figures are, however, not totally robust. Including patients with milder histological grades of coeliac disease would result in lower sensitivity.

■ *Tissue transglutaminase antibody (tTGA) test* is an alternative test which can be performed on IgA or IgG. The IgA version has no advantage over the EMA and there is no advantage in performing both. The IgG version would be useful in a patient known to have IgA deficiency.

■ *Intestinal biopsy.* Refer every patient in whom the diagnosis is suspected for consideration of whether biopsy is needed.

Table 54.1 Main grounds for testing for coeliac disease in the Oxfordshire study[3]

Grounds	Number of patients	Percentage with coeliac disease	95% confidence interval
Anaemia	125	12%	6–18%
Family history of coeliac disease	28	7%	0–17%
Malabsorption or diarrhoea	93	5%	1–10%
Chronic fatigue	329	1.8%	0.4–3.3%
A diagnosis of irritable bowel syndrome	132	0%	0–3%

Table 54.2 Value of the EMA in the diagnosis of coeliac disease according to the patient's pre-test risk

Patient's clinical picture	Probability before the assessment	EMA result	Likelihood ratio	Probability of coeliac disease
No known risk or symptoms	0.3%	Positive	97	23%
		Negative	0.03	<0.1%
Modest risk of coeliac disease because of anaemia	12%	Positive	97	93%
		Negative	0.03	0.4%

Follow each row from left to right to see how the EMA result alters the probability of coeliac disease.

■ *Investigations for nutritional deficiencies.* Full blood count, B_{12}, ferritin, serum albumin, calcium, alkaline phosphatase and DEXA bone scan. Iron and/or folate deficiency is present in 85%. Osteoporosis is common in longstanding cases and osteomalacia is not rare.

Complicating conditions

■ Dermatitis herpetiformis (an itchy blistering rash) complicates 2–5% of cases of coeliac disease.

■ Small bowel lymphoma is a complication and the risk of carcinoma of the small bowel, colorectum and oesophagus is increased.[1] Overall the risk of malignancy is five times that of the general population. Once the patient has been on a gluten-free diet for 5 years, the excess risk has disappeared.[4]

Example

A woman aged 55 falls and breaks her hip. She consults her GP following discharge from hospital. He arranges a bone density scan which shows severe osteoporosis. She has no risk factors for osteoporosis, other than being 3 years postmenopausal, and the GP orders further investigations. All are normal except her EMA which is positive.

The GP assesses the probability of this being coeliac disease. On questioning, the patient admits to tiredness but to no other symptoms. The GP does not consider that this alters the probabilities. The screen for nutritional deficiencies (above) is negative.

He cannot see how coeliac disease, if present, could cause osteoporosis without some other evidence of malabsorption. (In fact his common sense approach is mistaken here; osteoporosis is associated with coeliac disease, but it is not clear that the osteoporosis is always secondary to malabsorption.)

He returns to the predictive value of the EMA. With a population prevalence of 1 in 300 (0.3%), the positive EMA raises this to only 23% (Fig. 54.1).

He explains to her that coeliac disease may, or may not, be the cause of her osteoporosis, and that a specialist opinion, and possibly small bowel biopsy, are needed.

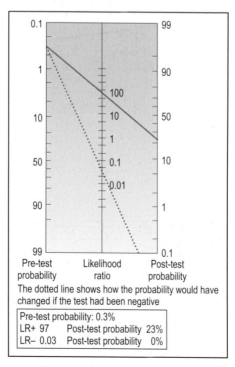

The dotted line shows how the probability would have changed if the test had been negative

Pre-test probability: 0.3%	
LR+ 97	Post-test probability 23%
LR– 0.03	Post-test probability 0%

Figure 54.1 The probability of coeliac disease before and after the EMA in the example above.

REFERENCES

1. British Society of Gastroenterology. *Guidelines for the management of patients with coeliac disease.* London: BSG, 2002. Online. Available: www.bsg.org.uk.

2. Rewers M. *Epidemiology of celiac disease: what are the prevalence, incidence and progression of celiac disease?* Gastroenterology 2005;128(4 Suppl 1):S47–S51.

3. Hin H, Bird G, Fisher P, et al. *Coeliac disease in primary care: case finding study.* BMJ 1999;318:164–167.

4. American Gastroenterological Association. *Medical position statement: celiac sprue.* Gastroenterology 2001;120:1522–1525.

5. Rostom A, Dube C, Cranney A, et al. *The diagnostic accuracy of serological tests for celiac disease: a systematic review.* Gastroenterology 2005;128(4 Suppl 1):S38–S46.

Colorectal carcinoma

KEY FACTS

- Colorectal cancer (CRC) is one of the commoner cancers; yet, in the UK, the patients of a single general practitioner will only develop one new colorectal cancer per year, despite the many patients who will present with lower bowel symptoms.
- Certain risk factors (age, a history of polyp or previous CRC, a family history, longstanding inflammatory bowel disease) increase the probability of CRC.

- Certain symptoms and signs will similarly contribute (altered bowel habit, rectal bleeding, weight loss, abdominal pain, a rectal or abdominal mass).
- A few investigations may be helpful in primary care (a haemoglobin, white cell count and erythrocyte sedimentation rate (ESR)).
- Using the above the GP can divide on a rational basis those who need referral, urgent referral or the offer of 'watchful waiting'.

A PRACTICAL APPROACH

- ★ Make an assessment of colonic symptoms and risk factors according to the risk of colorectal carcinoma attached to each.
- ★ Examine all patients with colonic symptoms for abdominal and rectal masses.
- ★ Check the haemoglobin, white blood cell count (WBC) and ESR in any patient where the results would alter a decision about referral.
- ★ Urgent referral is recommended in the UK for:
  - ■ Age ≥40 with rectal bleeding and altered bowel habit towards looser ± more frequent stool; or
  - ■ Age ≥60 with altered bowel habit towards looser ± more frequent stool; or

- ■ Age ≥60 with rectal bleeding and no anal symptoms; or
- ■ Right-sided lower abdominal mass consistent with bowel involvement; or
- ■ Palpable rectal (not pelvic) mass; or
- ■ Unexplained iron deficiency anaemia with haemoglobin ≤11 g/dl (men) or ≤10 g/dl (non-menstruating women).
- ★ Less urgent referral, or watchful waiting, will be appropriate for those whose symptoms and age carry lower risk.
- ★ Refer more readily the stronger the family history.

Incidence

The annual incidence is 0.05%, i.e. 1 in 2000 (although it varies with country). It is higher in men, in older people and in those with a positive family history, inflammatory bowel disease or untreated coeliac disease. A study from Exeter, UK, calculated that the risk of developing colorectal cancer over a 2-year period was 0.25% of adults aged 40 and over who attended primary care.[1]

The history

Only one study permits an evaluation of all relevant symptoms in the diagnosis of colorectal cancer in primary care. It is a case-control study conducted on patients aged 40 and over, in all 21 practices in Exeter.[1] While it suffers from the main weakness of a case-control study, that data were not collected prospectively, the fact that all cases of colorectal cancer in the area were identified meant that the authors were able to calculate positive likelihood ratios and positive predictive values for the most useful symptoms, signs and investigations. Predictive values are striking lower than in the studies from secondary care that had previously reported on the same symptoms. This is not surprising: GPs were selecting patients to refer to secondary care and those studies were bound to suffer from selection bias. Secondary care studies will therefore only be used in this chapter if they throw light on an issue not covered by the Exeter study.

The five most useful symptoms in the diagnosis of colorectal cancer are shown in Table 55.1.

Other points

- Most *combinations* of symptoms, signs and investigations further increased the risk of cancer but not as much as would be predicted if the post-test probability of cancer for one feature in Table 55.1 were used as the pre-test probability for another feature. The original article gives details of the predictive values for combinations of features.
- The *absence* of a symptom has little effect on the probability of colorectal cancer. This has been shown by studies from secondary care.[2] Negative likelihood ratios are not given in this section, and indeed they could not be calculated in the Exeter study because of its design.
- Increasing age increases the predictive value of almost all symptoms. This is shown in Table 55.2.
- 'Altered bowel habit' was not used as a symptom. A more precise definition (diarrhoea or constipation) is more useful. Altered bowel habit that alternates between firmer and looser, and between less frequent and more frequent stools carries a probability of cancer that is intermediate between the risk for diarrhoea and for constipation.[2,3] (see *Altered bowel habit*, p. 4).
- *Rectal bleeding*. The nature of the rectal bleeding influences the predictive value of the symptom (see *Rectal bleeding*, p. 225). Three specific descriptions are especially suggestive of cancer:
  (a) dark blood rather than bright blood (being less likely to be anal)
  (b) blood mixed with the stool (rather than on its surface or separate from it)
  (c) blood that is mixed with mucus.

Table 55.1 The predictive value of symptoms in the diagnosis of colorectal cancer based on a baseline risk of 0.25%[1]

Symptom	LR+	Probability of cancer
Rectal bleeding	10	2.4%
Weight loss	5.1	1.2%
Abdominal pain	4.4	1.1%
Diarrhoea	3.9	0.94%
Constipation	1.8	0.42%

LR+ = positive likelihood ratio.

Table 55.2 Effect of age on the predictive value of symptoms, signs and investigations[1]

Symptom	Age	Probability of cancer
Rectal bleeding	<70	1.4%
	≥70	4.8%
Weight loss	<70	0.74%
	≥70	2.5%
Abdominal pain	<70	0.65%
	≥70	2.0%
Diarrhoea	<70	0.63%
	≥70	1.7%
Constipation	<70	0.2%
	≥70	1.3%

- A study from Cheshire shows that all three of these are significant pointers towards cancer, although none of them alone is hugely significant (Table 55.3).[2]
- The presence of other pointers in the history increases the probability of colorectal carcinoma: a previous colorectal carcinoma or polyp or a family history (see below).

Significance of a family history of colorectal cancer

Colorectal cancer is so common that many patients with suspicious symptoms will have a family history. Most will have a single first-degree relative who developed cancer over the age of 45. Their risk will, at the most, be doubled. It is only a few who have one of the specific family histories that appreciably increase the risk (Table 55.4).

The patient's risk starts to rise about 10 years before the relative was diagnosed with cancer. Thus a 40-year-old whose sister developed CRC at that age has double the risk of CRC of the general population. The same person whose family history meets the criteria for hereditary non-polyposis colorectal cancer (HNPCC) has a risk that is 10 times that of the general population.

However, no studies have shown whether a family history helps in the assessment of a patient with colonic symptoms. The increase in lifetime risk for that patient may be more than offset by the patient's increased readiness to consult for minor colonic symptoms.

The predictive value of other risk factors for colorectal cancer

Age: rates of colorectal cancer in England and Wales in 1992, stratified by age, were:[5]

- Age <50: 4 per 100 000
- Age 50–69: 100 per 100 000
- Age >70: 300 per 100 000.

Inflammatory bowel disease increases the probability that a patient has colorectal cancer.

Ulcerative colitis (UC) carries a lifetime risk of colorectal cancer (CRC) of 3.7%,[6] which is a little under twice that of the general population. However, it is not the presence of UC but its duration which should influence the assessment of the probability of CRC:

- by 10 years the cumulative risk of CRC is 2%
- by 20 years the cumulative risk of CRC is 8%
- by 30 years the cumulative risk of CRC is 18%.

A person with a 30-year history of the disease therefore has a CRC risk that is nine times that of one with a 10-year history.[6]

However, no study has assessed whether the presentation with symptoms of altered bowel habit or rectal bleeding in a patient with UC is more, or less, likely to be due to cancer than in the general population, since these symptoms also occur in UC itself.

Crohn's disease carries an increased risk of CRC that has been estimated at double[7] and 6-fold[8] by

Table 55.3 The probability of cancer in patients referred to secondary care with colonic symptoms according to their description of the rectal bleeding.[2] The initial probability of cancer in this study was 5%

Symptom	Presence	LR (95% CI)	Probability of cancer
Rectal bleeding (all types)	Present	1.2 (1.1–1.4)	6%
	Absent	0.5 (0.3–0.7)	3%
Blood mixed with stool	Present	2.7 (1.9–3.9)	12%
	Absent	0.8 (0.7–0.9)	4%
Dark blood	Present	2.3 (1.0–5.5)	11%
	Absent	1.0 (0.9–1.0)	5%
Bloodstained mucus	Present	3.6 (2.8–4.7)	16%
	Absent	0.7 (0.6–0.8)	4%

Follow each row from left to right to see how different types of bleeding alter the probability of cancer.

different authors. The same doubt exists about whether the diagnosis of Crohn's disease increases or reduces the risk of CRC in a patient with colonic symptoms.

In *coeliac disease*, the risks of CRC and of small bowel lymphoma are increased, giving an overall cancer risk that is five times that of the population.[9] However, adherence to a gluten-free diet removes this excess risk.

Diabetes is associated with an increased risk of CRC (relative risk 1.3 (95% CI 1.2 to 1.4)), but not enough to influence a decision about the diagnosis of colonic symptoms.

The examination

The Exeter study identified two aspects of the examination which appear to be useful (Table 55.5).

Otherwise there are few data on the value of the examination in the diagnosis of colorectal cancer. There is a consensus that examination of the abdomen for a mass is worthwhile. The rectal examination may increase or reduce the probability of cancer. It may reveal benign anal pathology that explains the symptoms; it may show blood on the finger from above the anus;

Table 55.4 Lifetime risk of colorectal cancer in those with a family history if the disease[4]

Family history	Lifetime risk of colorectal cancer
Background lifetime risk	1:30 (1:50 risk of death)
One FDR aged >60 years	1:17
One FDR aged >45 years	1:15
One FDR and one SDR	1:12
One FDR age <45 years	1:10
Both parents any age	1:8.5
Two FDRs	1:6
Hereditary non-polyposis colorectal cancer (HNPCC)	1:3
Three FDRs	1:2
One FDR with familial adenomatous polyposis (FAP)	1:2

FDR = first-degree relative; SDR = second-degree relative.
HNPCC exists when three or more relatives have CRC; and one of them is an FDR of one of the others; and at least two generations are affected; and one was diagnosed before the age of 50.
HNPCC and FAP are autosomal dominant conditions which may also be associated with an increased incidence of ovarian, breast and endometrial carcinoma.

Table 55.5 The predictive value of signs in the diagnosis of colorectal cancer based on a baseline risk of 0.25%[1]

Signs	LR+	Probability of cancer
Abnormal rectal examination	18	4.0%
Abdominal tenderness	4.6	1.1%

or it may reveal a rectal carcinoma, more than half of which are palpable.[10]

The positive predictive values of the finding of a right-sided abdominal mass and a rectal mass can be calculated from the Bradford study.[11] A right-sided abdominal mass raises the probability of CRC in a patient referred urgently by the GP from 11% to 21% and a rectal mass raises it to 26%. They are, therefore, very useful signs; yet GPs detected them and used them to refer patients urgently in only about half of the cases in which they were present.

Investigations

Anaemia is one of the most powerful predictors of colorectal cancer (Table 55.6) yet GPs often fail to include it in the assessment of colonic symptoms. The Exeter study found it had the predictive values shown in Table 55.6.

Secondary care studies have found other investigations to be of value (Table 55.7).

Does the finding of occult blood usefully alter the probability of colorectal carcinoma?

The Exeter study found it the most valuable of all features examined, with a positive likelihood

ratio of 31, giving a probability of carcinoma of 7.1% if positive.[1] Other studies suggest that much depends on how many samples are tested.

- A prospective study of 802 patients with colorectal symptoms in which the patient tested two samples from each of three consecutive stools gave a sensitivity of 85.4% and a specificity of 91.4% for the detection of colorectal cancer.[13] This means that the test missed only 14.6% of colorectal cancers and gave a false positive in only 8.6% of cases. A positive test would raise the probability of cancer in this study from 4.2% to 30% (LR+ 9.9) and a negative would reduce it to 1% (LR– 0.16). These seem to be extremely useful figures in assessing the probability of cancer, until it is realised that they only apply if all six tests are performed.

- A much more common approach in primary care is for a single test to be performed on stool from the gloved finger at a single rectal examination. A study of 3121 asymptomatic patients aged 50 to 75, who were found to have a prevalence of colorectal cancer, a large polyp or high-grade dysplasia of 10.7%, were examined both by the testing of 6 samples of stool and by the testing of a single sample taken at rectal examination.[14] Testing of a single sample was of no value. The figures are shown in Table 55.8.

As a result of similar studies, the Scottish National Guideline[4] counsels against using testing

Table 55.6 The predictive value of different levels of anaemia in the diagnosis of colorectal cancer based on a baseline risk of 0.25%[1]

Haemoglobin level (g/L)	LR+	Probability of cancer
10–12.9	4.1	0.97%
<10	9.5	2.3%

These likelihood ratios apply equally to men and women.

Table 55.7 The value of investigations in the diagnosis of colorectal polyp or carcinoma.[12] The initial probability of cancer in this study was 5%

Investigation	LR+ (95% CI)	Probability according to the test result (95% CI)
Raised ESR (>30)	10 (2.8–35)	34% (17–57%)
Raised WBC (>10⁹/L)	7.5 (3.9–14)	28% (19–41%)

Table 55.8 Two methods of testing for occult blood in patients whose prior probability of carcinoma is 10.7%[14]

Investigation	Result	LR (95% CI)	Probability of carcinoma after the test (95% CI)
Six-sample occult blood	Positive	3.9 (3.0–5.0)	32% (24–38%)
	Negative	0.8 (0.8–0.9)	9% (8–10%)
Single sample at rectal examination	Positive	1.7 (1.0–2.9)	17% (9–25%)
	Negative	1.0 (0.9–1.0)	11% (9–12%)

Follow each row from left to right to see how different ways of testing for occult blood alter the probability of cancer.

for occult blood in the diagnosis of (as opposed to the screening for) colorectal cancer.

Referral

The UK NICE guidelines for the urgent referral of patients with suspected cancer illustrate the importance attached to combining symptoms:[10]
■ Age ≥40 with rectal bleeding and altered bowel habit towards looser ± more frequent stool
■ Age ≥60 with rectal bleeding and no anal symptoms
■ Age ≥60 with altered bowel habit towards looser ± more frequent stool
■ Right-sided lower abdominal mass consistent with bowel involvement

■ Palpable rectal (not pelvic) mass
■ Unexplained iron deficiency anaemia with haemoglobin ≤11 g/dl (men) or ≤10 g/dl (non-menstruating women).

In the first three categories, symptoms should have continued for at least 6 weeks.

These criteria have been shown to be useful in a study of urgent cancer referrals in Bradford Hospital NHS Trust over a 2-year period.[11] Of those with colorectal cancer, 73% met the criteria for urgent referral to a physician. The disappointment is that GPs appear to find the guidance hard to implement. Only 27% of those with cancer who met the criteria for urgent referral were referred urgently.

Example

A 50-year-old man presents with the history of a single profuse rectal bleed while away on holiday one week ago. The blood was bright; it continued on the toilet paper for two days thereafter and then stopped. He admits that for the last month his stool has been less frequent and harder to pass. He was straining at stool when he experienced the bleed.

The history is otherwise unremarkable.

The GP suspects an anal cause for the bleed. This seems to be confirmed when she finds no abdominal mass and rectally all she finds is a first-degree haemorrhoid.

Had she attempted to calculate the probabilities formally she would have been reassured that her decision was justified. His presentation with rectal bleeding at his age gives him a risk of carcinoma of 1.4%. The fact that the blood was bright and not mixed with stool or mucus reduces this slightly to, say, 1%. His constipation increases this slightly to, say, 2% (although she was thinking that it reduced his risk, by explaining the reason for the bleed). Overall, however, the evidence backs up her common sense assessment of the features that argue for and against the diagnosis of cancer.

She explains a dietary solution to his constipation, combined with advice about returning if symptoms continue.

REFERENCES

1. Hamilton W, Round A, Sharp D, et al. *Clinical features of colorectal cancer before diagnosis: a population-based case-control study.* Br J Cancer 2005;93:399–405.

2. Selvachandran S, Hodder R, Ballal M, et al. *Prediction of colorectal cancer by a patient consultation questionnaire and scoring system: a prospective study.* Lancet 2002;360:278–283.

3. Curless R, French J, William G, et al. *Comparison of gastrointestinal symptoms in colorectal carcinoma patients and community controls with respect to age.* Gut 1994;35:1267–1270.

4. Scottish Intercollegiate Guidelines Network. *Management of colorectal cancer: SIGN Guideline No. 67.* Edinburgh: SIGN, 2003. Online. Available: www.sign.ac.uk.

5. NHS Centre for Reviews and Dissemination. *The management of colorectal cancer.* Effective Health Care: University of York, 1997. Online. Available: www.york.ac.uk/inst/crd.

6. Eaden J, Abrams K, Mayberry J. *The risk of colorectal cancer in ulcerative colitis: a meta-analysis.* Gut 2001;48:526–535.

7. Jess T, Gamborg M, Matzen P, et al. *Increased risk of intestinal cancer in Crohn's disease: a meta-analysis of population-based studies.* Am J Gastroenterol 2005;100:2724–2729.

8. Eaden J. *Review article: colorectal carcinoma and inflammatory bowel disease.* Aliment Pharmacol Ther 2004;20 (Suppl 4):24–30.

9. British Society of Gastroenterology. *Guidelines for the management of patients with coeliac disease.* London: BSG, 2002. Online. Available: www.bsg.org.uk.

10. NICE. *Referral guidelines for suspected cancer.* London: National Institute for Health and Clinical Excellence, 2005. Online. Available: www.nice.org.uk. Reproduced with permission.

11. Allgar V, Neal R, Ali N, et al. *Urgent GP referrals for suspected lung, colorectal, prostate and ovarian cancer.* Br J Gen Pract 2006;56:355–362.

12. Fijten G, Starmans R, Muris J, et al. *Predictive value of signs and symptoms for colorectal cancer in patients with rectal bleeding in general practice.* Fam Pract 1995;12:279–286.

13. Leicester R, Lightfoot A, Millar J, et al. *Accuracy and value of the Hemoccult test in symptomatic patients.* BMJ 1983;286:673–674.

14. Collins J, Lieberman D, Durbin T, et al. *Accuracy of screening for fecal occult blood on a single stool sample obtained by digital rectal examination: a comparison with recommended sampling practice.* Ann Intern Med 2005;142:81–85.

Table 56.1 Questions to ask in the diagnosis of depression

	Suggested question	Criterion to score 1 point
1	Have you been feeling low lately?	Depressed mood most of the day nearly every day
2	Have you lost interest in your usual activities?	Markedly diminished interest or pleasure in almost all activities most of the day, nearly every day
3	How have you been sleeping?	Insomnia or hypersomnia nearly every day
4	Has your appetite or weight changed?	Substantial change in appetite nearly every day or unintentional weight loss or gain (e.g. 5% or more of body weight in 1 month)
5	Have you noticed a decrease in your energy?	Fatigue or loss of energy nearly every day
6	Have you felt more restless than usual or more slowed down than usual?	Psychomotor agitation or retardation nearly every day
7	Do you have trouble concentrating? Do you find it harder to make decisions than before?	Diminished ability to think or concentrate, or indecisiveness nearly every day
8	Are you feeling guilty or blaming yourself for things? How would you describe yourself to someone who had never met you before?	Feelings of worthlessness or excessive guilt nearly every day
9	Have you ever wished that you wouldn't wake up next morning?	Recurrent thoughts of death or suicide

Table 56.2 Value of the DSM questions in the diagnosis of major depression at different pre-test probabilities

Clinical picture	Probability before the assessment	Response to the DSM questions	Likelihood ratio (95% CI)	Probability of depression
Primary care attender	5%[1]	≥5	36 (20–68)	65%
		<5	0.28 (0.1–0.5)	1%
Patient 1 year post myocardial infarction	25%[4]*	≥5	36 (20–68)	92%
		<5	0.28 (0.1–0.5)	9%
Older person in residential care	48%[5]*	≥5	36 (20–68)	97%
		<5	0.28 (0.1–0.5)	21%

*These figures for depression do not distinguish major from minor depression.
Follow each row from left to right to see how the score alters the probability of depression.
Note how, while a higher pre-test probability of depression results in a higher post-test probability if the test is positive, it also means that a negative test is less successful in ruling out the diagnosis.

The symptoms must not be associated with a schizophrenic, or other psychotic, disorder and must not be due to substance abuse, including alcohol, or bereavement (although both of those circumstances can be associated with depression). See below for other possible diagnoses.

Scoring

● *A score of 5* or more with symptoms that have lasted 2 weeks (including depressed mood or loss of interest and causing significant impairment in functioning): this suggests *major depression*.

Antidepressants and/or counselling or psychotherapy are appropriate.

• *A score of 5 or more* with symptoms that have lasted at least 2 days but less than 2 weeks (including depressed mood or loss of interest and causing significant impairment in functioning): if present at least once a month for at least 1 year, this suggests *recurrent brief depression*. This diagnosis should not be made if it is linked to the menstrual cycle. What constitutes the most appropriate treatment is unclear.[14]

• *A score of 2 to 4* with symptoms that have lasted 2 weeks (including depressed mood or loss of interest and causing significant impairment in functioning): this suggests *minor depression*. Counselling or psychotherapy are more likely to be beneficial than antidepressants.

• *A score of 3 or 4* out of symptom numbers 1, 3, 4, 5, 7, 8, or a feeling of hopelessness, which have lasted at least 2 years (which must include question 1 and cause significant impairment in functioning): this suggests *dysthymia*. Antidepressants and/or counselling or psychotherapy are appropriate.

• The distinction between major and minor depression on the DSM-IV criteria should not be confused with mild, moderate and severe depression on the ICD-10 criteria,[15] where the scoring is out of 10, not 9, and includes an assessment of functioning, rather than a more rigid count of symptoms. The extra criterion is loss of confidence or self-esteem. These differences lead to the imperfect correlation between the two scores shown in Table 56.3.

Additional points

✱ *Assess the severity.* The questions suggested above are only the beginning. If the answer is yes, further questions will be needed to establish the severity of the symptom. Major depression may be mild, moderate or severe or associated with psychotic features.

✱ *Question all depressed patients about suicide.* The words used will depend on the culture of the patient. A typical sequence of questions, as follow-on to the answer yes to question 9, would be:

(a) Have you actually thought of killing yourself?

(b) Have you thought how you would do it?

(c) Have you thought when you would do it?

(d) Have you tried before?

Experience, but no quantitative studies, suggests that the more definite a plan, the more likely the patient is to attempt suicide. Attempts to predict the probability of suicide by scoring risk factors have failed.[17]

✱ *Assess whether a general medical disorder is present.* If it is, this does not invalidate the diagnosis of depression but makes the treatment of the medical disorder important as part of the management of the patient's depression.

✱ *Postnatal depression (PND)* is a special case. Use the Edinburgh Postnatal Depression Scale (see p. 464). A score of 11–12 out of 30 has a sensitivity

Table 56.3 Comparison of DSM-IV and ICD-10 definitions

ICD-10 definition	ICD-10 scores out of 10	Equivalent DSM-IV definition
Mild depression	2–3. The patient is distressed but able to continue functioning	Minor depression
Moderate depression	4 or more. The patient is likely to have great difficulty in continuing with normal activities	Minor or major depression
Severe depression	Several symptoms are marked and distressing, typically loss of self-esteem and ideas of worthlessness and guilt. Suicidal thoughts are common and a number of somatic symptoms are usually present. Hallucinations or delusions also mean that the episode is severe, regardless of other symptoms	Major depression

A further complication is that these scores from the 2003 version of ICD-10 (*The International Statistical Classification of Diseases and Related Health Problems 10th Revision*, 2003[15]) differ from those in the sister publication (*The ICD-10 Classification of Mental and Behavioural Disorders: Diagnostic Criteria for Research*, 1993[16]) in which mild depression requires a score of at least 4; moderate depression of at least 6 and severe depression at least 8.

of 76.7% and specificity of 92.5% for detecting PND.[18] This gives the following likelihood ratios: LR+ 10 (95% CI 8 to 14); LR– 0.25 (95% CI 0.2 to 0.4).

What if the patient has a physical illness which may itself be the cause of the somatic symptoms which contribute to the DSM score?

Use the score in the same way as in the patient without physical illness. A small Australian study suggests that false positives occurring for this reason are rare.[19] Forty-six patients with advanced physical disease were scored against the DSM criteria and underwent an unstructured interview, as the gold standard for depression. Even in this group, in whom the prevalence of somatic symptoms was high, the DSM score had a sensitivity of 88% (95% CI 79% to 97%) and a specificity of 93% (95% CI 86% to 100%). The alternative approach, of excluding the somatic questions from the score, improved the specificity to 100% (95% CI 97% to 100%) but dropped the sensitivity to 8% (95% CI 0% to 16%).

A mnemonic

Blenkiron has suggested the following as a way of remembering the 10 diagnostic features of depression according to the ICD-10 definition:[20]
Depressed mood
Energy loss/fatigue
Pleasure loss
Retardation or excitation
Eating changed – appetite/weight
Sleep changed
Suicidal thoughts
I'm a failure (loss of confidence)
Only me to blame (guilt)
No concentration
(Reproduced with permission of the BMJ Publishing Group from BMJ 2006;332:551.)

Exclude the possible alternative diagnoses[1]

- *Alcohol misuse.* If depression is diagnosed, check for *Alcohol misuse* (see p. 313).
- *Another substance-induced mood disorder*, e.g. on withdrawal from cocaine or amfetamines.
- *Mood disorder due to a specific condition* (e.g. hypothyroidism, multiple sclerosis, stroke) where the depression is the physiological, not psychological, result of the illness. Check the thyroid

function tests (TFTs) in women over 50 years old. The prevalence of biochemical hypothyroidism has been found to be as high as 5% in women aged 79,[21] although whether symptoms of tiredness or depression are useful in indicating which women are most likely to be hypothyroid is not clear.[22]

- *Depression due to medication*, e.g. CNS depressant drugs, reserpine, glucocorticoids and anabolic steroids.
- *Dementia*, where the patient may score as for depression, because of apathy, poor concentration, etc. (see p. 182). In dementia, the decline in cognitive function is likely to have preceded the apparent mood change.
- *Bipolar disorders* where the patient presents in a depressive phase.
- *Adjustment disorder with depressed mood.* Such patients have a psychosocial cause for their low mood and do not meet criteria for major depression. In bereavement, patients who do meet the criteria for major depression are considered to have an adjustment disorder unless the depression has continued for at least 2 months, or they include marked functional impairment, morbid preoccupation with worthlessness, suicidal thoughts, psychotic symptoms or psychomotor retardation.

Diagnosing depression in older patients

The Geriatric Depression Scale (GDS) has been developed for use in patients over 65. It removes the somatic symptoms of the DSM criteria and only requires the patient to give yes/no answers. A 5-item version has been shown to be as accurate as the earlier 15-item version.[23,24]

✱ Ask:
  1. Are you basically satisfied with your life?
  2. Do you often get bored?
  3. Do you often feel helpless?
  4. Do you prefer to stay at home rather than going out and doing new things?
  5. Do you feel pretty worthless the way you are now?

A 'yes' scores 1 except in question 1, where a 'no' scores 1.

Using a score of 2 or more as positive, this test has a sensitivity for detecting any depressive disorder of 94% (95% CI 91% to 98%) and a specificity of 81% (95% CI 75% to 87%); These give the probabilities in Table 56.4, which show that the GDS is a useful screening tool in any setting, because a negative test argues strongly against a diagnosis of depression.

Table 56.4 Value of the five-item GDS in the diagnosis of depression in an older person

Condition	Probability before the assessment	Score	Likelihood ratio	Probability of depression
Older person in the community	15%	Positive	4.9	46%
		Negative	0.1	2%
Older person in residential care	48%	Positive	4.9	82%
		Negative	0.1	8%

Follow each row from left to right to see how the GDS result alters the probability of depression.

* If the test is positive, conduct a diagnostic interview along the lines of the DSM-IV or ICD-10 criteria.

This author does not recommend the use of the Hamilton Depression Rating Scale[25] in the diagnosis of depression in primary care. It is designed to assess the severity of depression in a patient in whom depression has already been diagnosed. It is relatively long (being composed of 17 questions) and has been validated mainly in secondary care.

Diagnosing depression in adolescents

At any one time, about half of adolescents report moods which could be associated with depression, e.g. misery or wanting to be alone. Only 1% of mid-adolescent boys and 2% of girls suffer from a depressive illness.[26] Distinguishing between the two is especially difficult in a young person who is unwilling to talk.

* Ask the same questions as you would ask an adult in whom you suspect depression. Formal diagnostic instruments for diagnosing depression in adolescents have been devised but they all have their problems.[27]
* Look for objective signs of a depressive disorder:
  (a) a change in behaviour, e.g. avoiding school or preferring to be alone
  (b) physical signs, e.g. weight loss or the restlessness of agitated depression.
* In an adolescent who is unwilling to talk, ask with special sensitivity about delusions and hallucinations. ('Do you sometimes hear things, or have thoughts, that you prefer not to share with other people because they wouldn't believe you?') This may be the first presentation of a psychotic illness.
* Check for other mental disorders, such as anxiety or behavioural disorders. They often coexist with depression.
* Check whether substance abuse is complicating the picture, or is even the sole cause of the symptoms.

Example

A successful businesswoman, aged 55, presents with the fear that she is developing Alzheimer's disease. For the previous 6 months she has noticed difficulty in concentrating, that jobs take her longer than they used to, that she has lost interest in the firm. She brushes off a question about her mood with the comment that anyone would feel depressed if they thought they were becoming demented. She admits that she has thought a lot about what she would do if the diagnosis was confirmed; and that the answer is that she would kill herself. She has never been seriously ill and has always worked through minor illnesses.

A brief assessment of her mental function reveals no suggestion of dementia (see *Memory loss and dementia*, p. 181). Further questioning shows that she has lost interest in her usual pursuits, and that she is sleeping and eating poorly.

She scores 7 on the DSM scale. The GP decides that her pre-test probability was 25%, based on a population prevalence of 5% plus a sense he has that she is depressed: she has none of the alertness that he remembers from previous encounters. Her score takes the probability of depression to over 90%.

The GP explains this to her. She is initially dismissive, saying that she has nothing to be depressed about and anyway she regards mental illness as a failure of will. Then she says that her 'will' seems to have gone anyway, that she's not worth anything anymore. The GP, now even more confident of the diagnosis of depression, starts the process of helping her to 'allow herself' to be ill and to accept treatment.

REFERENCES

1. American Psychiatric Association. *Diagnostic and statistical manual of mental disorders, 4th edn,* text revision. Washington DC: American Psychiatric Association, 2000.

2. Arthur A, Jagger C, Lindesay J, et al. *Using an annual over-75 health check to screen for depression: validation of the short geriatric depression scale (GDS15) within general practice.* Int J Geriatr Psychiatry 1999;14:431–439.

3. Paul S, Dewey H, Sturm J, et al. *Prevalence of depression and use of antidepressant medication at 5-years poststroke in the North East Melbourne Stroke Incidence Study.* Stroke 2006;37:2854–2855.

4. Kaptein K, de Jonge P, van den Brink R, et al. *Course of depressive symptoms after myocardial infarction and cardiac prognosis: a latent class analysis.* Psychosom Med 2006;68:662–668.

5. Wegerer S, Hafner H, Mann A, et al. *Prevalence and course of depression among elderly residential home admissions in Mannheim and Camden, London.* Int Psychogeriatr 1995;7:479–493.

6. Henkel V, Mergl R, Kohnen R, et al. *Identifying depression in primary care: a comparison of different methods in a prospective cohort study.* BMJ 2003;326:200–201.

7. Pignone M, Gaynes B, Rushton J, et al. *Screening for depression in adults: a summary of the evidence for the US Preventive Services Task Force.* Ann Intern Med 2002;136:765–776.

8. Gilbody S, House A, Sheldon T. *Routinely administered questionnaires for depression and anxiety: systematic review.* BMJ 2001;322:406–409.

9. Gilbody S, House A, Sheldon T. *Screening and case finding instruments for depression (Cochrane Review).* The Cochrane Library, Issue 4, 2005. Chichester, John Wiley, 2005.

10. Whooley MA, Avins AL, Miranda J, et al. *Case-finding instruments for depression. Two questions are as good as many.* J Gen Intern Med 1997;12:439–445.

11. Arroll B, Goodyear-Smith F, Kerse N, et al. *Effect of the addition of a 'help' question to two screening questions on specificity for diagnosis of depression in general practice: diagnostic validity study.* BMJ 2005;331:884–886.

12. Williams JW Jr, Noël PH, Cordes JA, et al. *Is this patient clinically depressed?* JAMA 2002;287:1160–1170.

13. Spitzer RL, Kroenke K, Williams JB. *Validation and utility of a self-report version of PRIME-MD: the PHQ primary care study. Primary Care Evaluation of Mental Disorders. Patient Health Questionnaire.* JAMA 1999;282:1737–1744.

14. Pezawas L, Angst J, Gamma A, et al. *Recurrent brief depression – past and future.* Prog Neuropsychopharmacol Biol Psychiatry 2003;27:75–83.

15. WHO. *International statistical classification of diseases and related health problems, 10th Revision.* Geneva: World Health Organization, 2003. Online. Available: www.who.int/en (search on 'ICD-10').

16. WHO. *The ICD-10 classification of mental and behavioural disorders: diagnostic criteria for research.* Geneva: World Health Organization, 1993.

17. Wilkinson G. *Can suicide be prevented?* BMJ 1994;309:860–862.

18. Murray L, Carothers AD. *The validation of the Edinburgh Post-natal Depression Scale on a community sample.* Br J Psychiatry 1990;157:288–290.

19. Ellis G, Robinson J, Crawford G. *When symptoms of disease overlap with symptoms of depression.* Aust Fam Physician 2006;35:647–649.

20. Blenkiron P. *A mnemonic for depression (letter).* BMJ 2006;332:551.

21. Eden S, Sundbeck G, Lindstedt G, et al. *Screening for thyroid disease in the elderly. Serum concentrations of thyrotropin and 3,5,3'-triiodothyronine in a representative population of 79-year-old women and men.* Compr Gerontol 1988;2(Section A):40–45.

22. AHCPR. *Clinical Practice Guideline No.5: Depression in primary care: detection and diagnosis.* Rockville, Maryland: AHCPR, 1993.

23. Hoyl M, Alessi C, Harker J, et al. *Development and testing of a five-item version of the Geriatric Depression Scale.* J Am Geriatr Soc 1999;47:873–878.

24. Rinaldi P, Mecocci P, Benedetti C, et al. *Validation of the five-item Geriatric Depression Scale in elderly subjects in three different settings.* J Am Geriatr Soc 2003;51:694–698.

25. Hamilton M. *A rating scale for depression.* J Neurol Neurosurg Psychiatry 1960;23:56.

26. Harrington R. *Affective disorders.* In: Rutter M, Taylor E, eds. Child and adolescent psychiatry: modern approaches, 4th edn. Oxford: Blackwell Scientific, 2002:463–485.

27. Brooks S, Kutcher S. *Diagnosis and measurement of adolescent depression: a review of commonly utilized instruments.* J Child Adolesc Psychopharmacol 2001;11:341–376.

Diabetes and impaired glucose tolerance

Prevalences

- *Diabetes.* The prevalence depends on the population and the diagnostic criterion. Among US adults, it is 5.9% with a further 2.4% undiagnosed.[1]
- *Impaired glucose tolerance (IGT):* 15.6% of US adults aged 40 to 76.[2]
- *Impaired fasting glycaemia (IFG):* 9.7% of US adults aged 40 to 76[2] (of these, 16% have both IGT and IFG).

To make the diagnosis

* *Check the random blood glucose.*
  - *A level ≥11.1 mmol/L suggests diabetes.*

Confirm the diagnosis either by finding symptoms typical of diabetes, or repeat the test as a 2-hour blood glucose.
  - *A level <5.3 mmol/L makes diabetes unlikely.*[3]
  - *Levels between 5.3 and 11.1 mmol/L need further investigation with a fasting blood sugar. Since most patients will fall within this range, a fasting blood sugar is preferable as the initial investigation in a patient without typical symptoms.*

Or
* *Check the fasting blood glucose.*
  - *A level of 7 mmol/L or above suggests the diagnosis of diabetes. If there are also symptoms*

typical of diabetes, the diagnosis is established. If asymptomatic, repeat the fasting glucose. If still ≥7 mmol/L, the diagnosis is confirmed.

■ *A level of 6.1 to 6.9 mmol/L* indicates, at least, impaired fasting glycaemia (IFG). A 2-hour glucose is needed to distinguish between IFG, IGT and diabetes. A 2-hour glucose of 7.8–11.0 mmol/L signifies *impaired glucose tolerance (IGT). A 2-hour glucose ≥11.1 mmol/L suggests diabetes, which should be confirmed by a second test, unless typical symptoms are present.*

■ *A level of 5.3 to 6.0 mmol/L.* There are two options:

1. Re-screen as clinically indicated (e.g. in 3 years), as recommended by Diabetes UK;[4] or
2. Order a 2-hour blood glucose *in order to detect those with IGT or diabetes.* In a study of middle-aged Swedish women,[5] *not* proceeding to a 2-hour sugar in those with a fasting glucose of 6 mmol/L or below would have meant that 32 out of the 71 undetected diabetics were missed (45%). Performing a 2-hour glucose on all with a fasting glucose of 5.3 mmol/L or above would have detected a further 16, while still missing another 16 (23%).

However, such thoroughness comes at a cost. In the above study, only 1.9% of those with a fasting blood sugar <6.0 were found to be diabetic (Table 57.1). This represents a *number needed to test* of 53 (i.e. 53 middle-aged Swedish women with a fasting sugar <6.0 need to be tested with a 2-hour sugar to detect one with diabetes).

Table 57.1 shows that testing of patients with fasting blood glucose below 5.3 is even less rewarding.

Technicalities

These figures are for venous plasma. The 2-hour blood glucose should be taken after at least 3 days of an unrestricted carbohydrate diet and normal physical activity. The fast should be 8 to 14 hours. Water is permitted; smoking is not. The subject should drink 75 g of anhydrous glucose (= 82.5 g of glucose BP) in 250–300 ml water over 5 minutes. Blood is taken 2 hours after the start of the drink. Children should be given 1.75 g glucose per kg. Seventy-five grams of anhydrous glucose are found in 113 ml of Polycal (Nutricia Clinical).

Note also:

● The HbA_{1c} is not useful in the diagnosis of diabetes.[6]

● Urine testing for glucose in people who are asymptomatic is hardly worthwhile. A Danish study on 3041 individuals found that two urine tests missed 79% of patients with diabetes (sensitivity 21%; specificity 99%).[7]

Table 57.1 The probability of diabetes at different cut-off points for the fasting blood glucose when the pre-test probability is 3.9%[5]

Fasting blood sugar (mmol/L)	LR (95% CI)	Probability of diabetes
≥6.7	37 (21–64)	74%
<6.7	0.6 (0.5–0.8)	2.5%
≥6.0	18 (13–25)	42%
<6.0	0.5 (0.4–0.6)	1.9%
≥5.3	3.3 (2.9–3.9)	12%
<5.3	0.3 (0.2–0.5)	1.2%
≥4.8	1.6 (1.4–1.7)	6%
<4.8	0.3 (0.2–0.5)	1.2%

The predictive values are those for unselected middle-aged Swedish women not known to be diabetic who were found to have a prevalence of diabetes of 3.9% and of IGT of 27.9%. Diabetes was confirmed by the 2-hour glucose.

Symptoms typical of diabetes are:

- thirst and polyuria
- weight loss
- fatigue and malaise
- infections (bacterial or fungal)
- evidence of ketoacidosis.

Who should be screened?

Diabetes UK[4] recommends 3-yearly screening for those at high risk:

(a) Caucasians aged >40 or people from black, Asian and ethnic minority groups aged >25, with at least one of the following:

- a first-degree relative with diabetes
- overweight (body mass index > 25 kg/m^2) and sedentary
- macrovascular disease or hypertension.

(b) Women who have had gestational diabetes and who have tested normal postpartum and after 1 year.

(c) Women with polycystic ovary syndrome who are obese.

(d) Those known to have IGT or IFG.

A case can be made for the screening of other groups, e.g. men with erectile dysfunction (expected detection rate: diabetes 4.7%, IFG 12%[8]).

However, screening of everyone aged >45, as recommended by the American Diabetic Association, would, in a predominantly white UK population, detect only 0.2% with diabetes, IFG or IGT among those with no risk factors other than age, against 2.8% in those with at least one risk factor.[9]

The controversy over the biochemical criteria for the diagnosis of diabetes

The American Diabetes Association (ADA)[10] recommends that:

- The diagnosis of diabetes depends on a fasting glucose of ≥7 mmol/L.
- *Impaired fasting glycaemia* is present if the fasting glucose is 6.1–6.9 mmol/L.

The WHO criteria[3] remain that:

- The diagnosis of *diabetes* depends on a fasting sugar ≥7 mmol/L *or* a 2-hour glucose of 11.1 mmol/L or above.
- Impaired glucose tolerance (IGT) is present if the fasting plasma glucose is less than 7.0 mmol/L and a 2-hour glucose is 7.8–11.0 mmol/L.
- Gestational diabetes: the WHO definition is a fasting sugar of 7 mmol/L or above or a 2-hour sugar of 7.8 mmol/L or above, during pregnancy.

The ADA criteria are easier to use but they miss half the patients who would have been diagnosed as diabetic by the WHO criteria in the screening of a population. In a study of 936 Canadians of European, Chinese or South Asian origin,[6] the ADA criteria found that 3.1% had unsuspected diabetes, while the WHO criteria diagnosed 6.4% as diabetic. Furthermore, while the ADA criteria diagnosed 5.2% as having IFG, 15.2% were found to have IGT on the WHO criteria.

The importance of maximising the detection of 'minor' degrees of glucose intolerance is that they are associated with an increased risk of cardiovascular disease in their own right as well as an increased risk of diabetes.

REFERENCES

1. MMWR. *Prevalence of diabetes and impaired fasting glucose in adults – United States, 1999–2000.* Centre for Disease Control and Prevention, 2005. Online. Available: www.cdc.gov (search on 'impaired fasting glucose').

2. Rao S, Disraeli P, McGregor T. *Impaired glucose tolerance and impaired fasting glucose.* Am Fam Physician 2004;69:1961–1968.

3. World Health Organization. *Definition, diagnosis and classification of diabetes mellitus and its complications.* Geneva: WHO, 1999.

4. Diabetes UK. *Position Statement: early identification of people with type 2 diabetes:* Diabetes UK, 2002.

5. Larrson H, Ahren B, Lindgarde F, et al. *Fasting blood glucose in determining the prevalence of diabetes in a large, homogeneous population of Caucasian middle-aged women.* J Intern Med 1995;237:537–541.

6. Anand S, Razak F, Vuksan V, et al. *Diagnostic strategies to detect glucose intolerance in a multiethnic population.* Diabetes Care 2003;26:290–296.

7. Friderichsen B, Maunsbach M. *Glycosuric tests should not be employed in population screenings for NIDDM.* J Public Health Med 1997;19:55–60.

8. Sairam K, Kulinskaya E, Boustead G, et al. *Prevalence of undiagnosed diabetes mellitus in male erectile dysfunction.* BJU Int 2001;88:68–71.

9. Lawrence J, Bennett P, Young A, Robinson A. *Screening for diabetes in general practice: cross sectional population study.* BMJ 2001;323:548–551.

10. The Expert Committee on the Diagnosis and Classification of Diabetes Mellitus. *Report of the Expert Committee on the Diagnosis and Classification of Diabetes Mellitus.* Diabetes Care 1997;20:1183–1197.

Eating disorders

KEY FACTS

- Eating disorders are common in adolescent girls and young women and are largely undetected in primary care.
- Concern about anorexia nervosa usually arises because a young person is thin. In bulimia, the discovery of a patient bingeing, or spending too long in the toilet, or vomiting or purging suggests the diagnosis.

- Screening questions are helpful in detecting patients with a disorder but rely on the patient giving truthful answers.
- Once the patient's confidence has been obtained, questioning along the lines of the formal diagnoses of anorexia and bulimia allows a diagnosis to be made.

A PRACTICAL APPROACH

- Consider the possibility of an eating disorder in thin young women who seem *un*concerned about their thinness, or who show evidence of excessive concern over the hazards of eating, or who have infrequent periods.
- Consider the possibility of bulimia in young women of normal weight with repeated diarrhoea, vomiting or non-specific gastrointestinal symptoms.
- Use questions that get to the heart of the syndromes without seeming too

confrontational, e.g. 'Does food seem to dominate your life?' or 'Do you ever find yourself eating in secret?'
- Consider using the SCOFF questionnaire formally.
- If suspicion of an eating disorder remains, go into the history in more detail, with an examination and investigations once you have the patient's trust.

Definitions

Anorexia nervosa and bulimia have been strictly defined (see below) but they represent the extreme of a continuum of behaviour. Partial syndromes have also been recognised and may be called 'atypical eating disorders'. Many cases of both the full and partial syndromes are not recognised by the patients' doctors and sometimes patients have been referred for the

complications of the condition without the underlying condition having been diagnosed.[1]

Prevalence

In the population (of the Western industrialised world)

- *Anorexia nervosa*: 0.3% of young women,[2] 0.01% of young men[3]

Fibromyalgia

- There is general agreement that a syndrome exists, characterised by chronic widespread pain, often associated with the presence of tender spots and with depression, fatigue and other functional complaints.
- There is little agreement on a more precise definition.
- The accuracy of the history and examination cannot therefore be assessed and is dependent on the exclusion of other diagnoses.

A PRACTICAL APPROACH

- ★ In a patient with chronic widespread pain, make a diagnosis of fibromyalgia with two concurrent approaches:
  - (a) Look for positive pointers towards the condition: that the pain is felt in all four quadrants of the body; that, while the pain may vary from day to day, at any one time pain is consistently felt in certain well-defined locations. These places may also be tender.
  - (b) Look for alternative diagnoses, from the clinical assessment and from a limited battery of screening blood tests.

Prevalence

The point prevalence in the population is 2% (3.4% in women and 0.5% in men).[1] It is more common in older people, reaching a prevalence of 8% in women in their 70s.[2]

Using the wider definition of 'chronic widespread unexplained pain' (see below), it is present in 11.2% of the UK population.[3]

It often coexists with other rheumatological disorders; 20% of patients with rheumatological disorders also meet American College of Rheumatology (ACR) criteria for the diagnosis of fibromyalgia (FM).[4]

Definition

It is defined by the ACR as follows[5]:
1. a history of widespread pain for at least 3 months involving left and right sides and areas above and below the waist, and involving the axial skeleton (cervical spine, or thoracic spine, or anterior chest or lower back); and
2. where pressure on 11 out of 18 trigger points causes pain.

This definition seems to be supported by a Canadian study in which blinded examiners found that the tender point count was significantly associated with the presence of FM, with inter-rater and intra-rater reliability that was 'quite good'.[6]

Others, however, have pointed out the limitations of this definition.[7,8] Most patients with tender points do not have chronic widespread pain and 60% with chronic widespread pain have fewer than 11 tender points. It may be that a better definition of FM is 'chronic widespread unexplained pain', with the number of tender points merely indicating the severity of the condition.

Indeed, experts elicit different numbers of painful tender points in the same patients, and the presence or absence of trigger points varies from day to day. Furthermore, trigger points are associated with the presence of other functional symptoms independently of pain complaints, leading Croft and colleagues to argue that tender points are a measure of general distress.[9,10]

Other features of FM are fatigue, non-restorative sleep, mood alterations, non-neurological paraesthesiae, headache and stiffness. Fibromyalgia may be associated with depression, chronic fatigue syndrome and the irritable bowel syndrome.

Diagnosis from the history and examination

No studies have assessed the sensitivity and specificity of the history and examination in the diagnosis of fibromyalgia; indeed, such studies would be hard to conduct in the absence of a gold standard for the diagnosis.

There is a consensus that the syndrome of chronic widespread soft tissue pain is real, as is its association with more general symptoms, such as fatigue, headache and altered mood. *The diagnosis can be made in a patient with pain that is felt in all four quadrants of the body, that has been going on for months or years, and who may have the more general symptoms above, and provided the symptoms are not better explained by another condition.*

Blood tests

The only purpose of blood tests is to exclude other conditions with which fibromyalgia could be confused:

1. erythrocyte sedimentation rate or C-reactive protein to exclude inflammatory conditions, e.g. systemic lupus erthematosus or polymyalgia rheumatica
2. calcium and alkaline phosphatase to exclude osteomalacia and hypercalcaemia
3. thyroid function tests to exclude hypothyroidism
4. creatine kinase to exclude myopathy.

Example

A woman aged 55 presents with a complaint of 'pain all over' for about 3 months. She has complained over the years of tiredness, but it has never met the criteria of chronic fatigue syndrome nor has her GP been able to find any other cause. He considers her to be a 'somatiser' but is not clear how to establish that diagnosis.

At first her symptoms of pain seem to suggest another non-organic complaint. They are felt in all four limbs and in the neck and chest and back. They fluctuate during the day and may be different from one day to the next.

A brief examination reveals no arthritis and her back movements are normal for her age. However, as he palpates her upper back, for no better reason than to be seen to be conducting a thorough examination, he hits a tender spot just above the upper border of the scapula. He palpates elsewhere and finds that she is not tender except in well-defined and well-localised areas of the back of the neck, chest and back. These points are always where there is soft tissue. She never reports tenderness when he presses on a bony prominence.

The GP does not know enough about tender points to make a formal count, and is sceptical about such exactitude anyway, but recognises a consistency in the ones he has elicited.

He tells her that her symptoms suggest fibromyalgia but that he wants to take some blood to rule out some other, less likely, conditions. She is pleased to have a diagnosis, even though it will not lead to any specific treatment.

REFERENCES

1. Wolfe F, Ross K, Anderson J, et al. *The prevalence and characteristics of fibromyalgia in the general population.* Arthritis Rheum 1995;38:19–28.

2. McGurk C, Wilson D, Henry W. *Diagnosing fibromyalgia.* Practitioner 2001;245:1026–1038.

3. Croft P, Rigby A, Boswell R, et al. *The prevalence of chronic widespread pain in the general population.* J Rheumatol 1993;20:710–713.

4. Crofford L, Clauw D. *Fibromyalgia: where are we a decade after the American College of Rheumatology Classification Criteria were developed?* Arthritis Rheum 2002;46:1136–1138.

5. Wolfe F, Smythe H, Yunus M, et al. *The American College of Rheumatology 1990 criteria for the classification of fibromyalgia: report of the multicenter criteria committee.*

Arthritis Rheum 1990;33: 160–172.

6. Tunks E, McCain G, Hart L, et al. *The reliability of examination for tenderness in patients with myofascial pain, chronic fibromyalgia and controls.* J Rheumatol 1995;22:944–952.

7. Bandolier. *Fibromyalgia: diagnosis and treatment.* Bandolier 2001;August 2001:90–92.

8. Croft P. *Testing for tenderness: what's the point?* J Rheumatol 2000;27:2531–2533.

9. Croft P, Schollum J, Silman A. *Population study of tender point counts and pain as evidence of fibromyalgia.* BMJ 1994;309: 696–699.

10. Croft P. *Symptoms without pathology: should we try a little tenderness?* Rheumatology 2003;42: 815–817.

Food allergy

KEY FACTS

- Only a small minority of people who present with concern about food allergy have reactions that can be objectively confirmed on double-blind placebo-controlled food challenge.
- The history is central to the estimation of the probability of food allergy. From the history, an estimate of the pre-test probability prior to investigation can be estimated.

- Serum-specific IgE tests are the primary care investigation of choice in those in whom IgE-mediated food allergy is suspected. The choice of foods to be tested should be guided by the history.
- IgE-mediated food allergy requires total avoidance of the provoking foods, frequently for life. Dietetic assistance with the aim of providing detailed practical advice on avoidance strategies is often useful.

A PRACTICAL APPROACH

- ★ Decide whether the history suggests food allergy or a non-immunologically mediated food intolerance.
- ★ Confirm the suggestion of food allergy with a serological test directed at the allergen identified in the history.
- ★ If the history suggests that the problem is food intolerance, explain that allergy tests are unlikely to help: a positive test is more likely to be a false, than a true positive. Such individuals should be reassured that they are not food allergic. A period of abstinence from the offending food(s) should be advised, with periodic attempts at reintroduction.
- ★ Consider referral to a dietitian in those with unintended weight loss or nutritional deficiencies.

- ★ Refer to an allergist or organ-based specialist with an interest in allergy for skin prick testing and/or food challenge testing in cases of persistent diagnostic doubt.
- ★ In patients with life-threatening symptoms to food:
  (a) Refer to an allergy specialist.
  (b) Issue self-administered adrenaline (epinephrine) and provide a written management plan advising when, where and how to administer the adrenaline auto-injector.
  (c) Most fatal reactions to food occur in those with asthma. In those with coexistent asthma, ensure that asthma is optimally controlled.

be performed in an inpatient setting under clinical supervision.[4]

• *Serum-specific IgE* (sIgE). This is also known as the radioallergosorbent test (RAST). Measurement of food-specific serum IgE is the primary care investigation of choice for diagnosing IgE-mediated food allergy. These tests have the potential for both high sensitivity and specificity, depending on the cut-off values used (Table 60.3).[4] In general, specific serum IgE levels show a correlation with the outcome of positive oral food challenges for cow's milk and hen's eggs.[18]

• *Skin prick testing (SPT)*. The skin prick test is a very useful investigative technique that is performed by placing a drop of the allergen extract being evaluated (e.g. egg white protein) on the skin and then pricking the skin with a lancet.[19] The resulting wheal size is recorded approximately 15 minutes later, a wheal size of at least 3 mm greater than the diluent control being considered positive. The larger the wheal size, the greater the likelihood that the sensitisation being detected will be clinically significant.

• Skin prick tests are not recommended for use in suspected food allergy in primary care because of the risk of triggering a major systemic allergic reaction. However, a patient may attend with the diagnosis of allergy based on the results of a skin prick test performed elsewhere and the GP needs to understand the value and the limitations of the tests. The specificity is lower than that of serum IgE, 50% or less, and a positive skin test with a vague history often indicates the need for a food challenge (Table 60.4). Overall, only 40% of patients with a positive skin prick test will experience allergic symptoms if they ingest the food. In children older than 1 year, negative skin tests for major food allergens have high negative predictive accuracies, excluding IgE-mediated food allergy in most cases.

• *Atopy patch test (APT)*. APT is a patch test using protein allergens where the eczematous reaction is assessed. It tests the cellular aspect of the immune reaction. This test is particularly useful in those in whom non-IgE-mediated immunological reactions to food are suspected.[20] These tests will normally be performed by a dermatologist.

A suggested approach to a patient with possible food allergy

A logical systematic approach is recommended for those presenting with suspected food allergy. The clinical history is crucial in accurately securing the correct diagnosis.

Suggested schema for the clinical assessment

* Is there a personal or family history of allergic conditions such as eczema, hay fever or asthma?
* Explore what the patient means by 'food allergy'? Patients often use food allergy as a generic term that encompasses a broad range of symptoms triggered by certain foods.[17] This term should,

Table 60.4 The value of skin prick tests in the diagnosis of specific food allergies

Allergen	Prevalence[6,17]	Test result	Likelihood ratio (95% CI)	Post-test probability*
Cow's milk	2.5%	Positive	2.0 (1.9–2.0)	4.8%
		Negative	0.08 (0.07–0.09)	0.2%
Egg	1.3%	Positive	2.1 (2.0–2.1)	2.7%
		Negative	0.04 (0.03–0.04)	0.04%
Soya	1.1%	Positive	1.4 (1.4–1.5)	1.6%
		Negative	0.5 (0.5–0.5)	0.6%
Fish (including shellfish)	0.1%	Positive	2.1 (1.8–2.4)	2%
		Negative	0.2 (0.1–0.2)	0.01%
Peanut	0.8%	Positive	1.3 (1.2–1.3)	1%
		Negative	0.3 (0.3–0.4)	0.2%

Follow each row from left to right to see how the result of the skin prick test alters the probability of that particular food allergy. *These post-test probabilities are based solely on population prevalence and test result. In practice, the clinical picture must also be taken into account; see case examples at the end of the chapter.

however, be reserved for immunologically mediated abnormal reactions to foods.[1]

* Attempt to differentiate between immunological and non-immunological adverse reactions to food according to the following factors:[1]

  (a) The *precipitating food*: allergies are typically specific to a particular class of food. In IgE-mediated food allergy, common triggers include eggs, milk, peanuts and fish (including seafood); less common triggers include fruit, vegetables and tree nuts. A reaction will occur every time that food is ingested.

  (b) The *speed of the reaction*, which typically occurs within minutes of ingestion of the offending food(s).

  (c) The *type of reaction*, which may be local (angio-oedema, perioral itching and laryngeal oedema) or systemic (urticaria, rhinoconjunctivitis, wheezing, diarrhoea and vomiting, and, in some cases, anaphylaxis).[14]

* In contrast, in food intolerance, symptoms are typically non-specific and may occur in response to a range of foods.[6,21–23] A temporal relation between food intake and onset of symptoms is often difficult to establish. Detailed questioning typically shows that the offending foods are sometimes well tolerated.[14]

* Enquire if the patient has previously been investigated for food allergy.[14] Ask about the results of any food-specific skin prick tests and tests for specific IgE, and verify the concordance between symptoms and allergy tests. In some patients, food allergies will have been diagnosed on the basis of investigations of spurious value – for example, kinesiology or hair analysis.

* Also determine the minimum quantity of food that will cause an allergic reaction, any treatment received and the outcome.[1]

* Ask about the worst reaction. Is the patient at risk of food-induced anaphylaxis?

* Is the patient's diet nutritionally adequate? In children, assess and monitor height and weight gain.[14]

* In most cases there will be relatively little to find on examination at the time of presentation; however, examine for features suggestive of atopy: eczema, urticaria, rhinoconjunctivitis and asthma.

* Those presenting acutely may have any number of organ systems involved; the key hallmarks will be signs of inflammation: erythema, swelling and pruritus.

What to do after the clinical assessment

Suspected food intolerance

* Do not perform allergy tests in those with a history that strongly suggests food intolerance. Other differential diagnoses must, however, be considered and, if suspected, investigated appropriately.

* Reassure patients with a food intolerance that they do not have a food allergy. Advise them to abstain from the offending foods for a while, but encourage them to try, from time to time, to reintroduce them into their diet. In those with weight loss or dietary deficiencies, consider referral to a dietitian.

Suspected food allergy

* For those in whom IgE-mediated food allergy is suspected, or in those in whom you cannot safely exclude this diagnosis, request serum-specific IgE tests to the foods implicated. Indiscriminate testing to a range of foods is not recommended as these tests have low specificity. False positives will cause diagnostic confusion.

* IgE-mediated food allergy will require avoidance of the provoking foods. Help from a dietitian with detailed written advice on avoidance strategies is often useful.

* Refer patients with a history of IgE-mediated anaphylaxis to an allergy specialist.

Conclusion

Allergic problems are responsible for an estimated 12.5 million GP consultations per year.[24] Food allergy hospital admission rates have risen from 5 to 28 per million over a 10-year period.[25] The overwhelming majority of GPs felt that current allergy services within the NHS are poor, citing lack of suitable training for primary care staff and difficulties in accessing specialists as important barriers to improving standards of care.[26]

Example 1

A 19-year-old female presents complaining of having experienced swelling of the lips, tongue, flushing and wheezing within minutes of eating a seafood salad. This is her second similar reaction, the previous milder reaction having been triggered by seafood. She gives a strong family and personal history of atopic disorders, having personally experienced mild eczema and asthma since childhood.

The GP estimates that the history of the two episodes, her past history of atopy and the family history make the probability of allergy to seafood highly likely, say 80%.

RAST testing reveals a strongly positive reaction to prawns, but not to mussels, shrimps or oysters. With a specificity of 100%, this confirms the diagnosis of prawn allergy. It does not, however, rule out the possibility of other seafood allergies. The negative likelihood ratio of 0.75 (see Table 60.2) hardly reduces that below the population prevalence of 0.1%.

In view of the severity of the reaction, she is prescribed and shown how to use self-administered adrenaline (epinephrine) and is referred to a dietitian for detailed advice on avoiding prawns. Referral to an allergist is considered, but in view of the long distance to the nearest allergy centre, she opts not to be referred.

Example 2

A 25-year-old woman complains of a bloated feeling 1 to 2 hours after food. A previous doctor performed blood tests for allergy and found a positive specific IgE for wheat. She has excluded this from her diet but with no benefit and assumes she has additional food allergies. There are no pointers in her history or family history in favour of food allergy and the symptoms are very non-specific. The GP therefore estimates her pre-test probability of having wheat allergy to be no higher than the population prevalence of 0.3%. The positive test raises this to just 2% based on the figures from Table 60.3 (Fig. 60.1).

The GP tells her that he can be 98% certain that she does not have wheat allergy and that further tests, if positive, will be more likely to be false positives than true positives. However, while taking the history he has been able to come to a different diagnosis: that of irritable bowel syndrome. She reluctantly agrees to a trial of treatment for this.

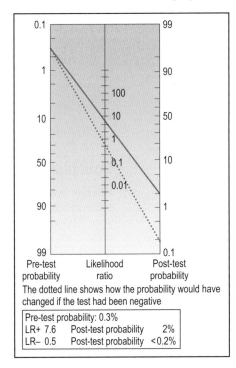

The dotted line shows how the probability would have changed if the test had been negative

Pre-test probability: 0.3%		
LR+ 7.6	Post-test probability	2%
LR– 0.5	Post-test probability	<0.2%

Figure 60.1 The probability of wheat allergy before and after the IgE test in example 2 above.

REFERENCES

1. James MH. *Food allergies.* Online. Available: http://www.emedicine.com/med/ 18 May 2005.

2. Sampson HA. *Food allergy.* JAMA 1997; 278:1888–1894.

3. Young E, Stoneham MD, Petruckevitch A, et al. *A population study of food intolerance.* Lancet 1994; 343:1127–1130.

4. Beyer K, Teuber SS. *Food allergy diagnostics: scientific and unproven procedures.* Curr Opin Allergy Clin Immunol 2005; 5:261–266.

5. McKevith B, Theobald H. *Common food allergies.* Nurs Stand 2005;19:39–42.

6. Sampson HA. *Food allergy accurately identifying clinical reactivity.* Allergy 2005;60(Suppl 79):19–24.

7. Grundy J, Matthews S, Bateman B, et al. *Rising prevalence of allergy to peanut in children: Data from 2 sequential cohorts.* J Allergy Clin Immunol 2002;110:784–789.

8. Devereux G. *The increase in allergic disease: environment and susceptibility. Proceedings of a symposium held at the Royal Society of Edinburgh, 4th June 2002.* Clin Exp Allergy 2003;33:394–406.

9. Tariq SM, Stevens M, Matthews S, et al. *Cohort study of peanut and tree nut sensitisation by age 4 years.* BMJ 1996;313:514–517.

10. Sheikh A, Walker S. *Food allergy.* BMJ 2002;325:1337.

11. Nestlé Infant Nutrition. *1 in 3 infants may be at a risk of developing an allergy.* Online. Available: at www.nestle.co.uk (search on 'Allergy Risk Chart') 30 May 2005.

12. Bindslev-Jensen C. *Food allergy.* BMJ 1998;316:1299–1302.

13. Sampson HA, Ho DG. *Relationship between food-specific IgE concentrations and the risk of positive food challenges in children and adolescents.* J Allergy Clin Immunol 1997;100:444–451.

14. Sheikh A, Walker S. *Ten-minute consultation: food allergy.* BMJ 2002;325:1337.

15. Walker S, Sheikh A. *Managing anaphylaxis: effective emergency and long-term care are necessary.* Clin Exp Allergy 2003;33:1015–1018.

16. Sampson HA. *Improving in-vitro tests for the diagnosis of food hypersensitivity.* Curr Opin Allergy Clin Immunol 2002;2:257–261.

17. Altman DR, Chiaramonte LT. *Public perception of food allergy.* J Allergy Clin Immunol 1996;97:1247–1251.

18. Celik-Bilgili S, Mehl A, Verstege A, et al. *The predictive value of specific immunoglobulin E levels in serum for the outcome of oral food challenges.* Clin Exp Allergy 2005;35:268–273.

19. Bock SA. *Diagnostic evaluation.* Pediatrics 2003;111:1638–1644.

20. Darsow U, Laifaoui J, Kerschenlohr K, et al. *The prevalence of positive reactions in the atopy patch test with aeroallergens and food allergens in subjects with atopic eczema: a European multicenter study.* Allergy 2004;59:1318–1325.

21. Sampson HA, Metcalfe DD. *Immediate reactions to foods.* In: Metcalfe DD, Sampson HA, Simon RA, eds. Food allergy: adverse reactions to foods and food additives. Boston: Blackwell Scientific Publications, 1991:100–112.

22. Dannaeus A, Ingunas M. *A follow-up study of children with food allergy: clinical course in relation to serum IgE and IgG antibody to milk, egg and fish.* Clin Allergy 1981;11:533–539.

23. Ford RPK, Taylor B. *Natural history of egg hypersensitivity.* Arch Dis Child 1982;57:649–652.

24. Gupta R, Sheikh A, Strachan DP, et al. *Burden of allergic disease in the UK: secondary analyses of national databases.* Clin Exp Allergy 2004;34:520–526.

25. Gupta R, Sheikh A, Strachan D, et al. *Increasing hospital admissions for systemic allergic disorders in England: analysis of national admissions data.* BMJ 2003;327:1142–1143.

26. Levy ML, Price D, Zheng X, et al. *Inadequacies in UK primary care allergy services: national survey of current provisions and perceptions of need.* Clin Exp Allergy 2004;34:518–519.

too close to 1 to be useful (dyspnoea on exertion, fatigue, weight gain and cough).

Diagnosis from the examination

The examination is of greater value than the history in deciding whether heart failure is present. Table 61.3 shows the value of different signs in its diagnosis.

Other signs seem to be encouraging but, in the meta-analysis referred to above,[7] failed to reach statistical significance (the abdominojugular reflex, the Valsalva manoeuvre, hypotension); or do not look as though they would ever prove helpful in this situation (a fourth heart sound, hypertension). Wheeze (LR+ 0.5) and ascites (LR+ 0.3) argue against the diagnosis of heart failure.

Another study[10] not included in the meta-analysis above, of patients referred from general practice for echocardiography with suspected heart failure, found that a displaced apex beat and a tachycardia were useful predictors of heart failure (Table 61.4).

Combinations of symptoms and signs have been shown to be highly specific for the diagnosis of heart failure (Table 61.5).

Overall, studies from secondary care show that the clinical evaluation is 62% sensitive and 76% specific for the detection of increased diastolic filling pressure and 85% sensitive and 66% specific for the detection of decreased ejection fraction.[11]

Table 61.3 Signs that increase the probability of heart failure in a patient presenting urgently with dyspnoea[7] based on an initial risk of heart failure of 50%

Signs	Presence	Likelihood ratio (95% CI)	Probability of heart failure
Third heart sound	Present	11 (5–25)	92%
	Absent	0.9 (0.9–0.9)	47%
Raised JVP*	Present	5.1 (3.2–7.9)	84%
	Absent	0.7 (0.6–0.8)	41%
Basal crackles	Present	2.8 (1.9–4.1)	74%
	Absent	0.5 (0.4–0.7)	33%
Any murmur	Present	2.6 (1.7–4.1)	72%
	Absent	0.8 (0.7–0.9)	44%
Leg oedema	Present	2.3 (1.5–3.7)	70%
	Absent	0.6 (0.5–0.9)	37%

Follow each row from left to right to see how signs alter the probability of heart failure.
*The relatively disappointing performance of the JVP is probably because physicians only estimate JVP correctly about half the time.[8] It can be more specific when examined in a cardiology service as part of a trial (sensitivity 17%, specificity 98%).[9]

Table 61.4 Value of signs in the diagnosis of impaired left ventricular function in patients referred from primary care for echocardiography with suspected heart failure[9] based on an initial risk of heart failure of 50%

Signs	Presence	Likelihood ratio (95% CI)	Probability of heart failure
Displaced apex beat	Present	16 (8.3–33)	94%
	Absent	0.3 (0.2–0.5)	23%
Tachycardia (>100 beats/min)	Present	2.8 (1.3–5.7)	74%
	Absent	0.8 (0.7–1.0)	44%

Follow each row from left to right to see how signs alter the probability of heart failure.

Table 61.5 Value of combinations of features of the history and examination in the diagnosis of heart failure in patients presenting in secondary care[9] based on an initial risk of heart failure of 50%

History and signs	Presence	Likelihood ratio	Probability of heart failure
A history of MI *and* one physical sign (a raised JVP *or* a gallop rhythm *or* crackles *or* oedema *or* a displaced apex beat)	Criteria met	9.7	91%
	Criteria not met	0.6	37%
A displaced apex beat *and* one other physical sign (a raised JVP *or* a gallop rhythm *or* crackles *or* oedema)	Criteria met	44	98%
	Criteria not met	0.6	37%

Follow each row from left to right to see how combinations of features alter the probability of heart failure.

Diagnosis from the investigations

ECG

The following are associated with heart failure:[12]
- Q waves
- T wave and ST segment abnormalities; the 'left ventricular (LV) strain pattern' is a depressed ST segment with an inverted T wave in leads V5 and V6
- left ventricular hypertrophy
- bundle branch block
- atrial fibrillation.

The sensitivity of the ECG in the diagnosis of heart failure depends on the expertise of the interpreter. It may reach 94%[13] or 97%.[14] However, the Breathing Not Properly Multinational Study (BNPMS), conducted in emergency departments, gives more typical statistics (sensitivity 58%, specificity 78%; LR+ 2.7, LR– 0.5).[15] Meta-analysis[11] suggests that anterior Q waves and left bundle branch block (LBBB) are the most useful ECG predictors of heart failure even though neither is specifically an ECG indicator of failure, while a later meta-analysis found that atrial fibrillation was the single most powerful predictor of heart failure (LR+ 3.8, LR– 0.8).[7] Other ECG changes (e.g. LV hypertrophy or LV strain pattern) are less specific.

Adding a BNP estimation to an abnormal ECG result does nothing to improve the sensitivity but does improve specificity.[16]

Chest X-ray

The following may, or may not, be present:[12]
- cardiomegaly
- pulmonary venous congestion, shown by, in increasing order of severity, upper lobe diversion,

fluid in the horizontal fissure and in the costophrenic angles (Kerley B lines), the 'bat's wing' appearance of frank pulmonary oedema, and pleural effusions, usually bilateral, occasionally unilateral.

The BNPMS[15] gives the figures for different CXR findings shown in Table 61.6. Note that the findings with the higher positive LRs tend to be associated with the higher (i.e. less useful) negative LRs. In other words, if a finding, when present, is helpful in confirming the diagnosis of heart failure, it tends to be unhelpful, when absent, in refuting it.

Plasma BNP or N-terminal proBNP (NTproBNP)

At a cut-off of 100 pg/ml, they have a sensitivity of 90% and a specificity of 75% (LR+3.7, LR– 0.1) for the diagnosis of heart failure.[15] They give information that is independent of the clinical indicators (above)[17] and have been shown to be useful in primary care[6] as well as the emergency hospital setting.[18] The likelihood ratios above show that the test is useful in the confirmation of heart failure but especially useful in refuting the diagnosis (LR– 0.1). Brain natriuretic peptide has an accuracy of 81% for the diagnosis of heart failure, which is greater than that of the physician's clinical judgement at 74%.[17] The Natriuretic Peptides in the Community Study[6] calculates that the number needed to test for N-BNP is 7; that is, it is necessary to measure N-BNP in 7 patients with suspected heart failure for the BNP results to alter the diagnosis in 1 patient. This makes it extraordinarily useful. However, a systematic review which examined the addition of BNP to ECG found that it increased specificity but not sensitivity.[16] This is disappointing because in primary care it is better to overdiagnose (and

Table 61.6 The value of different chest X-ray findings in the diagnosis of heart failure[15] based on an initial risk of heart failure of 50%

CXR finding	Presence	Likelihood ratio	Probability of heart failure
Cardiomegaly	Present	4.0	80%
	Absent	0.3	23%
Upper lobe diversion	Present	9.4	90%
	Absent	0.6	37%
Interstitial oedema	Present	13	93%
	Absent	0.7	41%
Alveolar oedema	Present	7.0	88%
	Absent	0.9	47%
Pleural effusion	Present	3.3	77%
	Absent	0.8	44%

Follow each row from left to right to see how X-ray findings alter the probability of heart failure.

not miss a case), than underdiagnose, the condition. Overdiagnosis can be corrected by the specialist; missed cases are less likely to have that opportunity.

Factors that can influence the BNP result[7]

False positives occur in:
- old age
- renal failure
- acute coronary syndrome
- cor pulmonale
- acute large pulmonary embolism
- high output cardiac states.

False negatives occur in:
- acute pulmonary oedema
- stable mild heart failure
- acute mitral regurgitation
- mitral stenosis
- atrial myxoma.

Combining clinical features and investigations

In clinical practice it is tempting to apply the likelihood ratios above, one after the other, using the previous post-test probability as the new pre-test probability, to arrive at the probability of heart failure for the individual patient. This would only be justified if the factors were independent of each other, and few studies have examined this aspect.

One that has is a study from Copenhagen[19] which found, on multivariate regression analysis, that three factors were independent predictors of the presence of systolic dysfunction:
- an ECG showing QRS or ST-T changes (LR+ 2.0, LR− 0.2)
- tachycardia where the resting supine heart rate was greater than the diastolic blood pressure (LR+ 3.8, LR− 0.6)
- a raised N-terminal atrial natriuretic peptide (>0.8 nmol/L) (LR+ 3.9, LR− 0.5).[20]

If these three pointers are present, their likelihood ratios can be used in sequence. If not, the GP must decide whether it seems likely that pointers would be independent of each other. Clearly it would be wrong to add the LR+ for one CXR finding to that of another; the one with the greater predictive power should be chosen. But adding the LR+ for a third heart sound to the CXR finding of a pleural effusion seems reasonable since they represent different pathophysiological events.

Another approach is suggested by Badgett and colleagues, in their systematic review.[11] They propose that if only one of the clinical features, including CXR and ECG, is present, the post-test probability of the diagnosis of heart failure is reduced (LR− = 0.1). If two are present, it is not greatly altered. If three or more are present, it is greatly increased (LR+ = 14). However, this approach ignores the fact that different features have different predictive power. Furthermore, these suggestions are based on secondary care data, based on studies of patients with suspected heart failure. The power of the positive findings may have already been 'used up' (see box below) because they were the reason why the GP or emergency physician suspected the diagnosis in the first place.

The concept of symptoms and signs being 'used up' is an important one when extrapolating from studies in secondary care to the situation in primary care. Assume that GPs are good at recognising a raised JVP and use it in their decision to refer patients with suspected heart failure. Most of the patients entering secondary care will have a raised JVP, whether they have heart failure or not; so it is less useful than it was in primary care as a discriminatory sign. If GPs *only* referred patients as having suspected heart failure if the JVP was raised, and patients only reached secondary care via GP referral, it would have lost *all* its value as a sign in secondary care.

Other investigations

Echocardiography. The measurement of left ventricular systolic ejection fraction is the gold standard for the diagnosis of left ventricular systolic heart failure, but it will miss the diagnosis of diastolic heart failure, which was present in 36.5% of patients with heart failure in the BNPMS.[21] These patients all had an ejection fraction >45%. To pick up those with diastolic heart failure, an echocardiogram analysing mitral inflow is needed, which has the following figures for the diagnosis of all types of heart failure in patients with acute dyspnoea: sensitivity 89%, specificity 93%; LR+ 12.7, LR− 0.1.[22]

The NICE guideline[13] calculates that echocardiography is only cost effective if performed on those with an abnormal ECG or BNP. Its role is to confirm the diagnosis, to decide between systolic and diastolic failure and look for valvular disease and for intracardiac shunts.

Diastolic (or non-systolic) heart failure

One-third of patients who present urgently with dyspnoea, and who are found to have congestive cardiac failure, have a systolic ejection fraction greater than 45%[21] (i.e. their heart failure is non-systolic).The BNP is still useful in separating diastolic heart failure from non-heart failure causes of dyspnoea, though with lower sensitivity than in patients with systolic heart failure. The sensitivity is 86% (using a cut-off of 100 pg/ml) and the specificity is considerably lower.[21]

This realisation of a type of heart failure with preserved systolic ejection fraction casts doubt on figures for the predictive value of symptoms and signs of heart failure arrived at with systolic ejection fraction as the gold standard. This reservation does not apply to those studies in which the final diagnosis included systolic and diastolic failure.[6,15,17,21,23]

Blood tests:

■ *Full blood count* is needed in the diagnosis of anaemia, which may be contributing to the heart failure. The clinical diagnosis of anaemia is not accurate (see p. 318).

■ *Creatinine and electrolytes.* Renal failure may mimic heart failure. Creatinine and electrolyte values will be important in guiding management decisions in heart failure.

■ *Thyroid function tests.* Heart failure is a feature of hyper- and hypothyroid states.

Peak flow or spirometry: may be helpful in ruling out a pulmonary cause for the patient's symptoms; or in showing that there is a pulmonary component as well as a cardiac one.

Other issues

Once the diagnosis of heart failure has been made, an attempt should be made to determine the aetiology

A study of a population of 151 000 in west London,[3] using non-invasive techniques, found the following aetiologies:

■ coronary heart disease 36%
■ unknown 34%
■ hypertension 14%
■ valvular disease 7%
■ atrial fibrillation alone 5%
■ others 5%.

The problem of diagnosing heart failure in a patient with chronic obstructive pulmonary disease (COPD)

Chronic obstructive pulmonary disease poses a problem in the diagnosis of heart failure because

7. Wang C, FitzGerald J, Schulzer M, et al. *Does this dyspneic patient in the emergency department have congestive heart failure?* JAMA 2005;294:1944–1956.

8. Cook D, Simel D. *Does this patient have abnormal central venous pressure?* JAMA 1996;275:630–634.

9. Davie A, Francis C, Caruana L, et al. *Assessing diagnosis in heart failure: which features are any use?* Q J Med 1997;90:335–339.

10. McGee S. *Evidence-based physical diagnosis.* Philadelphia: Saunders, 2001.

11. Badgett R, Lucey C, Mulrow C. *Can the clinical examination diagnose left-sided heart failure in adults?* JAMA 1997;277:1712–1719.

12. Davies M, Gibbs C, Lip G. *ABC of heart failure: investigation.* BMJ 2000;320:297–300.

13. The National Collaborating Centre for Chronic Conditions. *Chronic heart failure: a national clinical guideline for diagnosis and management in primary and secondary care.* London: Royal College of Physicians, 2003. Available online as NICE Clinical Guideline No. 5: www.nice.org.uk.

14. Hutcheon S, Gillespie N, Struthers A, et al. *B-type natriuretic peptide in the diagnosis of cardiac disease in elderly day hospital patients.* Age Ageing 2002;31:295–301.

15. Knudsen C, Omland T, Clopton P, et al. *Diagnostic value of B-type natriuretic peptide and chest radiographic findings in patients with acute dyspnea.* Am J Med 2004;116:363–368.

16. Davenport C, Cheng E, Kwok Y, et al. *Assessing the diagnostic test accuracy of natriuretic peptides and ECG in the diagnosis of left ventricular systolic dysfunction: a systematic review and meta-analysis.* Br J Gen Pract 2006;56:48–56.

17. McCullough P, Nowak R, McCord J, et al. *B-type natriuretic peptide and clinical judgement in emergency diagnosis of heart failure.* Circulation 2002;106:416–422.

18. Mueller C, Scholer A, Laule-Kilian K, et al. *Use of B-type natriuretic peptide in the evaluation and management of acute dyspnea.* N Engl J Med 2004;350:647–54.

19. Nielsen O, Hansen J, Hilden J, et al. *Risk assessment of left ventricular systolic dysfunction in primary care: cross sectional study evaluating a range of diagnostic tests.* BMJ 2000;320:220–224.

20. Meisner J, Hla A. *A combination of tests done in general practice could assess the risk for left ventricular systolic dysfunction.* Evidence-Based Medicine 2000;5:185.

21. Maisal A, McCord J, Nowak R, et al. *Bedside B-type natriuretic peptide in the emergency diagnosis of heart failure with reduced or preserved ejection fraction. Results from the Breathing Not Properly Multinational Study.* J Am Coll Cardiol 2003;41:2010–2017.

22. Logeart D, Saudubray C, Beyne P, et al. *Comparative value of Doppler echocardiography and B-type natriuretic peptide assay in the etiologic diagnosis of acute dyspnea.* J Am Coll Cardiol 2002;40:1794–1800.

23. Lainchbury J, Campbell E, Frampton C, et al. *Brain natriuretic peptide and N-terminal brain natriuretic peptide in the diagnosis of heart failure in patients with acute shortness of breath.* J Am Coll Cardiol 2003;42:728–735.

24. Rutten F, Moons K, Cramer M-J, et al. *Recognising heart failure in elderly patients with stable chronic obstructive pulmonary disease in primary care: cross sectional diagnostic study.* BMJ 2005;331:1379–1382.

62

Hypertension

KEY FACTS

- Since 2004, the accepted definition of hypertension has been a sustained blood pressure (BP) of 140/90 or above.
- Attention to the detail of BP measurement will reduce the number misdiagnosed.
- Random clinic readings are unreliable. Home and ambulatory readings may be more reliable but the readings must be adjusted for the fact that lower readings are consistently found outside the clinic setting.
- A limited number of investigations for an underlying cause are recommended. This approach will miss few treatable causes of hypertension provided abnormal urine or blood tests are followed up and provided patients uncontrolled on three or more drugs are referred.

A PRACTICAL APPROACH

- ★ Measure the blood pressure routinely in adults at least 5-yearly, increasing to annually in those in the high-normal range (i.e. systolic 130–139 or diastolic 85–89 mmHg).[1]
- ★ Arrange for the patient to measure his or her BP at home, or for ambulatory monitoring, if you suspect 'white coat hypertension' because of widely fluctuating levels or obvious unease at having the pressure taken.
- ★ If hypertension is found, examine for evidence of end-organ damage and of an underlying cause.
- ★ Repeat readings over 3 months unless evidence of end-organ damage or very high levels make treatment more urgent.
- ★ Perform a limited battery of investigations for an underlying cause.
- ★ Refer a patient for more detailed investigation if needing treatment under the age of 30, or if resistant to three antihypertensive drugs, or if hypertension is severe or worsens suddenly.

Background

- Hypertension is an arbitrary concept in which those with higher blood pressures are defined as suitable for treatment or surveillance. The diagnosis is therefore based on the patient's blood pressure (BP). Since an individual's blood pressure varies, both within one day and over weeks and months, repeated measurements under well-controlled conditions are needed, unless clinical examination shows unequivocal signs of hypertensive end-organ damage.

- Thirty-seven per cent of adults in the UK have hypertension, using the new UK definitions (Table 62.1).[2]

- The rule of halves was described in the USA in 1972.[3] It states that half of hypertensives are not known to have a raised BP; of those with known hypertension, half are not on treatment and half of

Table 62.1 Classification used by the British Hypertension Society (BHS), the European Society of Hypertension and the WHO, based on clinic readings[1]

Categories	Systolic BP	Diastolic BP
Optimal	<120	<80
Normal	120–129	80–84
High-normal	130–139	85–89
Mild hypertension (grade 1)	140–159	90–99
Moderate hypertension (grade 2)	160–179	100–109
Severe hypertension (grade 3)	≥180	≥110
Isolated systolic hypertension grade 1	140–159	<90
Isolated systolic hypertension grade 2	≥160	<90

NB. A patient should be allocated to the highest category for which he or she meets either the systolic or the diastolic criteria.

those on treatment are poorly controlled. Figures for the UK in 1998[2] showed that, using the new definitions (see below), half of those with hypertension knew they were hypertensive; of these, two-thirds were on treatment and a third of those were controlled. Even using a threshold and target of 160/95, 71% knew they had hypertension; of these, 59% were on treatment; and 65% of these were controlled.

Practicalities[1]

(a) *Patient positioning.* The patient should be seated, but in older patients and in diabetics check the blood pressure both standing and sitting, looking for postural hypotension. The arm should be at heart level and the patient relaxed and not talking.

(b) *The device* should be of known accuracy and recently checked.

(c) *The cuff* should cover at least 80% of the circumference of the upper arm. The standard adult cuff (bladder 12 cm wide and 18 cm long) is appropriate for those with an arm circumference 23 cm to 32 cm.

(d) *The measurement.* Measure the systolic and diastolic pressures (phase V) to the nearest 2 mm, on two occasions at least 1 minute apart. If phase V is zero, use phase IV. Use the second reading. If the two readings are markedly different from each other (>10 cm), take at least one more. Take the average. Repeated readings by a nurse give the most

reliable clinic results, occasional readings by a doctor the least.[4]

(e) *Timing.* In mild uncomplicated hypertension, do not accept the diagnosis until four readings have been taken over a 3-month period; 25% of blood pressures will settle in that time. However, those that settle to below treatment levels need lifelong annual follow-up. If the initial diastolic is >200/110 mmHg or there is evidence of end-organ damage, cardiovascular disease or diabetes, three readings over 2 weeks would be more appropriate. Consider immediate treatment if the pressure is >220/120.

Accuracy of blood pressure measurement

Does measurement of blood pressure at a routine clinic in primary care accurately measure blood pressure?

They tend to overestimate the blood pressure. A UK study[4] examined BP recordings in 200 patients who either had newly diagnosed hypertension, borderline hypertension or were established hypertensives poorly controlled on treatment. Using the mean daytime ambulatory BP measurement (ABPM) as the gold standard, with a cut-off of >135/85 mmHg considered to be raised, the last three clinic readings, using a cut-off of >140/90 as raised, had the following figures for the detection of raised blood pressure:

■ systolic: sensitivity 97%, specificity 14%; LR+ 1.1, LR– 0.2

■ diastolic: sensitivity 90%, specificity 35%; LR+ 1.4, LR– 0.3.

In other words, the clinic readings usually detected a raised level, when ABPM showed it was raised, but frequently overestimated as raised levels that ambulatory monitoring showed were normal. The weakness of the study is that it is not clear whether that level of ABPM is a reliable gold standard.

Home and ambulatory blood pressure measurement

● Hypertensives regularly record lower pressures at home or with ambulatory monitoring (ABPM) than in the clinic. Home readings are, on average, 5 mmHg lower than clinic readings and ambulatory monitoring readings are 15 mmHg lower.[5]

● 13% of patients show an exaggerated rise in BP when it is measured in the clinic ('white coat hypertension').[6]

● A similar number (9%) show the opposite phenomenon; that is, lower readings in the clinic than at home ('masked hypertension').[6]

● Cohort studies show that home readings predict prognosis better than clinic readings when there is a mismatch.[6–8]

● All randomised controlled trials (RCTs) of the benefits of antihypertensive treatment have been conducted using clinic readings. A recent RCT has shown that, while home monitoring can be useful in identifying those with white coat hypertension, its use in judging whether medication should be adjusted, in those in whom a decision to treat has been made, leads to undertreatment.[9] Until an RCT using home readings establishes the superiority of home readings in making the diagnosis and monitoring treatment, clinic levels should be used routinely.

✳ Consider asking a patient to record home levels if:

(a) levels are borderline and the decision about whether the patient is hypertensive is difficult

(b) white coat hypertension is suspected because of fluctuating readings, or obvious anxiety, in the clinic

(c) the patient has evidence of target organ damage which is greater than would be expected from the clinic baseline BP.

✳ If using home readings, adjust threshold levels down by 5 mmHg since the BHS thresholds refer to readings taken in clinic settings. Be aware that this is an approximation.

✳ For home readings, supply the patient with an automated machine that uses the upper arm and that prints or stores the results. Instruct the patient to become familiar with the machine and then to take two readings twice a day for 2 days, each time after sitting for 5 minutes. Take the average. Only ask for more readings if there are wide fluctuations or the eight readings show a tendency to decline towards the normal range over the 2 days. This gives a result akin to the reliability of ABPM.[10] Wrist and finger devices are inaccurate.

Examination for signs of end-organ damage

Look for hypertensive retinopathy and left ventricular hypertrophy, as well as evidence of associated macrovascular disease (absent foot pulses and evidence from the history of coronary heart disease, stroke or transient ischaemic attack).

Chest X-ray for cardiac enlargement is not recommended as a routine nor is ECG or urine microscopy and culture.[1]

The search for an underlying cause

Estimates of the proportion of patients with an underlying cause for their hypertension range from 0.1%[11] to 5%,[12] a variation largely explained by the variation in the screening tests used in different studies. The prevalence of secondary hypertension in secondary and tertiary care is inevitably higher. A US study of over 4000 patients in a hypertension referral centre found that 10.2% had an underlying cause as follows:

■ renovascular hypertension 3.1%

■ hypothyroidism 3.0%

■ renal insufficiency 1.8%

■ primary aldosteronism 1.4%

■ Cushing's syndrome 0.5%

■ phaeochromocytoma 0.3%.

Note:

1. In those with atherosclerosis, the prevalence of renovascular hypertension was 9.5% and renal insufficiency 8%.

2. Other estimates have produced far higher estimates of the prevalence of primary aldosteronism (5–13%)[13] even in primary care.[14]

No recent studies have examined the value of searching for secondary causes of hypertension in primary care. The pick-up is likely to be far less than that in the US study above. The British Hypertension Society Guidelines (BHS IV)[1] recommend a common sense approach which emphasises the clinical assessment and a limited number of investigations.

History:

   (a) drugs (NSAIDs, combined oral contraceptives, steroids)
   (b) lifestyle factors: excessive alcohol or salt intake, little exercise, obesity
   (c) personal or family history of renal disease
   (d) early onset (needing treatment <age 30).

Examination:

   (a) pulses for coarctation
   (b) cushingoid features (truncal obesity, striae)
   (c) abdominal bruit for renovascular disease.

Urine:

dipstick for protein and blood.

Blood:

creatinine and electrolytes. Refer if creatinine is >150 µmol/L or K$^+$ <3.2 mmol/L.[15]

Progress:

sudden onset or worsening; or resistance to three or more drugs.

Is there good evidence for this minimal approach?

The large cross-sectional study in primary care that would provide that evidence has not been performed. Indirect evidence exists from secondary care:

● *Renovascular hypertension.* In Finland, the selection of those with normal urine tests but with an onset <30 years old, or resistant to three or more drugs, produced a prevalence of a renovascular cause in 12%, i.e. these two criteria were useful in selecting those at high risk of renovascular hypertension.[16]

● *Primary aldosteronism.* Two screening tests for this condition are used in primary care:

   1. *Low serum potassium.* Estimates of the sensitivity of a low serum potassium in the detection of primary aldosteronism (PA) vary from 13%[17] to 74%.[18] Referral of patients with a low potassium will detect about half of those with PA.

   2. *Treatment resistance.* In Poland, 63% of those with primary aldosteronism were found to be resistant to three or more drugs.[18] Again, this seems to be a useful criterion for investigation.

Example

An asymptomatic man aged 42 is found to have a blood pressure of 170/100 on routine screening. His father was hypertensive but there is no other relevant history and examination is normal, as are urine dipstick tests and serum creatinine and electrolytes.

   He returns monthly for three more checks with the practice nurse. They are 160/80, 145/80 and 150/85, but when he sees the GP once more it is 180/100. He admits that he gets tense about having the pressure measured, especially by the GP when she is so busy.

The GP decides to send him home with an automated sphygmomanometer. When he returns, the GP learns that the initial home readings were around 145/90 but that they settled to 138/87.

   The GP is aware that this correlates with a clinic reading of approximately 143/92. She tells him that he has mild hypertension, which was hard to assess at first because of an element of white coat hypertension. However, it is so mild that increased exercise and changing his diet to more fruit and vegetables is all that is needed at this stage. Follow-up visits are set at 3-monthly initially, then 6-monthly.

REFERENCES

1. Williams B, Poulter N, Brown M, et al. *British Hypertension Society guidelines for hypertension management 2004 (BHS-IV).* J Hum Hypertens 2004;18:139–185.

2. Primatesta P, Brookes M, Poulter N. *Improved hypertension management and control: results from the Health Survey for England 1998.* Hypertension 2001;38:827–832.

3. Wilber J, Barrow J. *Hypertension: community problem.* Am J Med 1972;52:653–663.

4. Little P, Barnett J, Barnsley L, et al. *Comparison of agreement between different measures of blood pressure in primary care and daytime ambulatory blood pressure.* BMJ 2002;325:254–257.

5. Guidelines Committee. *European Society of Hypertension – European Society of Cardiology guidelines for the management of arterial hypertension.* J Hypertens 2003;21:1011–1053.

6. Bobrie G, Chatellier G, Genes N, et al. *Cardiovascular prognosis of 'masked hypertension' detected by blood pressure self-measurement in elderly treated hypertensive patients.* JAMA 2003;291:1342–1349.

7. Ohkubo T, Imai Y, Tsuji I, et al. *Home blood pressure measurement has a stronger predictive power for mortality than does screening blood pressure measurement: a population-based observation in Ohasama, Japan.* J Hypertens 1998;16:971–975.

8. O'Brien E, Coats A, Owens P, et al. *Use and interpretation of ambulatory blood pressure monitoring: recommendations of the British Hypertension Society.* BMJ 2000;320:1128–1134.

9. Staessen J, Den Hond E, Celis H, et al. *Antihypertensive treatment based on blood pressure measurement at home or in the physician's office: a randomized controlled trial.* JAMA 2004;291:955–964.

10. Brueren M, Schouten H, De Leeuw P, et al. *A series of self-measurements by the patient is a reliable alternative to ambulatory blood pressure measurement.* Br J Gen Pract 1998;48:1585–1589.

11. Omura M, Saito J, Yamaguchi K, et al. *Prospective study on the prevalence of secondary hypertension among hypertensive patients visiting a general outpatient clinic in Japan.* Hypertens Res 2004;27:193–202.

12. Akpunonu B, Mulrow P, Hoffman E. *Secondary hypertension: evaluation and treatment.* Dis Mon 1997;42:609–722.

13. Young W. *Minireview: primary aldosteronism – changing concepts in diagnosis and treatment.* Endocrinology 2003;144:2208–2213.

14. Lim P, Rodgers P, Cardale K, et al. *Potentially high prevalence of primary aldosteronism in a primary-care population (Research Letter).* Lancet 1999;353:40.

15. Goldenberg K, Snyder D. *Screening for primary aldosteronism: hypokalemia in hypertensive patients.* J Gen Intern Med 1986;1:368–372.

16. Helin K, Tikkanen I, von Knorring J, et al. *Screening for renovascular hypertension in a population with relatively low prevalence.* J Hypertens 1998;16:1523–1529.

17. Stowasser M, Gordon R, Gunasekera T, et al. *High rate of detection of primary aldosteronism, including surgically treatable forms, after 'non-selective' screening of hypertensive patients.* J Hypertens 2003;21:2149–2157.

18. Prejbisz A, Postula M, Cybulska I, et al. *The role of biochemical tests and clinical symptoms in differential diagnosis of primary aldosteronism.* Kardiol Pol 2003;58:17–26.

63

Hyperthyroidism

KEY FACTS

- The possibility of hyperthyroidism is raised by many different clinical situations: for instance, by non-specific symptoms (e.g. tiredness or fine tremor); and by other conditions of which hyperthyroidism is occasionally a cause (e.g. atrial fibrillation or osteoporosis).
- Despite the extraordinary reliability of modern thyroid function tests (TFTs), a clinical assessment is necessary to spot the occasional false positive and false negative, and to determine whether a patient has clinical or subclinical disease. Furthermore, a clear clinical diagnosis that the patient is euthyroid can sometimes mean that case-finding with TFTs is not needed.

A PRACTICAL APPROACH

* If the clinical picture raises the suspicion of hyperthyroidism, check the TFTs. Meanwhile, decide how strong the clinical picture is, either informally or with a formal Crooks score.
* If the free T_4 (FT_4) and free T_3 (FT_3) are raised and the TSH is low, this is the classical pattern of hyperthyroidism.
* If the FT_4 and FT_3 are normal and the TSH is low, there are several possibilities:
  (a) surreptitious ingestion of thyroxine in slimming pills
  (b) subclinical hyperthyroidism, seen in older people usually with multinodular goitre
  (c) serious concomitant illness.
* If the FT_4 and FT_3 are raised and the TSH is raised, there are several possibilities, all rare:
  (a) TSH-secreting pituitary tumour
  (b) amiodarone
  (c) acute psychiatric illness.
* If the clinical picture disagrees with the TFTs, repeat the test. If there is still disagreement, or the situation fits none of the above, seek specialist advice.

Prevalence

Prevalence in the general population is 0.3%, with 95% of cases occurring in women.[1]

Value of the history and examination in diagnosing hyperthyroidism

The classic symptoms and signs of hyperthyroidism have been well described. A review has summarised the likelihood ratios associated with each.[2] However, they are difficult to use because it is not clear whether they can be applied independently of each other. A way round this is to make an overall assessment, as described by Crooks, Murray and Wayne in 1959.[3] It may be used in two ways: either as a guide to the most discriminating symptoms (temperature, appetite and weight) and signs (goitre and hyperkinetic movements);

Table 63.1 The Crooks score for the diagnosis of hyperthyroidism[3]

Symptom	Positives	Negatives	Sign	Positives	Negatives
Dyspnoea on effort	+1		Palpable thyroid	+3	−3
Palpitations	+2		Thyroid bruit	+2	−2
Tiredness on exertion	+2		Exophthalmos	+2	
Prefers heat		−5	Lid retraction	+2	
Prefers cold	+5		Lid lag	+1	
Excessive sweating	+3		Hyperkinetic movements	+4	−2
Nervousness	+2		Fine tremor	+1	
Appetite increased	+3		Hot hands	+2	−2
Appetite decreased		−3	Moist hands	+1	−1
Weight increased		−3	Atrial fibrillation	+4	
Weight decreased	+3		Sinus rhythm pulse	<80	−3
				80–90	0
				>90	+3

From Crooks J et al. Statistical methods applied to the clinical diagnosis of thyrotoxicosis. QJM: An International Journal of Medicine 1959;28:211–234, by permission of Oxford University Press.

Table 63.2 The probability of hyperthyroidism, according to the Crooks score, at two different levels of initial risk

Initial risk of hyperthyroidism	Score	Likelihood ratio (95% CI)	Probability of hyperthyroidism
2%*	≥20	59 (11–335)	55%
	≥10	8.4 (4.5–16)	15%
	<10	0 (0–0.15)	0%
20%[†]	≥20	59 (11–335)	94%
	≥10	8.4 (4.5–16)	68%
	<10	0 (0–0.15)	0%

Follow each row from left to right to see how the initial risk and the score alter the probability of hyperthyroidism.
*An initial risk of hyperthyroidism of 2% might be suggested by the presentation of a young woman with a fine tremor.
[†]An initial risk of hyperthyroidism of 20% might be suggested by the presentation of a older woman with a fine tremor and a multinodular goitre.

or as a complete score from which the post-test probability can be calculated (Table 63.1).

Crooks and colleagues found that a score of 20 or over occurred in 45 out of 51 patients with hyperthyroidism and in 1 of 66 without it. A score of 10 or less occurred in none of 51 hyperthyroid patients and in 59 out of 67 euthyroid patients. Table 63.2 shows how these results translate into likelihood ratios and probabilities.

Note that:
(a) a confident clinical diagnosis is only possible in a patient whose baseline risk is already substantial

(b) while a score of 10 or below seems to rule out hyperthyroidism regardless of initial risk, the confidence intervals of the likelihood ratio mean that that post-test probability in the older woman with the multinodular goitre could be as high as 4% (although in the woman at lower risk it would be no higher than 0.3%).

However, *four cautions* should be noted:

1. Note how wide the confidence intervals are for statistics other than the sensitivity of a score of ≤10. This is because of the small numbers in Crooks' study.

2. The Crooks score was validated in secondary care using patients of 'doubtful' thyroid status, i.e. where the physician was in doubt about the patient's thyroid status. No studies have tested the score in primary care.

3. The problem with cut-off scores is that they do not allow for the 'barn door' clinical picture; that is, the clinical picture that is so strongly diagnostic of the condition that the diagnosis is virtually certain.

4. If a positive psychiatric diagnosis (mainly anxiety but also depressive illness) is made, it reduces the probability that the patient's symptoms are due to hyperthyroidism. This has been formalised in the Newcastle Index.[4]

Some sophistication is needed in the history taking:

* Avoid leading questions (e.g. ask 'Has your weight changed recently?' rather than 'Have you lost weight?'). A change of 7 lb or more over a period of up to one year is significant.

* Do not score a patient as having dyspnoea if the level of dyspnoea is appropriate for the patient's age or cardiovascular status.

* Only score a symptom as positive if there has been a recent change.

* If you plan to calculate the post-test probability, do not stop until the examination is complete. A score of 20 halfway through may end as a score below 20 at the end because of the possibility of negative scores.

* Beware of dismissing the diagnosis in patients over 60. Clinical evidence of hyperthyroidism may be missing in 1 in 4 cases.[5] In older patients, atrial fibrillation and weight loss were more likely to be present than in those <60, while increased appetite, heat intolerance, goitre, sweating and irritability are less likely to be present.[6]

Thyroid function tests

* Check the thyroid stimulating hormone (TSH).
* If the clinical picture is suggestive, check the FT_3 at this stage to save time.

A third generation TSH test has a sensitivity and specificity of >99%, giving an LR+ of 99 and an LR− of <0.01.[1] This means that a low TSH virtually rules in, and a normal TSH rules out the diagnosis of hyperthyroidism, but the FT_3 is required for confirmation because of the rare cases in which the TSH is misleading (see the box below). FT_3 is better than FT_4 because the latter would miss cases of T_3 toxicosis.

A falsely normal TSH (i.e. FT_3 raised and the patient is hyperthyroid) is found in TSH-secreting pituitary tumours and in thyroid hormone resistance (both very rare).

A falsely low TSH (i.e. FT_3 normal and patient is euthyroid) is found in severe concomitant illness, when the specificity of the low TSH in the diagnosis of hyperthyroidism falls to 95% and the LR+ falls to 20.[1] It also occurs in surreptitious thyroxine ingestion (e.g. in slimming pills), in pregnancy and with the use of high doses of glucocorticoids.

Diagnosing the cause of hyperthyroidism[7]

● *If thyroid eye disease, or thyroid receptor antibodies, are present*: this is likely to be Graves' disease, especially if the patient is aged <40. ('Thyroid eye disease' means proptosis, diplopia or conjunctival oedema, not the eye signs of lid retraction and lid lag.)

● *If one or more thyroid nodules are present*: the diagnosis is more likely to be toxic nodular goitre or a toxic adenoma, especially if the patient is aged >40. Refer for further investigation.

● *If the history is short (<1 month)*: consider transient or postpartum thyroiditis. A raised erythrocyte sedimentation rate supports the diagnosis of the former. If suspected, recheck the TSH and FT_3 after 6 weeks. If normal, no further action is needed.

● *Amiodarone* may cause true hyperthyroidism, as well as hypothyroidism, or it may result in the finding of a raised TSH in a euthyroid patient.

Subclinical hyperthyroidism

Definition. A low TSH in a patient with normal FT_3 and FT_4 and no symptoms of hyperthyroidism.

Prevalence. At 2% of the population, this is much lower than subclinical hypothyroidism.[8] Those with severely depressed TSH levels (<0.1 mU/L) are at increased risk of developing atrial fibrillation and osteoporotic fractures and deserve specialist assessment.[8] Patients with smaller degrees of TSH depression need annual surveillance.

Example

A 64-year-old man is admitted to hospital with congestive cardiac failure secondary to ischaemic heart disease and is found to be in atrial fibrillation (AF). His work-up includes thyroid function tests, which reveal a low TSH but normal FT_3 and FT_4. On discharge he is out of heart failure, though still in AF. He has an appointment to see the endocrinologist in 4 months' time; an earlier appointment is not available. He has been told by the hospital physician that his thyroid is overactive.

The GP goes over his history and, apart from the AF, finds no clinical pointers to hyperthyroidism. She is unconvinced that this is subclinical hyperthyroidism. His sex makes the probability 0.03%, raised to, say, 0.3% by the AF. The GP considers the ischaemic heart disease a much more likely cause of the AF. The LR+ of 20 in patients with severe concomitant illness and a low TSH only raises the probability of hyperthyroidism to 6% (Fig. 63.1). She repeats the thyroid function tests 3 months after discharge and finds them normal. She discusses the case with the endocrinologist, who is delighted to be able to cancel the appointment.

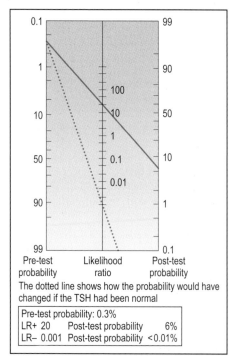

The dotted line shows how the probability would have changed if the TSH had been normal

Pre-test probability: 0.3%		
LR+ 20	Post-test probability	6%
LR− 0.001	Post-test probability	<0.01%

Figure 63.1 The probability of hyperthyroidism before and after the finding of a low TSH in the example above.

REFERENCES

1. Dolan JD, Wittlin SD. Hyperthyroidism and hypothyroidism. In: Black ER, Bordley DR, Tape TG, Panzer RJ, eds. *Diagnostic strategies for common medical problems,* 2nd edn. Philadelphia: American College of Physicians, 1999:473–483.

2. McGee S. *Evidence-based physical diagnosis.* Philadelphia: Saunders, 2001.

3. Crooks J, Murray IPC, Wayne EJ. *Statistical methods applied to the clinical diagnosis of thyrotoxicosis.* QJM 1959;28:211–234.

4. Gurney C, Hall R, Harper M, et al. *Newcastle Thyrotoxicosis Index.* Lancet 1970;2:1275–1278.

5. Davis PJ, David FB. *Hyperthyroidism in patients over the age of 60 years.* Medicine 1974;53:161–181.

6. Nordyke R, Gilbert F, Harada A. *Graves' disease: influence of age on clinical findings.* Arch Intern Med 1988;148:626–631.

7. Provan D, Krentz A. *Oxford handbook of clinical and laboratory investigation.* Oxford: Oxford University Press, 2002.

8. Surks M, Ortiz E, Daniels G, et al. *Subclinical thyroid disease: scientific review and guidelines for diagnosis and management.* JAMA 2004;291:228–238.

64

Hypothyroidism

- Scoring systems for the estimation of the probability of hypothyroidism based on the clinical picture have been developed. That of Billewicz rates symptoms according to their importance; others use a simpler count of the number of symptoms.
- The clinical assessment is important: it helps the physician to order thyroid function tests (TFTs) in those for whom they are appropriate, it allows a distinction between clinical and subclinical hypothyroidism, and it helps in the detection of situations in which the TFTs are misleading.
- A history of predisposing causes, the examination of the thyroid, the pattern of the TFTs and the thyroid autoantibody result usually allow the GP to diagnose the aetiology of the hypothyroidism.

A PRACTICAL APPROACH

- *If the clinical picture raises even a small suspicion of hypothyroidism, check the TFTs.* Most patients do not have the classical clinical picture. If an abnormal result is obtained, repeat the test after a wait of at least 2 weeks.
- *If the free T_4 (FT$_4$) and free T_3 (FT$_3$) are low and the thyroid stimulating hormone (TSH) is raised,* hypothyroidism is confirmed. If there are symptoms, it is overt, if not, it is subclinical.
- *If the FT$_4$ and FT$_3$ are low and the TSH is normal or low,* suspect secondary hypothyroidism. Consider referral for investigation of the hypothalamic/pituitary axis.

However, a commoner cause, especially if only the FT$_3$ is low, is the failure of peripheral conversion of FT$_4$ to FT$_3$ seen in any serious illness and in old age.
- *If the FT$_4$ and FT$_3$ are normal and the TSH is raised,* suspect subclinical hypothyroidism. Check anti-thyroid antibodies to decide on the prognosis and need for surveillance.
- *If the TSH is normal and the clinical picture is not suggestive of hypothyroidism:* hypothyroidism is effectively excluded.
- *If the situation fits none of the above,* seek specialist advice.

It is tempting to think that the diagnosis of hypothyroidism is completely resolved by the accuracy of modern thyroid function tests (TFTs). Unfortunately, three factors complicate the diagnosis:

1. The typical clinical picture is uncommon; non-specific complaints may not suggest the possibility of hypothyroidism to the doctor.
2. Subclinical hypothyroidism is common, especially in older women. The finding of

Menstrual changes and hypersomnia were not significantly more common in cases than controls and nor was coarser hair (because too few cases reported it for the difference to reach significance).

From this study, the most useful likelihood ratios proved to be those related to a simple count of symptoms. A change in seven or more symptoms had an LR+ of 8.7 (95% CI 3.8 to 20) and an unhelpful LR− of 0.7 (95% CI 0.6 to 0.8) while a change in three or more symptoms had an LR+ of 2.8 (95% CI 2.0 to 4.1) and an LR− of 0.5 (95% CI 0.4 to 0.7).

Summary of the implications of the clinical examination

If the clinical picture of hypothyroidism is strong (Billewicz score ≥+25), the correct diagnosis is very likely to be hypothyroidism. If the clinical picture is strongly against hypothyroidism (Billewicz score −30), the patient is almost certainly not hypothyroid. However, if the clinical picture is less clear (−29 to +24) the diagnosis could go either way.

If symptoms only are assessed, without, as in the Billewicz score, the examination being included, a score of 7 or more suggestive symptoms which have changed in the last year shifts the probabilities usefully in favour of the diagnosis while a low score shifts the probability only slightly against it.

The value of the history and examination is not in making a definitive diagnosis but in assisting the clinician to gauge the pre-test probability before performing thyroid function tests.

Does a family history of thyroid disease alter the probabilities?

The US study quoted above[5] found that a family history of thyroid disease was present in 42% of those who were hypothyroid but was also present in 18% of controls. This gave an LR+ of 2.5 (95% CI 1.6 to 4.0) and an LR− of 0.7 (95% CI 0.6 to 0.9). A family history therefore increases the probability of hypothyroidism slightly and its absence reduces it slightly. The value of the question lies more in gaining an understanding of what the patient's experience of thyroid disease might be, rather than in assisting with the diagnosis.

Thyroid function tests

* *Check the TSH.* If the clinical suspicion of hypothyroidism is strong, check the free T_4 at this stage to save time.

  A third generation TSH has a sensitivity and a specificity of 99%,[7] giving the likelihood ratios and probabilities at different levels of initial risk shown in Table 64.4.

  Caution: the TSH can be depressed by concomitant illness and is occasionally raised during recovery. During concomitant illness, its sensitivity remains high at 99% but its specificity falls to 95%.[7]

* *Check the free T_4 and free T_3.* Free T_4 is 90% sensitive and 90% specific, falling to 60% and 80% in a patient with concomitant illness, and free T_3

Table 64.4 The probability of hypothyroidism, according to the TSH

Initial risk of hypothyroidism	Likelihood ratio	Probability of hypothyroidism
1.5%	99	60%
	0.01	<0.1%
50%	99	99%
	0.01	1%

Follow each row from left to right to see how the TSH alters the probability of hypothyroidism.

The initial risk of 1.5% is that of the 70-year-old woman. A risk of 50% is that of a woman aged 70 with a Billewicz score of 20.

Note that the lower initial probability means that a raised TSH supports the diagnosis but does not prove it, while a normal result rules it out. Conversely, the higher initial probability means that the TSH rules the diagnosis in, if raised, but cannot totally rule it out if normal.

is 97% sensitive and 97% specific but becomes useless in a patient with concomitant illness (see box below).

The classic feedback loop. Put simply, thyroid function is controlled by the pituitary production of TSH, which in turn is regulated by feedback to the hypothalamus and the pituitary of plasma T_4 and T_3. If the thyroid gland fails, plasma T_4 and T_3 levels fall and so plasma TSH rises. In mild disease, this rise may return T_4 and T_3 levels to normal. If the hypothalamus or pituitary fails, free T_4, T_3 and TSH fall, or, at least, TSH is inappropriately low (while possibly within the normal range) for the low T_4 and T_3.

Sick euthyroid syndrome. Serious concomitant illness, and old age, can disturb this picture by reducing peripheral conversion of T_4 to T_3. Certain drugs; lithium, amiodarone, non-selective beta-blockers in high dosage and corticosteroids, can do the same. Free T_3 may be low but the patient has no thyroid disease; and TSH and free T_4 may be low because the failure of conversion of T_4 to T_3 in the hypothalamus and pituitary reduces TSH secretion.

Total T_4 and T_3 are unreliable because they are dependent on the concentration of thyroid binding proteins, which are raised in pregnancy, use of oral contraception and other drugs.

Misleading elevation of the TSH. The TSH may be artificially raised due to:

(a) the presence of heterophile antibody or antibody to thyroid hormone; they interfere with the test

(b) drugs: amiodarone, sertraline, cholestyramine; to add to the confusion, amiodarone can also cause true hypothyroidism

(c) recovery from concomitant illness

(d) rare congenital defects which may only be detected in adult life because the patient is clinically euthyroid[8]

(e) adrenal glucocorticoid insufficiency

(f) renal failure[9]

(g) undertreated hypothyroidism where the dose of thyroxine has been increased in the last 8 weeks.

What level of TSH is abnormal?

The normal range is usually quoted as 0.45 mU/L to 4.5 mU/L with a mean of 1.5 mU/L.[10] However, these cut-off points are arbitrary. Patients at the upper range of normal may have subclinical hypothyroidism; indeed, those with a TSH >2.5 mU/L have serum cholesterol levels higher than those with low-normal values, suggesting that some of them are hypothyroid.[9]

What is the cause of the hypothyroidism?

The *commonest causes* are:

(a) *autoimmune thyroiditis*: this is the cause in 60–70% of patients with hypothyroidism

(b) *previous surgery or radiotherapy*: 20–30% of cases of hypothyroidism fall into this category.

Other causes are uncommon or rare:

(a) *drugs*: amiodarone or lithium; anti-thyroid drugs, cytokines (e.g. interferon alpha)

(b) *congenital* hypothyroidism

(c) *very high iodine intake* (e.g. from water purifying tablets or contrast studies)

(d) *iodine deficiency* (though this is a common cause in areas of iodine deficiency)

(e) *thyroid blocking substances* in the diet (e.g. brassicas and cassava)

(f) The transient hypothyroidism of *viral thyroiditis*, or *postpartum thyroiditis*

(g) *Riedel's thyroiditis*

(h) secondary to *hypothalamic/pituitary failure*.

Deciding on the aetiology

* Check that the TFTs suggest primary hypothyroidism (i.e. that the TSH is raised). If not, refer for suspected hypothalamic/pituitary failure.

* Check that there is no history of surgery or radiotherapy to the neck.

* Check that the patient is not taking drugs that could suppress thyroid function.

* Check that the patient is not postpartum.

* Examine and refer if the thyroid is tender (acute thyroiditis), or hard (Riedel's thyroiditis).

* *Send blood for anti-thyroid antibodies.* They are almost always present in autoimmune thyroiditis, i.e. the sensitivity is almost 100%. However, they are not very specific: they are present in 10% of the healthy female population (giving LR+ 10 and LR– 0.01) and 2% of the male population (giving LR+ 49 and LR– 0.01). This means that they are

very useful in confirming a diagnosis already reached, as above. They should not be used to make a diagnosis of autoimmune thyroiditis in a patient who is euthyroid or in whom the clinical picture suggests another cause.

Subclinical hypothyroidism

Definition. Elevated TSH with a normal FT_4 in a patient with no clinical evidence of hypothyroidism. The elevated TSH should not be due to one of the causes in the box on p. 420.

Prevalence. This is high and rises with age. A US study found that 4.6% of the population, thought to be free from thyroid disease, had a raised TSH; in 4.3%, the hypothyroidism was subclinical.[11] In the UK, the Whickham study found a similar prevalence.[12] In those aged 65 and over, the prevalence is triple (1.7% overt, 13.7% subclinical).[11]

Of those with subclinical hypothyroidism, 2–5% progress to overt hypothyroidism each year.[10] The risk is higher in those with higher TSH levels and in those with anti-thyroid antibodies. A therapeutic trial of thyroxine is needed to see whether any symptoms are due to the condition or are coincidental. About 20% of patients report subjective improvement. If thyroxine is not given they need regular surveillance; only in 5% does the TSH revert to normal.[10]

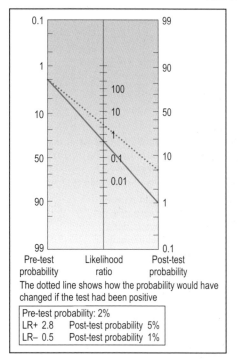

Figure 64.1 The probability of overt hypothyroidism after a score of 2 in the example below.

Example

A 72-year-old woman is found to have atrial fibrillation. Thyroid function tests are performed but, far from showing hyperthyroidism, they show a raised TSH and FT_3 and FT_4 that are borderline low. Her GP has to decide whether this is overt or subclinical hypothyroidism.

He questions her along the lines of the Billewicz score but finds himself unable to score her answers. She says she 'doesn't sweat and never has', her skin has 'always been dry' she's 'always hated the cold', she's deaf 'but isn't everyone my age?' etc. He decides to use the US criteria in which only a change in symptoms counts as positive. This works better and her score is only 2 (she is more tired and her memory is worse).

He calculates that this lowers the probability of hypothyroidism from the baseline of 2% for her age to 1% (Fig. 64.1). Examination adds nothing and he concludes that her hypothyroidism is subclinical.

He presents this patient's case to his partners at a clinical meeting and they question whether the formal scoring was worthwhile. He argues that it was. Without it he would have worried that her tiredness and deterioration in memory might be due to hypothyroidism. He might have been tempted into a trial of thyroxine and a positive placebo response might have meant that she was inappropriately treated long-term. As it is, he will monitor her without treatment.

REFERENCES

1. Helfand M, Redfern C. *Screening for thyroid disease: an update. American College of Physicians.* Ann Intern Med 1998;129:144–158.

2. McGee S. *Evidence-based physical diagnosis.* Philadelphia: Saunders, 2001.

3. Billewicz W, Chapman R, Crooks J, et al. *Statistical methods applied to the diagnosis of hypothyroidism.* Q J Med 1969;150:255–266.

4. Indra R, Patil S, Joshi R, et al. *Accuracy of physical examination in the diagnosis of hypothyroidism: a cross-sectional, double-blind study.* J Postgrad Med 2004;50:7–10.

5. Canaris G, Steiner J, Ridgway E. *Do traditional symptoms of hypothyroidism correlate with biochemical disease?* J Gen Intern Med 1997;12:544–550.

6. Doucet J, Trivalle C, Chassagne P, et al. *Does age play a role in clinical presentation of hypothyroidism?* J Am Geriatr Soc 1994;42:984–986.

7. Dolan JD, Wittlin SD. Hyperthyroidism and hypothyroidism. In: Black ER, Bordley DR, Tape TG, Panzer RJ, eds. *Diagnostic strategies for common medical problems,* 2nd edn. Philadelphia: American College of Physicians, 1999:473–483.

8. Dayan CM. *Interpretation of thyroid function tests.* Lancet 2001;357:619–624.

9. Roberts C, Ladenson P. *Hypothyroidism.* Lancet 2004;363:793–803.

10. Surks M, Ortiz E, Daniels G, et al. *Subclinical thyroid disease: scientific review and guidelines for diagnosis and management.* JAMA 2004;291:228–238.

11. Hollowell J, Staehling N, Flanders W, et al. *Serum TSH, T4, and thyroid antibodies in the United States population (1988–1994): National Health and Nutrition Examination Survey (NHANES III).* J Clin Endocrinol Metab 2002;87:489–499.

12. Tunbridge W, Evered D, Hall R, et al. *The spectrum of thyroid disease in a community: the Whickham survey.* Clin Endocrinol 1977;7:115–125.

Irritable bowel syndrome

KEY FACTS

- Diagnosis depends on:
  (a) the absence of alarm features in the history, examination and the full blood count; and
  (b) the presence of the characteristic clinical criteria.
- The diagnosis of irritable bowel syndrome (IBS) is supported by a positive family history and the presence of other conditions known to be associated with IBS.
- Irritable bowel syndrome is only one of the functional bowel disorders; however, it is the one whose diagnostic criteria have been tested. The term is often used incorrectly to mean all functional bowel disorders.

A PRACTICAL APPROACH

- * Search for alarm features. This must include an abdominal and rectal examination and a haemoglobin estimation.
- * Ask about a family history of functional bowel complaints.
- * Ask about a personal history of related disorders, such as fibromyalgia and chronic pelvic pain.
- * Examine the abdomen and rectum and order a haemoglobin.
- * Decide whether the symptoms meet the criteria for IBS or for one of the other functional bowel disorders.
- * If making a diagnosis of a functional bowel disorder, explain to the patient that such a diagnosis is, initially, tentative. Ensure you have the patient's understanding and agreement.

Prevalence, consultations, symptom pattern and underdiagnosis

- *Prevalence*: 9% to 12% of the population with a male/female distribution of 1 to 2.6.[1] Up to a quarter of women and a fifth of men have some kind of functional bowel disorder.[2]
- Of these, in the UK, half have consulted their GP in the last 6 months about the symptoms.[3] Those who do consult are more likely to have abdominal pain and diarrhoea but are also more likely to have adverse psychosocial factors.[4]
- Roughly a quarter of those with IBS have predominantly constipation, a quarter have predominantly diarrhoea and half have alternating symptoms.[5]
- Less than half of those who are discovered to suffer from IBS according to the Rome II criteria, on a postal survey, have been diagnosed as having IBS.[3]

The clinical assessment

* Ask about alarm symptoms and risk factors:[6]
  - rectal bleeding
  - anaemia
  - weight loss
  - persistent diarrhoea
  - severe constipation
  - travel history to locations with endemic parasitic diseases
  - fever
  - a family history of colorectal cancer, inflammatory bowel disease or coeliac disease
  - age >50 at onset.

The diagnostic utility of the first three of these alarm symptoms has been demonstrated (see the London study below).[7]

* *If there are alarm symptoms or signs*, refer for investigation.
* *Ask about other, non-gastroenterological symptoms* which would support the diagnosis, because they are more common in patients with IBS:
  - lethargy
  - insomnia
  - muscular pains
  - urinary frequency
  - dyspareunia
  - anxiety, depression and somatisation.[1]
* *Check for other related conditions.* Four syndromes have been identified as being more common in patients with IBS than would be expected[8] (with their prevalence vs. their prevalence in the general population):
  - fibromyalgia (32.5% vs. 2%)
  - chronic fatigue syndrome (14% vs. 0.4%)
  - chronic pelvic pain (35% vs. 14%) and
  - temporomandibular joint disorder (16% vs. 5%).
* *Ask about a family history* of functional abdominal pain or bowel dysfunction. If present, it more than doubles the likelihood of IBS in the patient.[9]
* *Examine* for organic pathology: look for an abdominal or rectal mass.[6] Tenderness on examination is of no diagnostic significance.
* *Check the haemoglobin* (see below).
* *If there are no alarm symptoms or signs*, check the patient's condition against the Rome II criteria (see below).
* *If the patient does not meet criteria for IBS*, check whether he or she meets the criteria for another functional bowel disorder (see below).[10]

* *If making a diagnosis of a functional bowel disorder, monitor the patient's progress* in order to confirm the diagnosis over time. Of those with an initial diagnosis of IBS, 2–5% will turn out to have organic disease over follow-up periods of 6 months to 6 years.[11] A failure to respond to IBS treatment should trigger referral.

The Rome II criteria for the diagnosis of IBS[10]

Abdominal discomfort or pain for 12 weeks or more in the last year with at least two of the following features:

1. relieved by defecation
2. onset associated with a change in the frequency of the stool
3. onset associated with a change in the form of the stool especially if any of the following are present:
   (a) abnormal stool frequency (>3 a day or <3 a week)
   (b) abnormal stool form
   (c) abnormal passage of stool (straining, urgency or a feeling of incomplete defecation)
   (d) mucus
   (e) a feeling of abdominal distension.

How reliable is a diagnosis based on the Rome criteria?

Moderately useful but not decisive. In the largest prospective study of 602 patients, with small or large bowel symptoms, referred to a gastroenterology clinic in London, the combination of a positive diagnosis using the Rome I criteria and the absence of three red flags (anaemia, weight loss and rectal bleeding) had a sensitivity of 71% and a specificity of 85%, for functional bowel disorders, giving the likelihood ratios and probabilities in Table 65.1.[7] (The Rome I criteria are the same as Rome II except that they require that two of the supporting criteria of Rome II are present on at least 25% of days or occasions.)

Note three points:
(a) 17% of those with organic disease met the Rome criteria. The criteria are thus not sufficient in the diagnosis of functional bowel disorders; they must be supplemented by the reasonable exclusion of organic disease.

Table 65.1 Value of the Rome criteria in the diagnosis of functional bowel disorders

Rome criteria for IBS	LR (95% CI)	Probability of functional bowel disorder
Criteria met	4.7 (3.6–6.4)	86%
Criteria not met	0.3 (0.3–0.4)	30%

The pre-test probability of functional bowel disorders among patients with bowel symptoms in this secondary care study was 56%.

(b) Thirty per cent of those who did not meet the Rome criteria still had a functional bowel disorder. The problem here is that this study, and others, refer to functional bowel disorders as IBS, ignoring the fact that there are five separate functional bowel disorders, and the Rome criteria are designed specifically for only one of them, namely IBS. By definition, the 30% had a functional bowel disorder other than IBS.

(c) The general practitioner should realise that these likelihood ratios may not apply to primary care. Furthermore, the pre-test probability of functional bowel disease in primary care will be much higher than in secondary care, and the post-test probabilities will be correspondingly higher too.

The removal of patients with alarm symptoms before applying the Rome criteria is important. In an earlier study of the diagnostic value of Manning's criteria in 361 patients,[12] *none of whom had been excluded because of alarm symptoms*, the sensitivity of the criteria for the diagnosis of IBS versus organic GI disease was 58%, and the specificity 42%, giving both LR+ and LR− of 1 (i.e. of no value either way). Manning's criteria were the first to attempt a positive diagnosis of IBS from the history and are not unlike the later Rome criteria.

This confidence in our ability to make a positive diagnosis based on the presence of the Rome criteria and the absence of red flags is new. Indeed, in 2002, the American College of Gastroenterology Functional Gastrointestinal Disorders Task Force recommended that, useful as they are for research purposes, the clinical utility of the Rome criteria is unproven and IBS should more simply be thought of as 'abdominal discomfort with altered bowel habit in the absence of structural and biochemical abnormalities'.[13] However, that verdict was reached before the publication of the latest research.[14]

The controversy about investigations in those with no pointers to organic disease

Possibilities:

1. *Order no tests.* The American College of Gastroenterology Functional GI Disorders Task Force finds that the evidence does not support the use of any tests in patients with suspected IBS since they are no more likely to have organic disease than the non-IBS population.[13] For instance, studies of lactose malabsorption in patients with a diagnosis of IBS are positive in 22–26%.[13] This equals the general population prevalence of 25%.

2. *Check at least the full blood count.*[15] Without a haemoglobin assay, one important 'red flag' for organic disease cannot be assessed. Other possible tests are thyroid function tests, endomysial antibodies, stool microscopy, a urinary screen for laxatives and visualisation of the lower bowel. However, the yield from each test is likely to be 1–2% positive only.[1] The only possible exception to this is testing for coeliac disease. One study in secondary care found that 5% of patients with a diagnosis of IBS had coeliac disease, against a population prevalence of 1%,[16] although a later study found only 0.5% with undetected coeliac disease.[17]

Functional bowel disorders other than IBS[10]

They all require that symptoms have been present for 12 weeks or more in the last year (not necessarily consecutively) or for 6 months in the case of functional abdominal pain syndrome.

Functional abdominal bloating:

1. a feeling of abdominal fullness, bloating, or visible distension; and
2. insufficient criteria for a diagnosis of another functional disorder.

Functional constipation (see *Constipation*, p. 37) at least two of the following:

1. straining in >1/4 defecations
2. lumpy or hard stools in >1/4 defecations
3. a sensation of incomplete evacuation in >1/4 defecations
4. a sensation of anorectal obstruction/blockage in >1/4 defecations

5. manual manoeuvres to facilitate >1/4 defecations (e.g. digital evacuation, support of the pelvic floor)
6. <3 defecations per week.

Functional diarrhoea (see *Diarrhoea*, p. 58):

1. liquid (mushy) or watery stools
2. present more than three-quarters of the time; and
3. no abdominal pain.

Functional abdominal pain syndrome:

1. continuous or nearly continuous abdominal pain; and
2. no, or only occasional, relation of pain with physiological events (e.g. eating, defecation or menses); and
3. some loss of daily functioning; and
4. the pain is not feigned; and
5. insufficient criteria for other functional GI disorders.

Note: In none of these functional disorders has the clinical utility of the Rome criteria been validated.

Example

A female mathematics teacher, aged 30, presents with a complaint of a bloated feeling in the abdomen. It has been present on and off for most of her adult life but over the last 3 months it has been there most days. Her stool varies but tends towards being looser than she thinks is normal. There is no history of bleeding, weight loss or fever, and no family history of bowel disorders.

The GP examines her abdominally and rectally and finds nothing wrong. His experience tells him that this is IBS; this is based on her age, the symptoms, the negative history and examination, and the high prevalence of the condition.

He embarks on an explanation of IBS and only then realises that the patient does not accept his diagnosis. Late, but not too late, he asks what she thinks she might have and learns that the consultation was prompted by a magazine article about coeliac disease. He agrees that he has chosen the most likely diagnosis without checking out other possibilities, and sends blood for a haemoglobin and endomysial antibodies (EMA).

She returns a week later to learn that the tests were normal. The GP has meanwhile looked up the Rome II criteria and scores her formally. He finds that her history is positive because her discomfort is relieved by defecation and because bouts of discomfort are associated with looser stool. In addition, most of the time she has a feeling of not being able to empty herself completely when defecating and her abdomen feels distended, thus meeting the stricter Rome I criteria.

Knowing that she will understand the concept of probability, he shows her how he calculates the probability that she has IBS using a nomogram (Fig. 65.1). He estimates her pre-test probability (after the normal blood tests) of IBS at 90%. The fact that she meets the Rome criteria raises this to 98%.

They both agree that the 2% chance that she has another disease (colorectal cancer, inflammatory bowel disease, EMA-negative coeliac disease) is so low that it does not justify the (largely) invasive investigations that would be necessary.

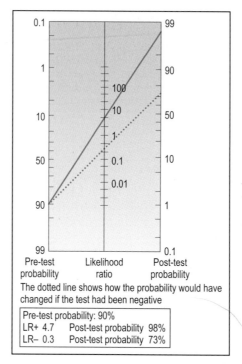

Figure 65.1 The probability of IBS before and after the application of the Rome criteria in the example on p. 426.

REFERENCES

1. Jones J, Boorman J, Cann P, et al. *British Society of Gastroenterology guidelines for the management of the irritable bowel syndrome.* Gut 2000;47(Suppl II):1–9.

2. Drossman D, Whitehead W, Camilleri M. *Irritable bowel syndrome: a technical review for practice guideline development.* Gastroenterology 1997;112:2120–2137.

3. Wilson S, Roberts L, A R, et al. *Prevalence of irritable bowel syndrome: a community survey.* Br J Gen Pract 2004;54:495–502.

4. Drossman D, McKee D, Sandler R, et al. *Psychosocial factors in the irritable bowel syndrome. A multivariate study of patients and nonpatients with irritable bowel syndrome.* Gastroenterology 1988;95:701–708.

5. Wilson S, Roberts L, Roalfe A, et al. *Prevalence of irritable bowel syndrome: a community survey.* Br J Gen Pract 2004;54:495–502.

6. Talley N. *When to conduct testing in patients with suspected irritable bowel syndrome.* Rev Gastroenterol Disord 2003;3 (Suppl 3):S18–24.

7. Tibble J, Sigthorsson G, Foster R, et al. *Use of surrogate markers of inflammation and Rome criteria to distinguish organic from nonorganic intestinal disease.* Gastroenterology 2002;123:450–460.

8. Whitehead W, Palsson O, Jones K. *Systematic review of the comorbidity of irritable bowel syndrome with other disorders: what are the causes and implications?* Gastroenterology 2002;122:1140–1156.

9. Kalantar J, Locke Gr, Talley N, et al. *Is irritable bowel syndrome more likely to be persistent in those with relatives who suffer from gastrointestinal symptoms? A population-based study at three time points.* Aliment Pharmacol Ther 2003;17:1389–1397.

10. Thompson W, Longstreth G, Drossman D, et al. *Functional bowel disorders and functional abdominal pain.* Gut 1999;45 (Suppl II):II 43–47.

11. El-Serag H, Pilgrim P, Schoenfeld P. *Systematic review: natural history of irritable bowel syndrome.* Aliment Pharmacol Ther 2004;19:861–870.

12. Talley N, Phillips S, Melton L, et al. *Diagnostic value of the Manning criteria in irritable bowel syndrome.* Gut 1990;31:77–81.

13. Brandt L, Bjorkman D, Fennerty M, et al. *Systematic review on the management of irritable bowel syndrome in North America.* Am J Gastroenterol 2002;97(11 (Suppl)):S7–26.

14. Lacy B. *Irritable bowel syndrome: new recommendations for diagnosis and treatment.* Arch Int Med 2003;163:1374–1375.

15. Paterson W, Thompson W, Vanner S, et al. *Recommendations for the management of irritable bowel syndrome in family practice.* Can Med Assoc J 1999;161:154–161.

16. Sanders D, Carter M, Hurlstone D, et al. *Association of adult coeliac disease with irritable bowel syndrome: a case-control study in patients fulfilling the ROME II criteria referred to secondary care.* Lancet 2001;358:1504–1508.

17. *Undetected coeliac disease rare in irritable bowel disease.* Annual meeting of the American College of Gastroenterology; 2006; Honolulu.

Lung cancer

- Rarities aside, no one symptom is strongly suggestive of lung cancer, although, of common symptoms, haemoptysis has the highest positive likelihood ratio.
- Combinations of symptoms increase the probability of lung cancer, as does the fact that the patient returns for a second or third consultation with haemoptysis, cough or loss of appetite. The presence of clubbing, thrombocytosis and abnormal spirometry are also useful predictors of cancer. However, most patients with cancer do not have these three confirmatory features.

- Chest X-ray (CXR) is extraordinarily useful in the diagnosis of lung cancer provided two points are understood:
  (a) shadowing thought to be due to pneumonia should be followed up with a repeat chest X-ray at 6 weeks
  (b) the sensitivity of the chest X-ray is only 77% (i.e. it will miss 23% of cancers). Patients with a clinical suspicion of cancer should be referred despite a normal chest X-ray.

A PRACTICAL APPROACH

(These are the UK guidelines; see text.)
* *Order an urgent CXR* for any patient with *haemoptysis* and for a patient with any of the following that is persistent and unexplained:
  (a) cough
  (b) chest and/or shoulder pain
  (c) dyspnoea
  (d) weight loss
  (e) chest signs
  (f) hoarseness
  (g) finger clubbing
  (h) features suggestive of metastasis from a lung cancer (e.g. brain, bone, liver or skin)
  (i) cervical/supraclavicular lymphadenopathy.

* *Refer urgently* if there is:
  (a) a CXR suggestive of lung cancer
  (b) persistent haemoptysis in a smoker or ex-smoker over 40 years of age
  (c) high suspicion of lung cancer despite a normal CXR.
* *Refer immediately* if there are:
  (a) signs of superior vena caval obstruction
  (b) stridor.
* Consider, with the patient's understanding and agreement, a policy of *watchful waiting*, in those with a normal CXR and less strong suspicion of cancer.

Prevalence

The incidence rises sharply with age. It is rare under the age of 40, with the most common age group at diagnosis being 70–74.[1] It is more common in men, with an incidence of 80/100 000/year in men and 38/100 000/year in women,[2] although this difference is likely to change as proportionally more women smoke.

Prevalence in primary care

A study from Exeter found that the risk of lung cancer in those age ≥40 consulting in primary care was 0.18% annually.[3] This means that a GP in the UK will see about one new case annually (see also *Haemoptysis*, p. 130).

The problem with diagnosis

Two studies show that the symptoms associated with lung cancer are common and rarely indicate cancer.

1. A Swedish study, in which 5200 patients aged >40, not known to have cancer, were asked about specific symptoms that could suggest cancer, found the following prevalences for those symptoms:[4]
   - cough for >1 month: 1%
   - shortness of breath: 1.8%
   - haemoptysis: 0.02%
   - chest pain on breathing deeply: 0.75%.

   None of these patients proved to have lung cancer.

   Note the rarity of the complaint of haemoptysis, hence its value as an indicator of cancer if it *is* reported (see below).

2. A Dutch study over 10 years found that 5% of primary care consultations are for cough.[5] With an annual incidence of lung cancer of only 60/100 000, very few of these will have carcinoma of the bronchus. Even if all those with lung cancer were to present with cough, the probability of any one patient with cough having lung cancer would be only 0.4%, giving a number needed to test (NNTest) to find one case of 250.

Is delayed diagnosis in primary care a significant problem?

The mean delay between presentation in primary care with the initial symptoms of lung cancer and referral for CXR has been reported to be 7 months.[6] It may be that recent initiatives have

reduced this figure. A study of 132 patients with lung cancer in Finland in 2001 found a mean delay from first GP consultation to referral of only 16 days,[7] and a Danish study in 2006 reported a median delay of only 32 days.[8]

Diagnosis from the history

The Exeter study analysed the predictive values in primary care of symptoms, signs and investigations by comparing the records of 247 patients with primary lung cancer with those of 1235 controls.[3] They found that some classical symptoms of lung cancer (hoarseness, stridor, superior vena cava obstruction and shoulder pain) were too rare to contribute sufficient numbers even in this large study. Other features were more common but none of them alone was able to rule in or rule out the diagnosis of cancer (Table 66.1).

An interesting point to emerge from the Exeter study is how repeat presentations with the same symptom add to the predictive power (Table 66.2).

Other symptoms have greater predictive power after a second presentation but the increase is less than those above. The reason for the increase in predictive power is easy to explain: most haemoptysis, for instance, will be the short-lived streak of blood in the mucus seen with an acute respiratory infection. Most of these will not return with further haemoptysis.

Using the above likelihood ratios

It is tempting to apply the likelihood ratios (LRs) in Table 66.1 sequentially, with the assumption that their predictive powers are independent of each other. An illustration of this approach is as follows: a patient with haemoptysis in primary care has, from the Exeter figures, a probability of cancer of about 2.4%. Using the nomogram on page xxiv, the additional complaint of weight loss will raise this probability to 13% and the further complaint of dyspnoea will raise it to 35%.

However, the Exeter study also examined specific combinations of symptoms (Table 66.3) and found that some of them could be combined in this way but others could not. For instance, haemoptysis and weight loss give a PPV of 9.2%, which is not unlike the 13% predicted from the nomogram. Similarly, haemoptysis and loss of appetite have a PPV >10% used sequentially on the nomogram and when examined in

Table 66.1 The predictive power of symptoms in the diagnosis of lung cancer based on a pre-test probability of 0.18%

Symptom	LR+ (95% CI)	Probability of lung cancer if the symptom is present	LR– (95% CI)
Haemoptysis	13 (7.9–22)	2.4%	0.8 (0.8–0.9)
Weight loss	6.2 (4.4–8.6)	1.1%	0.8 (0.7–0.8)
Loss of appetite	4.8 (3.3–7.0)	0.9%	0.8 (0.8–0.9)
Dyspnoea	3.6 (3.0–4.3)	0.7%	0.5 (0.4–0.6)
Chest or rib pain	3.3 (2.7–4.1)	0.8%	0.7 (0.6–0.8)
Fatigue	2.3 (1.9–2.9)	0.4%	0.8 (0.7–0.8)
Cough (first presentation)	2.2 (1.9–2.5)	0.4%	0.5 (0.4–0.6)
Cough (second presentation)	3.2 (2.6–3.9)	0.6%	0.7 (0.6–0.7)
Cough (third presentation)	4.2 (3.2–5.6)	0.8%	0.8 (0.7–0.8)

Figures calculated from Hamilton et al, 2005.[3] The post-test probabilities if the symptom is absent have not been listed because they hardly differ from the baseline risk. In other words, the absence of any one symptom does not usefully argue against the diagnosis of lung cancer.

Table 66.2 The predictive power of a second presentation with the same symptom in the diagnosis of lung cancer based on a pre-test probability of 0.18%[3]

Symptom	PPV – single presentation (95% CI)	PPV – second presentation (95% CI)
Haemoptysis	2.4% (1.4–4.1%)	17% (CI not calculated)
Cough	0.4% (0.3–0.5%)	0.6% (0.4–0.8%)
Loss of appetite	0.87% (0.6–1.3%)	1.7% (CI not calculated)

The PPV (positive predictive value) is the probability of lung cancer in the patient with this symptom. Confidence intervals were not calculated when controls had too few numbers to be meaningful.

Table 66.3 The predictive power of combinations of symptoms, signs and investigations in the diagnosis of lung cancer based on a pre-test probability of 0.18%[3]

Combination	Positive predictive value
Haemoptysis and loss of appetite	>10%
Haemoptysis and thrombocytosis	>10%
Haemoptysis and abnormal spirometry	>10%
Haemoptysis and loss of weight	9.2%
Loss of weight and thrombocytosis	6.1%
Haemoptysis and chest pain	5.0%
Haemoptysis and dyspnoea	4.9%
Fatigue and abnormal spirometry	4.0%

combination in the Exeter study. However, Table 66.3 shows that haemoptysis and dyspnoea give a PPV of only 4.9%, which is roughly half of the expected figure of 8% reached when the two LRs are applied sequentially on the nomogram.

Note that there are three combinations that *reduce* the positive predictive value below what would be expected from one symptom alone:
- dyspnoea and fatigue (odds ratio 0.28)
- loss of appetite and an age >70 (odds ratio 0.13)
- haemoptysis and cough (PPV 2.0% compared to 2.4% for haemoptysis alone).

Risk factors for lung cancer

Smoking. The odds ratio for a smoker, compared to a non-smoker, of developing the disease is 9.7 and for an ex-smoker 5.9. In other words, a smoker is roughly 10 times as likely to develop lung cancer as a non-smoker and an ex-smoker roughly five times as likely.

However, this does not mean that the probability of lung cancer can be increased 10-fold in a smoker who has symptoms. The Exeter study found that being a smoker doubled the probability over that in the whole group, while being a non-smoker more than halved it.[3] The reason for this (that the probability of cancer in a smoker with cough is double that of all those with cough, not multiplied by 10) is that the smoker is more likely to have a cough than a non-smoker. Smoking and cough are not independent predictors of lung cancer.
Age. Similarly, increasing age is a risk factor. In the Exeter study, only 14% of cancers were in patients under 60 years old. The 70s is the decade of highest risk, with 48% of patients aged between 70 and 79 at diagnosis.[3]

Diagnosis from the examination

Signs of pneumonia may lead to the diagnosis of lung cancer, but the Exeter study found that finger clubbing was the only sign that had independent predictive value in their study. At first sight it appears extraordinarily useful, with an LR+ of 55. However, so few patients had it (11 out of 247 with cancer) that its sensitivity is low (4%) and the 95% confidence interval for the LR+ is wide (7.1 to 420).

Investigations

Chest X-ray

Chest X-ray is the prime investigation ordered in primary care in patients suspected of having lung cancer. Two systematic reviews have failed to find evidence from which the predictive value of the CXR can be calculated.[1] However, a Danish case series has shown that the CXR was normal in 21% of patients who presented with symptoms subsequently shown to be due to lung cancer.[8] A UK cohort study has found that 23% of CXRs gave rise to no suspicion of malignancy; 10% were normal and 13% were abnormal but not thought to be suspicious.[9] These false negatives occur in small tumours, in central tumours and in tumours which are hidden by a simultaneous pneumonia. The current UK guideline urges doctors to refer patients urgently in whom the suspicion of cancer is strong, even when the CXR is normal.[1]

The pneumonia that fails to resolve

It is standard practice to repeat an abnormal CXR in a patient thought to have pneumonia, to search for an underlying carcinoma. Most follow-up X-rays are performed 4 weeks after the first X-ray, which is often too early, given that the median time to resolution of X-ray changes is 6 weeks.[6] There is no evidence from which the value of this practice can be calculated, nor whether it would be safe to confine such follow-up films to those with risk factors for lung cancer.

Other investigations

The Exeter study found two investigations (other than CXR) that were useful (Table 66.4). However, like clubbing, their value is limited by the fact that few patients were positive.

Referral

In the UK, the recommendations of the National Collaborating Centre for Acute Care have been adopted by the National Institute for Health and Clinical Excellence.[10] These are that *urgent referral for CXR* should be offered when the patient presents with:
- haemoptysis

or with any of the following that is unexplained and persistent (e.g. for more than 3 weeks):
- cough
- chest and/or shoulder pain

Table 66.4 The predictive power of investigations in the diagnosis of lung cancer based on a patient in whom the clinical assessment has raised the probability of cancer to 10%[3]

Symptom	Result	Likelihood ratio (95% CI)	Probability of lung cancer according to the test result
Thrombocytosis	Present	8.9 (5.2–15)	50%
	Absent	0.9 (0.8–0.9)	9%
Abnormal spirometry	Present	8.6 (4.5–16)	49%
	Absent	0.9 (0.9–0.9)	9%

Follow each row from left to right to see how the test result alters the probability of lung cancer.

- dyspnoea
- weight loss
- chest signs
- hoarseness
- finger clubbing
- features suggestive of metastasis from a lung cancer (e.g. brain, bone, liver or skin)
- cervical/supraclavicular lymphadenopathy.

Intervention should be considered more urgent in a patient with any of the above who has one or more risk factors for lung cancer:
- a current or ex-smoker
- chronic obstructive pulmonary disease due to smoking
- asbestos exposure
- a previous history of cancer, especially head and neck cancer.

Urgent referral to a chest physician is appropriate when any of the following are present:
- chest X-ray suggestive of lung cancer (including pleural effusion and slowly resolving consolidation)
- persistent haemoptysis in a smoker or ex-smoker over 40 years of age
- high suspicion of lung cancer despite a normal chest X-ray.

Immediate referral to a chest physician is appropriate when any of the following are present:
- signs of superior vena caval obstruction (swelling of face/neck with fixed elevation of jugular venous pressure) (consider immediate referral)
- stridor (consider immediate referral).

These criteria have been shown to be useful in a study of urgent cancer referrals in Bradford Hospital NHS Trust over a 2-year period.[11] Of those with lung cancer, 81% met the criteria for urgent referral to a physician (97% of them because of an abnormal CXR). The disappointment is that 64% of those with lung cancer who met the criteria were not referred urgently.

Example

A 72-year-old smoker presents with a complaint of cough for about a month. In fact he has produced phlegm daily for some years but he doesn't consider that a cough – just 'clearing his throat'. There are no other symptoms. The GP examines him and finds no signs in the chest and no nodes in the neck. She urges him to stop smoking, explaining that he has chronic bronchitis, and she reinforces this message by demonstrating that his spirometry shows a reduced FEV_1/FVC.

He returns 2 months later because of haemoptysis. An urgent CXR shows a mass at the left hilum. The GP arranges urgent referral but the lesion is found to be inoperable. The patient lodges a formal complaint against the GP for failure to refer at the first presentation.

By now the GP has done some research. She argues that the probability of lung cancer at the first presentation with cough was 0.4% (see above), increased to 0.8% by the fact that the patient was a smoker and to, say, 3% because of his age. She explains that she did not think that the NICE Guidelines for the Referral of Patients with Suspected Cancer applied to this situation because the cough was not unexplained; he had chronic bronchitis. She would have expected the patient to return if the cough continued and then she would have ordered an X-ray.

The tribunal found against the GP, on the grounds that they considered that the NICE guidelines did apply. His cough had changed and this change was unexplained. Furthermore, even if they accepted her calculations, a 3% risk of lung cancer was sufficient grounds to request an X-ray at first presentation. Had they also done their research they could have pointed out that his risk of lung cancer at first presentation was increased 3-fold by the abnormal spirometry, which the GP had mistakenly used to back up her diagnosis of chronic bronchitis, not realising that the finding of chronic bronchitis *increased* the patient's risk of his cough being due to cancer.

REFERENCES

1. National Collaborating Centre for Acute Care. *Diagnosis and treatment of lung cancer.* London: National Collaborating Centre for Acute Care, 2005. Online. Available: www. rcseng.ac.uk.

2. British Thoracic Society. *The burden of lung disease.* London: British Thoracic Society, 2001. Online. Available: www.brit-thoracic. org.uk.

3. Hamilton W, Peters T, Round A, et al. *What are the clinical features of lung cancer before the diagnosis is made? A population based case-control study.* Thorax 2005;60:1059–1065.

4. Carlsson L, Hakansson A, Nordenskjold B. *Common cancer-related symptoms among GP patients.* Scand J Prim Health Care 2001;19:199–203.

5. Okkes I, Oskam S, Lamberts H. *The probability of specific diagnoses for patients presenting with common symptoms to Dutch family physicians.* J Fam Pract 2002;51:31–36.

6. Summerton N. *Diagnosing cancer in primary care.* Oxford: Radcliffe Medical Press, 1999.

7. Salomaa E, Sallinen S, Hiekkanen H, et al. *Delays in the diagnosis and treatment of lung cancer.* Chest 2005;128:2282–2288.

8. Bjerager M, Palshof T, Dahl R, et al. *Delay in diagnosis of lung cancer in general practice.* Br J Gen Pract 2006;56:863–868.

9. Stapley S, Sharp D, Hamilton W. *Negative chest X-rays in primary care patients with lung cancer.* Br J Gen Pract 2006;56:570–573.

10. NICE. *Referral guidelines for suspected cancer.* London: National Institute for Health and Clinical Excellence, 2005. Online. Available: www.nice.org.uk. Reproduced with permission.

11. Allgar V, Neal R, Ali N, et al. *Urgent GP referrals for suspected lung, colorectal, prostate and ovarian cancer.* Br J Gen Pract 2006;56:355–362.

67

Meningitis

- In hospital-based studies, many patients with meningitis do not have the classic symptoms of headache, fever and drowsiness, nor the classic sign of neck stiffness. In primary care, where the patient may be seen within hours of the onset of the illness, those symptoms and signs may be even less common.
- A recent study has described three stages of meningococcal disease in children:
  - (a) the first 4–8 hours with fever, malaise, sore throat and runny nose
  - (b) a second stage when the child is more unwell with leg pains, abnormal skin colour and cold hands and feet
  - (c) the third stage when the child becomes even more unwell with the classic picture of meningitis or septicaemia.

The study does not help the GP decide whether to admit a child before the classic picture begins to emerge, because the early signs are all non-specific.

A PRACTICAL APPROACH

In the assessment of a patient with fever and/or headache:

- ★ Ask yourself, 'Is this person more ill than I would expect if this were one of the viral infections currently circulating in the community?' and
- ★ 'Is there evidence of a source of infection (e.g. respiratory or urinary tract) treatable in the community?'

If the patient is worryingly ill and no cause is obvious:

- ★ Ask about headache, neck pain, and ask the carer about episodes of confusion.
- ★ Look for fever, alertness, neck stiffness, rash and focal neurological signs.

- ★ Test for jolt accentuation. A positive test may not increase the probability of meningitis hugely but a negative test makes it unlikely.
- ★ Look also for the non-specific signs that could be associated with septicaemia or meningitis: thirst, diarrhoea, laboured breathing and, in children and young adults, mottled skin or pallor, cold hands and feet and leg pains.
- ★ If evidence of meningitis is found, admit as suspected meningitis.
- ★ If no evidence of meningitis is found but the patient is too ill to be reassured, admit as suspected septicaemia.
- ★ In borderline cases, review in 4 hours.

wards were tested for neck stiffness. It was present in 13% of the medical patients (the mean age of those in whom it was present was 72) and in 35% of the geriatric patients (the mean age of those in whom it was present was 81). None had meningitis. It is clear that in the older patient the potential for false positive tests is high (i.e. the specificity is low). Kernig's sign was found to be positive in 1.5% of medical patients and 12% of geriatric patients. This represents a higher specificity but, as shown above, its sensitivity is correspondingly lower.

Several features are absent from the above account which play a large part in the GP's assessment of a patient who may have meningitis. The patient with fever in whom there is no evidence of localised infection (e.g. respiratory or urinary), *and who seems to be more ill than other patients in the community with undiagnosed febrile illnesses*, should be admitted despite the absence of specific signs. The GP may prefer to admit the patient as a case of suspected septicaemia rather than as meningitis, although, in the case of meningococcal disease, both may be present. A qualitative study of GPs' attitudes to the diagnosis of meningitis shows that they are aware that they are likely to see a patient in the early stages of the disease when confirmatory signs are absent. Referral is often based on a sense that the patient is ill enough to need admission rather than on a precise diagnosis.[7]

Kernig's sign

With the patient lying supine, flex the hip to 90 degrees and then extend the knee. The test is positive if there is resistance to extension in a patient able to extend the knee fully when lying flat.

Brudzinski's sign

With the patient lying supine, flex the neck while watching the legs. The sign is positive if the patient pulls the knees up towards the chest, flexing the hips and knees.

Example

A 75-year-old man is admitted because of restlessness and confusion. He lives alone and the history is unclear but he seems to have become ill in less than 24 hours. He is afebrile. There is striking neck stiffness and a positive Kernig's sign. There are no focal neurological signs and no other relevant findings. The GP considers the neck stiffness and Kernig's sign to be due to cervical and lumbar spondylosis and admits him immediately to hospital with a diagnosis of acute confusional state of unknown cause. A lumbar puncture reveals pneumococcal meningitis. The case serves as a reminder that fever may be absent in older patients with infectious diseases.

REFERENCES

1. Attia J, Hatala R, Cook D, et al. *Does this adult patient have meningitis?* JAMA 1999;282:175–181.

2. McGee S. *Evidence-based physical diagnosis.* Philadelphia: Saunders, 2001.

3. Uchihara T, Tsukagoshi H. *Jolt accentuation of headache: the most sensitive sign of CSF pleocytosis.* Headache 1991;31:167–171.

4. Durand M, Calderwood S, Weber D, et al. *Acute bacterial meningitis in adults – a review of 493 episodes.* N Engl J Med 1993;328:21–28.

5. Thompson M, Ninis N, Perera R, et al. *Clinical recognition of meningococcal disease in children and adolescents.* Lancet 2006;367:397–403.

6. Puxty J, Fox R, Horan M. *The frequency of physical signs usually attributed to meningeal irritation in elderly patients.* J Am Geriatr Soc 1983;31:590–592.

7. Brennan C, Somerset M, Granier S, et al. *Management of diagnostic uncertainty in children with possible meningitis: a qualitative study.* Br J Gen Pract 1993;53:626–631.

Obstructive sleep apnoea

Definitions[1]

Obstructive sleep apnoea (OSA) is a condition in which the upper airway repeatedly collapses during sleep, causing apnoea for at least 10 seconds at a time.

Obstructive sleep hypopnoea or sleep disordered breathing is a related condition in which the patient continues to breathe but in which ventilation is reduced by at least 50% for at least 10 seconds at a time. The whole spectrum of the condition may be called *obstructive sleep apnoea/ hypopnoea syndrome (OSAHS)*.

Prevalence

Two per cent of middle-aged women and 4% of middle-aged men have OSA associated with daytime sleepiness.[2] One in 5 adults has at least mild OSAHS (5–15 episodes of apnoeic or hypopnoeic episodes per hour) and 1 in 15 has at least moderate OSAHS (15–30 episodes per hour).[3]

Significance

It is associated with hypertension, coronary heart disease, cardiac arrhythmias and an increase in mortality.[4] At least moderate OSAHS is associated with a 3-fold increase in risk of developing new hypertension over the next 4 years.[3]

Clinical diagnosis

* Suspect it when an adult complains of daytime sleepiness or interrupted sleep at night.
* Ask the patient (or partner) about what happens in the night:
  (a) Do you habitually snore or snort when asleep?
  (b) Do you sometimes stop breathing when asleep?
  (c) If so, does it happen at least five times an hour?
      Consider answers to these three questions to be positive if they apply to most or all days in the week.
* Ask the patient about daytime sleepiness:
  (a) Do you wake up unrefreshed, however long you have been asleep?
  (b) Do you feel excessively sleepy in the day?
  (c) Does this sleepiness interfere with daily living?
      Consider answers to these three questions to be positive if they apply to at least 2 days a week. The Epworth Sleepiness Scale (see box on p. 441) may be useful in deciding whether abnormal sleepiness is present.
● Patients who answer positively to all three questions about daytime sleepiness and who stop breathing for at least 10 seconds, 5 times an hour, may have OSAHS.[2] However, the above questions have not been validated as screening questions.
● The single most useful question is 'Do you have frequent pauses in your breathing when asleep on at least 3 nights a week?' A positive answer has a post-test probability of OSAHS of 49% in patients not previously suspected of having the condition.[5] It is not, however, a good screening question because its sensitivity is only 9%, possibly because of the difficulty patients, and their partners, have in knowing what is happening when they are asleep.
● The least useful question is 'Do you habitually snore?' since a quarter of women and half of all men acknowledge that they do.[5]
* Check for other predictive factors:

(a) male sex
(b) obesity
(c) thick neck
(d) age over 40
(e) overbite (the upper incisors overlap the lower incisors)
(f) narrow palatopharyngeal arch (the arch is at least half as narrow as the diameter of the tongue)
(g) a short crico-mental space (see below).

* Check that another cause for daytime sleepiness does not exist, e.g.:
  (a) lack of sleep (e.g. in shift workers)
  (b) poor quality sleep (e.g. due to caffeine, alcohol, anxiety, medication)
  (c) boredom
  (d) depression
  (e) sedatives
  (f) restless legs syndrome or other neurological conditions
  (g) narcolepsy.
* Examine the patient's build, mouth and throat, and measure the crico-mental space (see below)
  Several studies[6–8] have measured the predictive value of the above symptoms and signs in an attempt to guide the practitioner in the decision about referral. However, the statistics derived from these studies cannot be relied on in primary care, mainly because they have not been validated in that setting. The exception to this seems to be the measurement of the crico-mental space, because of its power in excluding OSAHS[8] (see below).

Examination of the crico-mental space[8]

Place something straight, e.g. a pencil, with one end on the cricoid cartilage. Swivel it up until the shaft of the pencil rests on the chin. Measure with a ruler the longest distance between the pencil and the skin of the neck. A distance of ≤1.5 cm increases the probability of OSA slightly. A distance of >1.5 cm virtually rules it out.

Scoring:
Crico-mental space ≤1.5 cm: LR+ 1.8 (95% CI 1.3 to 2.6); LR– 0.0 (95% CI 0.0 to 0.3).

Who should be referred for polysomnography?

Polysomnography assesses the number of apnoeic or hypopnoea episodes during sleep. It involves an overnight stay, and facilities would not cope with the demand if all snorers with daytime sleepiness were referred. For this reason an attempt to devise a clinical prediction rule for referral has been made. In a UK study, 71 patients referred by their GPs to a snoring clinic were assessed against the following criteria:[9]

1. Epworth Sleepiness Scale score ≥15 (see box)
2. body mass index (BMI) ≥28
3. at least two symptoms suggesting OSAHS:
   - ■ nocturnal choking *or*
   - ■ daytime sleepiness *or*
   - ■ morning headaches/a heavy head on waking
   (when no alcohol had been drunk the night before).

The presence of at least two out of the three criteria was found to be 93% sensitive and 60% specific for the finding on polysomnography of at least 15 episodes of apnoea per hour while asleep (LR+ 2.3; 95% CI 1.6 to 3.3; LR– 0.1; 95% CI 0.01 to 1.7). These are the patients who are most likely to benefit from treatment.

However, the patients in this study were those whom GPs had already decided to refer, and so were already highly selected. Furthermore, the numbers are small and the LR– is not statistically significant.

The Epworth Sleepiness Scale[10]

* Ask: 'How likely are you to doze off or fall asleep in the following situations, in contrast to just feeling tired? This refers to your usual way of life in recent times. Even if you have not done some of these things, try to work out how they would have affected you.'
  - Sitting and reading
  - Watching TV
  - Sitting inactive in a public place (e.g. a theatre or a meeting)
  - As a passenger in a car for an hour without a break
  - Lying down to rest in the afternoon when circumstances permit
  - Sitting and talking to someone
  - Sitting quietly after a lunch without alcohol
  - In a car, while stopped for a few minutes in traffic
* Score as follows:
  0 – would never doze
  1 – slight chance of dozing
  2 – moderate chance of dozing
  3 – high chance of dozing

A score >11 carries a high probability of a sleep problem, though not necessarily OSA, provided simple causes, e.g. lack of sleep or depression, have been excluded.

Example

A 45-year-old man is brought by his wife because of his snoring. He has always snored but it has worsened over the years so that, although she sleeps in another room, it wakes her through the walls. She can't comment on whether he stops breathing (saying 'I should be so lucky') but says that he's always falling asleep at home in the evening, and never manages to see more than 5 minutes of a TV programme. He admits, when questioned directly, that he often feels sleepy at work. He had put it down to the boredom of his job as a warehouseman.

The man is short, overweight, with a squat neck and a crico-mental space of 1.3 cm. He has no symptoms of COPD but his blood pressure that day is 160/95.

The GP adds up the pointers towards the diagnosis of OSA informally. She reckons that the snoring increases the probability of OSA from the baseline of 4% to 8%; that the complaint of daytime sleepiness increases this further to, say, 15%, and that his build and short crico-mental space increase this to 20%. She explains that this may be OSA, although it is probably not, and asks if he is willing to be referred to a sleep laboratory. He is not keen, although his wife is, taking something of a punitive delight in the thought that he might need pharyngeal surgery. They leave with an appointment for 2 weeks' time to see whether simple measures (less alcohol, wedging him on his side with pillows) have made a difference.

REFERENCES

1. Scottish Intercollegiate Guidelines Network. *Management of obstructive sleep apnoea/hypopnoea syndrome in adults.* Edinburgh: SIGN, 2003.

2. Young T, Palta M, Dempsey J, et al. *The occurrence of sleep-disordered breathing among middle-aged adults.* N Engl J Med 1993;328:1230–1235.

3. Shamsuzzaman A, Gersh B, Somers V. *Obstructive sleep apnoea: implications for cardiac and vascular disease.* JAMA 2003;290:1906–1914.

4. Wright J, Johns R, Watt I, Melville A, Sheldon T. *Health effects of obstructive sleep apnoea and the effectiveness of continuous positive airways pressure: a systematic review of the research evidence.* BMJ 1997;314:851–860.

5. Young T, Shahar E, Nieto FJ, et al. *Predictors of sleep-disordered breathing in community-dwelling adults.* Arch Intern Med 2002;162:893–900.

6. Pillar G, Peled N, Katz N, et al. *Predictive value of specific risk factors, symptoms and signs, in diagnosing obstructive sleep apnoea and its severity.* J Sleep Res 1994;3(4):241–244.

7. Kushida CA, Efron B, Guilleminault C. *A predictive morphometric model for the obstructive sleep apnea syndrome.* Ann Intern Med 1997;127:581–587.

8. Tsai WH, Remmers JE, Brant R, et al. *A decision rule for diagnostic testing in obstructive sleep apnea.* Am J Respir Crit Care Med 2003;167:1427–1432.

9. Lim P, Curry A. *The role of history, Epworth Sleepiness Scale Score and body mass index in identifying non-apnoeic snorers.* Clin Otolaryngol 2000;25:244–248.

10. Johns M. *Daytime sleepiness, snoring, and obstructive sleep apnea.* Chest 1993;103:30–36.

shows that the upper duodenum is patent but is not otherwise diagnostic; faeculent vomiting indicates a lower bowel obstruction.

3. *What toxins could be stimulating the CTZ?* These include:
   (a) drugs such as chemotherapeutic agents, those used in palliative care (e.g. opioids, drugs with anticholinergic properties), drugs for non-palliative care use (e.g. digoxin, anti-parkinsonian drugs, H_2 antagonists, iron supplements)
   (b) metabolic toxins (e.g. hypercalcaemia, uraemia, hepatic failure)
   (c) infections and septicaemia.

4. *Is there evidence of raised intracranial pressure,* particularly altered consciousness or delirium? Over what period did this develop?

5. *Is the person anxious?* Does the nausea or vomiting develop in certain contexts, e.g. prior to receiving chemotherapy? Is there pain and is it escalating in severity?

The examination

The examination again aims to distinguish between gut causes and cranial causes.

1. *Is there evidence of gut obstruction?* Low gut obstruction causes dehydration, abdominal distension, a succussion splash and tinkling bowel sounds. High gut obstruction may be complete or partial, and none of the above signs may be present. An epigastric mass may be present or there may be gross hepatomegaly compressing the stomach.

2. *Is there evidence of raised intracranial pressure?* Evidence from the examination includes altered conscious state (as shown by a lowered Confusion Assessment Scale[9]), papilloedema on fundoscopy and unequal pupil size. There may be focal neurological signs such as a cranial nerve palsy or hemiplegia indicating the presence of an intracranial mass lesion.

3. *Is there evidence of vestibular dysfunction?* Check for nystagmus, cerebellar dysfunction and evidence of middle ear pathology.

4. *Is there evidence of organ failure?* Consider uraemia if there is pallor or itch. Consider hepatic failure in patients with jaundice, and peripheral signs such as spider naevi, palmar erythema, liver flap, ascites, striae and testicular atrophy.

5. Is *there evidence of sepsis?* Look for fever, tachycardia (although this is almost universal in patients approaching death from any cause) and possible sites of infection (e.g. chest

rales, offensive cloudy urine or infected skin lesions).[10]

Investigations

* Check serum calcium (and creatinine and electrolytes) unless an obvious gastrointestinal cause has been found for the vomiting. Hypercalcaemia affects 10% to 20% of patients with advanced cancer, especially those with myeloma, and carcinomas of breast, lung, kidney and the head and neck.[11] It is not confined to those with bony metastases. It responds well to bisphosphonates and poorly to antiemetics, hence the importance of early diagnosis.

* Initiate antiemetic treatment without waiting for the results of the blood test. Try to identify the cause clinically. If the cause stimulates a specific part of the emetogenic pathway, choose an antiemetic that blocks the dominant neurotransmitter at the site of the dysfunction.[12] While this approach to management has not been proven to be superior to empirical treatment, it is no worse and intuitively attractive.[8] (See Table 69.2.)

* Consider investigations for reversible causes of vomiting if death is not considered imminent. Further tests would include full blood count, blood cultures if a leucocytosis is present, liver and renal function tests, urine microscopy and culture, and possibly a chest X-ray.

Who needs specialist referral?

Most patients with nausea can be controlled with one or perhaps two concomitant antiemetic agents that target different parts of the emetic process. Patients who are not readily controlled are best referred to palliative care specialists.

What if the initial assessment yields no strong clues as to the diagnosis?

See above. Treatment should not be delayed until a diagnosis is clear.

Constipation

Prevalence

Altered bowel habit is universal among palliative patients, as some or all of the prerequisites for defecation are affected: adequate diet, adequate fluid intake, normal peristalsis, adequate power of abdominal and pelvic musculature and perianal sensation.

Frank constipation due to medication is a risk in most patients, particularly with opioids and medications with an anticholinergic action impairing peristalsis.

Prognosis

The prognosis is rarely affected by constipation. However, rarely, severe constipation can lead to colonic perforation and peritonitis.[13]

The assessment in primary care

The main problem in primary care is that of not thinking to look for constipation. Having an accurate definition of what constitutes constipation is also important. Constipation relates to the effort required to pass bowel motions, plus or minus reduced frequency. It has to be distinguished from lower bowel obstruction.

The history
* Ask about the frequency of defecation, and whether the patient has to strain.
* Ask about pain on defecation (e.g. from an anal fissure).
* Ask about diarrhoea. Spurious, or overflow, diarrhoea is a sign of severe constipation. Motions are semi-formed with a pungent odour. Frequently they are passed without any sensation, soiling the patient.
* Ask about flatus. If large bowel obstruction is present, the passage of flatus is reduced or absent, and the patient complains of a distended abdomen, as well as nausea and vomiting in the later stages.

The examination
* Perform a rectal examination if constipation is suspected. In a normal examination, the rectum is empty and collapsed. In constipation, the examination may reveal copious soft faeces, a bolus of hard faeces, or a ballooned empty rectum.
* Examine the abdomen for a loaded colon.

Investigations
Most patients who have nursing support at home will have bowel movements recorded. Make a point of looking at these observations.

An abdominal X-ray (AXR) is not part of the work-up of constipation, but, if done for other reasons, a plain supine AXR will show colonic faecal loading. In obstruction, an erect film will show gas/fluid levels and distended loops of bowel proximal to the obstruction.

Other tests would only rarely yield useful results, e.g. hypercalcaemia.

Who needs specialist referral?
Patients whose constipation is not readily controlled will need referral to a domiciliary nursing team or specialist palliative care team. Patients in whom gut obstruction is suspected will require referral to the specialist palliative care team if this is considered a terminal event, or a surgeon if the patient has an otherwise reasonable prognosis.

Dyspnoea

Definition

Dyspnoea is the *subjective sensation* of breathlessness, and therefore not necessarily related to hypoxia or significant respiratory pathology. Assessing the meaning of the symptom to the patient is an important part of clinical assessment: some patients fear that dyspnoea means impending death or suffocation. While these can be realistic fears, they are usually not.

Prognosis

Dyspnoea can be longstanding or intermittent, and have minimal or no effect on prognosis. However, it can also escalate rapidly as a terminal event.

The assessment in primary care

The history
* Ask if the dyspnoea is longstanding, intermittent or of sudden onset.
  * If *longstanding*, is there a history of known respiratory disease such as emphysema, chronic bronchitis, chronic asthma, pulmonary fibrosis or malignant infiltration? Severe anaemia can present in this way.
  * If *intermittent*, what are the circumstances that bring the sensation on? Is there a relationship between dyspnoea and exertion, or with being in certain situations like attending a medical appointment?
  * If *of recent onset*, over what period did it arise? Dyspnoea arising over seconds or minutes suggests pulmonary embolus, cardiovascular compromise (e.g. myocardial infarct or paroxysmal tachycardia) or perhaps acute major airways obstruction. Spontaneous pneumothorax is unlikely in this population but has to be

considered. Dyspnoea arising over hours or a few days may be due to acute respiratory infection, heart failure or the development of a pleural effusion.

* Ask about cough and sputum and about pleuritic pain. They may point to a pulmonary cause for the dyspnoea.

The examination

* Observe the respiratory rate to determine whether the patient is tachypnoeic (for which the cause may be pulmonary, cardiac or psychological).
* Is the patient cyanotic? This would exclude a psychological cause.
* Is the patient tachycardic? (pulmonary, cardiac or psychological causes).
* Is there a fever? (indicating an infective cause).
* Is the jugular venous pressure raised? (indicating cardiac failure or catastrophic pulmonary embolus).
* Is there marked pallor? (indicating anaemia).
* Observe chest wall movement and the position of the trachea to determine if there is pathology localised to one side of the chest.
* Percuss and listen to the chest. Dullness suggests a large pleural effusion but is absent with a small one. A hyper-resonant percussion note may be heard with a pneumothorax. Auscultation will assist in identifying localised pathology or diffuse pathology, for example a lobar pneumonia or asthma.
* Examine the heart for signs of acute cardiac compromise: valvular lesions, gallop rhythms or the accentuated second sound of pulmonary embolism.

Investigations

* Use a pulse oximeter to determine oxygen saturation. Although there is little relationship between the sensation of dyspnoea and hypoxia, it may point to the appropriateness or otherwise of oxygen therapy.
* Consider a chest X-ray and/or CT scan for further information. A spiral CT scan for pulmonary embolus may be worthwhile if the patient has a reasonable prognosis and active treatment would be contemplated.

Who needs specialist referral?

Specialist referral may not be practicable in patients with sudden onset dyspnoea which appears to be a terminal event. It is better to treat the distress immediately. Patients experiencing less catastrophic dyspnoea may benefit from referral if the intensity of dyspnoea cannot be managed to the satisfaction of the patient. Patients with psychogenic dyspnoea may benefit from referral to a psychologist.

What if the initial assessment yields no strong clues as to the diagnosis?

Treatment of the symptom is the appropriate course of action.

Delirium

* Delirium is common. It is present in 40–60% of patients presenting to palliative care units.[14,15]
* Delirium in an ill patient is easily missed. In a study from Montreal, in which 10% of patients aged 65 and older presenting at an emergency department (ED) and requiring a stretcher had delirium, the ED physician missed the diagnosis of delirium in 65% of cases (although when the diagnosis of delirium was made, it was confirmed in 98% of cases).[16]
* *Prognosis.* Delirium in hospitalised cancer patients leads to increased morbidity and mortality as well as longer and costlier utilisation of health care services.[17] It is associated with impending death in up to 25% of inpatients.[18]

The assessment in primary care

* Delirium can be considered as acute brain failure. As in heart failure, it is a symptom, not a diagnosis. It can arise when the brain is hypoxic or hypoglycaemic; when it is distorted by intracranial lesions, or poisoned by external agents (Table 69.3).
* Delirium is obvious in some patients, who display restlessness, confused speech content and may describe visual hallucinations. However, other patients are disoriented and confused but display no outward signs. As the Montreal study (above) shows, active search for delirium is necessary in patients who are at risk.
* The Confusion Assessment Method (CAM) is a convenient screening tool. It states that the patient has delirium if:
  (a) there was an acute onset with a fluctuating course; and
  (b) there is inattention; and
  (c) there is either disorganised thinking or an altered level of consciousness.

It has a sensitivity of at least 94% and a specificity of at least 90% for the diagnosis of

Table 69.3 Causes of delirium

Inadequate oxygen delivery to the brain	Ischaemic or embolic stroke Transient ischaemic attack Myocardial infarction Tachy- or bradyarrhythmia Left ventricular failure Pneumonia Asthma Extensive pleural effusion Chronic obstructive pulmonary disease Pulmonary embolus Severe anaemia
Intracranial lesions	Cerebral secondaries, including peri-tumour oedema Intracranial (including intra-tumour) haemorrhage
Metabolic causes	Hypercalcaemia Hyponatraemia (e.g. inappropriate secretion of antidiuretic hormone) Uraemia Hepatic failure Septicaemia Tumour-mediated factors
Drugs	Opioids Overt anticholinergic drugs, e.g. atropine, hyoscine 'Covert' anticholinergic drugs, e.g. H_2 antagonists, antihistamines, antipsychotics, antidepressants Anti-parkinsonian drugs Steroids Alcohol and alcohol withdrawal
Pain	Unrecognised pain Urinary retention Constipation

delirium, when used by non-psychiatrists and compared to psychiatrists as the gold standard.[9]

- Approximately half of delirious patients have a reversible cause.[14] Psychoactive drugs, especially opioids, and dehydration are the most common reversible causes. Assume that there is more than one cause.

The history

* Check the history (from the family or carer) for the possible causes of delirium listed in Table 69.3. In palliative care, unrecognised pain is a frequent cause. Patients are often suffering from prior cognitive impairment, from more severe illness, and are likely to be older, and on psychoactive drugs.
* Check whether the patient is visually impaired or deaf. Sensory isolation can contribute to delirium as well as giving misleading results during the examination.

The examination

* Examine the patient for the possible causes listed in Table 69.3. Specifically check for dehydration, focal neurological signs, evidence of myocardial ischaemia (e.g. tachycardia or bradycardia) or of left ventricular failure. Look for pallor, signs of respiratory disease or infection. Check for urinary and faecal retention.

Investigations

The degree to which investigations are conducted depends on the patient's prognosis. If there is a reasonable prognosis, looking for reversible causes is justified. A typical regimen would include:

- full blood count (for anaemia or infection)
- biochemistry (for hyponatraemia, hypercalcaemia, uraemia or hepatic failure)

- chest X-ray (for infection, cardiac failure, COPD, pleural effusions or malignant infiltration)
- ECG (for tachyarrhythmia, or MI)
- CT brain scan (for cerebrovascular accident, intracerebral tumour, peri-tumour oedema)
- urine microscopy and culture (for infection)
- blood cultures if there is evidence of infection for which no source has been found.

Other tests would only rarely yield useful results.

Who needs specialist referral?

Established delirium is very difficult to manage at home, and referral to an inpatient unit will often be required.

What if the initial assessment yields no strong clues as to the diagnosis?

If a reversible cause is not identified, symptomatic treatment of delirium will be required.

REFERENCES

1. Jones RV, Hansford J, Fiske J. *Death from cancer at home: the carers' perspective.* BMJ 1993;306:249–251.

2. Addington Hall J, McCarthy M. *Dying from cancer: results of a national population-based investigation.* Palliat Med 1995;9:295–305.

3. Grande GE, Barclay SI, Todd CJ. *Difficulty of symptom control and general practitioners' knowledge of patients' symptoms.* Palliat Med 1997;11:399–406.

4. Merskey H, Bogduk N, eds. *Classification of chronic pain: descriptions of chronic pain syndromes and definitions of pain terms, 2nd edn.* Seattle: International Association for the Study of Pain, 1994.

5. Ashby MA, Fleming BG, Brooksbank M, et al. *Description of a mechanistic approach to pain management in advanced cancer. Preliminary report.* Pain 1992;51:153–161.

6. World Health Organization. *Cancer pain relief and palliative care: report of a WHO expert committee. Technical Report.* Geneva: World Health Organization; 1990. Report No. 804.

7. Loblaw DA, Perry J, Chambers A, Laperriere NJ. *Systematic review of the diagnosis and management of malignant extradural spinal cord compression: the Cancer Care Ontario Practice Guidelines Initiative's Neuro-Oncology Disease Site Group.* J Clin Oncol 2005;23:2028–2037.

8. Glare P, Pereira G, Kristjanson LJ, et al. *Systematic review of the efficacy of antiemetics in the treatment of nausea in patients with far-advanced cancer.* Support Care Cancer 2004;12:432–440.

9. Inouye S, Dyck CV, Alessi C, et al. *Clarifying confusion: the Confusion Assessment Method.* Ann Intern Med 1990;113:941–948.

10. Teasdale G, Jennett B. *Assessment of coma and impaired consciousness. A practical scale.* Lancet 1974;2:81–84.

11. Major P, Lortholary A, Hon J, et al. *Zoledronic acid is superior to pamidronate in the treatment of hypercalcemia of malignancy: a pooled analysis of two randomized, controlled clinical trials.* J Clin Oncol 2001;19:558–567.

12. Mannix KA. *Chapter 8.3.1. Palliation of nausea and vomiting. In:* Doyle D, Hanks G, Cherny N, Calman K, eds. Oxford textbook of palliative medicine, 3rd edn. Oxford: Oxford University Press; 2004.

13. Brombacher GD, Murray WR. *Emergency subtotal colectomy for chronic constipation.* Scott Med J 1998;43:21–22.

14. Lawlor PG, Gagnon B, Mancini IL, et al. *Occurrence, causes, and outcome of delirium in patients with advanced cancer: a prospective study.* Arch Intern Med 2000;160:786–794.

15. Nayeem K, O'Keeffe ST. *Delerium.* Clin Med 2003;3:412–415.

16. Elie M, Rousseau F, Cole M, et al. *Prevalence and detection of delirium in elderly emergency department patients.* Can Med Assoc J 2000;163:977–981.

17. Lawlor P, Fainsinger R, Bruera E. *Delirium at the end of life: critical issues in clinical practice and research.* JAMA 2000;284:2427–2429.

18. Rabinowitz T. *Delirium: an important (but often unrecognised) clinical syndrome.* Curr Psychiatry Rep 2002;4:202–208.

70

Penicillin allergy

KEY FACTS

- Only about 2% of patients who give a history
  of penicillin allergy develop an allergic reaction
  if given a further dose. This is because:
  (a) many of them had symptoms attributed to
      allergy that were not allergic

  (b) others had allergic reactions that were not
      type I (immediate) reactions and so were
      less likely to reoccur on subsequent
      exposure.

A PRACTICAL APPROACH

- * Try to ascertain whether the previous reaction
  was a type I reaction: occurring within 1 hour
  of exposure and having at least one element of
  an anaphylactic reaction.
- * If the history suggests a type I reaction, do not
  give a penicillin and, if obliged to use a
  cephalosporin, warn the patient of a possible
  reaction.
- * If there are no elements of a type I reaction in
  the history, explain that the risk of an allergic
  reaction is no higher than in the general
  population, that even a positive blood test or
  skin test would not alter that estimate hugely,
  and that penicillin may be given.

- * If the history is ambiguous in relation to a type I
  reaction, avoid penicillin if possible. In a patient
  in whom it is important to know the risk of
  allergy (e.g. where long-term prophylaxis with
  penicillin is being considered or the patient
  suffers from recurrent pyogenic ear infections),
  take blood for serum penicillin-specific IgE. If
  positive, continue to avoid using penicillin. If
  negative, refer to a specialist clinic for skin
  testing followed by a provocation test. If they
  are negative, penicillin can be recommended.

Background

A history of 'penicillin allergy' is common; yet it
is often ignored by doctors when prescribing
penicillin, usually without ill effects. A UK study
from general practice,[1] of over 3 million patients
given at least one course of penicillin, found 6212
(0.18%) who were recorded as having had an
allergic-type reaction to the first dose; 48.5% of
them were given a second course, which is only

slightly lower than the figure of 59.8% who had
no such history and were given a second course.
Fortunately, this apparent carelessness rarely
leads to harm. In the same study, 3014 patients
(0.15%) given two courses of penicillin were
recorded as having had an allergic-type reaction
after the first prescription; but of these, only 57
(1.9%) had a further allergic-type event after the
second prescription. The risk of an allergic-type
reaction in a patient with a history of penicillin

allergy is increased (odds ratio 11.2 (95% CI 8.6 to 14.6)), but in 98% of patients such a reaction does not reoccur.

The confusion is not surprising. Patients are usually given penicillin when they are thought to be suffering from an infection, and many different infective agents cause rashes. Also, reactions of the idiopathic type may be truly allergic but do not recur.

Prevalence

Estimates of the risk of a true allergic reaction to penicillin vary from 0.7% to 10%.[2] In the absence of a gold standard for the various types of penicillin allergy that are possible, such variation in rates is not surprising.

The immunology

■ *Immediate (type I) reactions* manifest as diffuse erythema, pruritus, urticaria, angio-oedema, bronchospasm and other anaphylactic manifestations. They occur in 0.004% to 0.015% of penicillin courses.[2] A history of atopy does not make such a reaction more likely but it may mean that, if it does occur, it is more severe.[3] They are IgE mediated and so blood tests for specific penicillin IgE and skin testing are usually positive. They usually occur within 1 hour, although some IgE-mediated reactions occur up to 72 hours after exposure. Re-exposure is certain to cause a further reaction.

■ *Late (type II, III, IV and idiopathic reactions)* occur >72 hours after exposure and are not IgE mediated. Almost all of them are idiopathic, i.e. the immune mechanism is unclear, and manifest as a maculopapular or morbilliform rash. It occurs in 1–4% of patients given penicillin and in 5.2–9.5% of those given ampicillin.[3] Blood tests for IgE and skin tests are usually negative. Re-exposure often does not cause a further rash, even when, after careful assessment, it has been concluded that the initial rash was allergic. In two studies, only 3.5–6.7% of such patients developed a rash after penicillin challenge and one-third of patients in the study with a rate of 6.7% had a type I reaction.[3]

■ *Exfoliative dermatitis and the Stevens–Johnson syndrome* due to penicillin are very rare but liable to recur with subsequent exposure and are absolute contraindications to its use.

How can the GP decide if the patient is allergic to penicillin?

The history

A meta-analysis of the value of a history of penicillin allergy, tested against the gold standard of a positive skin test, shows the limited value of such a history without further scrutiny.[3] A positive history has a likelihood ratio of 1.9 (95% CI 1.5 to 2.5) and a negative history a likelihood ratio of 0.5 (95% CI 0.4 to 0.6). This means that, using the mean figure of penicillin allergy of 2%, a patient with a history of penicillin allergy has a risk of having a true penicillin allergy, *as substantiated by a positive skin test*, of only 4%, which is not hugely different clinically from the risk that a patient without such a history will have; which is a risk of penicillin allergy of 1%.

A more recent study from Athens[4] found a vague history of penicillin allergy rather more suggestive of type I allergy than the meta-analysis above, with LR+ of 5.5 and LR– of 0.3. These patients, however, were referred within the Athens University Dermatological Hospital and their 'vague histories' may have been less vague than those encountered in other settings.

The crucial question

The discussion of the immunology above shows that the important question is not 'was the previous reaction allergic?' but 'was the previous reaction a type I allergic reaction?'

A reaction is more likely to be type I allergy to penicillin if:
■ the onset was <1 hour after exposure
■ the reaction had at least one feature suggesting an anaphylactic reaction, e.g. pruritus, urticaria, wheeze
■ the reaction was not better explained by the infection for which the penicillin was being given
■ no other medications were being taken which better account for the reaction
■ the reaction subsided within days of the discontinuation of the penicillin.

The Athens study quoted above found that a clear history suggesting a type I reaction predicted a positive skin test in 13 out of 18 patients, compared to a positive skin test in 5 out of 542 patients with no such history, giving a sensitivity of 72% and a specificity of 99%. This gives the likelihood ratios and probabilities in Table 70.1.[4] In contrast, a maculopapular rash following penicillin gave a probability

Table 70.1 Value of the history of a type I reaction in the diagnosis of penicillin allergy[4]

Probability before the assessment	History of a type I reaction	Likelihood ratio (95% CI)	Probability of penicillin allergy
3%	Present	78 (31–196)	72%
	Absent	0.3 (0.1–0.6)	1%

Follow each row from left to right to see how the history alters the probability of penicillin allergy as judged by a positive skin test.

of a positive skin test to penicillin of only 4% to 7%.[3]

Is it reassuring that the patient has had penicillin in the past without ill effect?

No, not if the patient has had a reaction subsequently. In a retrospective review of 151 anaphylactic deaths following penicillin administration, 70% had received penicillin previously.[2]

Serum penicillin-specific IgE assay

A blood test can measure IgE antibodies to penicillin. The predictive value of the test depends on which test, and what cut-off point, is used, as well as the time since the last exposure to the penicillin (since IgE levels fall as time passes without re-exposure). Studies suggest that serum IgE is highly specific for type I penicillin allergy (95% to 100%) but not very sensitive (41% to 74%).[5] These figures give likelihood ratios of the following orders: LR+ 10, LR– 0.5. In other words, a negative test hardly changes the probability of type I allergy. A positive test increases it: but if the pre-test probability was only 2% (because of a history of 'penicillin allergy' that had none of the features that would suggest a type I reaction), a positive test only raises that probability to 17%. The test would be most useful where the history was a little more worrying, perhaps because the patient describes a rash that, although not urticaria, was itchy. If the clinician assesses the pre-test probability of type I allergy at 20%, a positive IgE raises that to 71%. A negative would be still fairly unhelpful, lowering it only to 12%.

Skin tests

They are unnecessary in a patient with a clear history of anaphylactic symptoms following previous exposure to penicillin; and they are potentially misleading in a patient with a history not at all suggestive of type I allergy. They may be helpful in a patient with an ambiguous history. Exact positive predictive values for penicillin skin tests are not available because the necessary study would be unethical. In a study from the USA,[6] 9 patients who were skin test positive received penicillin; 2 (22%) developed a type I reaction. However, studies have been able to assess the negative predictive value of skin tests. Meta-analysis of 6739 patients with a history of penicillin allergy who were skin test negative, and who were given penicillin, found that only 7 (1.5%) developed a type I reaction on subsequent exposure to penicillin; a very useful negative predictive value of 98.5%. A further 0.63% developed a delayed reaction.[3]

A negative skin test is, therefore, useful in predicting that the probability of a reaction is so low that penicillin can be given with a risk of a reaction of only about 2%. This is consistent with other studies which have estimated the specificity of skin test at 97% to 99%.[5] Assessment of the test's sensitivity is more difficult and depends on the haptens used and their concentrations. If all four main haptens are used, a sensitivity of 70% can be achieved.[7]

Skin tests are only reliable if performed by competent personnel using specific protocols; conditions which are unlikely to be met in primary care.

The number needed to test (i.e. the number of patients with a history of penicillin allergy who need to be tested for one to be positive) has been estimated at 7.[3]

Does a patient with a history of penicillin allergy have an increased risk of an allergic reaction to a cephalosporin?

Yes, but only if the penicillin allergy is type I; and even then, third-generation cephalosporins may be safe.

- Studies suggest that the incidence of allergy in patients with a history of penicillin allergy, given a third- or fourth-generation cephalosporin, is of the order of 0–2%.[3] It has been suggested that the earlier higher figure of 10% was due to the greater cross-reactivity with older cephalosporins, and to contamination of cephalosporin drugs with penicillin in the early years of their production.

- However, a more recent study using a mixture of second- and third-generation cephalosporins has shown that, in patients in whom the diagnosis of a type I reaction to penicillin is clear, 11% have positive skin tests to cephalosporins.[8] The

assumption must be that they would develop an allergic reaction if given a cephalosporin. None of the 101 patients with negative skin tests developed a reaction to oral cefuroxamine and ceftriaxone.

- Finally, a study of 1170 children from Belgrade found cross-reactivity in 69% of penicillin allergic children skin tested for first- and second-generation cephalosporins but none for third-generation cephalosporins.[9] The latter would be the safer choice in a patient with significant suspicion of penicillin allergy when there is no time to perform IgE or skin tests.

Example

A boy aged 14 developed a generalised, non-itchy 'spotty' rash on the fifth day of a course of amoxicillin for a chest infection. A blood test was performed at a private laboratory and he was told he was allergic to penicillin. No further details are available. He now has had a splenectomy following a road traffic accident and is a candidate for penicillin prophylaxis. His clinician estimates that his history of rash is not at all suggestive of a type I allergic reaction. Even assuming that the IgE test was performed properly, a positive result merely raises the probability of a further serious reaction from an estimated 2% to

17% (Fig. 70.1). In other words, the chance of a type I reaction is less than 1 in 5. He is referred to a specialist who performs a prick test, followed by an intradermal test, both of which are negative. The probability of a type I reaction has now fallen back to 6%, still a little above that of the general population (Fig. 70.2). This is explained to the boy and his parents, and they are still concerned. A trial of oral penicillin is therefore undertaken with the boy under observation at the hospital for 2 hours. No reaction occurs and he and his parents decide to accept the offer of prophylactic penicillin.

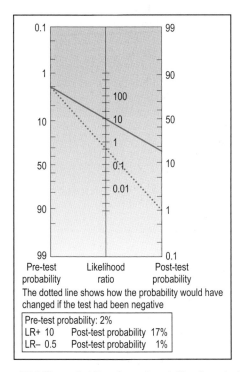

The dotted line shows how the probability would have changed if the test had been negative

Pre-test probability: 2%		
LR+ 10	Post-test probability	17%
LR− 0.5	Post-test probability	1%

Figure 70.1 The probability of type I penicillin allergy before and after the IgE test in the example above.

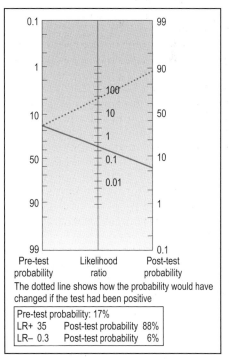

The dotted line shows how the probability would have changed if the test had been positive

Pre-test probability: 17%		
LR+ 35	Post-test probability	88%
LR− 0.3	Post-test probability	6%

Figure 70.2 The probability of type I penicillin allergy before and after the skin tests in the example above.

REFERENCES

1. Apter A, Kinman J, Bilker W, et al. *Represcription of penicillin after allergic-like events.* J Allergy Clin Immunol 2004;113:605–606.

2. Idsoe O, Guthe T, Willcox R, et al. *Nature and extent of penicillin side-reactions, with particular reference to fatalities from anaphylactic shock.* Bull World Health Organ 1968;38:159–188.

3. Salkind A, Cuddy P, Foxworth J. *Is this patient allergic to penicillin?* JAMA 2001;285:2498–2505.

4. Kalogeromitros D, Rigopoulos D, Gregoriou S, et al. *Penicillin hypersensitivity: value of the clinical history and skin testing in daily practice.* Allergy Asthma Proc 2004;25:157–160.

5. Torres M, Blanca M, Fernandez J, et al. *Diagnosis of immediate allergic reactions to beta-lactam antibiotics.* Allergy 2003;58:961–972.

6. Sogn D, Evans R 3rd, Shepherd G, et al. *Results of the National Institute of Allergy and Infectious Diseases Collaborative Clinical Trial to test the predictive value of skin testing with major and minor penicillin derivatives in hospitalized adults.* Arch Intern Med 1992;152:1025–1032.

7. Torres M, Romano A, Mayorga C, et al. *Diagnostic evaluation of a large group of patients with immediate allergy to penicillins: the role of skin testing.* Allergy 2001;56:850–856.

8. Romano A, Gueant-Rodriguez R-M, Viola M, et al. *Cross-reactivity and tolerability of cephalosporins in patients with immediate hypersensitivity to penicillins.* Ann Intern Med 2004;141:16–22.

9. Atanaskovic-Markovic M, Velickovic T, Gavrovic-Jankulovic M, et al. *Immediate allergic reactions to cephalosporins and penicillins and their cross-reactivity in children.* Pediatr Allergy Immunol 2005;16:341–347.

71

Pericarditis

KEY FACTS

- The possibility of pericarditis may be raised by a complaint of chest pain, or by the finding of a pericardial rub or of a raised jugular venous pressure (JVP).
- The symptoms of acute pericarditis are often non-specific, although typical symptoms (sharp chest pain, worse on lying down) are sometimes seen. Signs are usually absent, unless there is tamponade, but the ECG is characteristic.

- The cause of acute pericarditis may be obvious from the clinical context (e.g. myocardial infarction or chronic inflammatory disease) or revealed by a few screening tests.
- Constrictive pericarditis has no characteristic symptoms and, when the patient presents with right heart failure, the diagnosis is easily missed in primary care. However, the alert clinician might detect Friedreich's sign or Kussmaul's sign on examining the JVP.

A PRACTICAL APPROACH

- ⋆ Think specifically of the possibility of *acute pericarditis* when:
  - (a) the patient presents with chest pain associated with fever or malaise, and the pain is not obviously from the respiratory tract; or
  - (b) the patient develops a new chest pain in a situation, e.g. post myocardial infarction, when pericarditis occurs
  - (c) features of the history point towards the diagnosis (e.g. pain relieved by leaning forwards).
- ⋆ Listen for a rub and look for signs of tamponade but do not dismiss the diagnosis if they are absent.

- ⋆ Perform an ECG, looking for the characteristic ST elevation in all leads.
- ⋆ Make a decision about referral for imaging to assess the size of the effusion, and about admission in order to search for a cause, according to the situation.
- ⋆ Think specifically about *constrictive pericarditis* in a patient in right heart failure.
- ⋆ Look for the characteristic signs of a diminished apex beat, pulsus paradoxus, a pericardial knock, Friedreich's sign and Kussmaul's sign. However, even if these are not found, the patient will need specialist assessment to determine the aetiology of the heart failure.

Background

Prevalence. It is found in 1% of postmortems, almost always unsuspected clinically.[1]
Subtypes. Two distinct syndromes exist: *acute pericarditis*, which usually presents as chest pain; and *constrictive pericarditis*, which presents chronically as right-sided heart failure.

Acute pericarditis

The history

The pain is usually central and sharp, and may be worse on inspiration, because of inflammation of the adjacent pleura. It may be made worse by swallowing, as oesophageal peristalsis irritates the posterior pericardium. The pain is often worse on lying down and relieved by leaning forwards. It may radiate to the arms, left shoulder and neck. In other cases there is no more than a mild retrosternal discomfort.

Suspect it if:

1. there is a history of malaise or fever before the onset of chest pain. Viral infection is the commonest cause.
2. the patient has another condition which predisposes to pericarditis: acute myocardial infarction (MI) in the last few days, uraemia, recent chest irradiation, an autoimmune disorder (e.g. systemic lupus erythematosus (SLE)) or immunodeficiency.

The examination

If *a pericardial rub* is heard, the diagnosis is confirmed. It may be heard in systole and/or diastole and is often best heard at the end of expiration with the patient leaning forwards and holding the breath. It has a distinctive rasping or creaking quality. It may be present even in pericarditis with a large effusion, which raises doubt about whether it is really produced by the two pericardial surfaces rubbing together.

Signs of tamponade are, classically, Beck's triad (hypotension, quiet heart sounds and raised jugular venous pressure) and pulsus paradoxus. A meta-analysis found elevated neck veins in 100% of 121 cases of tamponade, a tachycardia (>100/min) in 81% to 100%, pulsus paradoxus (>10 mmHg) in 98%, hypotension (systolic <100 mmHg) in 58% to 100%, diminished heart sounds in 36% to 84% and a pericardial rub in 27%.[2]

In addition, the *y* descent of the jugular venous pulse is absent (see box).

Investigations

The ECG shows ST elevation in all chest leads, with an upward concave (saddle) pattern. In acute pericarditis, the ST elevation resolves over a few days to be followed by T wave inversion, which itself resolves. There are no pathological Q waves. If the patient is not admitted to hospital, arrange for imaging to assess the size of the pericardial effusion. A chest X-ray will only show an enlarged heart if >250 ml fluid has accumulated.[1] Smaller effusions are detectable on echocardiography. Only patients with small effusions, whose pain is controlled by an NSAID and with no sinister aetiology, can be managed without admission.

The pattern of the jugular venous pulse

* Inspect the internal jugular vein, distinguished by its inward movement – distinct from the outward thrust of the carotid pulse and from the more superficial up and down movement of the external jugular vein.
* Identify the two sharp inward movements of the internal jugular: the *x* descent, roughly in time with the carotid pulse, and the *y* descent which is seen during diastole. In the normal person, the *y* descent is smaller than the *x* or even absent.
* *The characteristic pattern of constrictive pericarditis* is the 'W' pattern, in which the *y* descent is as prominent as the *x*, so that two prominent descents are seen with each heartbeat (Friedreich's sign).
* *The characteristic pattern of tamponade* is an absent *y* descent in the presence of elevated venous pressure.

Caution is needed in interpreting a pulsus paradoxus

It is an exaggeration of a normal physiological event. Normal people can produce a pulsus paradoxus with vigorous respiration. The 95% upper limit of the fall in systolic pressure on inspiration in normal people is 12 mmHg.[2] Only a fall of >15 mmHg is likely to be palpable.

* Make sure the patient is breathing quietly.
* Inflate the blood pressure cuff above the systolic pressure then deflate it until the Korotkoff sounds appear. Hold the pressure there. If the sounds disappear with inspiration, there is a possibility that pulsus paradoxus is present.
* Deflate the cuff slowly in stages until the systolic pressure is reached at which the sounds are heard in inspiration as well as expiration. The difference between this level and the level at which the sounds first appeared is the depth of the paradox.

Searching for the cause of acute or subacute pericarditis

Definitive diagnosis is usually made in secondary care with sophisticated imaging techniques. However, a simple screen in primary care can identify the cause in some cases and, if the patient's condition is satisfactory, may avoid the need for referral.

A study of 204 patients found to have a pericardial effusion on echocardiography in Marseille, France found the following causes:[3]

- malignancy 15%
- viral infection 13%
- hypothyroidism 10%
- bacterial or fungal infection 3%
- SLE 3%
- rheumatoid arthritis 3%
- renal insufficiency 2%
- scleroderma 1%
- in the other half of patients, no diagnosis was reached.

The authors suggest that, in addition to clinical assessment, a simple work-up will almost double the clinical diagnosis rate:

- serology for Q fever and mycoplasma
- viral throat culture
- thyroid stimulating hormone
- anti-nuclear antibodies (although only high titres (>1/400) should be considered significant).

Note, however, that their method of recruitment meant that they did not see any patients with pericarditis associated with myocardial infarction: the commonest cause of pericarditis in primary care. This may be the pericarditis associated with transmural infarction seen in the first few days after infarction in 5–10% of patients, or the later post-infarct pericarditis (Dressler's syndrome) which presents more than one week after the infarct in up to 5% of patients and is associated with chest pain, fever and a raised erythrocyte sedimentation rate.[1]

Constrictive pericarditis

The symptoms and signs are those of chronic right heart failure. This is one of many conditions which will rarely be detected in primary care and forms part of the argument that every patient with heart failure should have the benefit of specialist assessment.

Signs are well described.[2] They are as follows:
Those found in right heart failure of any cause:

- an elevated JVP: sensitivity 98%
- oedema: sensitivity 63%
- hepatomegaly: sensitivity 87% to 100%.

Those more specific for constrictive pericarditis:

- decreased apical pulsation
- pulsus paradoxus >10 mmHg: sensitivity 17% to 43%; however, pulsus paradoxus >20 mmHg suggests tamponade, not constrictive pericarditis
- a pericardial knock (a sound heard in early diastole): sensitivity 28% to 94%
- Friedreich's sign (a 'W' pattern in the JVP): sensitivity 57% to 94%
- an elevated JVP which fails to fall with inspiration (Kussmaul's sign): sensitivity 50%.

Any ECG changes are usually non-specific and involve the T wave. Voltage may be low.

Chest X-ray may show pericardial calcification but is usually normal.

Example

A 35-year-old man was seen by a rheumatologist 2 days ago and the diagnosis of nodular rheumatoid arthritis made. Treatment with a disease-modifying antirheumatic drug (DMARD) is planned once the baseline blood test results are available.

He consults his GP because of central chest discomfort which had kept him awake during the previous night. He thought it was indigestion but antacids have not helped.

The GP suspected inflammation of the sternocostal joints but they are not swollen or tender. However, she is struck by the fact that he is clearly more uncomfortable the longer he lies down on her couch and better when sitting up. There is no evidence of heart failure, no rub and no pulsus paradoxus on formal testing. The apex beat feels normal. The ECG, however, shows the characteristic ST elevation of acute pericarditis.

She telephones the rheumatologist who agrees that there is no doubt about the diagnosis and no specific treatment other than analgesia and even more urgent commencement of a DMARD.

REFERENCES

1. Troughton R, Asher C, Klein A. *Pericarditis.* Lancet 2004;363: 717–727.

2. McGee S. *Evidence-based physical diagnosis.* Philadelphia: Saunders, 2001.

3. Levy P, Corey R, Berger P, et al. *Etiologic diagnosis of 204 pericardial effusions.* Medicine (Baltimore) 2003;82:385–391.

72

Pneumothorax

KEY FACTS

- Two clinical pictures exist:
  (a) sudden onset of pleuritic pain, and
      sometimes dyspnoea and cough, in a
      young man (or occasionally woman)
      (who often has a previous history)
  (b) sudden worsening of dyspnoea in an
      older person with COPD.

A PRACTICAL APPROACH

- ✱ Diagnose it according to the clinical picture:
  - ■ in the young person, the history will be
       very suggestive and examination
       confirmatory
  - ■ in the older person, the history will not
       usually suggest the diagnosis and only
       an examiner alert to the possibility of
       pneumothorax will detect it.
- ✱ Confirm the diagnosis with a
     posteroanterior (PA) chest X-ray.

Annual incidence

The annual incidence is 1 in 10 000.[1] This occurs
with two peaks in relation to age: one,
predominantly primary pneumothorax (i.e.
without underlying lung disease), in young
adults; the other in patients over 60.[2] The male:
female ratio is roughly 3:1.

The diagnostic problem

Primary pneumothorax in young patients is
usually suspected because of the characteristic
history (14 out of 15 in a series admitted to a
general hospital in Ireland).[1] However, in older
patients it is hard to diagnose. In the same series,
only 5 of 11 pneumothoraces in patients over 65
were suspected clinically. This was due to the
lack of typical symptoms in the older age group
and not to a difference in the size of the
pneumothorax between the two groups.

The history

Primary pneumothorax: the characteristic history is
of a tall young male smoker with a history of
pleuritic chest pain of sudden onset with
dyspnoea and cough. In young patients in the
Irish series, 13 out of 15 had pleuritic pain and in
all but one the onset was sudden. Only one had
dyspnoea. Between a third and a half of young
patients will give a history of a previous attack.

Secondary pneumothorax: the patient is usually
over 60 and known to suffer from COPD in 75%
of cases. Other common causes are tumour and
sarcoidosis.[3] In striking contrast to younger
patients, in the Irish series, only 2 out of 11 had
pleuritic pain when first seen, but 9 were
dyspnoeic.

Examination

The characteristic picture is of reduced movement
with reduced breath sounds on the affected side.
Percussion is hyper-resonant on that side and the
trachea may be deviated towards the normal side.
However, smaller pneumothoraces occur with no
physical signs.

The chest X-ray

The sensitivity and specificity approach 100%.
Very small pneumothoraces may be missed
(without much danger to the patient) and X-rays

in patients with extensive pulmonary disease may be hard to interpret. The British Thoracic Society Guidelines[4] no longer recommend a PA view in expiration. If the PA view is normal but clinical suspicion remains, they recommend a lateral or a lateral decubitus. The lateral view adds information in 14% of cases.[5]

REFERENCES

1. Liston R, McLoughlin R, Clinch D. *Acute pneumothorax: a comparison of elderly with younger patients.* Age Ageing 1994;23:393–395.

2. Gupta D, Hansell A, Nichols T, et al. *Epidemiology of pneumothorax in England.* Thorax 2000;55:666–671.

3. Weissberg D, Refaely Y. *Pneumothorax: experience with 1199 patients.* Chest 2000;117:1279–1285.

4. Henry M, Arnold T, Harvey J. *BTS guidelines for the management of spontaneous pneumothorax.* Thorax 2003;58 (Suppl 2):39–69.

5. Glazer H, Anderson D, Wilson B, et al. *Pneumothorax: appearances on lateral chest radiographs.* Radiology 1989;173:707–711.

Postnatal depression

KEY FACTS

- Three different clinical entities can present as low mood in the postpartum period: 'the blues', postnatal depression and puerperal psychosis. Careful questioning can usually distinguish them.
- Postpartum thyroiditis is an uncommon cause of low mood. Thyroid function tests are unlikely to be useful in the elucidation of depression unless there is a new goitre or other pointers towards hypothyroidism.

A PRACTICAL APPROACH

- ★ Screen all women at 6–8 weeks postpartum and assess them at any time if they feel low or have little interest in the baby.
- ★ Be on the alert for depression in those at high risk, especially those with previous mental or current physical health problems, or with inadequate support at home.
- ★ Use the Edinburgh Postnatal Depression Scale as a screening, but not a diagnostic, test. Further assessment is needed if it is positive.
- ★ If depression is suspected, check whether mother or baby is at risk of injury. Admission may be urgent.

Background

Postnatal depression is under-reported by patients, underdiagnosed by doctors and midwives, and under-treated.[1] Suicide is the second commonest cause of maternal death in the UK, causing 12% of such deaths.[2]

Prevalence

- About half of all women have 'the blues' postpartum. The prevalence peaks at 10 days postpartum. Mood is low but the condition is short-lived and characterised by emotional lability.[3]
- 10–15% of women have a depressive disorder within 3 months of delivery.[1] At 12 weeks, the prevalence is at its height and it has hardly fallen by 30 weeks.[4] In 3–5% of all women, the depression is moderate or severe and warrants consideration of antidepressants.[5]
- 0.1–0.2% of women will develop a puerperal psychosis.[2]

Current recommendations about screening

There is a lack of robust evidence to support unequivocally the use of routine postnatal screening for depression. The recommendations of guideline groups differ.

1. The Scottish guideline notes that, while evidence is lacking, many screening programmes have been implemented to screen for depression at 6 weeks and 3 months postpartum.[1] The Guideline Group comments that:

   ■ The Edinburgh Postnatal Depression Scale (EPDS)[6] may be administered by a trained professional (see below) as part of that screening process, but with the understanding that it is a screening, not a diagnostic, tool.

   ■ Clinical assessment is needed to establish the diagnosis. Between 30% and 70% of women who screen positive with the EPDS are not depressed.[5]

2. The UK National Screening Committee puts the point more strongly, recommending it as a checklist, not a screening tool, which may be used as part of the assessment of a woman's mood.[7]

Risk factors

Factors associated with an increased probability of developing depression in the year after childbirth are:

(a) perceived lack of social, emotional and practical support, particularly from a partner[8-10]

(b) physical health problems[11]

(c) exhaustion[12]

(d) infant factors: unsettled/'difficult' babies[13,14]

(e) negative life events[9,12,15]

(f) a previous psychiatric history, although this will only account for a small number of the women who experience depression.[16]

Making the diagnosis

* Screen all women at 6–8 weeks postpartum using the Edinburgh Postnatal Depression Scale (EPDS) (see below). The EPDS is not accurate if used in the few days after childbirth.[17] Other instruments are probably as good[18] but are less well validated in this setting. The screening needs to be introduced sympathetically, in a setting where the woman is comfortable, by a trained professional, and the woman needs to know what follow-up action is likely. Some women are comfortable completing the form themselves; others prefer to talk about the issues.[19]

* Assess all women postpartum in whom the possibility of depression is suggested at any stage by a report of low mood or lack of interest in things, especially if this extends to the baby.

* Note that a positive screen merely makes depression more likely, without proving it, and a negative screen makes it much less likely, without excluding it (see box below). A clinical assessment is still required, if depression is suspected, using questions like those below, to allow the mother to talk about her feelings:

(a) How are you feeling?

(b) How are you sleeping?

(c) How are you eating?

(d) How do you feel about the baby?

(e) How do you find being a mother?

* Alternatively, score the patient using the DMS-IV or ICD-10 diagnostic criteria for depression (see *Depressive illness*, p. 372).

* If the patient is depressed, assess whether she is at risk of self-harm or of harming the baby. Urgent admission may be needed. Severe depression, without danger of harm, needs urgent psychiatric assessment.

* Look for psychotic symptoms (delusions, hallucinations, disorganised speech or behaviour).

Thyroid disease mimicking depression

Hypothyroidism associated with postpartum thyroiditis may give rise to depressive symptoms. Thyroiditis occurs in 4–6% of women postpartum[20] but most are asymptomatic. A hyperthyroid state often precedes the hypothyroidism. Women who develop postpartum thyroiditis have a 20% risk of developing hypothyroidism within 4 years.[20]

* Check thyroid function tests in women with symptoms suggestive of hyper- or hypothyroidism (see *Hyperthyroidism* and *Hypothyroidism*, pp. 412 and 416).

The Edinburgh Postnatal Depression Scale

The EPDS (see box) was designed and validated as a questionnaire to be completed by the patient herself. However, it may be used as a prompt for direct questioning by the doctor.

The Edinburgh Postnatal Depression Scale

Instructions for users

1. The mother is asked to underline the response which comes closest to how she has been feeling in the previous 7 days.

2. All 10 items must be completed.

3. Care should be taken to avoid the possibility of the mother discussing her answers with others.

4. The mother should complete the scale herself, unless she has limited English or has difficulty with reading.

5. The EPDS may be used at 6–8 weeks to screen postnatal women. The child health clinic, postnatal check-up or a home visit may provide suitable opportunities for its completion.

The Edinburgh Postnatal Depression Scale–cont'd

Scoring the EPDS

- Response categories are scored 0, 1, 2 and 3 according to increased severity of the symptom.
- Items marked with an asterisk are reverse scored (i.e. 3, 2, 1 and 0). The total score is calculated by adding together the scores for each of the 10 items.
- Mothers who score above a threshold 12/13 are likely to be suffering from a depressive illness of varying severity. Nevertheless the EPDS score should not override clinical judgement. A careful clinical assessment should be carried out to confirm the diagnosis. The scale indicates how the mother has felt during the previous week, and in doubtful cases it may be usefully repeated after 2 weeks. The scale will not detect mothers with anxiety neuroses, phobias or personality disorders.

Introducing the scale to the patient

As you have recently had a baby, we would like to know how you are feeling. Please UNDERLINE the answer which comes closest to how you have felt IN THE PAST 7 DAYS, not just how you feel today. Here is an example, already completed.

I have felt happy:

    Yes, all the time

    <u>Yes, most of the time</u>

    No, not very often

    No, not at all

This would mean: 'I have felt happy most of the time' during the past week'. Please complete the other questions in the same way.

The scale

In the past 7 days:

1. I have been able to laugh and see the funny side of things:

    As much as I always could

    Not quite so much now

    Definitely not so much now

    Not at all

2. I have looked forward with enjoyment to things:

    As much as I ever did

    Rather less than I used to

    Definitely less than I used to

    Hardly at all

3. *I have blamed myself unnecessarily when things went wrong:

    Yes, most of the time

    Yes, some of the time

    Not very often

    No, never

4. I have been anxious or worried for no good reason:

    No, not at all

    Hardly ever

    Yes, sometimes

    Yes, very often

5. *I have felt scared or panicky for no very good reason:

    Yes, quite a lot

    Yes, sometimes

    No, not much

    No, not at all

6. *Things have been getting on top of me:

    Yes, most of the time I haven't been able to cope at all

    Yes, sometimes I haven't been coping as well as usual

    No, most of the time I have coped quite well

    No, I have been coping as well as ever

7. *I have been so unhappy that I have had difficulty sleeping:

    Yes, most of the time

    Yes, sometimes

    Not very often

    No, not at all

8. *I have felt sad or miserable:

    Yes, most of the time

    Yes, quite often

    Not very often

    No, not at all

9. *I have been so unhappy that I have been crying:

    Yes, most of the time

    Yes, quite often

    Only occasionally

    No, never

10. *The thought of harming myself has occurred to me:

    Yes, quite often

    Sometimes

    Hardly ever

    Never

Table 73.1 The value of the EPDS in the diagnosis of postnatal depression in unselected women, of whom 17.5% were found to have the condition[22]

Cut-off	Test result	Likelihood ratio (95% CI)	Post-test probability
>9	Positive	5.6 (3.7–8.4)	54%
	Negative	0.0 (0.0–0.3)	0%
>12	Positive	14 (6.9–29)	75%
	Negative	0.05 (0.01–0.3)	1%

Follow each row from left to right to see how the test result at that cut-off point alters the probability of postnatal depression.

Interpreting the results of the EPDS

A score of >9 is often reported to indicate possible depression, while a score >12 indicates probable depression.[1] These categories are an oversimplification. The probability of depression rises with each rise in score above 9.

Studies of unselected postpartum women have found sensitivities of 77%[21] to 95%[22] and specificities of 92%[21] to 93%[22] using a cut-off of >11 and >12 respectively. Table 73.1 shows how these figures from the second of those studies translate into likelihood ratios and probabilities at two different cut-off points.

A note for enthusiasts: why the EPDS had better likelihood ratios in subsequent studies than it did in the original study by the questionnaire's authors

The original study by Cox and colleagues found likelihood ratios for the two cut-off points as follows:

- cut-off >9: LR+ 1.9, LR– 0.1
- cut-off >12; LR+ 3.8, LR– 0.2.

These lower positive likelihood ratios in Cox's study, compared to Harris's in Table 73.1, are explained by spectrum bias. Cox's study was performed on women *in whom the midwife already suspected depression*. The power of the EPDS to distinguish depressed women from those without depression had therefore been diminished because some of the power of the scale had been 'used up' by the fact that all the women had already been judged to show some evidence of depression. This meant that the pre-test probabilities were higher in Cox's study than in Harris's (42% vs. 17.5%).

However, when the different likelihood ratios for a score >12 are used on those different pre-test probabilities, they result in remarkably similar post-test probabilities. In Cox's study (LR+ 3.8), a positive test raised the probability of depression from 42% to 73%; in Harris's study (LR+ 14)[22] a positive test raised the probability from 17.5% to 75%.

This confirms that the two studies agree. Their apparent differences are the result of differences in the samples studied.

Example

A 19-year-old single mother, living alone with her first baby, is visited by the GP at 3 weeks postpartum because the health visitor is concerned that the mother seems depressed. She has administered the EPDS and found a score of 13. Before visiting, the GP had checked this result on his nomogram, using Harris's figures, and found that, with a baseline risk of any depression of 12.5%, this positive score raised the probability of depression to 67% (Fig. 73.1). If he considers only moderate or severe depression, the baseline risk of 5% was raised to 42% (Fig. 73.2).

After a long interview, the GP has gathered more information. The patient seems low and seems to have no real interest in the baby. However, she is interested in other things, commenting that she hasn't been to a party for months, and that her friends don't seem interested in coming round any more. Her sleep, energy and appetite are hard to gauge because her schedules are upset by the baby, who wakes every 2 hours through the night. She seems to have no difficulty concentrating, her self-esteem is unimpaired and she's surprised by the GP's question about whether she has thought of harming herself or the baby. Asked whether she blames herself for anything she replies tartly 'only for not using a f . . . ing condom'.

The GP concludes that she is fed up because of the demands imposed on her by the baby. This puts her at risk of depression but she is not depressed. The health visitor agrees to continue to supervise her and to put her in touch with other single mothers of her own age.

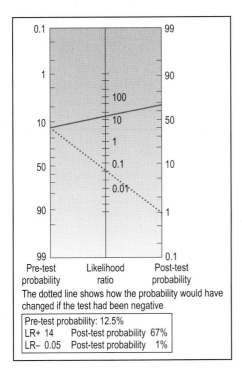

The dotted line shows how the probability would have changed if the test had been negative

Pre-test probability: 12.5%	
LR+ 14	Post-test probability 67%
LR– 0.05	Post-test probability 1%

Figure 73.1 The probability of depression before and after the EPDS in the example above.

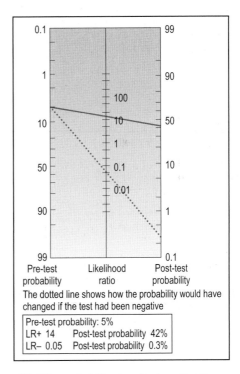

The dotted line shows how the probability would have changed if the test had been negative

Pre-test probability: 5%	
LR+ 14	Post-test probability 42%
LR– 0.05	Post-test probability 0.3%

Figure 73.2 The probability of moderate or severe depression before and after the EPDS in the example above.

REFERENCES

1. Scottish Intercollegiate Guidelines Network. *Postnatal depression and puerperal psychosis: a national guideline.* Edinburgh: SIGN, 2002.

2. Royal College of Obstetricians and Gynaecologists. *Why mothers die 1997–9: the fifth report of the Confidential Enquiries into Maternal Deaths in the United Kingdom.* London: RCOG, 2001.

3. Hapgood CC, Elkind GS, Wright JJ. *Maternity blues: phenomena and relationship to later post partum depression.* Aust N Z J Psychiatry 1988;22:299–306.

4. Stuart S, Couser G, Schilder K, et al. *Postpartum anxiety and depression: onset and comorbidity in a community sample.* J Nerv Ment Dis 1998;186:420–424.

5. Oates M. *Postnatal depression and screening: too broad a sweep?* Br J Gen Pract 2003;53:596–597.

6. Cox JL, Holden JM, Sagovsky R. *Detection of postnatal depression.* Br J Psychiatry 1987;150:782–786.

7. National Screening Committee UK. *Postnatal depression,* 2004. Online. Available: www.nsc.nhs.uk (choose 'National electronic Library for Screening' then search on 'postnatal').

8. Astbury J, Brown S, Lumley J, et al. *Birth events, birth experiences and social differences in postnatal depression.* Aust J Public Health 1994;18:176–184.

9. Paykel E, Emms E, Fletcher J, et al. *Life events and social support in puerperal depression.* Br J Psychiatry 1980;136:339–346.

10. Kumar R, Robson K. *A prospective study of emotional disorders in childbearing women.* Br J Psychiatry 1984;144:35–47.

11. Brown S, Lumley J. *Maternal health after childbirth: results of an Australian population based survey.* Br J Obstet Gynaecol 1998;105:156–161.

12. Small R, Brown S, Lumley J, Astbury J. *Missing voices: what women say and do about depression after childbirth.* J Reprod Infant Psychol 1994;12:89–103.

13. Miller A, Barr R, Eaton W. *Crying and motor behaviour of six-week-old infants and postpartum maternal mood.* Paediatrics 1993;92:551–558.

14. Murray L, Stanley C, Hooper R, et al. *The role of infant factors in postnatal depression and mother–infant interactions.* Dev Med Child Neurol 1996;38:109–119.

15. O'Hara M, Neunaber D, Zekoski E. *Social support, life events, and depression during pregnancy and the puerperium.* Arch Gen Psychiatry 1986;43:569–573.

16. Watson J, Elliot S, Rugg A, et al. *Psychiatric disorder in pregnancy and the first postnatal year.* Br J Psychiatry 1984;144:453–462.

17. Lee D, Yip A, Chan S, et al. *Postdelivery screening for postpartum depression.* Psychosom Med 2003;65(3):357–361.

18. Lee DTS, Yip ASK, Chiu HFK, et al. *Screening for postnatal depression: are specific instruments mandatory?* J Affect Disord 2001;63:233–238.

19. Shakespeare J, Blake F, Garcia J. *A qualitative study of the acceptability of routine screening of postnatal women using the Edinburgh Postnatal Depression Scale.* Br J Gen Pract 2003;53:614–619.

20. DTB. *The management of postnatal depression.* Drug Ther Bull 2000;38.

21. Murray L, Carothers AD. *The validation of the Edinburgh Post-natal Depression Scale on a community sample.* Br J Psychiatry 1990;157:288–290.

22. Harris P, Huckle P, Thomas R, et al. *The use of rating scales to identify post-natal depression.* B J Psychiatry 1989;154:813–817.

74

Prostate cancer

- Prostate cancer is a common cause of illness and death but most men with histological cancer remain asymptomatic.
- Lower urinary tract symptoms (LUTS) are usually the result of benign prostatic hypertrophy or detrusor instability. If a patient with LUTS is found to have prostate cancer it is probably coincidental.
- Digital rectal examination (DRE) is useful in the diagnosis of cancer but it is neither highly sensitive nor specific. It becomes less useful the older the patient, as non-malignant nodules become more common.
- Prostate specific antigen (PSA) is useful in the diagnosis of cancer; the higher the level the greater the predictive power. However, most patients with a raised level (traditionally >4 ng/ml) do not have cancer on biopsy, let alone clinically significant cancer. Like the DRE, the PSA becomes less useful the older the patient.
- Three factors contribute independently to an increased risk of cancer: an abnormal DRE, a raised PSA and a family history of prostate cancer.
- The degree of abnormality is important: a hard nodular prostate with induration of surrounding tissues, a PSA >50 and rising and a family history of three affected relatives would combine to give a very high risk of clinically significant cancer.

A PRACTICAL APPROACH

- ∗ When a patient presents with symptoms related to the lower urinary tract, perform a DRE as part of the clinical assessment. The evidence is not convincing that PSA should be part of that assessment, but UK guidelines recommend a PSA in this situation.[1]
- ∗ If the DRE suggests malignancy, or malignancy is suggested by some other feature of the history, such as haematuria, weight loss, bone pain, pelvic pain,[1] then order a PSA.
- ∗ Refer urgently for specialist assessment if either the DRE or the PSA suggests malignancy. However, if only the PSA is abnormal, check that the result is abnormal for that patient's age and that it is not artificially raised by prostatic inflammation or manipulation. If these are a possible cause, repeat the PSA after one month before taking action.

Prevalence

The prevalence depends on the age of the patient, the manner in which the diagnosis is made and the extent to which men are screened.

On histology at postmortem

Half of 50-year-old men; three-quarters of 85-year-old men.

Diagnosed in life

Incidence: 0.03% of the Swedish population per year;[2] 1% of European 80-year-olds per year.

Point prevalence of male population >40 years old: 0.35%.[3]

Point prevalence of those with lower urinary tract symptoms: 3%.[3]

Lifetime prevalence: 7% of European men;[4] 17% in the USA, where three-quarters of men over age 50 are screened.[5]

Lifetime risk of death from prostate cancer: 3%.[5]

The problems with studies of the accuracy of the diagnosis of prostate cancer are 2-fold

1. What constitutes a diagnosis of prostate cancer?
   - Is it a histological diagnosis on biopsy? With half of 50-year-old men having histological changes of cancer, this will detect too many men in whom those changes would never have led to illness.
   - Is it prostate cancer-related deaths in a defined period of follow-up? This will detect too few men, since not all will die from the disease.
   - Is it symptomatic prostate cancer developing in a defined period of follow-up? This is the outcome of most interest to patients, but the hardest to measure, and so the outcome least often used in studies.
2. Are the subjects in the trial similar to the patient to whom the results are to be applied?
   - Most trials are of the screening of asymptomatic men, or of men already referred to urological clinics, whereas the GP in the UK is usually trying to make a diagnosis in a patient who presents with symptoms in primary care.

The value of the history in the diagnosis of prostate cancer

It appears that, in most men who are diagnosed with cancer because of lower urinary tract symptoms (LUTS), the finding of cancer is incidental. Studies that appear to show that LUTS are associated with prostate cancer are too often confounded by a failure to control for age.[6] Even those that take all possible steps to avoid confounding cannot cope with the problem that the cancer may only be diagnosed because the men presented with coincidental LUTS.[3,4] Controls without LUTS may have a similar prevalence of cancer, but undiagnosed. A systematic review[6] found no evidence that prostate cancer presents with LUTS and determined that the complaint of LUTS does not justify screening for prostatic cancer with a PSA.

The situation is different when the patient presents with pelvic pain due to local spread or to bone pain from metastases. However, these are a small minority of the total with prostate cancer.

Digital rectal examination (DRE)

Every study of the value of DRE in the diagnosis of prostate cancer has confirmed its ability to shift the probability of cancer in a way that is statistically significant. The difficulty is in knowing how much the DRE result alters the probabilities. A meta-analysis has highlighted the difficulty with the evidence.[7] It has produced the summary figures shown in Table 74.1 but points out that there is marked heterogeneity between the 14 eligible studies. Sensitivities ranged from 38% to 79% and specificities from 38% to 79%. Using only the five good quality studies improved things but not much.

The explanation for the wide ranges of the value of a positive finding may lie in different spectra of patients, different examiner expertise, different definitions of abnormal and different intensities of investigation before the diagnosis was made or the possibility of cancer was dismissed.

Are GPs as good as urologists in distinguishing normal from malignant prostates?

It seems they can be. In a study in which a GP and a urologist examined the same 933 men, agreement was good on the six variables in which abnormalities were common: size, tenderness,

Table 74.1 The value of the DRE in the diagnosis of prostate cancer[7] based on a pre-test probability of 3%[3]

DRE	Likelihood ratio	Probability of cancer according to the DRE result
Positive	9.8	23%
Negative	0.4	1%

Table 74.2 Value of different PSA cut-offs in the diagnosis of histological prostate cancer, based on a prevalence of 22%[5]

PSA (ng/ml)	Sensitivity	Specificity	Whether above or below the cut-off	Likelihood ratio	Probability of cancer according to the PSA result
1.1	83%	39%	Above	1.4	28%
			Below	0.4	11%
2.1	53%	72%	Above	1.9	35%
			Below	0.6	15%
3.1	32%	87%	Above	2.5	41%
			Below	0.8	18%
4.1	20%	94%	Above	3.3	48%
			Below	0.8	19%
10.1	1%	99.7%	Above	3.0	46%
			Below	0.99	22%

Follow each row from left to right to see how the PSA result at that cut-off level alters the probability of cancer. Results for PSA levels >10 may be unreliable because <1% of subjects had such a level.

midline sulcus, symmetry, induration and nodularity (kappa = between 0.48 and 0.68).[8]
What constitutes an abnormal DRE?
A normal gland is smooth, symmetrical with a midline sulcus, and firm but not hard. In benign hypertrophy, the gland is enlarged but retains the characteristics of the normal gland. A gland suggestive of malignancy may be smooth with one or more nodules, or the whole gland may be enlarged, hard, irregular (craggy) with loss of the midline sulcus. If there has been spread outside the capsule, the gland will be fixed and definition between gland and surrounding tissue will be lost.

Prostate specific antigen (PSA)

As with DRE, there is agreement that a raised PSA is associated with prostate cancer but the degree of that association is in doubt. Sensitivities

of 57% to 99% and specificities of 59% to 97% are quoted.[9]

One of the difficulties has been the use of different cut-offs. This was examined in a study of 5587 men in the USA (the Prostate Cancer Prevention Trial) with initial PSA levels <3 ng/ml who were followed for 7 years, with prostatic biopsy if the level rose above 4, or at the end of the study in those cancer-free at that point (Table 74.2).[5]

As expected, increasing the cut-off leads to a falling sensitivity and a rising specificity. However, at no cut-off is the test very useful in a patient with a low pre-test probability, either in ruling in or in ruling out the disease.

The same study attempted to gauge the value of the PSA in the detection of those patients with higher-grade cancer, i.e. those in whom the cancer was likely to become clinically manifest. They chose a Gleason score of 7 or above to

Table 74.3 Value of different PSA cut-offs in the diagnosis of prostate cancer with a Gleason score ≥7. The prevalence of higher-grade cancer was 4.5%[5]

PSA (ng/ml)	Sensitivity	Specificity	Whether above or below the cut-off	LR	Probability of higher grade cancer
1.1	93%	37%	Above	1.5	7%
			Below	0.2	1%
2.1	76%	67%	Above	2.3	10%
			Below	0.4	2%
3.1	58%	82%	Above	3.2	13%
			Below	0.5	2%
4.1	40%	90%	Above	4.0	16%
			Below	0.7	3%
10.1	2.4%	99.5%	Above	4.8	18%
			Below	0.98	4%

Follow each row from left to right to see how the PSA result at that cut-off level alters the probability of higher-grade cancer.

signify higher-grade cancer. This gave similar figures for the likelihood ratios but very different post-test probabilities because of the lower baseline probability of higher-grade cancer (Table 74.3).

In primary care, the post-test probabilities are likely to be even lower than the above figures from secondary care, because the prevalence of disease tends to be lower.

PSA velocity

Another approach is to measure the rise of PSA over time. Many different ways of measuring velocity have been proposed, including a cut-off of a rise of 0.8 ng/ml per year, but the higher the cut-off the more specific the test. A study of 358 men with localised prostate cancer examined the value of a cut-off of 2 ng/ml/year in high- and low-risk men with cancer[10] (Table 74.4). Men with prostate cancer whose risk of death is already low, and who are found to have a PSA rise <2 ng/ml per year, have a 7-year risk of death approaching zero.

How do the DRE and the PSA results combine in the diagnosis of prostate cancer?

The Spanish Cooperative study of men referred with urological problems examined this thoroughly.[11] Their findings are interesting: an abnormal DRE predicts cancer especially if combined with a PSA >4. However, a PSA >4 in the presence of a normal DRE does not raise the probability of cancer (Tables 74.5 to 74.7). The prevalences of cancer given are those in the group of men to whom those criteria apply.

If the DRE is normal, a PSA >4 alters the probability of cancer very little (Table 74.6).

If the PSA is normal (<4) and the DRE is abnormal, the DRE finding is still useful (Table 74.7).

If the DRE is abnormal, an abnormal PSA further increases the probability of cancer. The LR+ is no more useful than the DRE alone but the LR– is more useful; i.e. if the DRE and PSA are both normal, the probability of cancer falls more (Table 74.6) than if only the DRE is abnormal (Table 74.7).

PSA interpretation

Normal values have been described for different age groups:[12]
- age <50: 2.5 ng/ml
- age 50–59: 3.0 ng/ml
- age 60–69: 4.0 ng/ml
- age 70+: 5.0 ng/ml.

However, the Prostate Cancer Prevention Trial quoted above has shown how arbitrary these cut-offs are and that it is better to see the PSA as a continuum with an increasing probability of cancer as it rises above 1.1 ng/ml.[5]

Table 74.4 Risk of death from prostate cancer over 7 years of follow-up in relation to PSA velocity before diagnosis

Risk of poor outcome	Rise of PSA (ng/ml/year)	7-year risk of prostate cancer death
High risk	>2	24%
	<2	4%
Low risk	>2	19%
	<2	0%

Initial risk of death was based on absolute PSA level, Gleason score and tumour category.

Table 74.5 Value of a PSA >4 in a man with a normal DRE. The prevalence of prostate cancer was 11%[11]

Sensitivity	Specificity	Test result	Likelihood ratio	Probability of cancer
95%	10%	Positive	1.05	11%
		Negative	0.5	6%

Table 74.6 Value of the DRE in a man with a normal PSA (<4). Prevalence of prostate cancer 12%[11]

Sensitivity	Specificity	Test result	Likelihood ratio	Probability of cancer
80%	44%	Positive	1.4	16%
		Negative	0.5	6%

Table 74.7 Value of a PSA >4 in a man with an abnormal DRE. The prevalence of prostate cancer was 44% (already high because of the abnormal DRE)[11]

Sensitivity	Specificity	Test result	Likelihood ratio	Probability of cancer
91%	34%	Positive	1.4	52%
		Negative	0.3	17%

Table 74.8 Effect of age on the predictive value of a PSA >4, based on a pre-test probability of cancer of 3%

	Sensitivity	Specificity	PSA result	Likelihood ratio	Probability of cancer
Men <60 years old	18%	98%	>4	9.0	22%
			≤4	0.8	2%
Men aged 60 and over	35%	88%	>4	2.9	8%
			≤4	0.7	2%

Follow each row from left to right to see how the PSA result in that age group alters the probability of prostate cancer. Three per cent is the pre-test probability of cancer in men with lower urinary tract symptoms in primary care.[3]

Table 74.9 Family history and risk of prostate cancer

Family history	Risk of prostate cancer
One first-degree relative diagnosed aged 70 or under	×2
Two relatives, of whom one was diagnosed aged 65 or under	×4
Three or more relatives	×7

Very high PSA levels are associated with high probabilities of cancer. In patients where the baseline risk of prostate cancer on needle biopsy is already high because of an age >50, the following figures apply:[13]

■ PSA 4–10: cancer risk 22%

■ PSA >10 or more: cancer risk 67%

■ PSA >60: usually indicates metastatic prostate cancer.

Several factors contribute to the unreliability of the PSA

■ The level varies from day to day and year to year. Repeat a borderline level in 2 weeks; the result can alter by up to 30%. Furthermore, a study from New York found that roughly half of those with a PSA >4 ng/ml had at least one normal reading over 4 years of follow-up without treatment.[14]

■ Double the result if the patient has been taking finasteride or dutasteride for 6 months or more.

■ Although rectal examination does not raise the PSA, more invasive manoeuvres (even catheterisation) can, as can urinary tract infection, prostatitis and benign prostatic hypertrophy. Postpone the PSA test for a month in these situations if they may resolve.[1]

Does age affect the reliability of the DRE and the PSA?

Yes; old age makes both less reliable.

■ *The specificity of DRE falls the older the patient.* Over the age of 65 the predictive value of the positive DRE is half that in a man under 65. Although cancer is more common in the older man, so also are non-malignant nodules.[9]

■ *The specificity of the PSA falls the older the patient.* Benign prostatic hypertrophy can raise the PSA and this becomes more common the older the patient. A study of 6691 American men screened with PSA found that, using a cut-off of 4.1 ng/ml, age had a major effect on the positive likelihood ratio (Table 74.8).[15]

Risk factors for cancer of the prostate

■ *Age.* Half of men age >50 have prostate cancer histologically but most are asymptomatic and will remain so. The proportion with cancer increases up to the age of 85 and beyond.

■ *Family history* increases the risk (Table 74.9).[16] A family history of cancers of the breast, ovary, bladder and kidney also increases the risk.

■ *Race.* African Americans have a rate that is double that of whites. Asian and Oriental men have the lowest rates.

Can these factors be used to predict prostate cancer? Analysis of the placebo arm of the Prostate Cancer Prevention Trial showed that family history was an independent predictor of cancer but that age and African American race were not (once DRE and PSA were already factored into the equation).[17] However, older age and African American race both predicted that, if cancer was diagnosed, it would be of a higher grade (i.e. a higher Gleason score).

An online calculator for the calculation of an individual's risk of prostate cancer based on these data (provided he is aged at least 50) is available on www.compass.fhcrc.org/edrnnci/bin/calculator/main.asp.

The patient's perspective

A positive PSA test may have adverse psychological effects even if the patient is found not to have carcinoma on biopsy. In a study from Boston, men who had a suspicious PSA followed by a negative biopsy were compared to controls with a normal PSA.[18] Six weeks later the biopsied group gave the following responses compared to the controls:

■ worried 'a lot' or 'some of the time' about developing prostate cancer: 40% vs. 8%

■ thought their chance of getting prostate cancer was more than average: 36% vs. 18%.

The effects were, however, not all bad. Following the false positive PSA, some men thought their lives had changed for the better: 31% vs. 13%. This phenomenon, that subjects had a feeling that they had something to be thankful for, is also seen in women following a suspicious mammogram with subsequent normal biopsy.

Example

A 65-year-old man is discharged from the emergency department following an episode of acute retention precipitated by a urinary tract infection. He is discharged after an overnight stay, once able to pass urine, but the GP subsequently receives a letter from the department saying that a PSA taken after catheterisation shows a level of 7 ng/ml and asks her to refer the patient to a urologist urgently.

The GP explains this to the patient but says she wants to repeat the test in 4 weeks, since the raised level may have been due to infection and the passage of a catheter. Meanwhile she suggests that she examine the patient rectally. The prostate is enlarged, compatible with benign prostatic hypertrophy, but is otherwise normal. The PSA level is now even more likely to be coming from a non-malignant gland. UK guidelines recommend urgent referral for a patient with a raised PSA[1] but this runs counter to her assessment of his risk. Even if his repeat level is raised, this only increases the risk, at his age, from a baseline of *clinically important* cancer of, say, 0.5%, to 2% as a result of the PSA (LR+ 3.3) which is just about cancelled out by the normal DRE (LR– 0.4). She does want to refer him, but not urgently, because of his episode of a UTI with retention and her finding of benign hypertrophy.

REFERENCES

1. NICE. *Referral guidelines for suspected cancer.* London: National Institute for Health and Clinical Excellence, 2005. Online. Available: www.nice.org.uk.

2. Mansson J, Bengtsson C. *Prostate cancer. From the general practitioner's point of view.* Neoplasma 1994;41:237–240.

3. Hamilton W, Sharp D, Peters T, et al. *Clinical features of prostate cancer before diagnosis: a population-based, case-control study.* Br J Gen Pract 2006;56:756–762.

4. Hamilton W, Sharp D. *Symptomatic diagnosis of prostate cancer in primary care: a structured review.* Br J Gen Pract 2004;54:617–621.

5. Thompson I, Ankerst D, Chi C, et al. *Operating characteristics of*

prostate-specific antigen in men with an initial PSA level of 3.0 ng/ml or lower. JAMA 2005;294:66–70.

6. Young J, Muscatello D, Ward J. *Are men with lower urinary tract symptoms at increased risk of prostate cancer? A systematic review and critique of the available evidence.* BJU Int 2000;85:1037–1048.

7. Hoogendam A, Buntinx F, de Vet H. *The diagnostic value of digital rectal examination in the primary care screening for prostate cancer: a meta-analysis.* Can Med Assoc J 1999;160:49–57.

8. Varenhorst E, Berglund K, Lofman O, et al. *Inter-observer variation in assessment of the prostate by digital rectal examination.* Br J Urol 1993;72:173–176.

9. Summerton N. *Diagnosing cancer in primary care.* Oxford: Radcliffe Medical Press, 1999.

10. D'Amico A, Renshaw A, Sussman B, et al. *Pretreatment PSA velocity and risk of death from prostate cancer following external beam radiation therapy.* JAMA 2005;294:440–447.

11. Cooperative Group for Diagnosis of Prostate Cancer. *A multicenter study on the detection of prostate cancer by digital rectal examination and prostate-specific antigen in men with and without urinary symptoms.* Eur Urol 1997;32:133–139.

12. Speakman M, Kirby R, Joyce A, et al. *British Association of Urological Surgeons. Guideline for the primary care management of male lower urinary tract symptoms.* BJU Int 2004;93:985–990.

13. Mokete M, Palmer A, O'Flynn K. *10 minute consultation: High result in prostate specific antigen test.* BMJ 2003;327:379.

14. Eastham J, Riedel E, Scardino P, et al. *Variation of serum prostate-specific antigen levels: an evaluation of year-to-year fluctuations.* JAMA 2003;289:2695–2700.

15. Punglia R, D'Amico A, Catalona W, et al. *Effect of verification bias on screening for prostate cancer by measurement of prostate-specific antigen.* N Engl J Med 2003;349:335–342.

16. Department of Health. *Department of Health Prostate Cancer Information Sheet, 2002.* Online. Available: www.dh.gov.uk (search on 'Prostate Cancer Information Sheet').

17. Thompson I, Ankerst D, Chi C, et al. *Assessing prostate cancer risk: results from the prostate cancer prevention trial.* J Natl Cancer Inst 2006;98:529–534.

18. McNaughton-Collins M, Fowler FJ, Caubet J, et al. *Psychological effects of a suspicious prostate cancer screening test followed by a benign biopsy result.* Am J Med 2004;117:719–725.

75

Pulmonary embolism

- The clinical picture of pulmonary embolus (PE) is neither sensitive nor specific for the diagnosis.
- The diagnosis becomes harder the older the patient; yet this is the age group most likely to have a PE.
- Despite these reservations, certain individual symptoms, signs, a normal chest X-ray (CXR) and an abnormal electrocardiogram (ECG) do argue in favour of PE. However, in many cases, the strongest factors in favour of a PE are risk factors for thromboembolism and the presence of a deep vein thrombosis (DVT), rather than specific signs and symptoms of PE.
- Clinical decision rules have been developed to divide patients into high, intermediate and low risk groups. These are useful in the assessment of the ability of a negative D-dimer test to exclude PE in a patient whose probability is already low. They do not provide sufficiently strong evidence for a GP who does not have access to a D-dimer test to rule out the diagnosis of PE.

- ★ Suspect a PE in any patient presenting with dyspnoea of sudden onset, or pleuritic chest pain or haemoptysis or collapse.
- ★ Refine the probability by considering:
  - (a) the risk of thromboembolism from the history
  - (b) whether a DVT is present
  - (c) whether there is hypotension, a raised jugular venous pressure (JVP), tachycardia or tachypnoea
  - (d) whether the ECG shows right ventricular strain
  - (e) whether there is another condition present which is a more likely explanation of the symptoms.
- ★ Be wary of using a formal scoring system derived from hospital series. Instead, use the items included in those scoring systems to make your own clinical assessment.
- ★ Admit any patient in whom the clinical picture raises the possibility of PE and in whom there is no more likely alternative diagnosis.

Incidence and background

- The annual incidence of pulmonary embolus (PE), based on autopsy findings, is thought to be 0.2%,[1] or 0.02% based on the clinical assessment of hospitalised patients.[2] Of the autopsy cases, only a third were diagnosed prior to autopsy. Conversely, only 1 in 5 patients referred with suspected PE has the condition.[3]

- The above figures point to the difficulty of diagnosing PE. The clinical picture and the ECG and X-ray findings are rarely specific, especially when

Table 75.1 The probability of DVT using the Wells score in primary care[9]		
Wells score	**Probability of DVT from Wells' study**	**Percentage with DVT (95% CI)**
3 or more	High	37.5% (35.6–39.4%)
1–2	Moderate	16.5% (15.4–17.6%)
≤0	Low	12.0% (10.9–13.1%)

the PE is small. Furthermore, it is uncommon, with only 1% of patients presenting to an emergency department with acute dyspnoea having a PE. Even when the presentation is one of pleuritic chest pain, the probability of PE is only 21%.[4]

● The classical clinical picture of PE (acute onset of pleuritic chest pain, dyspnoea and haemoptysis) is seen in only half of confirmed cases (55%; 95% CI 47% to 63%).[5] These symptoms are even more uncommon in older patients, who are more likely to present with collapse, even with emboli that are no bigger than those in younger patients.[6] When they do occur, these symptoms have a discriminatory power that is moderate at best (see below). Other symptoms have been omitted from this discussion either because they are too rare in PE or because they have no discriminatory power.

Questions to consider

Does the patient have risk factors for thromboembolism or evidence of a current deep vein thrombosis (DVT)?

Score the patient on the modified Wells score:[7,8]
  Score +1 for each of the following:
  (a) active cancer (treatment ongoing or given within the previous 6 months or at the stage of palliative care)
  (b) paralysis, paresis or recent plaster immobilisation of a lower limb
  (c) recently bedridden for ≥3 days or major surgery in the last 4 weeks
  (d) localised tenderness in the deep vein system in the calf and/or thigh
  (e) the entire leg is swollen
  (f) the calf circumference is >3 cm greater than the other side
  (g) unilateral pitting oedema
  (h) collateral superficial veins (other than varicose veins)
  (i) previous DVT.

Score minus 2 if an alternative diagnosis is at least as likely.

A study from primary care in the Netherlands of 1325 patients with suspected DVT found that 29% had a DVT.[9] The Wells score assisted with the diagnosis but only slightly (Table 75.1).

For a more detailed discussion of the diagnosis of DVT, see page 248.

Does the patient have symptoms, signs or an ECG or CXR suggestive of PE?

The classic triad of symptoms, pleuritic pain, dyspnoea and haemoptysis, occurs in a half to less than a third of patients.[10] A wider search for symptoms and signs is needed to avoid missing the diagnosis unnecessarily.

Table 75.2 shows the features significantly associated with a final diagnosis of PE in a study of 1090 consecutive patients with suspected PE in a Geneva emergency department.

Multivariate analysis shows that age, previous DVT or PE, tachycardia, and plate-like atelectasis and elevated hemidiaphragm on CXR are *independent* predictors of the presence of PE. This means that the likelihood ratios for these factors can be used one after the other, using the nomogram on page xxiv, to reach a final clinical probability of PE.

Note that the presence of chest pain argues *against* the diagnosis of PE; the absence of chest pain argues in its favour. The study did not separate pleuritic from other types of chest pain. The Pisa study (see Table 75.5) suggests that pleuritic pain is useful if analysed separately.

Wicki and colleagues in Geneva have used these criteria to formulate a scoring system; but it has not been validated in primary care, and is of limited use anyway. Even a low score carries a 10% risk of PE and would require further investigation.[11] A revised version of this score is described below (see Table 75.6). A further discouragement is that a study comparing clinical judgement to the use of a different score (the Wells score for PE) found that clinical judgement performed better in correctly identifying low-risk patients (of whom 19% still had a PE against 28% when 'low risk' was determined by the score).[12]

A smaller study from Vienna[13] found some additional signs to be useful in the confirmation of PE, although unhelpful in ruling it out (Table 75.3). Note that, in this study, a *normal* CXR is a powerful predictor of the *presence* of PE. Only 6% of those clinically suspected of having PE, and

Table 75.2 The value of symptoms, signs and investigations for PE in patients admitted to the emergency ward of the University Hospital Geneva,[11] based on a prevalence of 27%

Factor	Presence of the factor	Likelihood ratio (95% CI)	Probability of PE
Age ≥60	Present	1.6 (1.4–1.8)	37%
	Absent	0.5 (0.4–0.6)	16%
Previous DVT or PE	Present	2.6 (2.0–3.3)	49%
	Absent	0.8 (0.7–0.8)	23%
Dyspnoea	Present	1.2 (1.1–1.3)	31%
	Absent	0.6 (0.4–0.8)	18%
Haemoptysis	Present	2.4 (1.5–3.9)	47%
	Absent	0.9 (0.9–0.98)	25%
Chest pain	Present	0.8 (0.8–0.9)	23%
	Absent	1.7 (1.4–2.1)	39%
Tachycardia >100/min	Present	2.1 (1.7–2.5)	44%
	Absent	0.7 (0.6–0.8)	21%
Tachypnoea (>30/min)	Present	2.3 (1.7–3.1)	46%
	Absent	0.9 (0.8–0.9)	25%
Pleural effusion on CXR	Present	1.4 (1.1–1.8)	34%
	Absent	0.9 (0.8–0.98)	25%
Plate-like atelectasis on CXR	Present	2.1 (1.7–2.8)	44%
	Absent	0.8 (0.8–0.9)	23%
Elevated hemidiaphragm on CXR	Present	2.0 (1.5–2.6)	43%
	Absent	0.8 (0.8–0.9)	23%

Follow each row from left to right to see how the factor alters the probability of PE.

Table 75.3 Operating characteristics for signs and tests in the diagnosis of PE in patients presenting to secondary care in Vienna with suspected PE[13] where the prevalence of PE was 17%

Factor	Presence of the factor	Likelihood ratio (95% CI)	Probability of PE
Raised JVP	Present	2.4 (1.7–3.3)	47%
	Absent	0.4 (0.2–0.6)	13%
Systolic <100	Present	6.1 (2.7–14)	70%
	Absent	0.7 (0.6–0.9)	21%
Right axis deviation on ECG	Present	6.1 (2.7–14)	70%
	Absent	0.7 (0.6–0.9)	21%
Normal CXR	Present	6.1 (2.7–14)	70%
	Absent	0.7 (0.6–0.9)	21%

Follow each row from left to right to see how the factor alters the probability of PE.
NB. The similarity of the last six rows is not an error!

subsequently shown not to have it, had a normal CXR versus 34% of those with PE.

Other studies have found the ECG to have similar value to the Vienna study but the CXR to be less useful than those above. Two prospective studies found the value for ECG and CXR shown in Table 75.4.

However, tests in prospective studies in centres of excellence may perform better than those in the real world. The Geneva study is chosen here because it was conducted in a population in which the prevalence of PE was lower and the CXR signs chosen were less specialised.[11]

Above all, these differences show how dependent the statistics shown here are on the selection of patients and the expertise of the medical team. They can only be extrapolated very broadly to primary care.

An attempt has been made to assess the predictive power of combinations of symptoms and signs. However, while this increases the sensitivity, it results in a lower specificity than any of the symptoms or signs considered alone (Table 75.5). It is useful for ruling out PE but not for ruling it in.

Other studies have constructed scoring systems for the diagnosis of PE[13] but they tend to be too complex for primary care and include investigations that are not available to the GP. *A warning.* It must be stressed that the power of these findings in primary care is likely to be lower than stated for the following reasons:

(a) More patients will be suffering from small PEs and so are more likely to lack specific symptoms and ECG and CXR changes. Indeed, in most patients, these tests will be more useful in demonstrating another cause for the symptoms than in pointing towards a PE.

(b) They are derived from patients who present with suspected PE. Since two-thirds of patients with PE are undiagnosed and the above rules are inevitably derived from those who are diagnosed, they are likely to be least helpful in the patients most difficult to diagnose.

(c) GPs see patients with thromboembolism relatively rarely. Their skill in assessing signs and reading CXRs and ECGs will be less than that of clinicians in hospital studies.

Table 75.4 Operating characteristics for CXR and ECG in the diagnosis of PE in patients presenting to secondary care in Pisa, Italy,[14] and in the PIOPED study, USA,[15] with suspected PE, based on a prevalence of 25%

Test	Presence of the factor	Likelihood ratio (95% CI)	Probability of PE
Right ventricular overload on ECG[14]	Present	4.2 (3.0–5.9)	58%
	Absent	0.6 (0.5–0.7)	17%
CXR signs of PE*[14]	Present	6.1 (4.5–8.2)	67%
	Absent	0.2 (0.2–0.3)	6%
Normal CXR[15]	Present	1.3 (1.1–1.4)	30%
	Absent	0.5 (0.3–0.8)	14%

Follow each row from left to right to see how the factor alters the probability of PE.
*Oligaemia, amputation of hilar artery or consolidation compatible with infarction.

Table 75.5 Operating characteristics for symptoms in the diagnosis of PE in patients presenting to secondary care in Pisa, Italy, with suspected PE,[14] based on a prevalence of 25%

Symptom	Presence of the factor	Likelihood ratio (95% CI)	Probability of PE
Dyspnoea of sudden onset	Present	2.7 (2.2–3.2)	47%
	Absent	0.3 (0.2–0.4)	9%
Pleuritic chest pain	Present	1.5 (1.2–1.9)	33%
	Absent	0.8 (0.7–0.9)	21%
Loss of consciousness	Present	2.1 (1.4–3.0)	41%
	Absent	0.8 (0.8–0.9)	21%
At least one of the above three	Present	1.6 (1.5–1.8)	35%
	Absent	0.1 (0.1–0.2)	3%

Follow each row from left to right to see how the factor alters the probability of PE.

Investigations in secondary care

A negative D-dimer test can be useful in secondary care, if negative, in ruling out the need for further investigation in a patient whose probability of PE is already judged to be low.[16] An enzyme-linked immunosorbent assay (ELISA) test has a sensitivity of 95% (95% CI 85% to 100%) and an LR– of 0.1 (95% CI 0.03 to 0.6). A negative test in a patient with a pre-test probability that is low or moderate effectively rules out the diagnosis. Specificity is, however, poor at 45% (95% CI 38% to 53%) with an LR+ of only 1.7 (95% CI 1.5 to 2.0). A positive test, therefore, hardly contributes to the diagnosis.[17]

Pulmonary artery imaging is the definitive investigation, currently a computed tomography (CT) pulmonary angiogram.[18]

Some clinical prediction rules

1. The British Thoracic Society (BTS) has proposed a rule for the assessment of probability prior to investigation (see box).[19]

BTS prediction rule for the diagnosis of PE

A. Clinical features compatible with PE (e.g. tachypnoea, haemoptysis, pleuritic chest pain).
1. No other reasonable clinical explanation.
2. A major risk factor present (see above).
Score:

   A + 1 + 2 = high probability
   A + 1 or 2 = intermediate probability
   A only = low probability

Patients with low probability and a negative D-dimer may be discharged without further investigation. However, without access to the D-dimer test in primary care the GP cannot use the rule to exclude PE. Without it, even patients whose probability of PE is low need transfer to secondary care as quickly as possible.
2. The Christopher Study. A more complex clinical prediction rule plus D-dimer estimation has been shown to be effective in ruling out pulmonary embolism.[20] 1028 patients were scored as being unlikely to have PE and to have a negative D-dimer test. They were not investigated further and were not anticoagulated. Only 0.5% of these patients had a subsequent venous

thromboembolism. This study confirms the value of the negative D-dimer test.
3. The Revised Geneva Score has been developed in Switzerland.[21] Its strengths are that it does not depend on the absence of another reasonable clinical explanation (a subjective criterion) nor on the D-dimer result. Its weakness for primary care is that it was developed in patients admitted to emergency departments with suspected PE (i.e. acute onset of chest pain or shortness of breath without other obvious cause). In primary care, the decision about admission may be taken at an earlier stage – i.e. is this patient's acute chest pain or shortness of breath suggestive of PE or is another cause more likely? (see *Chest pain*, p. 33).

Furthermore, GPs are likely to decide that a patient with a low probability should still be referred if the probability of PE is as high as 8% (see Table 75.7).

What is striking from Tables 75.6 and 75.7 is that the risk of PE is at least moderate in a patient with acute chest pain or dyspnoea with no other reasonable explanation if there are sufficient risk factors, or there is evidence of a DVT, without any further pointers towards the diagnosis of PE.

Myths

Note that some signs, traditionally thought to be useful in ruling out PE, do not do so:
• A fever >38.5°C is traditionally thought to rule against the diagnosis of PE. The Geneva study shows that it does not influence the diagnosis either way (LR+ 0.8 (0.4 to 1.5), LR– 1.0 (0.98 to 1.04)).[11]
• Chest wall tenderness is usually thought to point to a musculoskeletal problem rather than a PE. This makes sense because a PE should have no effect on the parietal pleura, let alone on chest wall musculature. However, in one series in the emergency department, chest wall tenderness was found in 18% of patients with pleuritic pain, of whom 13% had a PE.[4] A Swiss study found that the presence of chest wall tenderness made no impact on the probability that the patient had a PE, with positive and negative likelihood ratios of 1.[22]
• A rub is traditionally thought to confirm that pleuritic pain is originating from the pleura. In PE, a rub is only present in 4% of those with pleuritic pain.[15]

Massive pulmonary embolism

Massive PE can give a deceptive clinical picture,[23] but exact diagnosis in primary care is less crucial

Table 75.6 The Revised Geneva Score for the diagnosis of pulmonary embolism[21]

Feature	Score
Age >65	1
Previous DVT or PE	3
Surgery or lower limb fracture in last month	2
Active malignancy (or cured within the last year)	2
Unilateral lower limb pain	3
Haemoptysis	2
Heart rate 75–94	3
Heart rate ≥95	5
Pain on deep palpation of lower limb and unilateral oedema	4

Table 75.7 Scoring the Revised Geneva Score[21] based on a prevalence of PE of 23% in patients in the emergency department with acute chest pain or dyspnoea

Score	PE risk	Probability of PE (95% CI)
0–3	Low	8% (5–12%)
4–10	Intermediate	28% (25–33%)
≥11	High	74% (61–83%)

because the patient is so clearly *in extremis*, with some of the following suggestive signs (tachycardia, tachypnoea, hypotension, right heart failure, cyanosis and loss of consciousness), that immediate admission is the only possible option. Patients less severely affected, but whose embolism is still defined as 'massive' by virtue of the obstruction of at least two lobar arteries, still do not present in the classical way. A US study of 90 such patients found that only 20% had the triad of dyspnoea, pleuritic pain and haemoptysis;[24] 80% had dyspnoea, often with a feeling of apprehension (in 61%), and 80% had chest discomfort but it was pleuritic in only 62%. Signs and investigations were more helpful, with tachypnoea in 88%, tachycardia in 63%, a gallop rhythm in 43%, an abnormal CXR in 85%, an abnormal ECG in 90% and a PaO_2 <90 mmHg in 99%.

Example

A man aged 50 presents with mild dyspnoea, which he had noticed on and off since the previous evening. He broke his leg recently and is still in a plaster cast.

The GP cannot examine the leg further because of the cast and so judges that his broken leg gives him a 16.5% probability of thromboembolism (from the Wells score), although she is aware that that implies a more precise estimate than is justified.

The complaint of dyspnoea raises the possibility of PE but does not raise that probability by much, in view of the LR+ of only 1.2 from the Geneva study (Fig. 75.1). However, this weak prediction of PE from the complaint of dyspnoea does not fit with her clinical experience. Perhaps the patients in the Geneva study had been admitted because of dyspnoea and so the value of the symptom had already been 'used up'.

She examines the chest and finds it clear but notes a slight fever. Her understanding of the non-specific nature of the presentation of PE and of the seriousness of missing the diagnosis makes her want to admit the patient to hospital, but this is January during a flu epidemic and she fears a sceptical response from the admitting physician. She is aware that the lack of more specific symptoms reduces the probability of PE. Using the three criteria from Pisa (sudden onset of dyspnoea, pleuritic pain and loss of consciousness) her patient's probability of PE has fallen to 2% (Fig. 75.2).

She orders an immediate ECG and, since radiography is available in the same building, a CXR. The ECG shows 'right heart strain', raising the probability from 2% to 8% (Fig. 75.3). The CXR is normal. She knows that different studies of the predictive value of the normal CXR show positive likelihood ratios of from 1 to 6; and that those figures were when the CXR was read by a radiologist, not a GP. She decides not to use the result to raise the probability of PE. The CXR was still worth doing: consolidation suggestive of pneumonia would have moved the diagnosis strongly away from PE. She telephones the admitting physician with enough grounds (unexplained dyspnoea in a patient at risk of PE because of a leg in plaster) to insist that hospital assessment is needed, even though she knows her patient probably does not have a PE.

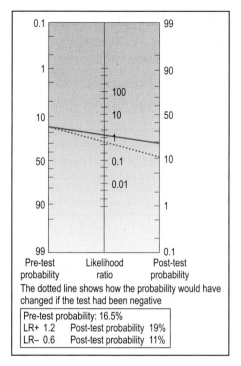

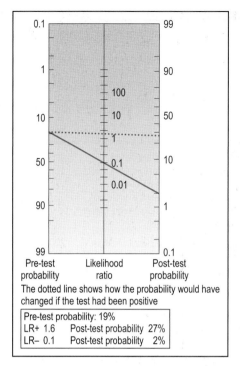

Figure 75.1 The probability of PE before and after applying the history of dyspnoea in the example on p. 482.

Figure 75.2 The probability of PE before and after applying the three Pisa criteria in the example on p. 482.

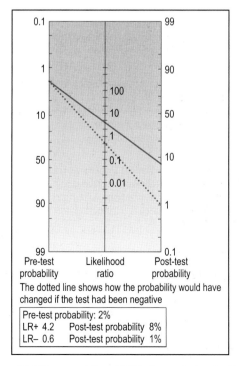

Figure 75.3 The probability of PE before and after the ECG result in the example on p. 482.

REFERENCES

1. Anish E, Mayewski R. Pulmonary embolism. In: Black E, ed. *Diagnostic strategies for common medical problems,* 2nd edn. Philadelphia: American College of Physicians, 1999.

2. Anderson FJ, Wheeler H, Goldberg R. *A population-based perspective of the hospital incidence and case-fatality rates of deep vein thrombosis and pulmonary embolism. The Worcester DVT Study.* Arch Intern Med 1991;151:933–938.

3. McGee S. *Evidence-based physical diagnosis.* Philadelphia: Saunders, 2001.

4. Hull R, Raskob G, Carter C, et al. *Pulmonary embolism in outpatients with pleuritic chest pain.* Arch Intern Med 1988;148:838–844.

5. Stein P, Henry J. *Clinical characteristics of patients with acute pulmonary embolism stratified according to their presenting syndromes.* Chest 1999;112:974–979.

6. Timmons S, Kingston M, Hussain M, et al. *Pulmonary embolism: differences in presentation between older and younger patients.* Age Ageing 2003;32:601–605.

7. Wells P, Anderson D, Bormanis J, et al. *Value of assessment of pretest probability of deep-vein thrombosis in clinical management.* Lancet 1997;350:1795–1798.

8. Wells P, Owen C, Doucette S, et al. *Does this patient have deep vein thrombosis?* JAMA 2006;295:199–207.

9. Oudega R, Hoes A, Moons K. *The Wells Rule does not adequately rule out deep venous thrombosis in primary care patients.* Ann Intern Med 2005;143:100–107.

10. Jones K, Raghuram A. *Investigation and management of patients with pleuritic chest pain presenting to the accident and emergency department.* J Accid Emerg Med 1999;16:55–59.

11. Wicki J, Perneger T, Junod A, et al. *Assessing clinical probability of pulmonary embolism in the emergency ward.* Arch Intern Med 2001;161:92–97.

12. Sanson B, Lijmer J, Mac Gillavry R, et al. *Comparison of a clinical probability estimate and two clinical models in patients with suspected pulmonary embolism.* Thromb Haemost 2000;83:199–203.

13. Stollberger C, Finsterer J, Lutz W, et al. *Multivariate analysis-based prediction rule for pulmonary embolism.* Thromb Res 2000;97:267–273.

14. Miniati M, Prediletto R, Formichi B, et al. *Accuracy of clinical assessment in the diagnosis of pulmonary embolism.* Am J Respir Crit Care Med 1999;159:864–871.

15. Stein P, Terrin M, Hales C, et al. *Clinical, laboratory, roentgenographic, and electrocardiographic findings in patients with acute pulmonary embolism and no pre-existing cardiac or pulmonary disease.* Chest 1991;100:598–603.

16. ACEP Clinical Policies Subcommittee on Suspected Pulmonary Embolism. *Clinical policy: critical issues in the evaluation and management of adult patients presenting with suspected pulmonary embolism.* Ann Emerg Med 2003;41:257–270.

17. Stein P, Hull R, Patel K, et al. *D-dimer for the exclusion of acute venous thrombosis and pulmonary embolism.* Ann Intern Med 2004;140:589–602.

18. The Board of the Faculty of Clinical Radiology. *Framework for primary care access to imaging – right test, right time, right place.* London: Royal College of Radiologists, 2006.

19. Robinson G. *Pulmonary embolism in hospital practice.* BMJ 2006;332:156–160.

20. Writing Group for the Christopher Study Investigators. *Effectiveness of managing suspected pulmonary embolism using an algorithm combining clinical probability, D-dimer testing, and computed tomography.* JAMA 2006;295:172–179.

21. Le Gal G, Righini M, Roy P-M, et al. *Prediction of pulmonary embolism in the emergency department: the Revised Geneva Score.* Ann Intern Med 2006;144:165–171.

22. Le Gal G, Testuz A, Righini M, et al. *Reproduction of chest pain by palpation: diagnostic accuracy in suspected pulmonary embolism.* BMJ 2005;330:452–453.

23. Bell W, Simon T, DeMets D. *The clinical features of submassive and massive pulmonary emboli.* Am J Med 1977;62:355–360.

24. Wenger N, Stein P, Willis P. *Massive acute pulmonary embolism.* JAMA 1972;220:843–844.

76

Restless legs syndrome

- Restless legs syndrome (RLS) is common, troublesome and underdiagnosed.
- It is more common in older people but, with a median age of onset of 27, is also common in the young, when the diagnosis is even less likely to be made.
- Most of those with distressing symptoms consult their GP but remain without a diagnosis.

A PRACTICAL APPROACH

- ★ Consider the possibility of RLS in every patient who complains of insomnia, daytime sleepiness or unpleasant feelings in the limbs that are worse at night.
- ★ Ask the four questions which are the criteria for the diagnosis of the syndrome.
- ★ If the diagnosis is made (from the history), look for the cause. Ask about a family history and look for associated diseases, for medication that may be responsible, and perform a few blood tests.
- ★ Confirm the diagnosis with a trial of a dopaminergic agent.

Prevalence

- Estimates range from 2% to 15% of the population.[1] A recent survey of over 15 thousand adults in the USA and Europe found that 7% reported all the diagnostic features of RLS listed below at some time in their lives, and 3% reported symptoms that were judged to be clinically meaningful (distressing symptoms at least twice weekly in the past year). Of these, 81% had discussed their symptoms with a primary care physician but only 6% of those reported that they had been diagnosed as having RLS.[2]
- RLS becomes more common with increasing age. However, it is often present in the young. The median age of onset is 27, though many are not diagnosed for 10 to 20 years.
- Patients often appear to complain about the insomnia and daytime sleepiness associated with RLS rather than restlessness of the legs. Thirteen per cent of the Dutch population who report daytime sleepiness meet criteria for RLS.[3]

Diagnosis

This is clinical and takes two parts:
1. *Is this RLS?* Diagnostic criteria have been proposed by the International RLS Study Group.[4] All the following must be present:
   (a) an urge to move the legs usually associated with uncomfortable or unpleasant sensations in the legs
   (b) symptoms begin or worsen during periods of rest or inactivity such as lying or sitting
   (c) symptoms are partially or totally relieved by movement, at least as long as the movement continues
   (d) symptoms are worse in the evening or at night.

   Note:
- If other symptoms are also present, they do not necessarily argue against the diagnosis. For instance, the restlessness may involve the arms in almost half of patients.[5]
- Examination is unlikely to add anything to a clear history, although it may reveal another condition that is mimicking RLS, e.g. peripheral neuropathy or Parkinson's disease.

- A response to dopaminergic therapy supports the diagnosis; indeed a lack of response argues strongly against the diagnosis.
- The diagnosis may be missed if the clinician depends on the patient to volunteer the above history. Many present with complaints of insomnia or tiredness, unaware that their restless legs are the cause.

2. *Is it primary or secondary RLS?* In primary RLS, there is usually a family history, with up to a half of cases transmitted as an autosomal dominant.[6] Secondary RLS may be found in a number of conditions, although in some the association may be by chance:

- iron, folate or vitamin B_{12} deficiency
- diabetes
- rheumatoid arthritis
- Parkinson's disease
- uraemia
- pregnancy
- medication use, e.g. antidepressants, calcium channel blockers or phenytoin.

Investigations are used to look for secondary causes of RLS: serum ferritin, red cell folate, serum B_{12}, fasting blood sugar, serum creatinine. No studies have determined the value of these investigations.

The diagnosis of RLS in the cognitively impaired is difficult because it depends on the history, which the patient may be unable to give. Five criteria for the diagnosis have been described, all of which should be present:[4]

1. signs of leg discomfort such as rubbing or kneading the legs and groaning while holding them
2. excessive motor activity of the lower limbs such as pacing, fidgeting, repetitive kicking, tossing and turning in bed, slapping the legs on the mattress, cycling movements, repetitive foot tapping, rubbing the feet together and inability to remain seated
3. signs of leg discomfort are exclusively present or worsen during rest or inactivity
4. signs of leg discomfort are diminished with activity
5. criteria 1 and 2 occur only in the evening or night or are worse at those times than during the day.

Example

A 45-year-old woman consults her GP because she has been threatened with disciplinary action at work for falling asleep at her reception desk. As the GP runs through his list of case-finding questions, he asks about her quality of sleep. She says it is poor. She wakes up frequently in the night and feels she can't get comfortable. She cannot be more specific. He asks about symptoms in the evening before she goes to bed. She says her husband complains that she is a terrible fidget. She'll sit down to watch TV but after a few minutes she'll have to get up again.

She gets up and walks about and the feeling goes off. Her husband says she fidgets in her sleep too. In fact, when she can finally be induced to describe the feelings in her legs, she meets all five criteria for the diagnosis of RLS.

She has no associated condition and her blood tests are normal. The GP's suspicion that this is primary RLS seems to be confirmed by her saying that her mother was a terrible fidget as well. She responds dramatically to a 4-week trial of pergolide.

REFERENCES

1. Allen R, Earley C. *Restless legs syndrome: a review of clinical and pathophysiologic features.* J Clin Neurophysiol 2001;18:128–147.

2. Allen R, Walters A, Montplaisir J, et al. *Restless legs syndrome prevalence and impact: REST General Population Study.* Arch Intern Med 2005;165:1286–1292.

3. Rijsman R, Neven A, Graffelman W, et al. *Epidemiology of restless legs in the Netherlands.* Eur J Neurol 2004;11:607–611.

4. Allen R, Picchietti D, Hening W, et al. *Restless legs: diagnostic criteria, special considerations, and epidemiology. A report from the restless legs diagnosis and epidemiology workshop at the National Institutes of Health.* Sleep Med 2003;4:101–119.

5. Chaudhuri K, Appiah-Kubi L, Trenkwalder C. *Restless legs syndrome.* J Neurol Neurosurg Psychiatry 2001;71:143–146.

6. Das P, Suman S. *Restless legs syndrome in older people.* Geriatr Med 2004;May:25–30.

77

Stable angina

KEY FACTS

- Angina is a clinical diagnosis made because of the occurrence of retrosternal pain brought on by exertion and relieved by rest. More detailed questioning and consideration of the presence of risk factors helps to confirm the diagnosis, or to rule it out in a patient whose history of chest pain does not suggest angina.
- Examination is unhelpful in the diagnosis of angina except that it may reveal the presence of risk factors, such as hypertension or absent peripheral pulses.
- Similarly, the resting ECG is only useful in displaying evidence of past infarction. However, the exercise ECG is useful in predicting that subsequent coronary angiography will be abnormal (though not in diagnosing or excluding angina).

A PRACTICAL APPROACH

- ★ Ask the traditional questions. Retrosternal chest pain brought on by exertion and relieved by rest has a probability of angina sufficiently high for the GP to refer the patient for cardiological assessment.
- ★ In patients with a less clear-cut history, check for risk factors: age, male sex, diabetes, smoking, hyperlipidaemia, stroke or peripheral vascular disease. The presence of one or more of these increases the probability of angina sufficiently to prompt referral unless another cause of the chest pain is more likely.
- ★ If the need for referral is still not clear, check three details:
  - ■ Does the pain always occur after the same degree of exertion?
  - ■ Does the pain occur at rest in ≤10% of attacks?
  - ■ Does the pain usually last <5 minutes?
  A negative answer to all three makes angina very unlikely unless the pre-test probability was unusually high.
- ★ Examine for associated conditions (e.g. hypertension, aortic stenosis, evidence of arterial disease elsewhere) and perform a baseline ECG.
- ★ Refer all patients with a reasonable suspicion of angina for a specialist assessment unless concomitant illness makes that inappropriate or the GP has the expertise, and access to exercise ECG testing, to assess the patient's suitability for invasive treatment.[1]

Table 77.1 Value of a positive response to the Rose Questionnaire, according to gender, in the diagnosis of angina confirmed on thallium scan[4]

Score	Sensitivity	Specificity	LR+ (95% CI)	LR– (95% CI)
Males	44%	77%	1.9 (1.5–2.5)	0.7 (0.6–0.9)
Females	41%	56%	0.9 (0.7–1.2)	1.0 (0.9–1.2)

Prevalence

In an urban practice in Oxford, the prevalence of angina was found to be 7.4% (95% CI 6.2 to 8.6%) of patients aged 45–74. The annual incidence of new diagnoses of angina in this age group was 1%. This age range comprises 30% of that practice's population, giving an overall prevalence of 2.2%.[2]

The history

Three questions are most useful:
1. Is the pain retrosternal?
2. Is it brought on by exertion?
3. Is it relieved within 10 minutes by rest or by glyceryl trinitrate (GTN)?

A typical history of angina is one in which the answers to all three questions are positive.

Unfortunately, when tested formally in secondary care, such a history is neither sensitive nor specific for coronary heart disease (CHD).

However, GPs are extraordinarily successful in ruling out the diagnosis of cardiac chest pain. A Swedish study, in which GPs assessed 532 patients presenting with chest pain, found that the GPs' clinical assessment achieved a sensitivity of 95% for the diagnosis of suspected CHD, although specificity was lower at 62%.[3] This means that the GPs' suspicion of CHD raised the probability from a baseline of 17% to only 34% (LR+ 2.5); but if the GPs excluded CHD, the probability fell from 17% to a usefully low 2% (LR– 0.09).

It is intriguing to know how GPs are so accurate in excluding CHD. Studies of the value of the history (all in secondary care) have failed to do so well. It may be that GPs' history taking is better than the questionnaire-type history of the studies; or that, as the first professional filter, they 'use up' the traditional history so that it cannot be used again in secondary care (see p. 403).

Table 77.2 The probability of CHD from the history[5]

No. of questions positive	Probability of CHD
Typical history	90%
Atypical history	50%
History suggests non-anginal chest pain	16%

The subjects were 4952 patients referred for coronary angiography because of chest pain in the 1970s.

Studies of the predictive value of the history in secondary care

A study from Rhode Island, USA found that the full Rose Questionnaire (which divides the three questions above into seven to gain more detail)[4] had the characteristics shown in Table 77.1 when applied to patients referred for exercise testing. In other words, by the time the patient reaches the cardiologist, the traditional history is almost useless in establishing the diagnosis, and, if absent, is completely useless in refuting it.

An earlier review of studies from secondary care was more encouraging, suggesting that the traditional history is useful in establishing the probability of coronary artery disease on subsequent coronary angiography (Tables 77.2 and 77.3).[5]

For a GP, the figure of 16% would be no reassurance. It would mean that if the GP relied on the history to exclude cardiac pain, 1 in 6 patients with cardiac pain would be missed.

A third study, from Guy's Hospital London,[6] has examined in detail the value of more detailed refinement of the history of pain by comparing the histories of 65 patients with chest pain (including, in 94% of them, chest pain on

Table 77.3 Value of the three questions concerning regularity, pain at rest and duration in the diagnosis of CHD in secondary care in patients with exertional chest pain,[6] based on a pre-test probability of CHD of 25%

Score	Likelihood ratio (95% CI)	Probability of angina
3 questions positive	3.9 (1.8–8.2)	57%
≥2 questions positive	3.2 (2.1–5.0)	52%
≥1 question positive	1.4 (1.2–1.6)	32%
0 questions positive	0.05 (0.01–0.4)	2%

The pre-test probability of CHD of 25% is that of a patient with chest pain in primary care.[7] The diagnosis of angina was made on coronary angiogram.

exertion) in whom the subsequent coronary angiogram was completely normal, with a group of 65 patients with chest pain whose angiograms showed significant stenosis. There were no important differences between the two groups in terms of site, radiation or quality of the pain (except that patients who indicated that the pain was felt over the heart were slightly more likely to have a normal angiogram).

Three questions have been found to be statistically significant in patients referred for angiography in the discrimination of cardiac from non-cardiac pain (Table 77.3):[6]

(a) *Regularity.* If you go uphill (or do whatever causes the pain) on 10 separate occasions, on how many do you get the pain? 'Cardiac' answer = 10.

(b) *Pain at rest.* Of 10 pains in a row, how many occur at rest? 'Cardiac' answer = <2.

(c) *Duration.* How many minutes does the pain usually last? 'Cardiac' answer = <5 minutes.

These results suggest that angina can be safely ruled out in a patient with chest pain not obviously anginal in nature, in whom the questions about regularity, rest pain and duration are negative, and who does not have strong risk factors for coronary heart disease.

Table 77.4 shows the value of individual symptoms in the Guy's Hospital study.[6] Note the fact that pain that is felt in relation to meals *increases* the probability that it is angina (see example below). Other questions that proved to have no discriminatory power were whether pain occurred at night or on lying down, whether pain was related to stress and whether GTN relieved the pain (without reference to speed of relief).

Several reservations should be stated about extrapolating the results of this study to primary care. The patients in this study were at the severe end of the spectrum, in that they were all considered to be candidates for angiography; the conclusions have not been validated in a further set of patients; and a normal angiogram does not exclude angina.

Adding consideration of risk factors to refine the probability of CHD

The main risk factors for angina are:
- male sex
- increasing age
- past history of CHD, peripheral vascular disease or stroke
- family history
- diabetes
- smoking
- hypertension
- hyperlipidaemia
- lack of exercise.

The review mentioned above showed how the probability of angina depends on the pre-test probability in terms of age and sex (Table 77.5). It appears that risk factors for CHD are almost as useful as specific questions about the pain.

A different review of secondary care studies found that the risk factors of diabetes, smoking or hyperlipidaemia increased the probability of coronary artery disease hugely.[8] The increase was most significant clinically in patients in whom the possibility of CHD would otherwise have been dismissed. Examples are shown in Table 77.6.

Table 77.4 The association of individual symptoms with abnormal coronary angiography in patients with chest pain,[6] based on a pre-test probability of angina of 25%

Symptom	Presence of symptom	Likelihood ratio (95% CI)	Probability of angina
Pain is not felt over the heart	Present	1.7 (1.3–2.4)	36%
	Absent	0.5 (0.3–0.7)	14%
Pain lasts 5 minutes or less	Present	2.4 (1.7–3.4)	44%
	Absent	0.2 (0.1–0.4)	6%
Pain lasts 30 minutes or less	Present	1.2 (1.0–1.3)	29%
	Absent	0 (0.0–0.9)	0%
Relief from GTN within 5 minutes	Present	2.2 (1.4–3.3)	42%
	Absent	0.5 (0.4–0.7)	14%
Pain on exertion occurs every time	Present	2.0 (1.5–2.8)	40%
	Absent	0.4 (0.2–0.6)	12%
Pain is felt at rest in less than 10% of episodes	Present	2.4 (1.7–3.5)	45%
	Absent	0.4 (0.2–0.7)	12%
Pain in relation to meals	Present	2.7 (1.1–6.4)	47%
	Absent	0.8 (0.7–0.97)	21%

Follow each row from left to right to see how that feature of the history alters the probability of angina.
The pre-test probability of CHD of 25% is that of a patient with chest pain in primary care.[7] The diagnosis of angina was made on coronary angiogram.

Table 77.5 The probability of angina according to the patient's age and sex[5]

	Probability of angina in a man aged 60–69	Probability of angina in a woman aged 60–69	Probability of angina in a man aged 40–49	Probability of angina in a woman aged 40–49
Typical history	94%	91%	87%	55%
Atypical history	67%	54%	46%	13%
History suggests non-anginal chest pain	28%	19%	14%	3%

Table 77.6 The probability of angina, in patients with chest pain *not* suggestive of angina, according to the risk factors of diabetes, smoking and hyperlipidaemia[8]

Patient	Probability of angina with no risk factors	Probability of angina with at least 1 risk factor
Woman aged 35	1%	19%
Man aged 35	3%	35%

Table 77.7 The probability of angina according to the degree of ST depression on exercise testing,[6] based on a pre-test probability of angina of 25%

ST depression	Likelihood ratio	Probability of a positive angiogram
<0.5 mm	0.2	6%
≥0.5 mm	3.7	55%
≥1.0 mm	5.9	66%
≥1.5 mm	21	88%
≥2.0 mm	33	92%

The presence of risk factors in patients at higher risk because of their age is less important because they would be investigated anyway. In this study, a man aged 65 with chest pain not suggestive of angina had a probability of CHD of 49%. The fact that the presence of risk factors raised this to 69% would make no difference to the management in primary care.

Investigations

The value of the resting ECG is limited. Any abnormality between attacks signifies past myocardial damage and so only indirectly increases the probability that chest pain is due to angina. A meta-analysis of three studies[7] found that *any* abnormality on the ECG had an LR+ of 1.53 (95% CI 1.01 to 2.33) and an LR– 0.74 (95% CI 0.48 to 1.15), figures that mean that the ECG is virtually worthless in the diagnosis of angina. Its value is as a baseline against which subsequent changes can be measured. In the rare event, in primary care, that an ECG is recorded during an attack, a horizontal or downsloping ST segment depression of at least 1 mm in two or more adjacent leads is significant (as it would be during an exercise ECG).

Exercise ECG testing is more helpful in the prediction of an abnormal coronary angiogram. Comparing exercise testing results to coronary artery disease, proven angiographically, gives the figures in Table 77.7.[5] These figures show that ST depression is useful both in predicting the presence of coronary artery stenosis and in ruling it out if absent. It is not, however, appropriate for primary care where the GP must make a decision about referral on the basis of the history alone (see below).

Is an exercise test useful in primary care in the *diagnosis* of coronary heart disease?

In the UK, the exercise ECG is reserved for an assessment of the need for coronary angiography when the diagnosis of ischaemic heart disease has been made. It is not considered sufficiently sensitive to be used in making that diagnosis. In other health care systems, however, primary care access to exercise testing is used in the diagnosis of CHD.[3] Meta-analysis gives the following summary figures for exercise testing in the diagnosis of CHD: sensitivity 68%, specificity 77%; LR+ 3.0, LR– 0.4.[9] This relatively poor performance leads to worse outcomes and, in some groups, higher costs than echocardiography, single photon emission computed tomography (SPECT) or coronary angiography.[9]

These findings seem to be borne out by a prospective study from primary care in Sweden.[3] Exercise tests were performed on 181 patients with clinically suspected CHD, sufficiently stable not to need emergency referral to hospital. The test permitted the diagnosis of 12 with CHD and the diagnosis of 127 as not having CHD, but the diagnosis was still in doubt in 42. These primary care diagnoses were not tested against a gold standard but, from the likelihood ratios above, it seems inevitable that a firm diagnosis of CHD can only be made following exercise testing in patients in whom the clinical suspicion of the presence or absence of CHD was already substantial.

This conclusion was also reached in an English study which examined the use of open access exercise electrocardiography by 47 GPs. The GPs used the test primarily to confirm their impression that the patient did not have CHD.[10] In 5 out of 110 tests, the results were strongly positive but the GPs were so sure the patient did not have CHD that they were not referred to a cardiologist.

Exercise ECGs may be helpful in primary care in countries with limited access to a cardiologist, but unnecessary in a country in which all patients with suspected CHD will be referred for a cardiological opinion anyway.

Example

A man aged 64 reported episodes of retrosternal pain that only came on about half an hour after the main meal of the day. It was relieved by an antacid. He denied that exercise could bring on the pain. The GP diagnosed reflux oesophagitis.

Two days later the patient telephoned to report that he was now having chest pain on all mild exertion. The clinical diagnosis was now clearly unstable angina (see *Acute coronary syndrome*, p. 289).

The GP realised she had failed to take a sufficiently detailed history on the first occasion. In fact, the pain came on half an hour after supper, as he climbed three flights of stairs to the bedroom. He would pause on the stairs to take the antacid, giving him the impression that the antacid had relieved the pain, when in fact it was the rest. He therefore had a positive answer to all three initial questions (Is it retrosternal? Is it brought on by exertion? Is it relieved by rest?) and a positive answer to two of the three subsidiary questions (Does it occur at rest? Does it last <5 minutes?) and had a high probability of angina.

The GP was still puzzled by the fact that climbing the stairs at other times did not bring on the pain, until she realised that the explanation lay with the meal. Diversion of blood to the splanchnic circulation plus exertion was more likely to bring on angina than more vigorous exertion on an empty stomach.

REFERENCES

1. DOH. *The National Service Framework for coronary heart disease.* London: Department of Health, 2000.

2. Gill D, Mayou R, Dawes M, Mant D. *Presentation, management and course of angina and suspected angina in primary care.* J Psychosom Res 1999;46:349–358.

3. Nilsson S, Scheike M, Engblom D, et al. *Chest pain and ischaemic heart disease in primary care.* Br J Gen Pract 2003;53:378–382.

4. Garber C, Carleton R, Heller G. *Comparison of 'Rose Questionnaire Angina' to exercise thallium scintigraphy: different findings in males and females.* J Clin Epidemiol 1992;45:715–720.

5. Diamond G, Forrester J. *Analysis of probability as an aid in the clinical diagnosis of coronary-artery disease.* N Engl J Med 1979;300:1350–1358.

6. Cooke R, Smeeton N, Chambers J. *Comparative study of chest pain characteristics in patients with normal and abnormal coronary angiograms.* Heart 1997;78:142–146.

7. Mant J, McManus R, Oakes R, et al. *Systematic review and modelling of the investigation of acute and chronic chest pain presenting in primary care.* Health Technology Assessment: NHS R&D HTA Programme, 2004. Online. Available: www.ncchta.org.

8. Snow V, Barry P, Fihn S, et al. *Evaluation of primary care patients with chronic stable angina: guidelines from the American College of Physicians.* Ann Intern Med 2004;141:57–64.

9. Garber A, Solomon N. *Cost-effectiveness of alternative test strategies for the diagnosis of coronary artery disease.* Ann Intern Med 1999;130:719–728.

10. Paul V, Sulke A, Norris A. *Open access exercise electrocardiography: does it improve the management of cardiovascular disease in the community?* J R Soc Med 1990;83:143–145.

Thrombophilia

- Roughly 10% of the population have thrombophilia, almost all of it inherited.
- About half of people with venous thromboembolism have thrombophilia.
- There are arguments in favour, and against, making the diagnosis of thrombophilia. Once a patient has had a deep vein thrombosis, prophylactic measures against further thrombosis should be taken at times of risk, so a formal diagnosis of thrombophilia would usually not make any difference to management.

A PRACTICAL APPROACH

- * Consider the diagnosis in every patient with venous thromboembolism (VTE).
- * Explain to the patient that the occurrence of one episode of VTE means that the risk of another one is increased. Explain the situations in which prophylaxis will be needed (e.g. if undergoing surgery or immobilised).
- * Order a thrombophilia screen, or refer to a haematologist, if the benefits of discovering that the patient has thrombophilia (i.e. more intensive prophylaxis) seem to outweigh the disadvantages (e.g. anxiety and difficulties with life insurance).

Definition

The presence of a long-term increased risk of venous thromboembolism (VTE).

Prevalence

- Nine per cent of the population have a heritable thrombophilia, most of them (5% of the population) the heterozygous factor V Leiden mutation. Among patients with VTE, 38% to 63% will have a heritable thrombophilia.[1]
- Acquired thrombophilia may be due to another condition in which an antiphospholipid antibody is produced, as in systemic lupus erythematosus (SLE), or to exogenous oestrogen, as in oral contraception and hormone replacement therapy (HRT), or to malignancy, obesity or to another inflammatory condition. These are different in principle from the specific risk factors for thrombosis, immobility, trauma and surgery, which may also exist.

Who should be referred?

- * Consider referring the following for investigation for thrombophilia:[2]
  - (a) VTE aged under 40
  - (b) recurrent VTE or superficial thrombophlebitis
  - (c) unusual VTE, e.g. mesenteric vein thrombosis
  - (d) skin necrosis in association with venous thrombosis
  - (e) those with a VTE and a first-degree relative who has had a VTE
  - (f) recurrent fetal loss (×3)
  - (g) unexplained neonatal thrombosis.
- * In borderline cases, consider screening the patient with a full blood count, prothrombin time (PT), activated partial thromboplastin time (APTT) and a thrombin clotting time. These will detect most patients with thrombophilia. However, laboratory tests will not detect all patients with thrombophilia; new genetic defects are still being discovered.[3] Conversely, many patients with a laboratory diagnosis of thrombophilia never have a thrombosis. Such is the complexity of full

investigations that referral to a haematologist is usually wise in those in whom it would make a difference to future management.

* Consider the implications of the diagnosis carefully before recommending testing. It will cause anxiety, and will have implications for life insurance, without providing most patients with any useful prophylaxis. An estimate of the benefit of screening women for the factor V Leiden mutation before they take combined oral contraception found a number needed to test of 2 million; that is, 2 million women would need to be tested in order to save one life per year from pulmonary embolism.[3]

Example

A 50-year-old English man marries a Thai woman but after a few months in England she returns to Thailand. He stays behind but arranges to visit her every 6 months. Two days after the first flight to Bangkok he develops a deep vein thrombosis (DVT). He flies back to Bangkok 6 months later, by now off warfarin but wearing a support stocking, and develops a second DVT.

On his return, he discusses the future with his GP who explains that it is very likely that, despite a negative family history, he has an underlying predisposition to venous thrombosis. Because of the complexity of full investigations and the fact that the patient wants to continue to fly to Thailand, the GP refers him to a haematologist, and plans to keep him on warfarin until a future plan is decided.

REFERENCES

1. BHF. *Thrombophilia*. London: British Heart Foundation Factfile, 2002. Online. Available: www.bhf.org.uk.

2. DTB. *Management of patients with thrombophilia*. Drug Ther Bull 1995;33:6–8.

3. Walker I, Greaves M, Preston F. *Investigation and management of heritable thrombophilia*. Br J Haematol 2001;114:512–518. Online. Available: www.bcshguidelines.com.

Index